Emerging Applications, Perspectives, and Discoveries in Cardiovascular Research

Ashim Malhotra
Pacific University, USA

Shivani Soni
California State University, Fullerton, USA & Chapman University, USA & Alabama State University, USA

A volume in the Advances in Medical Diagnosis, Treatment, and Care (AMDTC) Book Series

IGI GLOBAL
DISSEMINATOR OF KNOWLEDGE

www.igi-global.com

Published in the United States of America by
IGI Global
Medical Information Science Reference (an imprint of IGI Global)
701 E. Chocolate Avenue
Hershey PA, USA 17033
Tel: 717-533-8845
Fax: 717-533-8661
E-mail: cust@igi-global.com
Web site: http://www.igi-global.com

Library of Congress Cataloging-in-Publication Data

Names: Malhotra, Ashim, 1977- editor. | Soni, Shivani, 1975- editor.
Title: Emerging applications, perspectives, and discoveries in cardiovascular research / Ashim Malhotra and Shivani Soni, editors.
Description: Hershey PA : Medical Information Science Reference, [2017] | Includes bibliographical references.
Identifiers: LCCN 2016053529| ISBN 9781522520924 (hardcover) | ISBN 9781522520931 (ebook)
Subjects: | MESH: Cardiovascular Diseases | Biomedical Research | Biomedical Technology
Classification: LCC RC669 | NLM WG 120 | DDC 616.10072--dc23 LC record available at https://lccn.loc.gov/2016053529

This book is published in the IGI Global book series Advances in Medical Diagnosis, Treatment, and Care (AMDTC) (ISSN: Pending; eISSN: Pending)

British Cataloguing in Publication Data
A Cataloguing in Publication record for this book is available from the British Library.

For electronic access to this publication, please contact: eresources@igi-global.com.

Advances in Medical Diagnosis, Treatment, and Care (AMDTC) Book Series

ISSN:Pending
EISSN:Pending

Mission

Advancements in medicine have prolonged the life expectancy of individuals all over the world. Once life-threatening conditions have become significantly easier to treat and even cure in many cases. Continued research in the medical field will further improve the quality of life, longevity, and wellbeing of individuals.

The **Advances in Medical Diagnosis, Treatment, and Care (AMDTC)** book series seeks to highlight publications on innovative treatment methodologies, diagnosis tools and techniques, and best practices for patient care. Comprised of comprehensive resources aimed to assist professionals in the medical field apply the latest innovations in the identification and management of medical conditions as well as patient care and interaction, the books within the AMDTC series are relevant to the research and practical needs of medical practitioners, researchers, students, and hospital administrators.

Coverage

- Emergency Medicine
- Critical Care
- Medical Testing
- Cancer Treatment
- Alternative Medicine
- Experimental Medicine
- Disease Prevention
- Medical Procedures
- Chronic Conditions
- Patient Interaction

IGI Global is currently accepting manuscripts for publication within this series. To submit a proposal for a volume in this series, please contact our Acquisition Editors at Acquisitions@igi-global.com or visit: http://www.igi-global.com/publish/.

The Advances in Medical Diagnosis, Treatment, and Care (AMDTC) Book Series (ISSN Pending) is published by IGI Global, 701 E. Chocolate Avenue, Hershey, PA 17033-1240, USA, www.igi-global.com. This series is composed of titles available for purchase individually; each title is edited to be contextually exclusive from any other title within the series. For pricing and ordering information please visit http://www.igi-global.com/book-series/advances-medical-diagnosis-treatment-care/129618. Postmaster: Send all address changes to above address.

Titles in this Series

For a list of additional titles in this series, please visit: www.igi-global.com

Healthcare Community Synergism between Patients, Practitioners, and Researchers
Valerie C. Bryan (Florida Atlantic University, USA) and Jennifer Lynne Bird (Florida Atlantic University, USA)
Medical Information Science Reference • copyright 2017 • 348pp • H/C (ISBN: 9781522506409) • US $210.00 (our price)

Transformative Healthcare Practice through Patient Engagement
Guendalina Graffigna (Catholic University of the Sacred Heart, Italy)
Medical Information Science Reference • copyright 2017 • 382pp • H/C (ISBN: 9781522506638) • US $215.00 (our price)

Promoting Patient Engagement and Participation for Effective Healthcare Reform
Guendalina Graffigna (Catholic University of the Sacred Heart of Milan, Italy)
Medical Information Science Reference • copyright 2016 • 357pp • H/C (ISBN: 9781466699922) • US $220.00 (our price)

Effective Methods for Modern Healthcare Service Quality and Evaluation
Panagiotis Manolitzas (Technical University of Crete, Greece) Evangelos Grigoroudis (Technical University of Crete, Greece) Nikolaos Matsatsinis (Technical University of Crete, Greece) and Denis Yannacopoulos (Piraeus University of Applied Sciences, Greece)
Medical Information Science Reference • copyright 2016 • 315pp • H/C (ISBN: 9781466699618) • US $190.00 (our price)

Handbook of Research on Trends in the Diagnosis and Treatment of Chronic Conditions
Dimitrios I. Fotiadis (University of Ioannina, Greece)
Medical Information Science Reference • copyright 2016 • 659pp • H/C (ISBN: 9781466688285) • US $385.00 (our price)

Dr. Ashim Malhotra dedicates this book to his family: his mother, Sunil, and father, Amrit Malhotra, and his late grandmother Savitri Batra.

Editorial Advisory Board

Table of Contents

Detailed Table of Contents

This chapter focuses on effect of genetic variation on the cardiovascular disease therapies, mechanism involved and need for personalized medicine.

Infective endocarditis although uncommon infectious disease but can cause significant mortality and morbidity. This chapter focuses on advances made in diagnosis and therapies to combat drug resistant micro-organisms.

The cardiology diagnostics including technology, new biomarkers, genetics markers (with potential of being diagnostic tools) have been improved significantly in recent years. This chapter focuses on these advancements and its effect on diagnosis, therapy and prevention of heart disease.

Traditional immunosuppressive drugs after heart transplantation is still in practice but new generation of immunosuppressive medicine holds better promise and the focus of discussion in this chapter.

Preface

ADDRESSING CHALLENGES IN CARDIOVASCULAR SCIENCES: THE NEED FOR THIS WORK

Investigation into the mechanisms of cardiovascular diseases and the development of novel translational and alternative methods for their treatment has come to a head recently with 399,899 articles published in the field, with 221,494 or approximately 55% just in the previous decade. These advancements are not limited to being focused on enhancing comprehension of molecular and genetic mechanisms underlying cardiovascular pathology, but also include rapid advancements in the manufacture and process technology for diagnosis and treatment of cardiovascular disease. The emphasis on manufacture and process technology improvements includes classic topics such as 1) advances in material sciences, 2) application of nanotechnology, 3) novel pharmaceutical drug formulation strategies, 4) novel drug delivery processes including targeted drug delivery, and 5) integration of tissue engineering and artificial reconstruction into therapy. Interestingly, from an academic point-of-view, these topics have remained isolated in discrete research areas, preventing much-needed collaboration which would enable furtherance of the entire field of the cardiovascular sciences.

Moreover, in recent years, research into natural products and alternative medical therapies for the treatment of cardiovascular disease have gained popularity and scientific support. Instances include public support especially for systems of the medicine inspired by the ancient Eastern practitioners, such as those of Chinese herbal medicine and acupuncture, or the Indian Ayurveda. However, there is a need for adopting an integrative, synthesis-based and comprehensive approach that merges fields as disparate as engineering and technology on the one hand, and alternative medicine on the other, to enable the emergence of new ideas for the development of therapeutic strategies to address this prominent killer group of diseases. However, the broad scope of such an endeavor has largely resulted in challenging the development of such an effort.

The current work has emerged from the overwhelming need to survey and contextualize the rapid and discipline-specific advancements in basic, clinical, applied, and technological sciences that are collectively changing our understanding of, and therapeutic approach to, cardiovascular disease. Titled "Recent Advancements in Cardiovascular Diseases", our current effort purports to encompass all these areas by experts in the field, with each book section dedicated to exploring these ideas as a separate chapter.

THE INTENDED IMPACT OF THIS BOOK

We believe that our comprehensive approach and general treatment of the subject of cardiovascular diseases will be of benefit to a broad readership, including professionals practicing in the field, postdoctoral fellows, graduate students, medical school and pharmacy school students, and researchers. It is our contention and earnest desire that the exploration and presentation of the various aspects of cardiovascular diseases in this work will have the impact of presenting these advancements in light of multi-party, diversified, and disparate perspectives. We are confident that this will ensure a comprehensive survey and synthesis of information in the field of cardiovascular science.

OBJECTIVES OF THE CURRENT WORK

Recent findings in the field of cardiovascular sciences and diseases include those in the fields of cardiomyopathy, myocardial infarction, ischemia-reperfusion injury, arrhythmias, hypertension and related disorders to name just a few. Coupled with emerging technologies in research, transplant medicine, and organ system biology, these advancements have created an urgent need for an edited collection of manuscripts from scientific disciplines as diverse as pharmaceutics, pharmaceutical formulation, organic and medicinal chemistry, microfabrication, molecular biology, pharmacology, pharmacokinetics and transplant medicine in one publication. The overarching goal of this book is to highlight the strengths and future potential of this new interdisciplinary approach to cardiovascular science by bringing a comprehensive and thorough review of this new and fast-evolving field; its advantages and disadvantages, and future perspectives. Our main goal though this publication is to make the foundational cardiovascular sciences, therapy, alternative and complimentary therapy, and the social and administrative sciences as they pertain to cardiovascular diseases, a group of inter-related disciplines with dynamic cross-talk. Our objective is to impart knowledge to a diverse audience so that experts in one field can easily explore disparate topics, including those outside the confines of their expertise.

WHO SHOULD USE THIS BOOK?

This book offers to be an easy-to-comprehend interface between different disciplines of science, as applicable to cardiovascular materials, thus benefiting the synthetic chemists and engineers to study the biological context and vice versa. It will also be advantageous to graduate students to plan their research proposals in the field of nanotechnology as it will be a concise overview of past, present and ongoing research in the field. It can also target researchers who can get a comprehensive review of all topics of interest (e.g., how research on a particular nanoparticle started, pros and cons and ongoing modifications which can substantially help in shaping their research).

TOPICAL COVERAGE AND CONTENT EMPHASIS

The current work is broadly divided into five sections, arranged in a logical progression from the foundational sciences which underlie the molecular mechanisms that modulate physiology and etiology of disease to clinical, diagnostic, and later, the social perspectives of cardiovascular disease. Also, included is a discussion of alternative and complementary medical approaches to the treatment of cardiovascular disorders.

The first section introduces the latest advancements in our understanding of the cardiovascular diseases with an emphasis on basic foundational sciences. Accordingly, chapters in this section are focused on recent discoveries in molecular physiology, etiology, and pathology in the field of cardiovascular sciences.

Section 1: Six chapters are included in this section, beginning with Matthews and Schweighardt's chapter on exploring the role of natriuretic peptides in the development of heart disease and strategies based on employing this knowledge to inform therapy. The next two chapters explore the impact of signaling transduction on cardiovascular function, such as epithelial permeability (chapter by Tauseef, Aquil, and Mehta) and the multiple cellular and physiological processes regulated by the general and ubiquitous transcriptional factor Nuclear Factor-κB (chapter by Mishra). Chapter 4 discusses the role of the cardinal ion that modulates the electrophysiology of the heart: the all-important calcium and its storage and trafficking in the cells of the cardiovascular system (chapter by Bose). Following, an exploration of signal transduction pathways and their effect on ionic movement, the focus shifts to an analysis of organelle contribution, specifically the regulation of the biogenesis of the mitochondria and its impact on the physiology and pathophysiology of the heart (chapter by Malhotra and Soni). The last chapter in this section, Chapter 6, examines disorders of platelets by identifying new discoveries in the etiology and pathophysiological mechanisms of platelet diseases (chapter by Karim and Khasawneh).

Section 2: There are five chapters in Section 2. In general, these chapters examine the latest discoveries in the field of cardiovascular sciences from a clinical perspective. The section opens with Chapter 7, which introduces the pathophysiology and etiology of myocardial infarction and explores the recent innovations in this field (chapter by Chapalamadugu, Gudla, and Tipparaju). To account for the effect of the possible differences in the genetic make-up of individuals on the development of heart disease, Dornblaser, Worby and Brazeau outline the underlying pharmacogenomics of cardiovascular diseases and therapy in Chapter 8. Turner and Schwartz expand the clinical focus by elaborating on relatively rare infectious diseases, in particular, infectious endocarditis in Chapter 9. The following chapter takes a sweeping look at some of the main advancements in recent times in the diagnosis, including newer technologies and strategies for diagnostic techniques in cardiovascular diseases (chapter by Li, Fang, Huang, Lu, Zhang, and Yao). Finally, the last chapter in this section presents an examination of the advancements in drugs, therapeutic strategies, and treatment of heart transplantation, with an emphasis on the role of immunosuppression in successful heart transplants (chapter by Li, Li, Nwankwo, Huang, Zhang, Lanzhou, and Lanzhou).

Section 3: Titled "Recent Technological Advancements in Cardiovascular Sciences", Section 3 presents the latest information regarding improvements in process technology as it applies to devices and drug delivery, including targeted delivery systems. Chapter 12 outlines advancements in coronary stents technology (chapter by Sengupta), while Chapter 13 explores the use of nanotechnology for the creation of targeted drug delivery systems (chapter by Patel and Pathak).

Section 4: Following an examination of the recent discoveries in cardiovascular science, clinical perspectives, and technological advancements, we wished to examine lesser-known complementary, alternative and natural therapies for cardiovascular disorders that are both popular in the public eye and scientifically promising. Chapter 14 focuses on the use of alternative and complementary therapies for the treatment of hypertension (chapter by Shatnawi, Shafer, Ahmed, and Elbarbry), while Chapter 15 discusses the potential uses for the polyphenolic phytochemicals resveratrol which is present in red wine and has been shown to be effective in overcoming some of the deleterious changes that occur at the molecular and physiological level in cardiovascular disease (chapter by Powell, Zhang, Bowman, and Choudhury).

Section 5: The last section, Section 5, is titled "Recent Ideas in Social and Applied Cardiovascular Sciences" and covers a broad area of innovation and recent changes in aspects related to the social causality of cardiovascular disease (chapter by Min) and the forensic assessment of death due to cardiovascular disease. We felt the need to add this section based on the observation that treatment of cardiovascular diseases does not occur in a vacuum. In fact, both patient care and the assessment of therapeutic outcome in patients depends on upon a multitude of factors including social derivatives, which must be kept in mind, to the best possible extent while either designing therapy or assessing overall impact.

We are confident and hopeful that readers will find our approach interesting and will gain from the multiplicity of perspectives presented in this book. If this book facilitates and encourages the seeking of additional reading from fields different from original, the book would have attained its primary objective - that of promoting the integration of knowledge across the various disciplines that feed into the general umbrella of the cardiovascular sciences.

Ashim Malhotra

Portland, Oregon
September 26, 2016

Acknowledgment

Dr. Shivani Soni wishes to acknowledge the constant support of her husband Dr. Amandeep Salhotra, her son Mr. Shivam Salhotra and dearest friends Ms. Rosalind (Kim) Wilson and Dr. Gulnaz Javan.

Section 1

Discoveries in Cardiovascular Sciences:

Molecular Pharmacology and Pathophysiology Perspectives

Chapter 1
The Role of Natriuretic Peptides in the Pathophysiology and Treatment of Heart Failure

Jennifer L. Mathews
St. John Fisher College, USA

Anne Schweighardt
St. John Fisher College, USA

ABSTRACT

The pathophysiology of heart failure is due in part to compensatory mechanisms utilized to maintain cardiac output. Neurohormonal responses include activation of the renin-angiotensin-aldosterone and sympathetic nervous systems leading to vasoconstriction, increased blood volume through reabsorption of sodium and water, and increased myocardial contractility and heart rate. Prolonged activation of these systems often results in a maladaptive response and a further reduction in cardiac output (Colucci, 2015). Natriuretic peptides counterbalance the neurohormonal systems by antagonizing the actions of renin-angiotensin-aldosterone, promoting vasodilation and natriuresis. In hypervolemic states atrial myocytes are stretched resulting in the release of atrial natriuretic peptide (ANP). Ventricular cells secrete brain-type natriuretic peptide (BNP) in response to the high ventricular filling pressures (de Sa, 2008). The natriuretic peptides are degraded enzymatically by neprilysin. Plasma concentrations of ANP and BNP can be used as markers for the diagnosis of heart failure (Grewal, 2004). The kidneys also produce a natriuretic peptide, urodilatin, and new studies suggest a role for this peptide in the pathophysiology and treatment of heart failure (Anker, 2015). The natriuretic peptides can be targeted therapeutically for the treatment of heart failure. Nesiritide, a recombinant preparation of human B-type natriuretic peptide (BNP), is FDA approved and has been available for several years for treatment of acute decompensations of heart failure, but has received limited use due to cost and adverse effect profile. Ularatide, a synthetic analog of urodilatin, is currently in phase three clinical trials. In addition, the FDA has recently approved an angiotensin receptor blocker-neprilysin inhibitor that has shown mortality benefit.

DOI: 10.4018/978-1-5225-2092-4.ch001

INTRODUCTION

The pathophysiology of heart failure is due in part to compensatory mechanisms aimed at maintaining cardiac output (Colucci, 2015). Prolonged activation of these systems often results in a maladaptive response and a further reduction in cardiac output (Colucci, 2015). Natriuretic peptides counterbalance the neurohormonal systems by antagonizing the actions of renin-angiotensin-aldosterone and promoting vasodilation and natriuresis (de Sa, 2008). The natriuretic peptides can be targeted for the treatment of heart failure and current clinical trials aim to introduce novel compounds with therapeutic benefits over medications currently on the market.

BACKGROUND

Heart failure (HF) is a complex condition which effects 5.7 million people in the United States, or approximately 10 out of every 1,000 individuals over the age of 65 (Lloyd-Jones, 2002). Newly diagnosed cases of HF are expected to increase 46% by 2030 (Heidenreich, 2013). Heart failure occurs equally in men and women and is more prevalent in African Americans and Hispanics followed by Caucasians and Asian Americans (Lloyd-Jones, 2002; Bahrami, 2008).

Risk factors for HF include: cigarette smoking, hypertension, obesity, diabetes and dietary sodium intake (He 2001; 2002). Seventy-five percent of patients with HF have pre-existing hypertension and the lifetime risk for people with blood pressure (BP) >160/90 mmHg is double that of those with BP <140/90 mmHg (Lloyd-Jones, 2002).

Significant healthcare dollars are spent on the diagnosis and treatment of HF. Total cost for HF has been estimated to be over $30 billion and projections show that by 2030 the total cost of HF will increase to $69.7 billion or $244 for every US adult (Heidenreich, 2013). On average, patients with HF take 6 medications and 78% have at least two hospital admissions per year (English, 1995). Heart failure is the most common hospital discharge diagnosis among individuals served by Medicare and more Medicare dollars are spent for the diagnosis and treatment of heart failure than for any other diagnosis (Massie, 1997).

The cardiac dysfunction that underlies HF is often chronic and irreversible, interspersed with episodes of acute decompensation. Current drug therapies aim to manage symptoms associated with the syndrome. Despite advances in treatment the 5-year mortality rate for HF has remained high at 50% (Roger, 2004).

PATHOPHYSIOLOGY OF HEART FAILURE

Heart failure begins with myocardial damage which can often be attributed to ischemic heart disease, hypertension or diabetes (Mozaffarian, 2016). The impaired myocardial fibers may be unable to contract (systolic HF) or relax (diastolic HF).

Cardiovascular Parameters

With each heartbeat, a volume of blood from the left ventricle is ejected into the aorta and the same happens from the right ventricle into the pulmonary artery. The amount of blood pumped out of the ventricles in 1 minute is cardiac output (CO) and is the product of heart rate (HR) and stroke volume (SV) (Marieb, 2013). CO is normally 4-8 L/min (Carlsson, 2012).

Stroke volume is the amount of blood pumped from each ventricle with 1 heartbeat and is typically between 60-100 ml/beat. In clinical practice CO is frequently indexed to body surface area and termed cardiac index, expressed as (L/min) per body surface area (m^2) and normally ranges from 2.6 to 4.2 L/min/m^2 (Carlsson, 2012).

Changes to CO can be directly affected by both SV and HR. There are three factors which impact stroke volume: preload, afterload and contractility (Figure 1). Preload is the degree of myocardial stretch at the end of diastole (Marieb, 2013). The higher the preload the higher the SV as determined by the Frank-Starling law of the heart. The length-tension relationship is directly impacted by the amount of venous return and the subsequent stretching of the cardiac muscle (Marieb, 2013). Afterload is the pressure that needs to be overcome for the heart to eject the blood. There is an inverse relationship between afterload and ventricular function (Kemp, 2013). As pressure increases the force of contraction decreases which results in a decreased stroke volume (Kemp, 2013; Marieb, 2013). Afterload is typically constant, but can be impacted in people with hypertension as this increases the back pressure of the arterial blood (Marieb, 2013). Contractility is the inotropic state of the heart independent of the preload and the afterload. Contractility is directly related to the amount of available calcium required for the actin and myosin interaction (Marieb, 2013). Sympathetic nervous stimulation increases contractility of the heart by increasing calcium.

Increasing heart rate is also a mechanism to increase cardiac output. Activation of the sympathetic nervous system causes the release of norepinephrine. Norepinephrine binds to β_1-adrenergic receptors in the heart impacting the conduction system, resulting in the SA node firing more rapidly (Marieb, 2013).

It is also important to note the importance of mean arterial pressure (MAP), the product of CO and total peripheral resistance (TPR). As described, HF results in a decrease in CO which in turn leads to a decrease in MAP and tissue perfusion (Kemp, 2012). Several mechanisms are used physiologically to return MAP to normal including the neurohormonal activation and ventricular remodeling (Kemp, 2012). While initially these mechanisms provide support to the physiological functions of the heart, the long-term consequences are maladaptive and worsen HF.

Figure 1. The factors affecting cardiac output (CO)
Adapted from Kemp (2012)

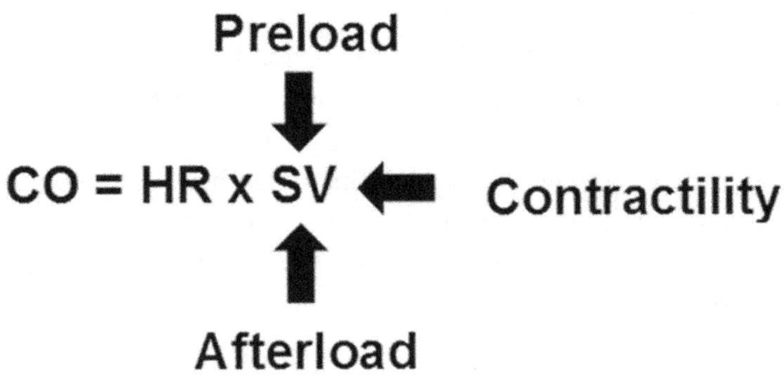

Compensatory Mechanisms

Sympathetic Nervous System

Sympathetic nervous system (SNS) and subsequent neurohormonal activation play important roles in the early compensatory mechanisms aimed at maintaining MAP (Marieb, 2013). A decrease in MAP activates the baroreceptor reflex and increased release of catecholamines (norepinephrine and epinephrine). This results in increased heart rate and contractility (β1 receptors), vasoconstriction (α1), and activation of the RAAS pathway (β1) (Chaggar, 2009). These mechanisms increase SV and TPR and ultimately, MAP. Long-term sympathetic stimulation results in arrhythmias, and tachycardia (Chaggar, 2009).

Excessive sympathetic activity is also associated with cardiac myocyte apoptosis, hypertrophy, and focal myocardial necrosis (Golan, 2012). With prolonged SNS activation alterations in the size, shape, structure, and function of the ventricle occurs (Curry, 2000). As remodeling occurs, there are changes in ventricular mass, composition, volume and geometry (Curry, 2000). Chronic pressure overload causes concentric hypertrophy, increasing wall thickness and decreasing cavity size (Golan, 2012). This pattern of remodeling also decreases left ventricular compliance increasing diastolic pressure (Golan, 2012). Chronic volume overload results in eccentric hypertrophy, resulting in chamber enlargement (Golan, 2012). This remodeling accommodates increased volumes without subsequent increases in atrial or ventricular diastolic pressures (Golan, 2012). The remodeling process in HF is progressive and eventually becomes detrimental not only to the ability of the heart to pump effectively, but also results in myocardial apoptosis (Kemp, 2012).

Renin-Angiotensin-Aldosterone System

In response to sympathetic activation and reduced renal blood flow, from a decreased MAP, the juxtaglomerular cells of the kidneys secrete renin (Rea, 2008). Renin hydrolyzes angiotensinogen in the liver to make angiotensin I. In the lungs, circulating angiotensin I is converted to angiotensin II by angiotensin-converting enzyme (ACE). Angiotensin II then promotes the release of aldosterone. The end results are sodium reabsorption, vasoconstriction of renal efferent arterioles, and secretion of vasopressin.

Vasopressin (ADH)

Vasopressin is synthesized in the hypothalamus and secreted by the posterior pituitary gland (Golan, 2012). When MAP decreases there is a corresponding increase in vasopressin release (Rea, 2008). Water permeability in the collecting duct of the kidney is regulated by vasopressin resulting in insertion of aquaporins into the apical membrane and subsequent reabsorption of water, increasing blood volume and MAP (Rea, 2008).

Sympathetic nervous system activation results in increased heart rate, contractility, and increased intravascular volume all aimed at maintaining CO (Golan, 2012). Systemic vasoconstriction overrides local vascular control to ensure adequate tissue perfusion of vital tissues (Golan, 2012). Consequently, this results in increased preload and afterload resulting in increased myocardial oxygen demand (Golan, 2012).

Natriuretic Peptides

There are other neurohormonal mechanisms at work in HF, including the natriuretic peptides. Natriuretic peptides antagonize the actions of renin-angiotensin-aldosterone, promote vasodilation, increase natriuresis, and inhibit ventricular remodeling (de Sa, 2008). In hypervolemic states atrial myocytes are stretched resulting in the release of atrial natriuretic peptide (ANP) (de Sa, 2008). Ventricular cells secrete brain-type natriuretic peptide (BNP) in response to the high ventricular filling pressures (de Sa, 2008). The kidneys also produce a natriuretic peptide, urodilatin (Anker, 2015). All are degraded enzymatically by neprilysin. Elevated BNP, in particular, is thought to be one of the first signs of HF and is used to follow the progression of disease (Grewal, 2004). Elevated N-terminal pro-BNP levels are associated with a high risk of all-cause mortality in people with HF (van den Broek, 2011). These hormones play a significant role in regulating the pathophysiology of HF and represent novel therapeutic targets for treatment.

CLINICAL PARAMETERS

Left Ventricular Dysfunction

Left ventricular (LV) dysfunction can be divided into two categories: systolic and diastolic dysfunction. Most people with HF (70%) have systolic dysfunction (Kemp, 2012). This is a result of impaired contractility and the quality of heart as a pump is compromised. Diastolic dysfunction results from impaired filling while contractility is often normal. Whether or not a patient with HF has systolic or diastolic dysfunction is often determined based on the ejection fraction (EF). Ejection fraction is the fraction of blood ejected by the ventricle relative to its end diastolic volume. In most cases, the term EF refers to left ventricular ejection fraction (LVEF). Normal EF is between 50% and 70%. If the EF is ≤40%, it is systolic dysfunction and if it is ≥40%, it is diastolic dysfunction (Kemp, 2012).

The leading cause of LV systolic dysfunction is loss of functional myocardium due to myocardial infarction (MI) which impairs the contractile machinery required for the heart to pump effectively (Copstead, 2010). Both systolic and diastolic dysfunction can also be the result of uncontrolled hypertension or ischemic heart disease.

Left ventricular dysfunction causes an increase in the amount of blood in the ventricle and a subsequent increase in both end systolic (ESV) and end diastolic volumes (EDV), resulting in an increase in LV end diastolic pressure (LVEDP) (Kemp, 2012). This increased pressure in the LV results in elevations in left atrial pressures as well as increased pressure in the capillaries of the lungs (Kemp, 2012). The clinical signs and symptoms associated with left ventricular dysfunction can be attributed to these elevated pressures (Figure 2).

Right Ventricular Dysfunction

Right ventricular dysfunction is usually a result of LV dysfunction. As the RV fails there is an increase in the amount of blood within the ventricle, which in turn leads to elevated pressures in the right atria and vena cava (Kemp, 2012) (Figure 3). The clinical signs and symptoms associated with right ventricular dysfunction can be seen in the liver, the gastrointestinal tract, and the lower extremities (Kemp, 2012).

Figure 2. Left-sided heart failure
Adapted from Copstead (2010)

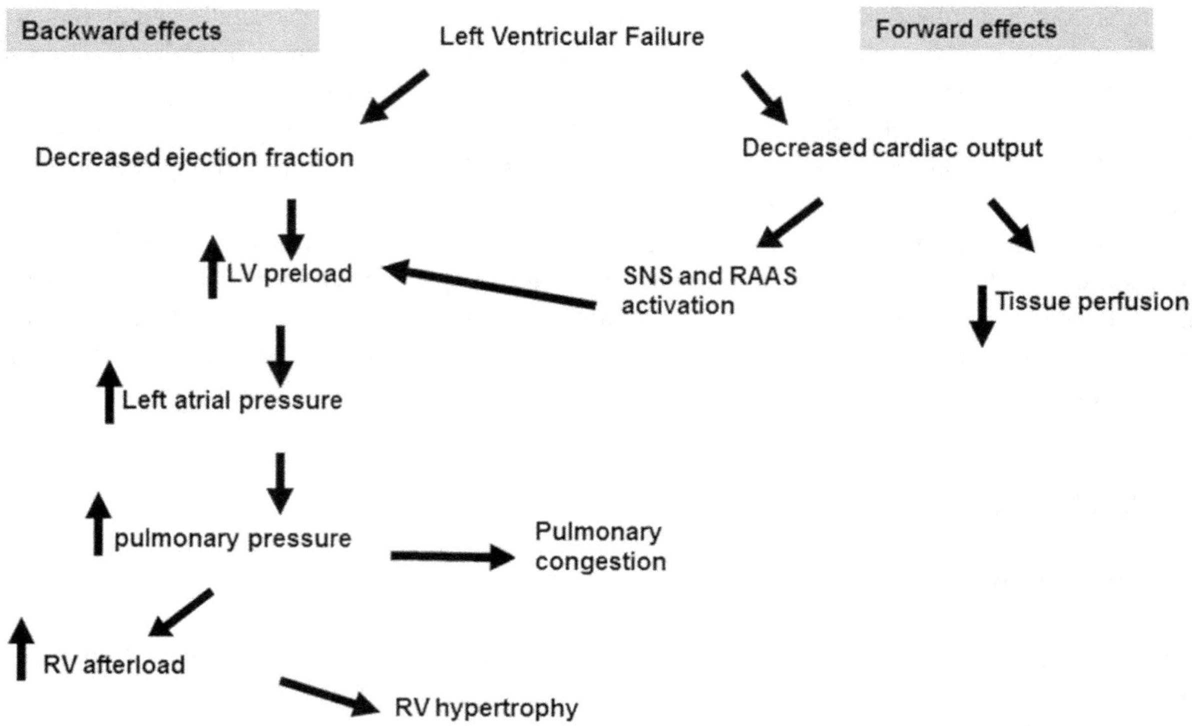

Figure 3. Right-sided heart failure
Adapted from Copstead (2010)

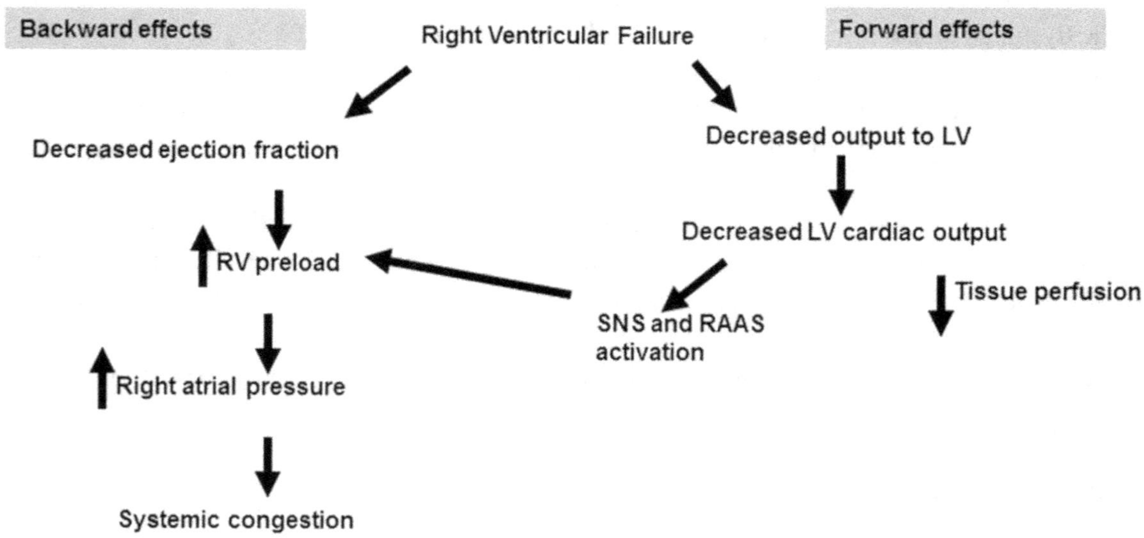

Signs and Symptoms

Left-Sided HF

The signs and symptoms of LV dysfunction are all the result of increased left atrial and pulmonary capillary pressures (Table 1). Dyspnea, cough, and wheezing result from increased hydrostatic pressure in the pulmonary capillary bed forcing fluid out into the interstitial and alveolar spaces (Copstead, 2010, Kemp 2012). Additional pulmonary dysfunction will be produced as the LV fails.

Right-Sided HF

The RV and LV function in series, as the left ventricle fails this will eventually increase the stress on the RV (Copstead, 2010) and signs and symptoms will begin to occur (Table 1). Elevated right atrial pressure results in lower extremity edema, as well as ascites (Kemp, 2012). As CO continues to decrease metabolic demands are not being met. Blood flow will be conserved for vital organs such as the brain and heart. As blood flow is diverted nausea and lack of appetite may occur as blood is shifted from the gastrointestinal tract to the more vital organs (Kemp, 2012).

Classification and Disease Progression

Heart failure classification is commonly based on two different systems (Table 2). The New York Heart Association (NYHA) classification system places people in one of four classes based upon the physical disability caused by their HF. The American College of Cardiology (ACC) and the American Heart Association (AHA) system emphasizes the progression of HF including risk factors and structural changes. There are some overlaps between the ACC/AHA system and the NYHA system.

Treatment Standards

The goals of therapy are to improve symptoms, maintain myocardial function, and reduce mortality. Many treatment options currently available target the SNS and neurohormonal responses described above (Table 3). Importantly, new investigational therapies must also be considered.

Table 1. Right- and left-sided HF signs and symptoms and signs

	Clinical Symptoms	Clinical Signs
Right-sided HF	abdominal pain, anorexia, fatigue, nausea, bloating, swelling	peripheral edema, jugular venous distention, abdominal-jugular reflux, hepatomegaly, splenomegaly, ascites
Left-sided HF	dyspnea on exertion, orthopnea, cough, fatigue, restlessness, confusion, hemoptysis	basilar rales, pulmonary edema, S3 gallop, pleural effusion, Cheyne-Stokes respiration

Adapted from (Copstead, 2010; Kemp, 2012)

Table 2. Heart failure stage and class

ACC/AHA Stage	Description	NYHA Class	Description	Clinical Clues
A	At high risk for HF but without structural heart disease or symptoms of HF		None	Coronary artery disease, hypertension, diabetes, dyslipidemia, family history of cardiomyopathy
B	Structural heart disease but without signs or symptoms of HF	I	Asymptomatic	Left ventricular hypertrophy (ECG or echo), valvular disease, past MI
C	Structural heart disease with prior or current symptoms of HF	II-III	Symptomatic with minimal or moderate exertion	Dyspnea, fatigue, exercise intolerance, prior HF hospitalization
D	Refractory HF requiring specialized interventions	IV	Symptomatic at rest	End-stage, awaiting transplant, receiving palliative care

Adapted from (Hunt, 2009; Farrell, 2002)

Table 3. Therapeutics by class

Drug Class	Mechanism of Action	Hemodynamic Effect	Examples
Drugs with Proven Mortality Reduction			
β-blockers[1]	competitive antagonists at β-adrenergic receptors	decreased afterload decreased preload	carvedilol bisoprolol metoprolol
ARBs[2]	competitive antagonists at angiotensin I receptors	decreased preload decreased afterload	valsartan candesartan
ACE inhibitors[3]	inhibit angiotensin II generation	decreased preload decreased afterload	enalapril captopril
Aldosterone antagonist	competitive antagonist at aldosterone receptor	decreased preload	spironolactone eplerenone
Drugs Used for Symptom Management			
Diuretics	inhibit renal sodium absorption	preload	furosemide hydrochlorothiazide
Organic nitrates	venous smooth muscle relaxation	decreased preload	nitroglycerin isosorbide dinitrate
PDE3 inhibitors[4]	Inhibit PDE, increase β-adrenergic effects	increased contractility decreased preload decreased afterload	inamrinone milrinone
Inotropes	Inhibit Na^+/K^+ ATPase; increase intracellular Ca^{2+},	increased contractility	digoxin

[1]beta-adrenergic receptor blockers,[2]angiotensin II receptor blockers, [3]angiotensin converting enzyme inhibitors, [4]phosphodiesterase class 3 inhibitors

NEW HORIZONS: NATRIURETIC PEPTIDES IN THE TREATMENT OF HF

Management of heart failure using current modalities of ACE inhibitors, ARBs, β-blockers, and aldosterone antagonists is well established (Hunt 2009). Current research focused on the development of therapeutic natiuretic peptides is most advanced on ularitide, carperitide, nesiritide, and via neprilysin inhibition. The natriuretic peptides counterbalance many of the neurohormonal mechanisms related to the pathology of heart failure. Multiple agents are currently available for modulation of endogenous natriuretic peptides either through administration of synthetic analogs or by inhibition of enzymes that responsible for the breakdown of natriuretic peptides.

Ularitide

Ularitide is a synthetic form of the natiuretic peptide urodilantin (Mitrovic, 2005; Mitrovic, 2006). To date, two phase II studies have been completed and published, a phase III study has completed enrollment of participants and is awaiting publication.

The SIRIUS I trial randomized 24 NYHA class III-IV HF patients to receive placebo or 24 hour continuous infusion of ularitide 7.5, 15, or 30 ng/kg/min (Mitrovic, 2005). Patients had a mean age of 66 (± 12 years) and were primarily male (n=18). At time of admission to the study, patients had dyspnea at rest or with minimal physical activity and a mean cardiac index (CI) of 1.91 ±0.34, pulmonary capillary wedge pressure (PCWP) elevated to 26 ±6 mmHg, and right atrial pressure (RAP) of 11 ±4 mmHg. Hemodynamic parameters were measured prior to study drug initiation and at 6, 24, and 30 hours. Additionally, NT-proBNP and cGMP were measured at identical time points and at 6 hours patients were asked to self-assess dyspnea. Patients were allowed to continue taking baseline cardiovascular medications as well as loop diuretics and inotropic infusions at the discretion of the study investigators. Eleven of 12 patients in the placebo and 7.5 ng/kg/min group required loop diuretics, while only three of 12 patients in the combined 15 and 30 ng/kg/min group required loop diuretics. PCWP was decreased relative to placebo in the 30 ng/kg/min group at 6 and 24 hours, and returned to baseline at 30 hours without showing evidence of rebound. All patients including placebo reported either no change or mild to marked improvement in their self-reported dyspnea scales. Urine output was similar among groups, with the placebo and 7.5 ng/kg/min group received more loop diuretic. Serum creatinine was increased in the 7.5 ng/kg/min group while other groups showed a decrease in serum creatinine. NT-proBNP levels were decreased at 24 and 30 hours in both the 15 and 30 ng/kg/min group. All patients completed the study, two patients died 8 and 20 days after completion of the study. Adverse effects were limited to hypotension observed in three patients, two required interruption of infusion for one hour. No significant changes were noted in EKGs or relevant lab values.

A second phase two study, the SIRIUS II trial randomized 221 HF patients to receive identical dosing regimens as the SIRIUS I trial with similar primary endpoints (Mitrovic, 2006). Patients were predominantly male (78.3%) and were all white. At time of enrollment, more than 90% of patients had an ejection fraction of less than 40%. During the study drug infusion, PCWP was statistically decreased in the 15 ng/kg/min and the 30 ng/kg/min group compared to both placebo and the 7.5 ng/kg/min group. This was difference was significant among all groups at the 6 hour mark and persisted through the 24 hour mark. Patient self-assessment of dyspnea was statistically significantly improved in all groups at both the 6 and 24 hour marks. Only one patient in the placebo arm reported worsening of dyspnea. Both CI and systemic vascular resistance (SVR) were improved in the 15 and 30 ng/kg/min groups starting at the one hour mark and persisting through the 24 hour mark. Loop diuretics were given at investigator discretion and were given less frequently in the 15 ng/kg/min arm. Mean urine output was consistent between treatment groups and at the end of the infusion serum creatinine (SCr) was unchanged in all groups with the exception of the 15 ng/ml/min group which had a decreased SCr. Creatinine clearance decreased at 48 and 72 hours except in the 15 ng/kg/min group. A small number of patients in all of the ularitide arms required a temporary interruption of the ularitide infusion due to hypotension, similarly one patient in each of the active treatment arms discontinued study drug due to hypotension. A numerically lower number of patients died in the ularitide treated groups through day 30. Additionally, median hospital length of stay was numerically but not statistically shorter in the 15 and 30 ng/kg/min groups compared to placebo and 7.5 ng/kg/min.

Currently, ularitide is being tested in a multicenter, multinational, double blind, placebo controlled trial (O'Connor, 2016; Thomas, 2015). This study will enrolled 2157 patients of both genders, aged 18-85 years old, presenting with acutely decompensated heart failure with elevated levels of NT-proBNP and worsening symptoms of dyspnea at rest. Patients must have a systolic blood pressure of 116 to 180 mmHg and estimated glomerular filtration rate (eGFR) measured by modification of diet in renal disease (MDRD) of greater than 25 ml/min/1.73m^2 (O'Connor, 2016). Patients were randomized to receive ularitide 15 ng/kg/min or placebo in the setting of standard background pharmacotherapy. The study has two co-primary outcomes; cardiovascular mortality for duration of trial and a composite outcome consisting of a global assessment of the patient, need for additional interventions, and all-cause mortality. As of this writing, results of this study have not been released, however, the FDA has granted fast track approval status for this drug (Thomas, 2016).

Clinical studies of ularitide are currently limited to the acutely decompensated patients with signs and symptoms of volume overload. Data suggests that ularitide may have a diuretic sparing effect in this setting, and may have a role in preserving tenuous renal function (Mitrovic, 2006).

Carperitide

Carperitide, a synthetic analog of ANP is currently only available in Japan. There have been few trials in heart failure patients, two of which are only available in Japanese. Two large trials released after approval of the drug in Japan are both prospective, open label studies.

Suwa et. al. enrolled 3852 patients with a mean EF of 46.9% and PCWP of 15.6 mmHg in an open label prospective trial of carperitide dose adjusted at investigators discretion to a maximum approved dosage of 0.2 mcg/kg/min (Suwa, 2005). Efficacy was defined as percentage of patients assessed by the attending physician on a subjective scale as either improved or markedly improved. The primary safety outcome was defined as BP lowering to less than 90 mmHg or a decrease of 20 mmHg from baseline. Approximately 55% of patients were rated as improved or markedly improved. Hypotension was the most commonly reported adverse effect however, the study population reported fluctuation in renal function and electrolyte abnormalities. Limited data were available regarding concomitant drug therapy.

Nomura et al, enrolled 1932 patients with a mean LVEF of 45.5% to receive either carperitide monotherapy or carperitide in combination with medications including diuretics, nitrates, calcium channel blockers, vasopressors, PDE III inhibitors (Nomura, 2008). Patients that were considered to have received carperitide monotherapy were allowed to receive a bolus dose of diuretics, nitrates, calcium channel blockers, morphine, or digoxin. 83.2% of patients responded to carperitide monotherapy, 16.8% required either additional agents or discontinuation of carperitide due to adverse effects. Hypotension was the most commonly occurring adverse effect (3 patients), followed by AMI, HF, ventricular tachycardia, renal failure, cerebral infarction, shock, and acute renal failure.

Significant limitations of both studies include the non-randomized design, observational nature, use of subjective surrogate endpoints, and lack of control group. Further, both studies were performed exclusively in Japanese medical centers, severely limiting the generalizability of the results.

Nesiritide

Nesiritide was FDA approved in 2001 (FDA 2016). The VMAC trial, one of the original trials used for FDA approval, reflected improvement in patient reported dyspnea scales and decreases in PCWP (Young 2002). Subsequent to these trials, pooled data reflect increased rates of worsening renal function and early death (Sackner-Berstein, Kowalski, Fox, & Aaronson, 2005; Sackner-Bernstein, Skopicki, & Aaronson, 2005). Due to this data, the ASCEND–HF study, a large, double-blind, placebo controlled trial was designed to compare nesiritide plus standard of care to standard of care alone.(O'Connor et al., 2011) This multinational study enrolled 7141 patients, 7007 received either study drug or placebo. Median duration of nesiritide or placebo infusion was 41 hours and approximately 90% of patients in both arms received a loop diuretic, 6% received an inotropic agent, and 15% received a vasodilator. This study had co-primary endpoints, change in dyspnea at 6 and 24 hours and a composite end point of heart failure rehospitalization and all-cause mortality for 30 days. Due to conflicting views between United States and European regulators, there were two predefined strategies for reaching statistical significance for dyspnea scores. For the United States regulators, both the 6 and 24 hour dyspnea scores had have a p value of $\leq$0.005 or either the 6 or 24 hour dyspnea score had to have a p value of $\leq$0.0025. While there was a small numerical difference in the number of patients reporting markedly or moderately better dyspnea scores (42.1% in the placebo group versus 44.5% in the nesiritide group) the p value at 6 and 24 hours was 0.03 and 0.007, this did not achieve the predefined statistical significance. The composite endpoint of death or rehospitalization for heart failure did not achieve statistical significance ($p = 0.31$). Multiple subgroup analyses were predefined, the results consistently did not achieve statistical significance. Consistent with previous studies, patients receiving nesiritide experienced hypotension (28.6% vs 16.4%).

The initial publication ASCEND-HF study did not directly address the concerns with renal function associated with the use of nesiritide (O'Connor, 2011). An additional analysis of the ASCEND-HF data was completed comparing urine output and loop diuretic dose (Gottlieb, 2013). Complete data was available for 4881 patients. No significant difference was noted for either parameter, even with analysis of multiple subgroups.

These two studies taken together suggest a limited role for nesiritide for the management of patients with acute decompensated heart failure (Gottlieb, 2013; O'Connor, 2011).

Angiotensin Receptor Neprilysin Inhibitor

The newest medication targeting natriuretic peptides is sacubitril which is combined with valsartan. Although not a natriuretic peptide, sacubitril inhibits neprilysin allowing for increased exposure to endogenous natriuretic peptides. The PARADIGM-HF study randomized 8,399 patients with HFrEF to receive sacubitril in combination with valsartan or enalapril after consecutive run-in phases with enalapril and sacubitril/valsartan (McMurray, 2014). The majority of patients enrolled in this study were receiving appropriate standard of care. The primary endpoint was a composite of death from a cardiovascular cause or a first hospitalization for heart failure. The primary endpoint occurred in 21.8% of the patients in the treatment group compared to 26.5% of patient in the placebo group ($p<0.001$). This change was seen at each interim analysis, after the third interim analysis it was recommended to stop the trial as prespecified criteria for benefit had been met. Analysis of mortality was also statistically significant, with 13.3% of patients dying in the sacubitril/valsartan group versus 16.5% in the placebo group ($p<0.001$) Fewer patients in the sacubitril/valsartan group had elevated serum creatinine or elevated potassium and more patients in the enalapril group stopped medication due to adverse effects. This study led to rapid approval of the combination of sacubitril/valsartan by the FDA. While the PARADIGM-HF study does reflect both clinical and statistical significance, some of the methodology has been criticized. The most significant criticism arises from the dose of enalapril used in the placebo arm. The maximum recommended dose of enalapril is 20 mg twice daily (Yancy 2013). PARADIGM-HF patients achieved a mean goal of 18.9 mg of enalapril daily (McMurray, 2014). While the maximum recommended dose of enalapril is significantly higher, the mean dose of enalapril achieved in previous heart failure clinical trials is 16.6 mg (Yancy, 2013).

Current heart failure guidelines have not been updated to reflect the approval of sacubitril/valsartan combination (Yancy, 2013). The Institute for Clinical and Economic Review has evaluated the combination of sacubitril and valsartan and determined there was a moderate degree of certainty that there is incremental to substantial benefit and that on an individual basis, the cost/QALY gained were below generally accepted thresholds (Ollendorf, 2015). The concern arises when analyzed from a population basis, the cost of the combination drug therapy would need to be discounted by approximately 20% to avoid exceeding existing thresholds.

CONCLUSION

HF remains a complex syndrome which is difficult to manage. A significant number of people in the United States have been diagnosed with HF which brings with it a heavy financial burden on the medical system as well as high rates of morbidity and mortality. Much of the pathophysiology associated with HF is related to compensatory mechanisms aimed at maintaining CO to meet the metabolic demands of the body. Many of the current medications used for the treatment of HF target these mechanisms, and are primarily managing symptoms. New research has suggested a key role for the natriuretic peptides in counterbalancing the compensatory mechanisms of HF and represent novel therapeutic targets for treatment which would ideally improve survival rates among patients with HF.

REFERENCES

Anker, S. D., Ponikowski, P., Mitrovic, V., Peacock, W. F., & Filippatos, G. (2015). Ularitide for the treatment of acute decompensated heart failure: From preclinical to clinical studies. *European Heart Journal*, *36*(12), 715–723. doi:10.1093/eurheartj/ehu484 PMID:25670819

Bahrami, H., Kronmal, R., Bluemke, D. A., Olson, J., Shea, S., Liu, K., & Lima, J. A. et al. (2008). Differences in the incidence of congestive heart failure by ethnicity: The Multi-Ethnic Study of Atherosclerosis. *Archives of Internal Medicine*, *168*(19), 2138–2145. doi:10.1001/archinte.168.19.2138 PMID:18955644

Carlsson, M., Andersson, R., Bloch, K. M., Steding-Ehrenborg, K., Mosen, H., Stahlberg, F., & Arheden, H. et al. (2012). Cardiac output and cardiac index measured with cardiovascular magnetic resonance in healthy subjects, elite athletes and patients with congestive heart failure. *Journal of Cardiovascular Magnetic Resonance*, *14*(1), 51. doi:10.1186/1532-429X-14-51 PMID:22839436

Chaggar, P. S., Malkin, C. J., Shaw, S. M., Williams, S. G., & Channer, K. S. (2009). Neuroendocrine effects on the heart and targets for therapeutic manipulation in heart failure. *Cardiovascular Therapeutics*, *27*(3), 187–193. doi:10.1111/j.1755-5922.2009.00094.x PMID:19689618

Colucci, W. S. (2015). *Pathophysiology of heart failure: Neurohormonal adaptations*. UpToDate®. Retrieved March 6, 2016 from http://www.uptodate.com/contents/pathophysiology-of-heart-failure-neurohumoral-adaptations

Copstead, L.-E., & Banasik, J. L. (2010). Determinants of cardiac output. In *Pathophysiology* (pp. 419–421). St. Louis, MO: Saunders Elsevier.

Curry, C. W., Nelson, G. S., Wyman, B. T., Declerck, J., Talbot, M., Berger, R. D., & Kass, D. A. et al. (2000). Mechanical dyssynchrony in dilated cardiomyopathy with intraventricular conduction delay as depicted by 3D tagged magnetic resonance imaging. *Circulation*, *101*(1), E2. doi:10.1161/01.CIR.101.1.e2 PMID:10618315

de Sa, D. D., & Chen, H. H. (2008). The role of natriuretic peptides in heart failure. *Current Cardiology Reports*, *10*(3), 182–189. doi:10.1007/s11886-008-0032-2 PMID:18489861

English, M. A., & Mastrean, M. B. (1995). Congestive heart failure: Public and private burden. *Critical Care Nursing Quarterly*, *18*, 1–6. PMID:7719944

Farrell, M. H., Micale-Foody, J., & Krumholz, H. M. (2002). β-blockers in heart failure. *Journal of the American Medical Association*, *287*(7), 890–897. doi:10.1001/jama.287.7.890 PMID:11851583

FDA/Center for Drug Evaluation and Research. (2016). *FDA Approved Drug Products: Natrecor*. Retrieved on March 11, 2016, from http://www.accessdata.fda.gov/scripts/cder/drugsatfda/index.cfm?fuseaction=Search.DrugDetails

Golan, D. E., Tashjian, A. H., Armstrong, E. J., & Armstrong, A. W. (2012). Integrative cardiovascular pharmacology: hypertension, ischemic heart disease, and heart failure. In *Principles of Pharmacology* (pp. 437–463). Philadelphia, PA: Lippincott Williams & Wilkins.

Gottlieb, S. S., Stebbins, A., Voors, A. A., Hasselblad, V., Ezekowitz, J. A., Califf, R. M., & Hernandez, A. F. et al. (2013). Effects of nesiritide and predictors of urine output in acute decompensated heart failure: Results from the ASCEND-HF (acute study of clinical effectiveness of nesiritide and decompensated heart failure). *Journal of the American College of Cardiology*, *62*(13), 1177–1183. doi:10.1016/j.jacc.2013.04.073 PMID:23747790

Grewal, J., Chandavimol, M., & Ignaszewski, A. (2004). B-type natriuretic peptide: A new marker for congestive heart failure. *BCMJ*, *46*(1), 24–29.

He, J., Ogden, L. G., Bazzano, L. A., Vupputuri, S., Loria, C., & Whelton, P. K. (2001). Risk factors for congestive heart failure in US men and women: NHANES I epidemiologic follow-up study. *Archives of Internal Medicine*, *161*(7), 996–1002. doi:10.1001/archinte.161.7.996 PMID:11295963

He, J., Ogden, L. G., Bazzano, L. A., Vupputuri, S., Loria, C., & Whelton, P. K. (2002). Dietary sodium intake and incidence of congestive heart failure in overweight US men and women: First national health and nutrition examination survey epidemiologic follow-up study. *Archives of Internal Medicine*, *162*(14), 1619–162. doi:10.1001/archinte.162.14.1619 PMID:12123406

Heidenreich, P. A., Albert, N. M., Allen, L. A., Bluemke, D. A., Butler, J., Fonarow, G. C., & Trogdon, J. G. et al. (2013). Forecasting the impact of heart failure in the United States: A policy statement from the American Heart Association. *Circulation: Heart Failure*, *6*(3), 606–619. doi:10.1161/HHF.0b013e318291329a PMID:23616602

Hunt, S., Abraham, W. T., & Chin, M. H. (2009). Focused update incorporated into the ACC/AHA 2005 guidelines for the diagnosis and management of heart failure in adults: A report of the american college of cardiology foundation/american heart association task force on practice guidelines developed in collaboration with the international society for heart and lung transplantation. *Journal of the American College of Cardiology*, *53*(15), e1–e90. doi:10.1016/j.jacc.2008.11.013 PMID:19358937

Kemp, C. D., & Conte, J. V. (2013). The pathophysiology of heart failure. *Cardiovascular Pathology*, *21*(5), 365–371. doi:10.1016/j.carpath.2011.11.007 PMID:22227365

Lloyd-Jones, D. M., Larson, M. G., Leip, E. P., Beiser, A., DAgostino, R. B., Kannel, W. B., & Levy, D. et al. (2002). Lifetime risk for developing congestive heart failure: The Framingham Heart Study. *Circulation*, *106*(24), 3068–3072. doi:10.1161/01.CIR.0000039105.49749.6F PMID:12473553

Marieb, E. N., & Hoehn, K. (2013). The cardiovascular system: the heart. In *Human anatomy and physiology* (pp. 658–691). Boston, MA: Pearson.

Massie, B. M., & Shah, N. B. (1997). Evolving trends in the epidemiologic factors of heart failure: Rationale for preventive strategies and comprehensive disease management. *American Heart Journal*, *133*(6), 703–712. doi:10.1016/S0002-8703(97)70173-X PMID:9200399

McMurray, J. J., Packer, M., Desai, A. S., Gong, J., Lefkowitz, M. P., Rizkala, A. R., & Zile, M. R. et al. (2014). Angiotensin-neprilysin inhibition versus enalapril in heart failure. *The New England Journal of Medicine*, *371*(11), 993–1004. doi:10.1056/NEJMoa1409077 PMID:25176015

Mitrovic, V., Luss, H., Nitsche, K., Forssmann, K., Maronde, E., Fricke, K., & Meyer, M. et al. (2005). Effects of the renal natiuretic peptide urodilantin (ularitide) in patients with decompensated chronic heart failure: A double-blind, placebo-controlled, ascending-dose trial. *American Heart Journal*, *150*(6), 1239.e1–1239.e8. doi:10.1016/j.ahj.2005.01.022 PMID:16338265

Mitrovic, V., Seferovic, P. M., Simeunovic, D., Ristic, A. D., Miric, M., Moiseyev, V. S., & Meyer, M. et al. (2006). Haemodynamic and clinical effects of ularitide in decompensated heart failure. *European Heart Journal*, *27*(23), 2823–2832. doi:10.1093/eurheartj/ehl337 PMID:17074775

Mozaffarian, D., Benjamin, E. J., Go, A. S., Arnett, D. K., Blaha, M. J., Cushman, M., & Turner, M. B. et al. (2016). Heart disease and stroke statistics—2016 update: A report from the American Heart Association. *Circulation*, *133*(4), e1–e324. doi:10.1161/CIR.0000000000000366 PMID:26673558

Nomura, F., Kurobe, N., Mori, Y., Hikita, A., Kawai, M., Suwa, M., & Okutani, Y. (2008). Multicenter prospective investigation on the efficacy and safety of carperitide as a first-line drug for acute heart failure syndrome with preserved blood pressure: COMPASS: Carperitide Effects Observed Through Monitoring Dyspnea in Acute Decompensated Heart Failure Study. *Circulation Journal, 72*(11), 1777–1786. doi:10.1253/circj.CJ-07-0760 PMID:18832779

O'Connor, C., & Peacock, W. F. (2016). *Efficacy and safety of ularitide for the treatment of acute decompensated heart failure (TRUE-AHF).* Retrieved on March 11, 2016 from https://clinicaltrials.gov/ct2/show/study/NCT01661634#locn

OConnor, C. M., Starling, R. C., Hernandez, A. F., Armstrong, P. W., Dickstein, K., Hasselblad, V., & Califf, R. M. et al. (2011). Effect of nesiritide in patients with acute decompensated heart failure. *The New England Journal of Medicine, 365*(1), 32–43. doi:10.1056/NEJMoa1100171 PMID:21732835

Ollendorf, D. A., Sandhu, A. T., Chapman, R., Heidenreich, P. A., Russo, E., Shore, K. K., …Pearson, S. D. (2015). *CardioMEMS HF System (St. Jude Medical) and sacubitril/valsartan (Entresto, Norvatis) for Management of Congestive Heart Failure: effectiveness, Value and Value Based Price Benchmarks.* Retrieved March 11, 2016, from http://ctaf.org/sites/default/files/u148/CHF_Draft_Report_091115.pdf

Rea, M. E., & Dunlap, M. E. (2008). Renal hemodynamics in heart failure: Implications for treatment. *Current Opinion in Nephrology and Hypertension, 17*(1), 87–92. doi:10.1097/MNH.0b013e3282f357da PMID:18090676

Roger, V. L., Weston, S. A., Redfield, M. M., Hellermann-Homan, J. P., Killian, J., Yawn, B. P., & Jacobsen, S. J. (2004). Trends in heart failure incidence and survival in a community-based population. *Journal of the American Medical Association, 292*(3), 344–350. doi:10.1001/jama.292.3.344 PMID:15265849

Sackner-Bernstein, J. D., Kowalski, M., Fox, M., & Aaronson, K. D. (2005). Short-term risk of death after treatment with nesiritide for decompensated heart failure: a pooled anyalysis of randomized controlled trials. *JAMA, 293,*(15) 1900-1905.

Sackner-Bernstein, J. D., Skopicki, H. A., & Aaronson, K. D. (2005). Risk of worsening renal function with nesiritide in patients with acutely decompensated heart failure. *Circulation, 111*(12), 1487–1491. doi:10.1161/01.CIR.0000159340.93220.E4 PMID:15781736

Suwa, M., Seino, Y., Nomachi, Y., Matsuki, S., & Funahashi, K. (2005). Multicenter prospective investigation of the efficacy and safety of carperitide for acute heart failure in the real world of therapy. *Circulation Journal, 36*(3), 283–290. doi:10.1253/circj.69.283 PMID:15731532

Thomas, N., & Walsh, K. (2015). *Ularitide received FDA Fast Track designation for the treatment of acute decompensated heart failure.* Retrieved on March 11, 2016, from http://www.cardiorentis.com/de/media/index.php

van den Broek, K. C., Defilippi, C. R., Christenson, R. H., Seliger, S. L., Gottdiener, J. S., & Kop, W. J. (2011). Predictive value of depressive symptoms and B-type natriuretic peptide for new-onset heart failure and mortality. *The American Journal of Cardiology, 107*(5), 723–729. doi:10.1016/j.amjcard.2010.10.055 PMID:21316507

Vincent, J.-L. (2008). Understanding cardiac output. *Critical Care (London, England)*, *12*(4), 174. doi:10.1186/cc6975 PMID:18771592

Yancy, C. W., Jessup, M., Bozkurt, B., Butler, J., Casey, D. E. Jr, Drazner, M. H., & Wilkoff, B. L. et al. (2013). 2013 ACCF/AHA guideline for the management of heart failure: A report of the American college of Cardiology Foundation/American Heart Association Task Force on practice guidelines. *Circulation*, *128*(16), e240–e327. doi:10.1161/CIR.0b013e31829e8807 PMID:23741058

Young, J. B., Abraham, W. T., Stevenson, L. W., Horton, D. P., Elkayam, U., & Bourge, R. C. (2002). Intravenous nesiritide vs nitroglycerin for treatment of decompensated congestive heart failure: A randomized controlled trial. *Journal of the American Medical Association*, *287*(12), 1531–1540. PMID:11911755

Chapter 2
Signaling Mechanisms Regulating Vascular Endothelial Barrier Function

Mohammad Tauseef
Chicago State University, USA & University of Illinois at Chicago, USA

Madeeha Aqil
University of Illinois at Chicago, USA

Dolly Mehta
University of Illinois at Chicago, USA

ABSTRACT

During inflammatory conditions, such as sepsis, myocardial infarction and acute respiratory distress syndrome, endothelial cell-cell junctions start to disrupt because of the internalization of the junctional proteins such as vascular endothelial (VE) cadherin. This leads to the formation of minute inter-endothelial gaps, and the infiltration of protein-rich fluid and immune cells in the interstitial space. If remains unchecked, the persistent buildup of edema underlying the endothelial lining sets the stage for the serious life-threatening complications and ultimately leads to the multi-organ failure and death. Thus, to determine the molecular mechanisms underlying the opening and resolution phase of the gap formation, will provide an insight to better understand the pathology of the cardiovascular and pulmonary inflammatory disorders. In this chapter, we will discuss about how the signaling mechanisms activated by the known inflammatory molecules increase endothelial permeability.

Acronyms:

ALI: Acute Lung Injury
ARDS: Acute Respiratory Distress Syndrome
IEJs: Inter Endothelial Junctions
AJs: Adherens Junctions

DOI: 10.4018/978-1-5225-2092-4.ch002

LPS: Endotoxin Lipopolysaccharide
TEER: Tansendothelial Electrical Resistance
PAR1: Protease Activated Receptor 1
MYLK: Myosin Light Chain Kinase
FAK: Focal Adhesion Kinase
RACK1: Receptor for Activated C Kinase 1
ROCK: Rho kinase
PIP_2: $_P$hosphoinositol 4, 5-bisbiphosphate
IP_3: Inositol 1, 4, 5 triphosphate
DAG: Diacylglycerol
STIM1: Stromal Interaction Molecule 1
SOC: Store Operated Ca^{2+}
SOCE: Store Operated Ca^{2+} Entry ROCE: Receptor Operated Ca^{2+} Entry TRPC Channel: Transient Receptor Potential Canonical Channel
SPHK1: Sphingosine Kinase 1
S1P: Sphingosine 1 Phosphate
CRAC Channel: Ca^{2+} Release Activated Ca^{2+} Channel
OAG: 1-Oleoyl-2-Acetyl-*sn*-Glycerol
PECAM1: Platelet Endothelial Cell Adhesion Molecule-1

INTRODUCTION

Vascular endothelium forms the inner most lining of the blood vessels, regulates variety of biological processes such as angiogenesis, wound healing, cell growth and host defense mechanisms (Chavez, Smith, & Mehta, 2011; Gong et al., 2015; Komarova, Mehta, & Malik, 2007; Mehta, 2012; Mehta & Malik, 2006; Rajput et al., 2016; Sukriti, Tauseef, Yazbeck, & Mehta, 2014; Tauseef et al., 2016; Tauseef et al., 2012). Maintenance of uninterrupted endothelial barrier function is pre-requisite for the tissue fluid homeostasis, vessel tone and prevention of the activation of pathological coagulation cascade (Chavez et al., 2011; Komarova et al., 2007; Mehta, 2012; Mehta & Malik, 2006; Sukriti et al., 2014; Tauseef et al., 2016; Tauseef et al., 2012). However, endothelium is permeable to certain molecules ranging from the sizes 0.1 nm to 11.5 nm in diameters (Chavez et al., 2011; Komarova et al., 2007; Mehta & Malik, 2006; Sukriti et al., 2014). During physiological conditions, endothelium transport molecules such as ions and water molecules, using two different mechanisms (Chavez et al., 2011; Komarova et al., 2007; Mehta & Malik, 2006; Sukriti et al., 2014; Vandenbroucke, Mehta, Minshall, & Malik, 2008): i) Transcellular pathway (Chavez et al., 2011; Mehta & Malik, 2006; Sukriti et al., 2014) ii) Paracellular pathway (Chavez et al., 2011; Mehta & Malik, 2006; Sukriti et al., 2014). Molecules, which are greater than 3 mm radii, such as albumin, IgG, etc., are transported across the endothelium via transcellular transport mechanism (Komarova et al., 2007; Mehta & Malik, 2006; Sukriti et al., 2014; Vandenbroucke et al., 2008). This transport mechanism is also called vesicular transport or transcytosis (Mehta & Malik, 2006; Predescu, Predescu, & Malik, 2007). However, molecules , which are smaller than 3mm in sizes, for example, glucose molecules, water molecules and ions; transportation is mediated via paracellular mechanism through the inter endothelial junctions (IEJs) (Chavez et al., 2011; Komarova et al., 2007; Mehta & Malik, 2006; Sukriti et al., 2014; Vandenbroucke et al., 2008).

A Transcellular pathway is regulated by a tight coordination between proteins such as caveolae, dynamin and intersectin (Chavez et al., 2011; Komarova et al., 2007; Mehta & Malik, 2006; Predescu et al., 2007; Predescu, Predescu, Timblin, Stan, & Malik, 2003; Sukriti et al., 2014). Caveolae are flasked shaped vesicles, which are composed of proteins called caveolin 1 (Chavez et al., 2011; Mehta & Malik, 2006; Predescu et al., 2007; Zhao et al., 2009). Caveolin 1 forms the key structural and signaling molecule of caveolae (Chavez et al., 2011; Predescu et al., 2007; Sukriti et al., 2014). Dysfunctioning of caveolin 1 in the endothelial cells has been linked to some of the serious cardiovascular and pulmonary disorders, such as pulmonary hypertension (Maniatis et al., 2008; Zhao & Malik, 2009; Zhao et al., 2009). Caveolin 1 also negatively regulates endothelial nitric oxide synthase (eNOS) (Mehta & Malik, 2006; Zhao & Malik, 2009; Zhao et al., 2009). Caveolin1 knockout mice displayed increase endothelial barrier permeability because of the dismantling of IEJs in capillaries and venules (Chavez et al., 2011; Mehta & Malik, 2006; Sukriti et al., 2014; Zhao & Malik, 2009; Zhao et al., 2009).

Paracellular pathway is tightly regulated complex interplay between various junctional proteins, such vascular endothelial cadherins (VE cadherins) (Chavez et al., 2011; Dejana, Orsenigo, Molendini, Baluk, & McDonald, 2009; Giannotta, Trani, & Dejana, 2013; Komarova et al., 2007; Mehta & Malik, 2006) and catenins (β-catenin, p120 catenin) in the endothelial cells. These junctional proteins bind endothelial cells together and form adherens junctions (AJs). In healthy endothelium, VE-cadherin is linked through its cytoplasmic domain to p120-catenin and β-catenin or plakoglobin (γ-catenin), to provide a basic organization of AJs. (Chavez et al., 2011; Dejana, Orsenigo, et al., 2009; Giannotta et al., 2013; Komarova et al., 2012; Komarova et al., 2007; Mehta & Malik, 2006; Rajput et al., 2013; Sukriti et al., 2014; Thennes & Mehta, 2012; Vandenbroucke St Amant et al., 2012) (Figure 1). Besides catenins and cadherins, molecular motors such as actin and myosin machinery play an integral role in the functioning of paracellular transport mechanism in the endothelial cells (Figure 1). Endothelial cell-to-cell junctions are not only maintain integrity of AJs, but they are also required to initiating intracellular signaling processes to prevent an uncontrolled cell growth, lumen formation, cell polarity and interactions with pericytes and smooth muscle cells (Chavez et al., 2011; Dejana, Orsenigo, et al., 2009; Giannotta et al., 2013; Gong et al., 2015; Komarova et al., 2007; Mehta & Malik, 2006; Sukriti et al., 2014; Thennes & Mehta, 2012). Therefore, conditions that disrupt endothelial junctions might not only increase vascular permeability by opening intercellular gaps but also change the endothelial cell responses to their environment and to the surrounding cells (Chavez et al., 2011; Daneshjou et al., 2015; Dejana, Orsenigo, et al., 2009; Giannotta et al., 2013; Gong et al., 2015; Komarova et al., 2007; Mehta & Malik, 2006; Sukriti et al., 2014; Thennes & Mehta, 2012).

During physiological conditions both transcellular and paracellular pathways work with each other to maintain endothelial barrier homeostasis, immune regulation and to preserve the normal tissue-oncotic pressure (Chavez et al., 2011; Mehta & Malik, 2006; Sukriti et al., 2014; Tauseef et al., 2008; Thennes & Mehta, 2012; Vandenbroucke et al., 2008). However, during inflammatory conditions, for example, during septicemia, activation of proinflammatory signaling cascades leads to the generation of potent inflammatory mediators such as thrombin, endotoxin Lipopolysaccharide (LPS), tumor necrosis factor α (TNF α) and vascular endothelial growth factor (VEGF), which through activation of their corresponding receptors, initiate endothelial barrier dysfunction (Bates & Harper, 2002; Daneshjou et al., 2015; Gong et al., 2015; Liu, Yu, Yu, & Kou, 2015; Mehta & Malik, 2006; Paria et al., 2004; Sukriti et al., 2014; Tauseef et al., 2008; Tauseef et al., 2012; Uhlig et al., 2014; Vandenbroucke et al., 2008). Endothelial dysfunction is the earliest step in the disorganization of IEJs. This disorganization ultimately leads to increase in endothelial permeability and accumulation of tissue edema (Daneshjou et al., 2015; Gong et al., 2014; Gong et al., 2015; Knezevic, Tauseef, Thennes, & Mehta, 2009; Tauseef et al., 2008; Tiruppathi et al., 2014; Vandenbroucke et al., 2008).Excessive accumulation of fluid along with albumin and inflammatory cells underneath the breached endothelium, sets the stage of inflammatory disorders such acute lung injury and acute respiratory distress syndrome, which has no treatment so far (Gong et al., 2014; Gong et al., 2015; Knezevic et al., 2009; Tauseef et al., 2008; Tauseef et al., 2012; Tiruppathi et al., 2014).

Pulmonary Endothelial Barrier Permeability

Studies suggest that proinflammatory mediators such as thrombin, histamine and endotoxin LPS increase pulmonary endothelial permeability by opening of the IEJs (Ashina et al., 2015; Gong et al., 2015; Rajput et al., 2016; Schmidt et al., 2013; Tauseef et al., 2008; Tauseef et al., 2012; Tiruppathi, Ahmmed, Vogel, & Malik, 2006). IEJs are composed of adheres junctions (AJs), tight junctions (TJs) and junctional adhesion molecules (JAMs) (Chavez et al., 2011; Dejana, Orsenigo, et al., 2009; Giannotta et al., 2013; Knezevic et al., 2009; Mehta & Malik, 2006; Tiruppathi et al., 2014; Tran et al., 2015; Wang, Li, Cho, & Malik, 2014). These junctional proteins along with cell contractile cytoskeleton machinery, initiate a complex signaling mechanisms to regulate paracellular permeability pathways (Chavez et al., 2011; Komarova et al., 2007; Mehta & Malik, 2006; Tiruppathi et al., 2014; Tran et al., 2015; Vandenbroucke et al., 2008). In the endothelium, AJs play a prominent role in the formation and regulation of barrier function (Komarova et al., 2007; Sukriti et al., 2014; Thennes & Mehta, 2012). Also, vascular-endothelium (VE) cadherin constitute a major cadherin in the assembly of endothelial barrier and regulate paracellular permeability pathway (Dejana, Orsenigo, et al., 2009; Giannotta et al., 2013; Gong et al., 2014; Gong et al., 2015) (Figure 1). Endothelial cells are linked to each other through these cadherin molecules. Hence, if any signaling pathway affects the VE-cadherin molecules, will disturb the endothelial barrier integrity, and may lead to increase in endothelial permeability (Daneshjou et al., 2015; Dejana, Orsenigo, et al., 2009; Giannotta et al., 2013; Gong et al., 2014; Mehta & Malik, 2006) (Figure 1).

Permeability increasing factors or inflammatory agonists induce minute gaps between endothelial cells and thus allow cells and protein rich fluid to pass across the endothelial monolayer (Chava, Tauseef, Sharma, & Mehta, 2012; Kini, Chavez, & Mehta, 2010; Knezevic et al., 2009; Komarova et al., 2012; Minshall et al., 2010; Singh et al., 2007; Tauseef et al., 2008). In acute inflammatory insults, increasing in endothelial permeability is reversible; however, in chronic inflammation, as happens during sepsis, the persistent increase in permeability leads to perturbation of gas exchange process and multi organ failure (Mehta & Malik, 2006; Pierrakos, Karanikolas, Scolletta, Karamouzos, & Velissaris, 2012; Rajput et al., 2016; Sukriti et al., 2014; Tauseef et al., 2012). The molecular mechanisms that initiate disturbances in the endothelial monolayer, and produce minute gap in between the endothelial cells, are still not clearly defined. However, recent studies from our laboratory as well as from other laboratories suggest the role excessive cytosolic calcium (Ca^{2+}) entry induced by inflammatory mediator in the endothelial cells, is the initial trigger in the induction of endothelial permeability (Ahmmed et al., 2004; Cioffi, Barry, & Stevens, 2010; Mehta et al., 2003; Samapati et al., 2012; Singh et al., 2007; Sundivakkam et al., 2012; Sundivakkam, Natarajan, Malik, & Tiruppathi, 2013; Tauseef et al., 2016; Tauseef et al., 2012; Tiruppathi et al., 2002) (Figure 2). Small GTPases, phosphatases and kinases, by regulating the phosphorylation and internalization of VE-cadherin, controls the junctional stability and vascular permeability (Chavez et al., 2011; Dejana, Tournier-Lasserve, & Weinstein, 2009; Giannotta et al., 2013; Mehta et al., 2003; Mehta & Malik, 2006; Schmidt et al., 2013; Thennes & Mehta, 2012). Besides, different types of vessel beds for example, veins, arteries, capillaries and lymphatics, display heterogeneity and therefore differ in terms of vascular permeability at the basal level and in response to edemagenic agents (Aird, 2012; Ofori-Acquah, King, Voelkel, Schaphorst, & Stevens, 2008; Regan & Aird, 2012; Stevens, 2011; Sukriti et al., 2014). Vascular endothelial cells of coronary, pulmonary and skeletal muscle form more restrictive barrier. However, vascular beds of kidney, liver and lymphatics formed discontinuous and permeable endothelial barrier (Mehta & Malik, 2006; Ofori-Acquah et al., 2008; Stevens, 2011). Measurement of coefficient of vascular endothelial permeability (K_{fc}), a sensitive marker of endothelial permeability, using isolated perfused lung preparations under basal conditions in experimental animals, demonstrated huge permeability variabilities across the arterial versus venous sites (Chavez et al., 2011; Mehta & Malik, 2006; Stevens, 2011). For example, permeability observed at the microvascular site was 42%, while at arterial bed approximately 19% and venous site approximately 37% (Mehta & Malik, 2006; Ofori-Acquah et al., 2008; Stevens, 2011; Sukriti et al., 2014). These studies suggest that arterial vascular bed constitute more restrictive barrier than venous area. More interestingly, the pulmonary micro vascular endothelial barrier is about four times tighter than the barrier formed by arterial or venous endothelial cells (Mehta & Malik, 2006; Ofori-Acquah et al., 2008; Stevens, 2011). Finally, measurement of endothelial barrier function *in vitro* using tansendothelial electrical resistance (TEER) technique showed that microvascular endothelial cells display tighter barrier as compare to large artery's endothelial cells (Chavez et al., 2011; Mehta & Malik, 2006; Sukriti et al., 2014). These observations suggest that there are many more regulators that dictate endothelial permeability and will ultimately behave accordingly in response to inflammatory mediators. To understand the molecular signaling pathways regulating endothelial barrier function at basal level as well as during inflammatory conditions are primers in the development of rationale therapeutic to treat vascular inflammatory conditions.

Signaling Mechanisms Regulating Endothelial Barrier Disruption

AJs have a central role in the regulation of endothelial barrier function (Komarova et al., 2007; Mehta, 2012). Multiple signaling pathways are involved in the induction of endothelial permeability (Beckers et al., 2015; Daneshjou et al., 2015; Dejana, Orsenigo, et al., 2009; Kini et al., 2010; Tauseef et al., 2012; Tiruppathi et al., 2006). However, increase in endothelial cells cytoskeleton contraction followed by disassembly of AJs are the main events taken place after challenging the cells with inflammatory agonists and cytokines (Beckers et al., 2015; DebRoy et al., 2014; Tauseef et al., 2012). In the following section we describe in detail how the activated inflammatory signaling pathways modulate the plasticity of AJs, leading to the mounting of endothelial permeability.

PAR-1 Activation Increases Endothelial Barrier Permeability

Thrombin, a procoagulant serine protease, increases endothelial permeability by activating predominantly its receptor, protease activated receptor (PAR)-1 on the endothelial cell surface (Tauseef et al., 2008; Vogel et al., 2000; Vogel & Malik, 2012). PAR-1 is activated by its ligation, which thrombin-dependent proteolytic cleavage of the PAR-1 extracellular extension (between Arg-41 and ser-42) (Knezevic et al., 2009; Tauseef et al., 2008; Vogel et al., 2000). Thus, resulting tethered ligand bind and activate PAR-1 receptor to initiate downstream signaling leads to increase in endothelial permeability (Knezevic et al., 2009; Tauseef et al., 2008). Studies show that thrombin increased endothelia permeability within few minutes and reversal of response occurred within two hours after removal of the agonist (Knezevic et al., 2007; Mehta & Malik, 2006; Mehta, Ravindran, & Kuebler, 2014; Uhlig et al., 2014; van Nieuw Amerongen, Draijer, Vermeer, & van Hinsbergh, 1998). However, in the continuous presence of agonist, recovery still occurs within two hours (Chava et al., 2012; Knezevic et al., 2007; Tauseef et al., 2008). This suggests that either desensitization of PAR-1 or activation of endogenous signaling pathways leads to the restoration disrupted endothelial barrier function. *In vivo* studies show that PAR-1 deleted mice are protected from thrombin induced increase in pulmonary vascular permeability, which further suggest a role of PAR-1 signaling in the increase in endothelial permeability (Mehta & Malik, 2006; Vogel et al., 2000).

PAR-1 is a seven-transmembrane heterotrimeric G protein coupled receptor (Mehta & Malik, 2006; Vogel et al., 2000; Vogel & Malik, 2012). Upon activation by thrombin, PAR-1 induces the breakdown of α- subunits of G_q and $G_{12/13}$ from the $G_{\beta\gamma}$ dimer. G_q and $G_{12/13}$ induce endothelial permeability via activating myosin light chain kinase (MYLK) and RhoA pathways (discussed below) by inducing endothelial contraction (Birukova et al., 2004; Mehta et al., 2003) (Knezevic et al., 2009; Mehta & Malik, 2006; Singh et al., 2007; Vogel et al., 2000; Vogel & Malik, 2012). However, the downstream signaling consequences following the $G_{\beta\gamma}$ subunit activation, are not well studied, and are one of the active areas of research in our laboratory. Knezevic et al. using *in vitro* cell culture and *in vivo* genetic knockout mouse models showed that $G_{\beta\gamma}$ subunit restores endothelial barrier function following the activation of barrier disruptive PAR-1 receptor activation (Knezevic et al., 2009). Using siRNA approach, Knezevic et al. (2009) found that knocking down of $G_{\beta\gamma}$ subunit in the endothelial cells prevented the reannealing of endothelial barrier function (Knezevic et al., 2009). This study discovered that during unperturbed endothelial barrier function, $G_{\beta\gamma}$ subunit remained associated with receptor for activated C kinase 1 (RACK1). However, upon stimulation of PAR-1 receptor with thrombin, $G_{\beta\gamma}$ subunit dissociated from RACK1, and interacted with tyrosine kinases, Fyn and focal adhesion kinase (FAK), a required step to activate of FAK in order to reseal disrupted endothelial monolayer (Knezevic et al., 2009). Upon depletion of RACK1, they found that $G_{\beta\gamma}$ subunit was able to activate FAK and endothelial barrier resolution, suggest RACK1 is upstream of $G_{\beta\gamma}$. Moreover, Fyn knockdown halted the $G_{\beta\gamma}$ subunit mediated recovery of endothelia monolayer, emphasizes that Fyn is required to activate FAK in the endothelial cells (Knezevic et al., 2009). Lastly, upon interaction with AJs, FAK stabilizes AJ assembly and thus, tightens the endothelial barrier. Thus, Knezevic et al. identified hitherto unknown novel signaling pathway to recover endothelial barrier function during the face of inflammatory milieu (Knezevic et al., 2009).

MYLK Activation and Role of Actin-Myosin Machinery in the Dismantling of AJs

The first and foremost event during the initiation of endothelial permeability is rounding of endothelial cells due to the activation of contractile machinery (Holinstat et al., 2006; Komarova et al., 2007; Shi et al., 1998; Singh et al., 2007; Sukriti et al., 2014; Tiruppathi et al., 2006). It happens through the formation of the stress fibers (Beckers et al., 2015; Chava et al., 2012; Mehta & Malik, 2006; Rajput et al., 2013). Stress fibers are composed of bundles of polymerized actin and myosin filaments (Beckers et al., 2015; Komarova et al., 2007; Mehta & Malik, 2006; Rajput et al., 2013). These fibers attain characteristic shape following the stimulation of endothelial cells with inflammatory mediators (Beckers et al., 2015; Rajput et al., 2013). This actin-myosin mediated endothelial contraction is initiated by myosin light chain kinase (MYLK). MYLK is a Ca^{2+}-calmodulin dependent enzyme (Beckers et al., 2015; Mirzapoiazova et al., 2011; Tauseef et al., 2012; Usatyuk et al., 2012; Wainwright et al., 2003). It exists in two isoforms- the muscle type, which presents in smooth muscle cells; and a non-muscle type, expressed in non-muscle cells including endothelial cells (Mehta & Malik, 2006; Tauseef et al., 2012; Usatyuk et al., 2012). Upon activation, following the cytosolic Ca^{2+} entry induced by inflammatory agonist such as thrombin, MYLK phosphorylates regulatory myosin light chain (MLC) on ser-19 (monophosphorylation) or ser-19/thr-18 (diphosphorylation) (Mirzapoiazova et al., 2011; Schmidt et al., 2013; Sukriti et al., 2014; Tauseef et al., 2012; Wainwright et al., 2003). These events take place with few seconds to minutes. Therefore, phosphorylation of MLC, especially, diphosphorylation of MLC, is a pre-requisite event in the initiation of endothelial contraction (Mehta & Malik, 2006; Mehta et al., 2014; Mirzapoiazova et al., 2011; Sukriti et al., 2014; Vogel & Malik, 2012). Interestingly, mice only lacking non-muscle isoform of MYLK, found protected from LPS induced pulmonary vascular permeability and inflammation (Rossi, Velentza, Steinhorn, Watterson, & Wainwright, 2007; Wainwright et al., 2003). Furthermore, pharmacological inhibition of MYLK using ML-7 prevented increase in endothelial permeability (Chavez et al., 2011; Garcia, Davis, & Patterson, 1995; Mehta & Malik, 2006). Mice injected with ML-7 or cultured human endothelial cells pretreated with ML-7 were found protected against LPS induced endothelial permeability (Chavez et al., 2011; Garcia et al., 1995). Besides, MYLK inhibition also prevented LPS induced renal endothelial cell dysfunction in *in vivo* mouse model (Chavez et al., 2011; Wu, Guo, Chen, Wang, & Cunningham, 2009). These findings demonstrating the potential role of MYLK in the disassembly of AJs by mediating endothelial cell rounding, and thus reveal a tempting target to develop a drug against inflammatory induced increased in endothelial permeability.

Role of Rho Family of GTPases in the Regulation of Endothelial Permeability

Similarly to MYLK, RhoA GTPase also demonstrated regulation of vascular permeability in response to variety of inflammatory stimuli in endothelial cells (Beckers et al., 2015; Mehta et al., 2003; Schmidt et al., 2013). RhoA GTPase induces vascular permeability by activating its downstream effector Rho kinase (ROCK) (Beckers et al., 2015). Upon activation, ROCK phosphorylates myosin light chain phosphatase (MYLP or PP1) regulatory subunit, and suppresses its activity. Inhibition of MYLP activity downstream of the activation of ROCK, leads to the prolongation of the activity of MYLK, which basically maintained endothelial cells in their contractile state (Beckers et al., 2015; Mehta & Malik, 2006). And this eventually leads to the long lived endothelial permeability and setting up the stage for inflammation (Mehta & Malik, 2006). In contrast to RhoA activation, another GTPase, Rac1, when activated tightens the endothelial barrier function by stabilizing AJs (Chavez et al., 2011; Tauseef et al., 2008; Vandenbroucke et al., 2008). For example, inhibiting the Rac1 function using specific Rac1 inhibitor, clostridium sordelli toxin, induced AJs destabilizing and promotion of endothelial barrier leakiness (Schlegel et al., 2008). Using *in vivo* mouse model, research findings demonstrated that a very fine balance between RhoA and Rac1 activity is required to maintain AJs stability (Schmidt et al., 2013; Tauseef et al., 2008). It was further demonstrated that endothelial focal adhesion kinase (FAK) maintains vascular endothelial barrier function by suppressing the RhoA signaling (Mehta, 2012; Schmidt et al., 2013; Thennes & Mehta, 2012). However, upon deletion of FAK in the mouse lung endothelial cells, switch the GTPase dynamics, and RhoA up regulated, while suppression in the activity of Rac1 (Schmidt et al., 2013). This led to the increase in endothelial permeability and lung edema formation (Schmidt et al., 2013). It has been observed that under the setting of increased in endothelial permeability, RhoA and Rac1 are basically opposed each other's activation (Schmidt et al., 2013). For example, during the disruption of endothelial permeability in response to myriad of inflammatory agonist, RhoA activity is increased while Rac1 decreased (Schmidt et al., 2013). However, during the recovery phase, reverse phenomena have taken place (Schmidt et al., 2013; Tauseef et al., 2008). It is not very well understood how RhoA suppresses Rac1 activity, and thus induced vascular permeability. It has been demonstrated that activation of FilGAP, a recently discovered filamin A (FLNa)-binding Rho GTPase-activating protein, also targets Rac1, and suppresses its activation. Ohta et al. 2006, demonstrated in a very elegant manner that activation of RhoA associated protein kinase kinase (ROCK) phosphorylated FilGAP and thus induced its GTPase activity (Ohta, Hartwig, & Stossel, 2006). Upon activation, FilGAP inhibited Rac1 and, thus prevented Rac1 induced lemilopodia formation (Ohta et al., 2006). Moreover, overexpression of dominant-negative FilGAP constructs, which lacks GAP activity or knockdown of endogenous FilGAP using small interference RNA (siRNA) leads to the lamellopdia formation and enhanced cell spreading. Furthermore, knockdown of endogenous FilGAP abrogated ROCK-dependent suppression of lamellae. On the other hand, forced expression of FilGAP induces cell contractility and bleb formation; and a ROCK-specific inhibitor suppresses bleb formation (Ohta et al., 2006). This study showed that how RhoA via activation of FilGAP switched off Rac activity and thus induced endothelial permeability (Ohta et al., 2006). Besides established role of Rac1 in the prevention of endothelial barrier function via inducing cells spreading, Kouklis et al., demonstrated that Cdc42, another Rho family GTPase prevented endothelial permeability (Kouklis, Konstantoulaki, Vogel, Broman, & Malik, 2004). They found that induction of endothelial permeability following the stimulation of thrombin, leads to the activation of Cdc42 (Kouklis et al., 2004). Interestingly, they observed that mice and endothelial cells over-expressing Cdc42, displayed resistance towards increasing in endothelial permeability (Kouklis et al., 2004). To further explore the role of activated Cdc42 in the reannealing of AJs, Kouklis et.al. overexpressed dominant negative Cdc42 mutant (N17Cdc42) in the endothelial cells (Kouklis et al., 2004). They found that over expression of N17Cdc42, delayed formation of VE cadherin and thus prevented restoration of vascular endothelial permeability (Kouklis et al., 2004). These findings identify the critical role of Cdc42 in restoring AJs assembly and endothelial permeability (Kouklis et al., 2004).

Excessive Intracellular Calcium (Ca^{2+}) and Endothelial Permeability

Ca^{2+} is an ubiquitous second messenger in almost all cell types including endothelial cells (Ahmmed et al., 2004; Di, Mehta, & Malik, 2016; Mehta et al., 2003; Singh et al., 2007; Tauseef et al., 2016; Tiruppathi et al., 2006). It regulates number of physiological and pathological cell processes such as cell division, blood vessel formation and maintenance of AJs (Bates & Harper, 2002; Li et al., 2011; Mehta & Malik, 2006; Tauseef et al., 2016). However, it is the excessive uncontrolled cytosolic Ca^{2+} entry following the activation of inflammatory signaling pathways leads to the deleterious disruption of endothelial barrier function and tissue edema (Singh et al., 2007; Tauseef et al., 2016; Tauseef et al., 2012). Resting levels of intracellular Ca^{2+} in endothelial cells varies between 40 to 100 nM. However, stimulation of endothelial cells with inflammatory mediators such as thrombin, oxidants, growth factors and histamine increase Ca^{2+} levels to 1 to 2 µM within few seconds (Singh et al., 2007; Tauseef et al., 2012; Tiruppathi et al., 2006; Tiruppathi et al., 2002). Extracellular Ca^{2+} is required in the maintenance of AJs. Increase in free intracellular Ca^{2+} activates downstream contractile cell machinery leads to the cell rounding and opening of AJs (Singh et al., 2007; Tauseef et al., 2016; Tiruppathi et al., 2002). Thus, Ca^{2+} acts as a switch, as its concentration in the cytosol regulate endothelial cell activity (Singh et al., 2007). Affords are going on in our laboratory as well as in other laboratories to better understand the tight regulation of Ca^{2+} signaling in endothelial cells (Tauseef et al., 2016; Tauseef et al., 2012).

Ca^{2+} entry activating pro-inflammatory stimuli upon stimulating their receptors on the endothelial cell surface leads to the phospholipase $(PLC)_{\beta}$ or PLC_{γ} mediated hydrolysis of phosphoinositol 4, 5-bis-biphosphate (PIP_2) into inositol 1, 4, 5 triphosphate (IP_3) and diacylglycerol (DAG) (Figure 2) (Mehta & Malik, 2006; Sukriti et al., 2014; Tauseef et al., 2012; Tiruppathi et al., 2006). IP_3, via activating its receptor, inositol triphosphate receptor (IP_3R) at the surface of endoplasmic rectum (ER), induces ER Ca^{2+}store depletion (Mehta & Malik, 2006; Sukriti et al., 2014). The ER store depletion is sensed by another ER resident monomeric protein, stromal interaction molecule 1 (STIM1) (DebRoy et al., 2014; Gudermann & Steinritz, 2013; Lee et al., 2010; Shinde et al., 2013; Zeng et al., 2008). Once activated by the ER Ca^{2+} release, STIM1 protein, which presents as a monomeric unit, immediately polymerizes to form a STIM1 cluster, called puncta formation (Gandhirajan et al., 2013; Gudermann & Steinritz, 2013; Lee et al., 2010). The whole STIM1 cluster moves near to the plasma membrane to interact with plasmalemma Ca^{2+} channels, called store operated Ca^{2+} (SOC) channels (Gudermann & Steinritz, 2013; Lee et al., 2010; Zeng et al., 2008) (Figure 2). This leads to the activation of store operated Ca^{2+}entry (SOCE) (Gudermann & Steinritz, 2013; Lee et al., 2010; Zeng et al., 2008). On the other side, DAG activates another type of Ca^{2+} entry pathway called receptor operated Ca^{2+}entry (ROCE), which is independent of the ER Ca^{2+}store depletion (Pocock, Foster, & Bates, 2004; Singh et al., 2007; Tauseef et al., 2012). The transient receptor potential canonical (TRPC) channels are involved in the regulation of SOCE and ROCE in endothelial cells (Birnbaumer, 2009; Dietrich & Gudermann, 2011; Earley & Brayden, 2015; Tauseef et al., 2012). The endothelial cells express TRPC1, TRPC4, TRPC6 and TRPC7. TRPC1 and TRPC4 constitute the components of SOC channels, while TRPC6 and TRPC7 composed ROC channels (Birnbaumer, 2009; Sukriti et al., 2014) (Figure 2). Furthermore, TRPC1, TRPC4 and TRPC6 have been shown to be important mediators of increasing in endothelial permeability and inflammation in response to inflammatory agonists (DebRoy et al., 2014; Tauseef et al., 2016; Tauseef et al., 2012; Tiruppathi et al., 2002). Initial studies suggest that the blocking the TRPC1 channel using anti-TRPC1 antibody reduced Ca^{2+} entry and prevented increase in endothelial permeability in response to thrombin (Jho et al., 2005). Overexpression of TRPC1 channel enhanced cytosolic Ca^{2+}entry, stress fiber formation and thereby increased in endothelial permeability (Jho et al., 2005; Sukriti et al., 2014). To understand the relevance of TRPC channel mediated Ca^{2+}entry in the regulation of vascular permeability during *in vivo* setting, it was observed that deletion of TRPC4 channel in mice reduced pulmonary vascular permeability to about 50% following the injection of protease activation receptor (PAR1) agonist peptide (Tiruppathi et al., 2002). Mehta et al. demonstrated the role of RhoA mediated actin fibers re-organization in the activation of TRPC1 channel mediated Ca^{2+} entry in the endothelial cells (Mehta et al., 2003). Furthermore, Ahmmed et al. showed that PKC_{α} phosphorylates at serine/threonine residues on the TRPC1 protein to induce Ca^{2+}entry (Ahmmed et al., 2004). Inhibition of PKC_{α} using siRNA prevented Ca^{2+}entry and endothelial permeability (Ahmmed et al., 2004). MYLK has also been shown to regulate SOCE in endothelial cells (Garcia et al., 1995). Inhibition of MYLK using ML-7 suppressed SOCE in endothelial cells (Garcia et al., 1995; Mehta & Malik, 2006). Tauseef et al. demonstrated that TRPC1-mediated cytosolic Ca^{2+} entry induces lung vascular permeability by altering VE-cadherin cell-surface expression, and thus, disrupting AJs stability (Tauseef et al., 2016) (Figure 3). Sphingosine-1-phosphate (S1P), is a phospholipid, is generated in endothelial cells via phosphorylation of sphingosine by sphingosine kinase 1 (SPHK1) enzyme (Sammani et al., 2010; Tauseef et al., 2016; Tauseef et al., 2008). Upon generation, S1P tightens the endothelial barrier, and prevents increase in endothelial permeability via Rac1 activation signaling pathway (Proia & Hla, 2015; Sammani et al., 2010; Tauseef et al., 2008). Tauseef et al. showed that TRPC1 deleted mouse lung endothelial cells were protected from thrombin induced barrier disruption (Tauseef et al., 2016) (Figure 3). Moreover, TRPC1 deleted cells displayed increased activity of SPHK1 and increased generation of S1P (Tauseef et al., 2016). They also observed increased accumulation of VE-cadherin at the inter-endothelial cell junctions, under basal conditions (Tauseef et al., 2016) (Figure 3). TRPC1 deleted mice displayed increased survival in response to lethal dose of endotoxin LPS. Altogether, present study suggests that TRPC1 channel modulate VE-cadherin expression in the endothelial cells through regulation of sphingosine kinase (SPHK1)-induced sphingosine 1 phosphate (S1P) generation (Tauseef et al., 2016). Thus, the study identified TRPC1 channel as a novel drug target for up-regulating S1P levels particularly in the setting of increase in vascular permeability as observed during sepsis and in diabetes induced vasculopathies (Tauseef et al., 2016).

STIM1 protein, originally was discovered as a tumor suppressor protein, has been identified and characterized as an important regulator of SOCE in endothelial cells (DebRoy et al., 2014; Gandhirajan et al., 2013; Lee et al., 2010; Sukriti et al., 2014). STIM1 senses ER Ca^{2+} stores, and upon ER Ca^{2+}depletion, it activates SOCE via interaction with SOC channels (Bird et al., 2009; DebRoy et al., 2014; Lee et al., 2010) (Figure 2). STIM1 contains several motifs or domains that are important in the activation of SOCE (Bird et al., 2009; Cahalan, 2009; Lee et al., 2010; Yuan et al., 2009). The STIM1 N-terminal EF hand domain has Ca^{2+} binding site, sterile α motif or SAM domain, a single transmembrane domain (TM), an Ezrin-radixin-moesin (ERM) domain, a serine-proline-rich domain (S/P-region) and a lysine rich domain (Bird et al., 2009; Cahalan, 2009; Cao et al., 2015; Cioffi et al., 2010; Gudermann & Steinritz, 2013; Sukriti et al., 2014; Yuan et al., 2009). When the ER store is filled Ca^{2+}, EF hand remains bind with Ca^{2+}ions, and STIM1 exists as monomer (Cao et al., 2015; Cioffi et al., 2010; Lee et al., 2010; Yuan et al., 2009). Upon store deletion, the EF hand and SAM domain from different STIM1 proteins come near with each other and form aggregates, called puncta (Bird et al., 2009; Cahalan, 2009; Cao et al., 2015; Cioffi et al., 2010; Gudermann & Steinritz, 2013; Lee et al., 2010; Yuan et al., 2009). These puncta ultimately moves near the plamsmamembrane to interact with SOC channels to induce SOCE (Bird et al., 2009; Cao et al., 2015; Lee et al., 2010; Yuan et al., 2009). STIM1 protein induces SOCE via interacting with TRPC1, TRPC4, TRPC5 and ORAI channels. These channels are important constitutes of SOC as well as Ca^{2+}release activated Ca^{2+} (CRAC) channels (Cao et al., 2015; Cioffi et al., 2010; Gudermann & Steinritz, 2013; Lee et al., 2010). In the recent published study, Sundivakkam et al. showed that SOCE activated p38 MAP kinase, which phosphorylated STIM1 and suppressed SOCE in endothelial cells (Sundivakkam et al., 2013). On the other hand, Vasauskas et al. demonstrated in human endothelial cells that calcinuerin, a phosphatase, by dephosphorylating the STIM1 activates SOCE (Vasauskas, Chen, Wu, & Cioffi, 2014). These studies identified an auto regulatory pathway of controlling SOCE, and thus provide us a better understanding how to regulate uncontrolled Ca^{2+} signaling in endothelial cells during inflammatory conditions.

STIM2, an isoform of STIM1, also expresses in endothelial cells (Cahalan, 2009; Sukriti et al., 2014). Unlike STIM1, STIM2 doses not regulate SOCE, but it has a role in the regulation of cytosolic Ca^{2+}in the basal conditions (Brandman, Liou, Park, & Meyer, 2007; Cahalan, 2009; Hogan, Lewis, & Rao, 2010). Overexpression of STIM2 in non-endothelial cell such as in HEK cells and jurkat cells prevented SOCE and CRAC activity, respectively (Brandman et al., 2007; Cahalan, 2009; Hogan et al., 2010; Sukriti et al., 2014). The role of STIM2 in the prevention of STIM1 induced SOCE needs to be evaluated in endothelial cells. Thus, in future STIM2 may emerge as potential drug target to regulate SOCE during inflammatory conditions (Cahalan, 2009; Hogan et al., 2010).

Besides SOC channels, ROC channel such as TRPC6 has emerged as an important regulator of vascular endothelial permeability under the condition of septicemia and reactive oxygen production during pulmonary inflammation (Tauseef et al., 2012; Weissmann et al., 2012). TRPC6 channel is highly expressed in mammalian lung and lung endothelial cells. Singh et al. using 1-Oleoyl-2-acetyl-*sn*-glycerol (OAG), a cell membrane permeable analog of DAG and an specific activator of TRPC6 channel, showed that TRPC6 increased permeability in human pulmonary artery endothelial cells through increasing cytosolic Ca^{2+} entry (Singh et al., 2007). Tauseef et. al. 2012, showed that TRPC6 plays a central role in signaling both LPS-induced lung vascular permeability and inflammation (Tauseef et al., 2012). The study found that LPS induced DAG production in endothelial cells to activate TRPC6 channel (Tauseef et al., 2012). Activated TRPC6 induced MYLK activity that by stimulating actomyosin cross-bridging mediates endothelial cell contraction leading to increased lung vascular permeability (Tauseef et al., 2012). Additionally, activated MLCK promoted the interaction of myeloid differentiation primary response gene (MyD88) with interleukin receptor-1 associated kinase 4 (IRAK-4), is involved in triggering NF-kB signaling and pulmonary inflammation downstream of TLR4 activation (Tauseef et al., 2012). Thus, TRPC6 channel acted as a central molecule, relying dual signaling pathways in regulating MYLK mediated lung vascular permeability and TLR4 signaling in endothelial cells (Tauseef et al., 2012).

In another recent study published by Weber et al., demonstrated that TRPC6 mediated Ca^{2+} entry was required to induce transendothelial migration (TEM) of neutrophils (Weber et al., 2015). They showed that increased in free cytosolic Ca^{2+} concentration mediated my TRPC6 channel, induced TEM of neutrophils (diapedesis) down-stream of Platelet endothelial cell adhesion molecule-1 (PECAM1) homophilic interactions (Weber et al., 2015). They further discovered that TRPC6 interacted with PECAM and thus, facilitated polymorphonuclear leukocytes (PMN) TEM (Weber et al., 2015). Overexpression of dominant-negative TRPC6 or knockdown of TRPC6 in endothelial cells prevented PMN apically over the junction, while selective activation of endothelial TRPC6 with hyperforin 9 induced TEM even in the absence of PECAM. Mice lacking TRPC6 channel exhibited a profound defect in neutrophil TEM with no effect on leukocyte trafficking in a croton oil-mediated acute ear inflammation (Weber et al., 2015). Thus, they identified endothelial TRPC6 channel as a regulator of PECAM mediated TEM of neutrophils, suggests a potential therapeutic implication in the treatment of vascular inflammation (Weber et al., 2015).

Role of SPHK1-SP1 Signaling Pathway in the Regulation of Endothelial Barrier Function

Sphingosine kinase (SPHK) presents in the endothelial cells in two isoforms-SPHK1 and SPHK2 (Chavez et al., 2011; Christensen et al., 2016; Huang et al., 2013; Tauseef et al., 2016; Tauseef et al., 2008; Wadgaonkar et al., 2009). Both SPHK1 and SPHK2 are bioactive enzymes, and catalyze conversion of membrane phospholipid, sphingosine into sphingosine 1 phosphate (S1P) (Christensen et al., 2016; Huang et al., 2013). S1P has been identified as one of the most potent endothelial protective agent against variety of inflammatory insults (Blaho et al., 2015; Christensen et al., 2016; Huang et al., 2013; Proia & Hla, 2015; Singleton, Dudek, Chiang, & Garcia, 2005; Tauseef et al., 2016). Besides tightening the endothelial barrier function, S1P is also involved in cell survival, vascular tone regulation; cell proliferation and migration pathways (Chavez et al., 2011; Mehta & Malik, 2006; Proia & Hla, 2015). Deletion of individual SPHK isoforms (SPHK1 and SPHK2) did not show any marked phenotypic changes in the mice models (Tauseef et al., 2008). However, deletion of both genes leads to the mouse embryonic lethality within E13.3 due vascular defects and hemorrhage, particularly in the region brain (Mizugishi et al., 2005). SPHK1 isoform is involved in the regulation of cell proliferation, migration and pro-survival signals, while SPHK2 has been shown to inhibit DNA synthesis and induce apoptosis (Chavez et al., 2011; Mizugishi et al., 2005; Tauseef et al., 2016).

SPHK1 maintains endothelial barrier function by generating an anti-inflammatory phospholipid, S1P.(Blaho et al., 2015; Huang et al., 2013; Proia & Hla, 2015; Sammani et al., 2010; Singleton et al., 2005; Tauseef et al., 2016; Tauseef et al., 2008). SPHK1 deleted mice failed to resolve lung vascular permeability following the exposure to nebulized LPS (Tauseef et al., 2008). Prakash et al. demonstrated that inhibition of SPHK1 in macrophages increased their sensitivity toward Mycobacterium smegmatis infection (Prakash et al., 2010). Di et al. showed that SPHK1-deleted neutrophils produced high amount of oxidants upon exposing them to LPS, that leads to sever pulmonary inflammation and increased mortality in SPHK1 deleted mice (Di et al., 2010); however, as SPHK2 was expressed in SPHK1 deleted mice, neither it did compensate nor it provided any kind of protection in above mentioned vascular defects observed in SPHK1 null mice (Di et al., 2010; Tauseef et al., 2008). This reveals the specificity of SPHK1 in the regulation of endothelial barrier function (Tauseef et al., 2008).

S1P signals its effects via activating its receptors, sphingosine 1 phosphate receptors ($S1PR_{1-5}$), formerly known as endothelial differentiation gene or Edg receptors (Chavez et al., 2015; Tauseef et al., 2016; Tauseef et al., 2008). Among the 5 S1PR, S1P1R1 is a high affinity S1P receptor (Chavez et al., 2015; Mehta, Konstantoulaki, Ahmmed, & Malik, 2005). S1P induces endothelial barrier tightening signaling via binding to S1PR1 on endothelial cells (Chavez et al., 2015; Mehta, Konstantoulaki, Ahmmed, & Malik, 2005). Effect of S1P on the endothelial barrier function is very rapid, as observed during the increase in transendothelial electrical resistance (TEER) (Chavez et al., 2015; Tauseef et al., 2008). Upon knocking down of S1PR1 in endothelial cells using siRNA approach, S1P failed to enhance endothelial barrier, indicates role of S1PR1 in the maintenance of AJs in endothelial cell (Chavez et al., 2015; Chavez et al., 2011; Tauseef et al., 2008). Using *in vivo* mouse models, studies showed that infusion of S1P prevented LPS- or PAR1-receptor activation induced pulmonary edema formation (Chavez et al., 2011; Natarajan et al., 2013; Tauseef et al., 2008). S1P analog, FTY720, suppressed LPS mediated microvascular permeability (Natarajan et al., 2013; Peng et al., 2004; Xiong & Hla, 2014). Altogether, research findings strongly suggest the potent vascular protective mechanisms offered by S1P during increased in endothelial permeability conditions (Chavez et al., 2011; Natarajan et al., 2013; Peng et al., 2004; Xiong & Hla, 2014).

In order to establish signaling activated downstream of activation of S1PR1 by S1P, studies have identified the role of Rac1 in tightening the endothelial barrier (Abbasi & Garcia, 2013; Mehta et al., 2005; Tauseef et al., 2008; Xiong & Hla, 2014). S1P1 failed to enhance endothelial barrier following the transduction of dominant negative Rac1 mutant in the cells (Mehta et al., 2005). On the similar lines, Tauseef et al. showed that knocking down of SPHK1 using siRNA inhibited the basal Rac1 activity, leading to lower down than normal TEER resistances (Tauseef et al., 2008).

S1P enhanced endothelial barrier function by the formation of cortical actin rings as well increase recruitment of VE-cadherin at inter-endothelial junctions (Abbasi & Garcia, 2013). Moreover, S1P increase FAK activity and thus leads to the tightening of endothelial barrier (Chavez et al., 2011; Sun et al., 2009). Recent studies also suggest induction of nitric oxide production in the vascular endothelium following the S1P challenge. Activation of S1PR1 by S1P activated phosphatidylinositol 3-kinase, which phosphorylates nitric oxide synthase (NOS) in a protein kinase B/Akt- dependent manner, induces NO generation in the endothelium (Igarashi, Bernier, & Michel, 2001). S1P mediated NO production tightens the endothelial cell-cell connections leads to enhance barrier function (Chavez et al., 2011; Igarashi et al., 2001).

SUMMARY

This review discussed the role of signaling mechanisms, involved in the disruption of endothelial barrier via affecting the integrity of AJs. It particularly focused on how excessive cytosolic Ca^{2+} entry leads to the activation of RhoA and MYLK signaling pathways and disassembles AJs, and thereby inducing endothelial permeability during inflammatory conditions. It also described important endogenous signaling pathways such as SPHK1-S1P signaling cascade, activated during the increase in endothelial permeability, such as during the activation of PAR-1 receptor signaling, in order to restore endothelial barrier function. Finally, it discussed in endothelial cell context the roles of Rac1, Cdc42 and FAK that how they regulate endothelial barrier function and activated their signaling in order to reanneal disrupted endothelial barrier. These signaling molecules are potential drug targets, and if we develop therapeutics against these molecules, especially TRPC channels, we hope to bring rationale treatment of inflammatory vascular diseases. Endothelial dysfunction is the earliest step in almost every vascular disorder initiated by myriad of diseases such as diabetes mellitus, myocardial ischemia and infraction, acute lung injury, acute respiratory distress syndrome, cancer and sepsis. If endothelial permeability persists, it may lead to the development of life threatening edema, as in the case of acute respiratory distress syndrome. So, if endothelial dysfunction is treated at an early stage of cardiovascular disease by preventing or restoring endothelial barrier dysfunction, we strongly believe that the high rate of morbidity and mortality can significantly be lowered down.

REFERENCES

Abbasi, T., & Garcia, J. G. (2013). Sphingolipids in lung endothelial biology and regulation of vascular integrity. *Handb Exp Pharmacol,* (216), 201-226. doi: 10.1007/978-3-7091-1511-4_10

Ahmmed, G. U., Mehta, D., Vogel, S., Holinstat, M., Paria, B. C., Tiruppathi, C., & Malik, A. B. (2004). Protein kinase Calpha phosphorylates the TRPC1 channel and regulates store-operated Ca2+ entry in endothelial cells. *The Journal of Biological Chemistry*, *279*(20), 20941–20949. doi:10.1074/jbc.M313975200 PMID:15016832

Aird, W. C. (2012). Endothelial cell heterogeneity. *Cold Spring Harb Perspect Med*, *2*(1), a006429. doi:10.1101/cshperspect.a006429 PMID:22315715

Ashina, K., Tsubosaka, Y., Nakamura, T., Omori, K., Kobayashi, K., Hori, M., & Murata, T. et al. (2015). Histamine Induces Vascular Hyperpermeability by Increasing Blood Flow and Endothelial Barrier Disruption In Vivo. *PLoS ONE*, *10*(7), e0132367. doi:10.1371/journal.pone.0132367 PMID:26158531

Bates, D. O., & Harper, S. J. (2002). Regulation of vascular permeability by vascular endothelial growth factors. *Vascular Pharmacology*, *39*(4-5), 225–237. doi:10.1016/S1537-1891(03)00011-9 PMID:12747962

Beckers, C. M., Knezevic, N., Valent, E. T., Tauseef, M., Krishnan, R., Rajendran, K., & van Nieuw Amerongen, G. P. et al. (2015). ROCK2 primes the endothelium for vascular hyperpermeability responses by raising baseline junctional tension. *Vascular Pharmacology*, *70*, 45–54. doi:10.1016/j.vph.2015.03.017 PMID:25869521

Bird, G. S., Hwang, S. Y., Smyth, J. T., Fukushima, M., Boyles, R. R., & Putney, J. W. Jr. (2009). STIM1 is a calcium sensor specialized for digital signaling. *Current Biology*, *19*(20), 1724–1729. doi:10.1016/j.cub.2009.08.022 PMID:19765994

Birnbaumer, L. (2009). The TRPC class of ion channels: A critical review of their roles in slow, sustained increases in intracellular Ca(2+) concentrations. *Annual Review of Pharmacology and Toxicology*, *49*(1), 395–426. doi:10.1146/annurev.pharmtox.48.113006.094928 PMID:19281310

Birukova, A. A., Smurova, K., Birukov, K. G., Kaibuchi, K., Garcia, J. G., & Verin, A. D. (2004). Role of Rho GTPases in thrombin-induced lung vascular endothelial cells barrier dysfunction. *Microvascular Research*, *67*(1), 64–77. doi:10.1016/j.mvr.2003.09.007 PMID:14709404

Blaho, V. A., Galvani, S., Engelbrecht, E., Liu, C., Swendeman, S. L., Kono, M., & Hla, T. et al. (2015). HDL-bound sphingosine-1-phosphate restrains lymphopoiesis and neuroinflammation. *Nature*, *523*(7560), 342–346. doi:10.1038/nature14462 PMID:26053123

Brandman, O., Liou, J., Park, W. S., & Meyer, T. (2007). STIM2 is a feedback regulator that stabilizes basal cytosolic and endoplasmic reticulum Ca2+ levels. *Cell*, *131*(7), 1327–1339. doi:10.1016/j.cell.2007.11.039 PMID:18160041

Cahalan, M. D. (2009). STIMulating store-operated Ca(2+) entry. *Nature Cell Biology*, *11*(6), 669–677. doi:10.1038/ncb0609-669 PMID:19488056

Cao, X., Choi, S., Maleth, J. J., Park, S., Ahuja, M., & Muallem, S. (2015). The ER/PM microdomain, PI(4,5)P(2) and the regulation of STIM1-Orai1 channel function. *Cell Calcium*, *58*(4), 342–348. doi:10.1016/j.ceca.2015.03.003 PMID:25843208

Chava, K. R., Tauseef, M., Sharma, T., & Mehta, D. (2012). Cyclic AMP response element-binding protein prevents endothelial permeability increase through transcriptional controlling p190RhoGAP expression. *Blood*, *119*(1), 308–319. doi:10.1182/blood-2011-02-339473 PMID:22049513

Chavez, A., Schmidt, T. T., Yazbeck, P., Rajput, C., Desai, B., Sukriti, S., & Mehta, D. et al. (2015). S1PR1 Tyr143 phosphorylation downregulates endothelial cell surface S1PR1 expression and responsiveness. *Journal of Cell Science*, *128*(5), 878–887. doi:10.1242/jcs.154476 PMID:25588843

Chavez, A., Smith, M., & Mehta, D. (2011). New insights into the regulation of vascular permeability. *Int Rev Cell Mol Biol*, *290*, 205–248. doi:10.1016/B978-0-12-386037-8.00001-6 PMID:21875566

Christensen, P. M., Liu, C. H., Swendeman, S. L., Obinata, H., Qvortrup, K., Nielsen, L. B., & Christoffersen, C. et al. (2016). Impaired endothelial barrier function in apolipoprotein M-deficient mice is dependent on sphingosine-1-phosphate receptor 1. *The FASEB Journal*, *30*(6), 2351–2359. doi:10.1096/fj.201500064 PMID:26956418

Cioffi, D. L., Barry, C., & Stevens, T. (2010). Store-operated calcium entry channels in pulmonary endothelium: The emerging story of TRPCS and Orai1. *Advances in Experimental Medicine and Biology*, *661*, 137–154. doi:10.1007/978-1-60761-500-2_9 PMID:20204728

Daneshjou, N., Sieracki, N., van Nieuw Amerongen, G. P., Conway, D. E., Schwartz, M. A., Komarova, Y. A., & Malik, A. B. (2015). Rac1 functions as a reversible tension modulator to stabilize VE-cadherin trans-interaction. *The Journal of Cell Biology*, *209*(1), 181. doi:10.1083/jcb.20140910803202015c PMID:25847538

DebRoy, A., Vogel, S. M., Soni, D., Sundivakkam, P. C., Malik, A. B., & Tiruppathi, C.DebRoy. (2014). Cooperative signaling via transcription factors NF-kappaB and AP1/c-Fos mediates endothelial cell STIM1 expression and hyperpermeability in response to endotoxin. *The Journal of Biological Chemistry*, *289*(35), 24188–24201. doi:10.1074/jbc.M114.570051 PMID:25016017

Dejana, E., Orsenigo, F., Molendini, C., Baluk, P., & McDonald, D. M. (2009). Organization and signaling of endothelial cell-to-cell junctions in various regions of the blood and lymphatic vascular trees. *Cell and Tissue Research*, *335*(1), 17–25. doi:10.1007/s00441-008-0694-5 PMID:18855014

Dejana, E., Tournier-Lasserve, E., & Weinstein, B. M. (2009). The control of vascular integrity by endothelial cell junctions: Molecular basis and pathological implications. *Developmental Cell*, *16*(2), 209–221. doi:10.1016/j.devcel.2009.01.004 PMID:19217423

Di, A., Kawamura, T., Gao, X. P., Tang, H., Berdyshev, E., Vogel, S. M., & Malik, A. B. et al. (2010). A novel function of sphingosine kinase 1 suppression of JNK activity in preventing inflammation and injury. *The Journal of Biological Chemistry*, *285*(21), 15848–15857. doi:10.1074/jbc.M109.075549 PMID:20299461

Di, A., Mehta, D., & Malik, A. B. (2016). ROS-activated calcium signaling mechanisms regulating endothelial barrier function. *Cell Calcium*, *60*(3), 163–171. doi:10.1016/j.ceca.2016.02.002 PMID:26905827

Dietrich, A., & Gudermann, T. (2011). TRP channels in the cardiopulmonary vasculature. *Advances in Experimental Medicine and Biology*, *704*, 781–810. doi:10.1007/978-94-007-0265-3_41 PMID:21290327

Earley, S., & Brayden, J. E. (2015). Transient receptor potential channels in the vasculature. *Physiological Reviews*, *95*(2), 645–690. doi:10.1152/physrev.00026.2014 PMID:25834234

Gandhirajan, R. K., Meng, S., Chandramoorthy, H. C., Mallilankaraman, K., Mancarella, S., Gao, H., & Madesh, M. et al. (2013). Blockade of NOX2 and STIM1 signaling limits lipopolysaccharide-induced vascular inflammation. *The Journal of Clinical Investigation*, *123*(2), 887–902. doi:10.1172/JCI65647 PMID:23348743

Garcia, J. G., Davis, H. W., & Patterson, C. E. (1995). Regulation of endothelial cell gap formation and barrier dysfunction: Role of myosin light chain phosphorylation. *Journal of Cellular Physiology*, *163*(3), 510–522. doi:10.1002/jcp.1041630311 PMID:7775594

Giannotta, M., Trani, M., & Dejana, E. (2013). VE-cadherin and endothelial adherens junctions: Active guardians of vascular integrity. *Developmental Cell*, *26*(5), 441–454. doi:10.1016/j.devcel.2013.08.020 PMID:24044891

Gong, H., Gao, X., Feng, S., Siddiqui, M. R., Garcia, A., Bonini, M. G., & Malik, A. B. et al. (2014). Evidence of a common mechanism of disassembly of adherens junctions through Galpha13 targeting of VE-cadherin. *The Journal of Experimental Medicine*, *211*(3), 579–591. doi:10.1084/jem.20131190 PMID:24590762

Gong, H., Rehman, J., Tang, H., Wary, K., Mittal, M., Chaturvedi, P., & Malik, A. B. et al. (2015). Corrigendum. HIF2alpha signaling inhibits adherens junctional disruption in acute lung injury. *The Journal of Clinical Investigation*, *125*(3), 1364. doi:10.1172/JCI81377 PMID:25729855

Gudermann, T., & Steinritz, D. (2013). STIMulating stress fibers in endothelial cells. *Science Signaling*, *6*(267), pe8. doi:10.1126/scisignal.2004051 PMID:23512987

Hogan, P. G., Lewis, R. S., & Rao, A. (2010). Molecular basis of calcium signaling in lymphocytes: STIM and ORAI. *Annual Review of Immunology*, *28*(1), 491–533. doi:10.1146/annurev.immunol.021908.132550 PMID:20307213

Holinstat, M., Knezevic, N., Broman, M., Samarel, A. M., Malik, A. B., & Mehta, D. (2006). Suppression of RhoA activity by focal adhesion kinase-induced activation of p190RhoGAP: Role in regulation of endothelial permeability. *The Journal of Biological Chemistry*, *281*(4), 2296–2305. doi:10.1074/jbc.M511248200 PMID:16308318

Huang, L. S., Berdyshev, E., Mathew, B., Fu, P., Gorshkova, I. A., He, D., & Natarajan, V. et al. (2013). Targeting sphingosine kinase 1 attenuates bleomycin-induced pulmonary fibrosis. *The FASEB Journal*, *27*(4), 1749–1760. doi:10.1096/fj.12-219634 PMID:23315259

Igarashi, J., Bernier, S. G., & Michel, T. (2001). Sphingosine 1-phosphate and activation of endothelial nitric-oxide synthase. differential regulation of Akt and MAP kinase pathways by EDG and bradykinin receptors in vascular endothelial cells. *The Journal of Biological Chemistry*, *276*(15), 12420–12426. doi:10.1074/jbc.M008375200 PMID:11278407

Jho, D., Mehta, D., Ahmmed, G., Gao, X. P., Tiruppathi, C., Broman, M., & Malik, A. B. (2005). Angiopoietin-1 opposes VEGF-induced increase in endothelial permeability by inhibiting TRPC1-dependent Ca2 influx. *Circulation Research*, *96*(12), 1282–1290. doi:10.1161/01.RES.0000171894.03801.03 PMID:15920022

Kini, V., Chavez, A., & Mehta, D. (2010). A new role for PTEN in regulating transient receptor potential canonical channel 6-mediated Ca2+ entry, endothelial permeability, and angiogenesis. *The Journal of Biological Chemistry*, *285*(43), 33082–33091. doi:10.1074/jbc.M110.142034 PMID:20705603

Knezevic, N., Roy, A., Timblin, B., Konstantoulaki, M., Sharma, T., Malik, A. B., & Mehta, D. (2007). GDI-1 phosphorylation switch at serine 96 induces RhoA activation and increased endothelial permeability. *Molecular and Cellular Biology*, *27*(18), 6323–6333. doi:10.1128/MCB.00523-07 PMID:17636025

Knezevic, N., Tauseef, M., Thennes, T., & Mehta, D. (2009). The G protein betagamma subunit mediates reannealing of adherens junctions to reverse endothelial permeability increase by thrombin. *The Journal of Experimental Medicine*, *206*(12), 2761–2777. doi:10.1084/jem.20090652 PMID:19917775

Komarova, Y. A., Huang, F., Geyer, M., Daneshjou, N., Garcia, A., Idalino, L., & Malik, A. B. et al. (2012). VE-cadherin signaling induces EB3 phosphorylation to suppress microtubule growth and assemble adherens junctions. *Molecular Cell*, *48*(6), 914–925. doi:10.1016/j.molcel.2012.10.011 PMID:23159740

Komarova, Y. A., Mehta, D., & Malik, A. B. (2007). Dual regulation of endothelial junctional permeability. *Science's STKE*, *re8*(412), •••. doi:10.1126/stke.4122007re8 PMID:18000237

Kouklis, P., Konstantoulaki, M., Vogel, S., Broman, M., & Malik, A. B. (2004). Cdc42 regulates the restoration of endothelial barrier function. *Circulation Research, 94*(2), 159–166. doi:10.1161/01.RES.0000110418.38500.31 PMID:14656933

Lee, K. P., Yuan, J. P., Hong, J. H., So, I., Worley, P. F., & Muallem, S. (2010). An endoplasmic reticulum/plasma membrane junction: STIM1/Orai1/TRPCs. *FEBS Letters, 584*(10), 2022–2027. doi:10.1016/j.febslet.2009.11.078 PMID:19944100

Li, J., Cubbon, R. M., Wilson, L. A., Amer, M. S., McKeown, L., Hou, B., & Beech, D. J. et al. (2011). Orai1 and CRAC channel dependence of VEGF-activated Ca2+ entry and endothelial tube formation. *Circulation Research, 108*(10), 1190–1198. doi:10.1161/CIRCRESAHA.111.243352 PMID:21441136

Liu, H., Yu, X., Yu, S., & Kou, J. (2015). Molecular mechanisms in lipopolysaccharide-induced pulmonary endothelial barrier dysfunction. *International Immunopharmacology, 29*(2), 937–946. doi:10.1016/j.intimp.2015.10.010 PMID:26462590

Maniatis, N. A., Shinin, V., Schraufnagel, D. E., Okada, S., Vogel, S. M., Malik, A. B., & Minshall, R. D. (2008). Increased pulmonary vascular resistance and defective pulmonary artery filling in caveolin-1-/- mice. *American Journal of Physiology. Lung Cellular and Molecular Physiology, 294*(5), L865–L873. doi:10.1152/ajplung.00079.2007 PMID:18192592

Mehta, D. (2012). Focal adhesion kinase regulation of endothelial barrier function, apoptosis, and neovascularization. *Microvascular Research, 83*(1), 1–2. doi:10.1016/j.mvr.2011.10.001 PMID:22036672

Mehta, D., Ahmmed, G. U., Paria, B. C., Holinstat, M., Voyno-Yasenetskaya, T., Tiruppathi, C., & Malik, A. B. et al. (2003). RhoA interaction with inositol 1,4,5-trisphosphate receptor and transient receptor potential channel-1 regulates Ca2+ entry. Role in signaling increased endothelial permeability. *The Journal of Biological Chemistry, 278*(35), 33492–33500. doi:10.1074/jbc.M302401200 PMID:12766172

Mehta, D., Konstantoulaki, M., Ahmmed, G. U., & Malik, A. B. (2005). Sphingosine 1-phosphate-induced mobilization of intracellular Ca2+ mediates rac activation and adherens junction assembly in endothelial cells. *The Journal of Biological Chemistry, 280*(17), 17320–17328. doi:10.1074/jbc.M411674200 PMID:15728185

Mehta, D., & Malik, A. B. (2006). Signaling mechanisms regulating endothelial permeability. *Physiological Reviews, 86*(1), 279–367. doi:10.1152/physrev.00012.2005 PMID:16371600

Mehta, D., Ravindran, K., & Kuebler, W. M. (2014). Novel regulators of endothelial barrier function. *American Journal of Physiology. Lung Cellular and Molecular Physiology, 307*(12), L924–L935. doi:10.1152/ajplung.00318.2014 PMID:25381026

Minshall, R. D., Vandenbroucke, E. E., Holinstat, M., Place, A. T., Tiruppathi, C., Vogel, S. M., & Malik, A. B. et al. (2010). Role of protein kinase Czeta in thrombin-induced RhoA activation and inter-endothelial gap formation of human dermal microvessel endothelial cell monolayers. *Microvascular Research, 80*(2), 240–249. doi:10.1016/j.mvr.2010.04.007 PMID:20417648

Mirzapoiazova, T., Moitra, J., Moreno-Vinasco, L., Sammani, S., Turner, J. R., Chiang, E. T., & Garcia, J. G. et al. (2011). Non-muscle myosin light chain kinase isoform is a viable molecular target in acute inflammatory lung injury. *American Journal of Respiratory Cell and Molecular Biology*, *44*(1), 40–52. doi:10.1165/rcmb.2009-0197OC PMID:20139351

Mizugishi, K., Yamashita, T., Olivera, A., Miller, G. F., Spiegel, S., & Proia, R. L. (2005). Essential role for sphingosine kinases in neural and vascular development. *Molecular and Cellular Biology*, *25*(24), 11113–11121. doi:10.1128/MCB.25.24.11113-11121.2005 PMID:16314531

Natarajan, V., Dudek, S. M., Jacobson, J. R., Moreno-Vinasco, L., Huang, L. S., Abassi, T., & Garcia, J. G. et al. (2013). Sphingosine-1-phosphate, FTY720, and sphingosine-1-phosphate receptors in the pathobiology of acute lung injury. *American Journal of Respiratory Cell and Molecular Biology*, *49*(1), 6–17. doi:10.1165/rcmb.2012-0411TR PMID:23449739

Ofori-Acquah, S. F., King, J., Voelkel, N., Schaphorst, K. L., & Stevens, T. (2008). Heterogeneity of barrier function in the lung reflects diversity in endothelial cell junctions. *Microvascular Research*, *75*(3), 391–402. doi:10.1016/j.mvr.2007.10.006 PMID:18068735

Ohta, Y., Hartwig, J. H., & Stossel, T. P. (2006). FilGAP, a Rho- and ROCK-regulated GAP for Rac binds filamin A to control actin remodelling. *Nature Cell Biology*, *8*(8), 803–814. doi:10.1038/ncb1437 PMID:16862148

Paria, B. C., Vogel, S. M., Ahmmed, G. U., Alamgir, S., Shroff, J., Malik, A. B., & Tiruppathi, C. (2004). Tumor necrosis factor-alpha-induced TRPC1 expression amplifies store-operated Ca2+ influx and endothelial permeability. *American Journal of Physiology. Lung Cellular and Molecular Physiology*, *287*(6), L1303–L1313. doi:10.1152/ajplung.00240.2004 PMID:15347566

Peng, X., Hassoun, P. M., Sammani, S., McVerry, B. J., Burne, M. J., Rabb, H., & Garcia, J. G. et al. (2004). Protective effects of sphingosine 1-phosphate in murine endotoxin-induced inflammatory lung injury. *American Journal of Respiratory and Critical Care Medicine*, *169*(11), 1245–1251. doi:10.1164/rccm.200309-1258OC PMID:15020292

Pierrakos, C., Karanikolas, M., Scolletta, S., Karamouzos, V., & Velissaris, D. (2012). Acute respiratory distress syndrome: Pathophysiology and therapeutic options. *J Clin Med Res*, *4*(1), 7–16. doi:10.4021/jocmr761w PMID:22383921

Pocock, T. M., Foster, R. R., & Bates, D. O. (2004). Evidence of a role for TRPC channels in VEGF-mediated increased vascular permeability in vivo. *American Journal of Physiology. Heart and Circulatory Physiology*, *286*(3), H1015–H1026. doi:10.1152/ajpheart.00826.2003 PMID:14551041

Prakash, H., Luth, A., Grinkina, N., Holzer, D., Wadgaonkar, R., Gonzalez, A. P., & Kleuser, B. et al. (2010). Sphingosine kinase-1 (SphK-1) regulates Mycobacterium smegmatis infection in macrophages. *PLoS ONE*, *5*(5), e10657. doi:10.1371/journal.pone.0010657 PMID:20498849

Predescu, S. A., Predescu, D. N., & Malik, A. B. (2007). Molecular determinants of endothelial transcytosis and their role in endothelial permeability. *American Journal of Physiology. Lung Cellular and Molecular Physiology*, *293*(4), L823–L842. doi:10.1152/ajplung.00436.2006 PMID:17644753

Predescu, S. A., Predescu, D. N., Timblin, B. K., Stan, R. V., & Malik, A. B. (2003). Intersectin regulates fission and internalization of caveolae in endothelial cells. *Molecular Biology of the Cell*, *14*(12), 4997–5010. doi:10.1091/mbc.E03-01-0041 PMID:12960435

Proia, R. L., & Hla, T. (2015). Emerging biology of sphingosine-1-phosphate: Its role in pathogenesis and therapy. *The Journal of Clinical Investigation*, *125*(4), 1379–1387. doi:10.1172/JCI76369 PMID:25831442

Rajput, C., Kini, V., Smith, M., Yazbeck, P., Chavez, A., Schmidt, T., & Mehta, D. et al. (2013). Neural Wiskott-Aldrich syndrome protein (N-WASP)-mediated p120-catenin interaction with Arp2-Actin complex stabilizes endothelial adherens junctions. *The Journal of Biological Chemistry*, *288*(6), 4241–4250. doi:10.1074/jbc.M112.440396 PMID:23212915

Rajput, C., Tauseef, M., Farazuddin, M., Yazbeck, P., Amin, M. R., Avin Br, V., & Mehta, D. et al. (2016). MicroRNA-150 Suppression of Angiopoetin-2 Generation and Signaling Is Crucial for Resolving Vascular Injury. *Arteriosclerosis, Thrombosis, and Vascular Biology*, *36*(2), 380–388. doi:10.1161/ATVBAHA.115.306997 PMID:26743170

Regan, E. R., & Aird, W. C. (2012). Dynamical systems approach to endothelial heterogeneity. *Circulation Research*, *111*(1), 110–130. doi:10.1161/CIRCRESAHA.111.261701 PMID:22723222

Rossi, J. L., Velentza, A. V., Steinhorn, D. M., Watterson, D. M., & Wainwright, M. S. (2007). MLCK210 gene knockout or kinase inhibition preserves lung function following endotoxin-induced lung injury in mice. *American Journal of Physiology. Lung Cellular and Molecular Physiology*, *292*(6), L1327–L1334. doi:10.1152/ajplung.00380.2006 PMID:17307813

Samapati, R., Yang, Y., Yin, J., Stoerger, C., Arenz, C., Dietrich, A., & Kuebler, W. M. et al. (2012). Lung endothelial Ca2+ and permeability response to platelet-activating factor is mediated by acid sphingomyelinase and transient receptor potential classical 6. *American Journal of Respiratory and Critical Care Medicine*, *185*(2), 160–170. doi:10.1164/rccm.201104-0717OC PMID:22246702

Sammani, S., Moreno-Vinasco, L., Mirzapoiazova, T., Singleton, P. A., Chiang, E. T., Evenoski, C. L., & Garcia, J. G. et al. (2010). Differential effects of sphingosine 1-phosphate receptors on airway and vascular barrier function in the murine lung. *American Journal of Respiratory Cell and Molecular Biology*, *43*(4), 394–402. doi:10.1165/rcmb.2009-0223OC PMID:19749179

Schlegel, N., Burger, S., Golenhofen, N., Walter, U., Drenckhahn, D., & Waschke, J. (2008). The role of VASP in regulation of cAMP- and Rac 1-mediated endothelial barrier stabilization. *American Journal of Physiology. Cell Physiology*, *294*(1), C178–C188. doi:10.1152/ajpcell.00273.2007 PMID:17989211

Schmidt, T. T., Tauseef, M., Yue, L., Bonini, M. G., Gothert, J., Shen, T. L., & Mehta, D. et al. (2013). Conditional deletion of FAK in mice endothelium disrupts lung vascular barrier function due to destabilization of RhoA and Rac1 activities. *American Journal of Physiology. Lung Cellular and Molecular Physiology*, *305*(4), L291–L300. doi:10.1152/ajplung.00094.2013 PMID:23771883

Shi, S., Verin, A. D., Schaphorst, K. L., Gilbert-McClain, L. I., Patterson, C. E., Irwin, R. P., & Garcia, J. G. et al. (1998). Role of tyrosine phosphorylation in thrombin-induced endothelial cell contraction and barrier function. *Endothelium*, *6*(2), 153–171. doi:10.3109/10623329809072202 PMID:9930649

Shinde, A. V., Motiani, R. K., Zhang, X., Abdullaev, I. F., Adam, A. P., Gonzalez-Cobos, J. C., & Trebak, M. et al. (2013). STIM1 controls endothelial barrier function independently of Orai1 and Ca2+ entry. *Science Signaling*, *6*(267), ra18. doi:10.1126/scisignal.2003425 PMID:23512989

Singh, I., Knezevic, N., Ahmmed, G. U., Kini, V., Malik, A. B., & Mehta, D. (2007). Galphaq-TRPC6-mediated Ca2+ entry induces RhoA activation and resultant endothelial cell shape change in response to thrombin. *The Journal of Biological Chemistry*, *282*(11), 7833–7843. doi:10.1074/jbc.M608288200 PMID:17197445

Singleton, P. A., Dudek, S. M., Chiang, E. T., & Garcia, J. G. (2005). Regulation of sphingosine 1-phosphate-induced endothelial cytoskeletal rearrangement and barrier enhancement by S1P1 receptor, PI3 kinase, Tiam1/Rac1, and alpha-actinin. *The FASEB Journal*, *19*(12), 1646–1656. doi:10.1096/fj.05-3928com PMID:16195373

Stevens, T. (2011). Functional and molecular heterogeneity of pulmonary endothelial cells. *Proceedings of the American Thoracic Society*, *8*(6), 453–457. doi:10.1513/pats.201101-004MW PMID:22052919

Sukriti, S., Tauseef, M., Yazbeck, P., & Mehta, D. (2014). Mechanisms regulating endothelial permeability. *Pulm Circ*, *4*(4), 535–551. doi:10.1086/677356 PMID:25610592

Sun, X., Shikata, Y., Wang, L., Ohmori, K., Watanabe, N., Wada, J., & Garcia, J. G. et al. (2009). Enhanced interaction between focal adhesion and adherens junction proteins: Involvement in sphingosine 1-phosphate-induced endothelial barrier enhancement. *Microvascular Research*, *77*(3), 304–313. doi:10.1016/j.mvr.2008.12.004 PMID:19323978

Sundivakkam, P. C., Freichel, M., Singh, V., Yuan, J. P., Vogel, S. M., Flockerzi, V., & Tiruppathi, C. et al. (2012). The Ca(2+) sensor stromal interaction molecule 1 (STIM1) is necessary and sufficient for the store-operated Ca(2+) entry function of transient receptor potential canonical (TRPC) 1 and 4 channels in endothelial cells. *Molecular Pharmacology*, *81*(4), 510–526. doi:10.1124/mol.111.074658 PMID:22210847

Sundivakkam, P. C., Natarajan, V., Malik, A. B., & Tiruppathi, C. (2013). Store-operated Ca2+ entry (SOCE) induced by protease-activated receptor-1 mediates STIM1 protein phosphorylation to inhibit SOCE in endothelial cells through AMP-activated protein kinase and p38beta mitogen-activated protein kinase. *The Journal of Biological Chemistry*, *288*(23), 17030–17041. doi:10.1074/jbc.M112.411272 PMID:23625915

Tauseef, M., Farazuddin, M., Sukriti, S., Rajput, C., Meyer, J. O., Ramasamy, S. K., & Mehta, D. (2016). Transient receptor potential channel 1 maintains adherens junction plasticity by suppressing sphingosine kinase 1 expression to induce endothelial hyperpermeability. *The FASEB Journal*, *30*(1), 102–110. doi:10.1096/fj.15-275891 PMID:26316271

Tauseef, M., Kini, V., Knezevic, N., Brannan, M., Ramchandaran, R., Fyrst, H., & Mehta, D. et al. (2008). Activation of sphingosine kinase-1 reverses the increase in lung vascular permeability through sphingosine-1-phosphate receptor signaling in endothelial cells. *Circulation Research*, *103*(10), 1164–1172. doi:10.1161/01.RES.0000338501.84810.51 PMID:18849324

Tauseef, M., Knezevic, N., Chava, K. R., Smith, M., Sukriti, S., Gianaris, N., & Mehta, D. et al. (2012). TLR4 activation of TRPC6-dependent calcium signaling mediates endotoxin-induced lung vascular permeability and inflammation. *The Journal of Experimental Medicine*, *209*(11), 1953–1968. doi:10.1084/jem.20111355 PMID:23045603

Thennes, T., & Mehta, D. (2012). Heterotrimeric G proteins, focal adhesion kinase, and endothelial barrier function. *Microvascular Research*, *83*(1), 31–44. doi:10.1016/j.mvr.2011.05.004 PMID:21640127

Tiruppathi, C., Ahmmed, G. U., Vogel, S. M., & Malik, A. B. (2006). Ca2+ signaling, TRP channels, and endothelial permeability. *Microcirculation (New York, N.Y.)*, *13*(8), 693–708. doi:10.1080/10739680600930347 PMID:17085428

Tiruppathi, C., Freichel, M., Vogel, S. M., Paria, B. C., Mehta, D., Flockerzi, V., & Malik, A. B. (2002). Impairment of store-operated Ca2+ entry in TRPC4(-/-) mice interferes with increase in lung microvascular permeability. *Circulation Research*, *91*(1), 70–76. doi:10.1161/01.RES.0000023391.40106.A8 PMID:12114324

Tiruppathi, C., Soni, D., Wang, D. M., Xue, J., Singh, V., Thippegowda, P. B., & Malik, A. B. et al. (2014). The transcription factor DREAM represses the deubiquitinase A20 and mediates inflammation. *Nature Immunology*, *15*(3), 239–247. doi:10.1038/ni.2823 PMID:24487321

Tran, K. A., Zhang, X., Predescu, D., Huang, X., Machado, R. F., Gothert, J. R., & Zhao, Y. Y. et al. (2015). Endothelial beta-Catenin Signaling Is Required for Maintaining Adult Blood-Brain Barrier Integrity and CNS Homeostasis. *Circulation*. doi:10.1161/CIRCULATIONAHA.115.015982

Uhlig, S., Yang, Y., Waade, J., Wittenberg, C., Babendreyer, A., & Kuebler, W. M. (2014). Differential regulation of lung endothelial permeability in vitro and in situ. *Cellular Physiology and Biochemistry*, *34*(1), 1–19. doi:10.1159/000362980 PMID:24977477

Usatyuk, P. V., Singleton, P. A., Pendyala, S., Kalari, S. K., He, D., Gorshkova, I. A., & Natarajan, V. et al. (2012). Novel role for non-muscle myosin light chain kinase (MLCK) in hyperoxia-induced recruitment of cytoskeletal proteins, NADPH oxidase activation, and reactive oxygen species generation in lung endothelium. *The Journal of Biological Chemistry*, *287*(12), 9360–9375. doi:10.1074/jbc.M111.294546 PMID:22219181

van Nieuw Amerongen, G. P., Draijer, R., Vermeer, M. A., & van Hinsbergh, V. W. (1998). Transient and prolonged increase in endothelial permeability induced by histamine and thrombin: Role of protein kinases, calcium, and RhoA. *Circulation Research*, *83*(11), 1115–1123. doi:10.1161/01.RES.83.11.1115 PMID:9831706

Vandenbroucke, E., Mehta, D., Minshall, R., & Malik, A. B. (2008). Regulation of endothelial junctional permeability. *Annals of the New York Academy of Sciences*, *1123*(1), 134–145. doi:10.1196/annals.1420.016 PMID:18375586

Vandenbroucke St Amant, E., Tauseef, M., Vogel, S. M., Gao, X. P., Mehta, D., Komarova, Y. A., & Malik, A. B. (2012). PKCalpha activation of p120-catenin serine 879 phospho-switch disassembles VE-cadherin junctions and disrupts vascular integrity. *Circulation Research*, *111*(6), 739–749. doi:10.1161/CIRCRESAHA.112.269654 PMID:22798526

Vasauskas, A. A., Chen, H., Wu, S., & Cioffi, D. L. (2014). The serine-threonine phosphatase calcineurin is a regulator of endothelial store-operated calcium entry. *Pulm Circ*, *4*(1), 116–127. doi:10.1086/675641 PMID:25006427

Vogel, S. M., Gao, X., Mehta, D., Ye, R. D., John, T. A., Andrade-Gordon, P., & Malik, A. B. et al. (2000). Abrogation of thrombin-induced increase in pulmonary microvascular permeability in PAR-1 knockout mice. *Physiological Genomics*, *4*(2), 137–145. PMID:11120874

Vogel, S. M., & Malik, A. B. (2012). Cytoskeletal dynamics and lung fluid balance. *Compr Physiol*, *2*(1), 449–478. doi:10.1002/cphy.c100006 PMID:23728978

Wadgaonkar, R., Patel, V., Grinkina, N., Romano, C., Liu, J., Zhao, Y., & Natarajan, V. et al. (2009). Differential regulation of sphingosine kinases 1 and 2 in lung injury. *American Journal of Physiology. Lung Cellular and Molecular Physiology*, *296*(4), L603–L613. doi:10.1152/ajplung.90357.2008 PMID:19168577

Wainwright, M. S., Rossi, J., Schavocky, J., Crawford, S., Steinhorn, D., Velentza, A. V., & Watterson, D. M. et al. (2003). Protein kinase involved in lung injury susceptibility: Evidence from enzyme isoform genetic knockout and in vivo inhibitor treatment. *Proceedings of the National Academy of Sciences of the United States of America*, *100*(10), 6233–6238. doi:10.1073/pnas.1031595100 PMID:12730364

Wang, Z., Li, J., Cho, J., & Malik, A. B. (2014). Prevention of vascular inflammation by nanoparticle targeting of adherent neutrophils. *Nature Nanotechnology*, *9*(3), 204–210. doi:10.1038/nnano.2014.17 PMID:24561355

Weber, E. W., Han, F., Tauseef, M., Birnbaumer, L., Mehta, D., & Muller, W. A. (2015). TRPC6 is the endothelial calcium channel that regulates leukocyte transendothelial migration during the inflammatory response. *The Journal of Experimental Medicine*, *212*(11), 1883–1899. doi:10.1084/jem.20150353 PMID:26392222

Weissmann, N., Sydykov, A., Kalwa, H., Storch, U., Fuchs, B., Mederos y Schnitzler, M., & Dietrich, A. et al. (2012). Activation of TRPC6 channels is essential for lung ischaemia-reperfusion induced oedema in mice. *Nature Communications*, *3*, 649. doi:10.1038/ncomms1660 PMID:22337127

Wu, X., Guo, R., Chen, P., Wang, Q., & Cunningham, P. N. (2009). TNF induces caspase-dependent inflammation in renal endothelial cells through a Rho- and myosin light chain kinase-dependent mechanism. *American Journal of Physiology. Renal Physiology*, *297*(2), F316–F326. doi:10.1152/ajprenal.00089.2009 PMID:19420112

Xiong, Y., & Hla, T. (2014). S1P control of endothelial integrity. *Current Topics in Microbiology and Immunology*, *378*, 85–105. doi:10.1007/978-3-319-05879-5_4 PMID:24728594

Yuan, J. P., Zeng, W., Dorwart, M. R., Choi, Y. J., Worley, P. F., & Muallem, S. (2009). SOAR and the polybasic STIM1 domains gate and regulate Orai channels. *Nature Cell Biology*, *11*(3), 337–343. doi:10.1038/ncb1842 PMID:19182790

Zeng, W., Yuan, J. P., Kim, M. S., Choi, Y. J., Huang, G. N., Worley, P. F., & Muallem, S. (2008). STIM1 gates TRPC channels, but not Orai1, by electrostatic interaction. *Molecular Cell*, *32*(3), 439–448. doi:10.1016/j.molcel.2008.09.020 PMID:18995841

Zhao, Y. Y., & Malik, A. B. (2009). A novel insight into the mechanism of pulmonary hypertension involving caveolin-1 deficiency and endothelial nitric oxide synthase activation. *Trends in Cardiovascular Medicine*, *19*(7), 238–242. doi:10.1016/j.tcm.2010.02.003 PMID:20382348

Zhao, Y. Y., Zhao, Y. D., Mirza, M. K., Huang, J. H., Potula, H. H., Vogel, S. M., & Malik, A. B. et al. (2009). Persistent eNOS activation secondary to caveolin-1 deficiency induces pulmonary hypertension in mice and humans through PKG nitration. *The Journal of Clinical Investigation*, *119*(7), 2009–2018. doi:10.1172/JCI33338 PMID:19487814

APPENDIX

Figure 1. Signaling mechanisms regulating endothelial barrier function and integrity. Activation of PAR-1 receptor using thrombin increases intracellular Ca^{2+} entry. Ca^{2+} upon interaction with calmodulin (CaM) activates non muscle-myosin light chain kinase (MLCK) in endothelial cells. MYLK upon activation, phosphorylates (P) myosin light chains (MLCs). This leads to increase in actin-myosin interaction, endothelia cell contraction, and disruption of endothelial barrier integrity (left). During the recovery phase, sphingosine 1-phosphate (S1P) binds with, and activate its receptor, sphingosine 1 phosphate receptor 1 (S1PR1). This initiates formation of cortical actin and tightening of endothelial cell-cell junctions (right). Vascular endothelial cadherin (VE-cadherin) is the integral component in the formation of adherens junction (AJs) in endothelial cells. Other junctional proteins such as catenins (α, β, γ, and p120) provide junctional stability through their linkages with the actin cytoskeleton in the cytosol. The stability of junctional proteins is required in the maintenance of uninterrupted barrier function.

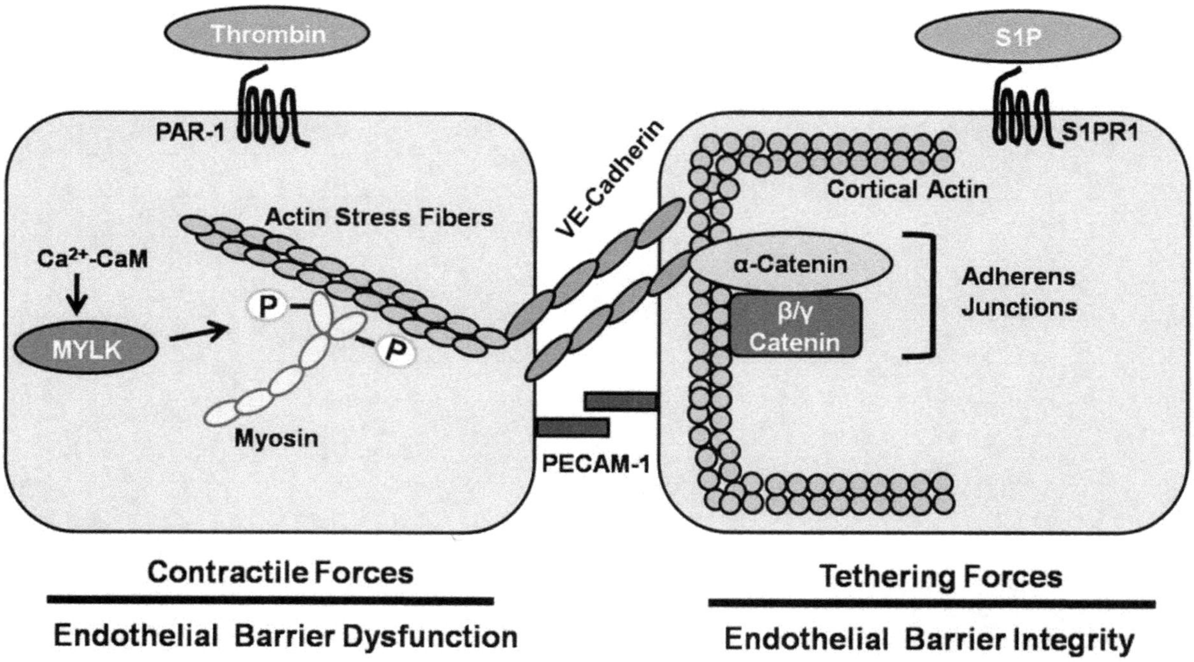

Figure 2. Signaling mechanisms activating transient receptor potential canonical channel mediated calcium entry in the endothelial cells. Agonists such as thrombin or vascular endothelial growth factor (VEGF) activate their corresponding receptors, G-protein coupled receptor (PAR-1) or receptor tyrosine kinase (RTK), generate inositol triphosphate (IP_3) and diacylglycerol (DAG). IP_3 binding to its receptor, IP_3R induces endoplasmic reticulum (ER) Ca^{2+} store release into the cytoplasm of the cell. This ER store depletion activates ER Ca^{2+} sensor, STIM1 and aggregation of STIM1, called punctae. Puntae move near to the plasma membrane and induces store operated Ca^{2+} entry (SOCE) via activation of TRPC1 and TRPC4 channels in the endothelial cells. DAG directly activates the receptor-operated channel (TRPC6) independent of ER store depletion.

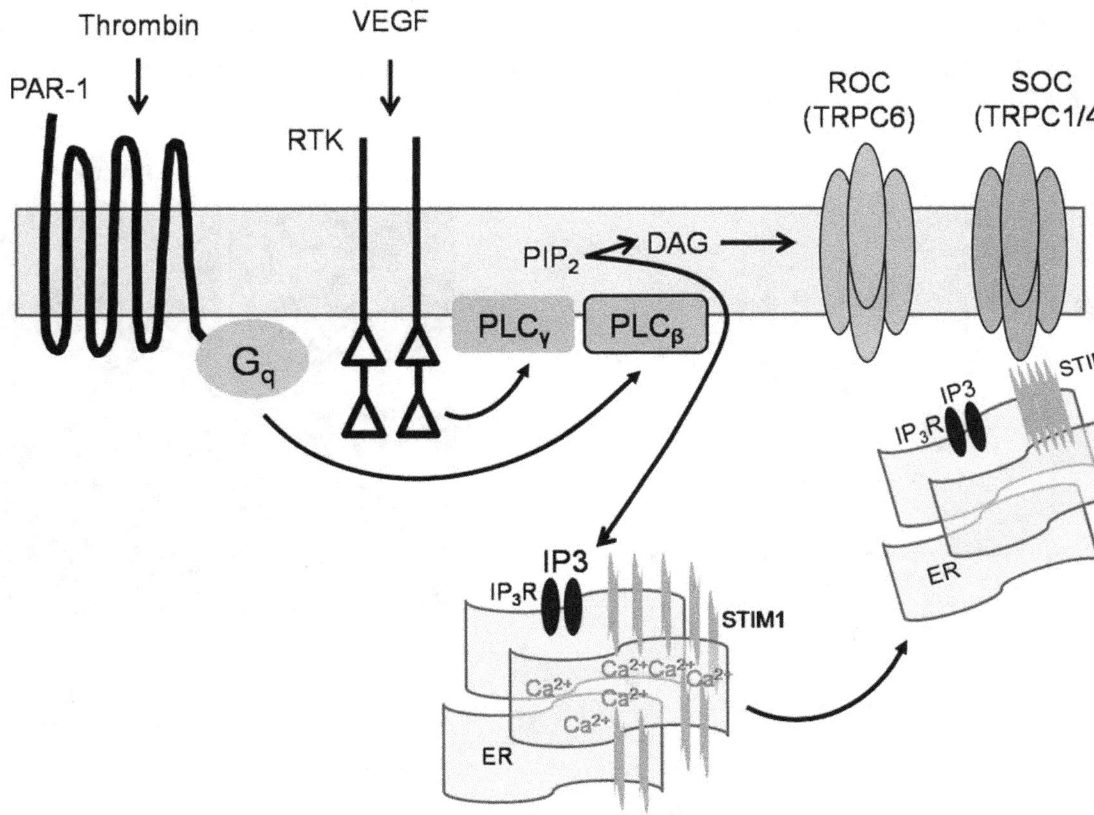

*Figure 3. Deletion of TRPC1 channel prevents thrombin induced increased in endothelial permeability by enhancing cell-surface VE-cadherin expression. (A) Lung endothelial cells were isolated from WT or TRPC1 deleted mice, grown to confluence in gold plated electrodes. Changes in transendothelial electrical resistance (TEER) in a real time were recorded following the stimulation of cells with thrombin. * TEER normalized values lower than TRPC1 deleted endothelial cells compared to wild type (WT) cells; $P < 0.05$. (B) Mouse lung endothelial cells were stained with anti–VE-cadherin antibody to evaluate VE-cadherin cell-surface intensity and interendothelial gap formation after 5 min thrombin challenge of WT or TRPC1-deleted endothelial cells. (C-D). Means ± SD of VE-cadherin pixel intensity and interendothelial gap formation from at least 10 individual cells per experiment. Each experiment was repeated at least 3 to 4 times. *Values different than WT endothelial cells without thrombin or TRPC1 deleted endothelial cells; **values different than WT endothelial cells after thrombin stimulation or no thrombin stimulation; $P < 0.05$. Arrows indicate gap formation in WT endothelial cells after thrombin stimulation.*
Adapted from Tauseef et al. FASEB J, 30(1), 102-110. doi: 10.1096/fj.15-275891; with permission

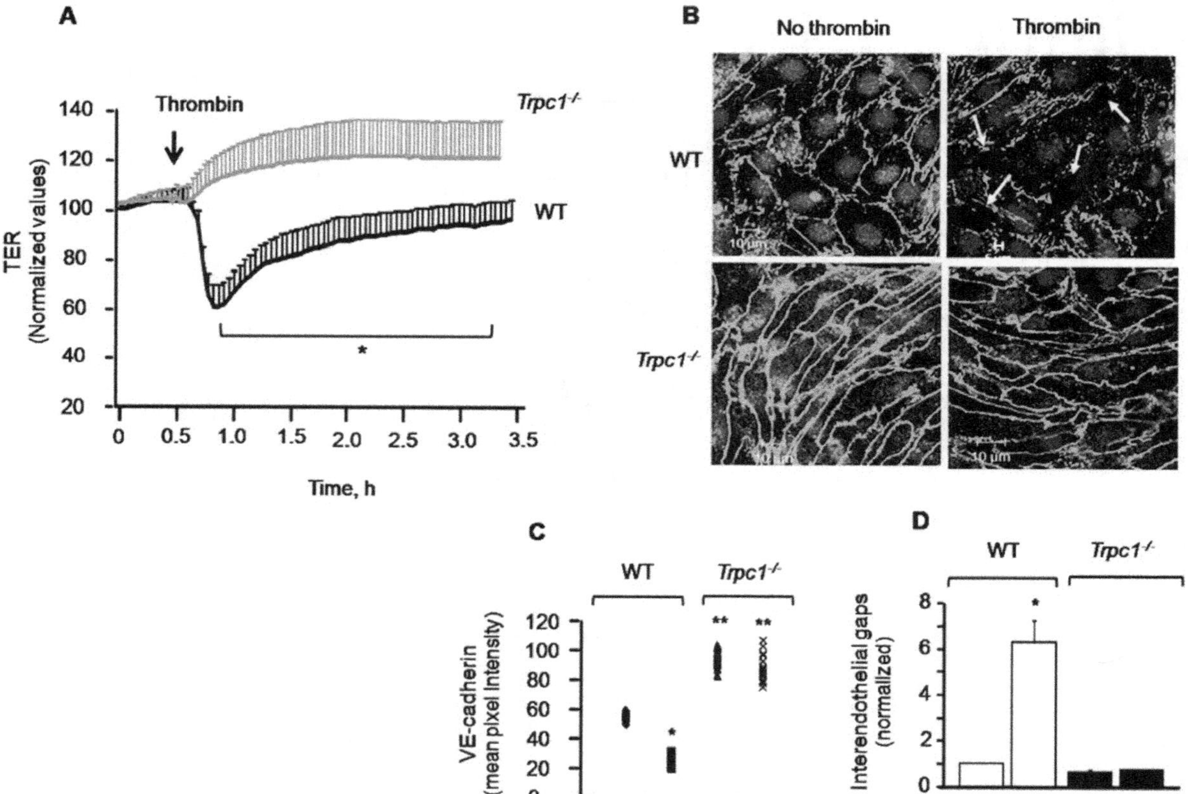

Chapter 3
Potential Role of Nuclear Factor κB in Cardiovascular Disease:
An Update

Rakesh K. Mishra
Feinstein Institute for Medical Research, USA

ABSTRACT

Lung and Cardiovascular disease creating a major health burden in developed countries and primary cause of deaths. Although treatments have progressed, the development of novel treatments for patients with cardiovascular diseases remains a major research goal. Despite modern advances in pharmacological and interventional cardiology, cardiovascular disease still remains a leading cause of morbidity and mortality in all over the world. The nuclear factor (NF)-κB super family of transcription factors has been implicated in the regulation of immune cell maturation, cell survival, and inflammation in many cell types, including cardiac myocytes. Recent studies have shown that NF-κB is cardioprotective during acute hypoxia and reperfusion injury. NF-kB regulates the gene expression of major pro-inflammatory cytokines (TNF-a, IL-b), chemokines [macrophage inflammatory protein (MIP-2), cytokine-induced neutrophil chemoattractant (CINC)], and adhesion molecules (ICAM-1, E selectin) (2), all of which play a major role in lung injury. However, prolonged activation of NF-κB appears to be detrimental and promotes heart failure by eliciting signals that trigger chronic inflammation through enhanced elaboration of cytokines. In this review, we summarize progresses in understanding the NF-kB pathway in lung and cardio-vascular disease development as well as in modulating NF-kB for prevention and therapy.

INTRODUCTION

Over the past few years, the transcription factor nuclear factor (NF)-kB and the proteins that regulate it have emerged as an importance signaling system in human physiology and in an increasing number of disease pathogenesis. Ranjan Sen and David Baltimore (Sen & Baltimore, 1986) identified a DNA-binding factor that has since been found to be ancient and evolutionarily conserved and to be linked to many biological pathways. It influences cellular development, innate and adaptive immune responses,

DOI: 10.4018/978-1-5225-2092-4.ch003

the induction of inflammatory mediators and wound repair, and, when dysregulated, can lead to various forms of cancer, autoimmunity and chronic inflammatory syndromes this factor is NF-κB (Baltomore, 1986, Pages 705-716).The NF-κB family controls multiple processes, including immunity, inflammation, cell survival, differentiation and proliferation, and regulates cellular responses to stress, hypoxia, stretch and ischemia (Evans etal, 2010). It is therefore not surprising that NF-κB has been shown to influence numerous cardiovascular diseases including atherosclerosis, myocardial ischaemia/reperfusion injury, ischaemic preconditioning, vein graft disease, cardiac hypertrophy and heart failure (Hopkins, Ouchi, Shibata & Walsh, 2007). The function of NF-κB is largely dictated by the genes that it targets for transcription and varies according to stimulus and cell type (Morgan & Liu, 2011,page 103–115). Thus NF-κB has divergent functions and can protect cardiovascular tissues from injury or contribute to pathogenesis depending on the cellular and physiological context. The present book chapter will focus on recent studies on the function of NF-κB in the lung and cardiovascular system.

Nuclear Factor-κB Signaling

NFκB comprises a family of transcription factors first described as B-lymphocyte-specific nuclear proteins, essential for transcription of immunoglobulin kappa (κ) light chains. Mammalian cells contain five NFκB subunits—relA (p65), relB, c-rel, p50 and p52, that exist in an inactive form in the cytoplasm bound to three inhibitory proteins (IκBα, IκBβ and IκBε) (Evans etal, 2010). In most cell types, NF-kB proteins are sequestered in the cytoplasmic compartment, associated with members of the inhibitor of kB (IkB) family (IkBa, IkBb and IkBe). In response to multiple stimuli such as inflammatory cytokines, bacterial lipopolysaccharide (LPS), viral infection or stress, IkBs are phosphorylated on two critical serine residues. This modification triggers their ubiquitination and destruction via the proteasome degradation machinery. As a consequence, free NF-kB enters the nucleus and activates transcription of a variety of genes participating in immune and inflammatory responses, cell adhesion, growth control and regulation of apoptosis (Ghosh et al, 2009, Jones et al, 2003, Tiruppathi et al, 2014).

Pro-inflammatory cytokines produced by macrophages, T cells and other immunologic cells exert their actions on target cells by transactivating NF-kB (Karin & Ben, 2000, page 621–663). These cells express receptors for the pro-inflammatory cytokines, IL-1b and TNF-a, and they also contain the IKK complex that is crucial for signal transduction. Cells such as leukocytes, vascular endothelial and smooth muscle cells, cardiomyocytes and fibroblasts therefore respond to pro-inflammatory cytokines by NF-kB activation (Ghosh et al 2004; Baeuerle et al, 1998; Baldwin et al, 1996; Maniatis et al, 1995). Also, NF-kB activation induces the expression of pro-inflammatory cytokines in a positive feedback loop.

The NF-kB pathway is used not only by pro-inflammatory cytokines but also by microbial products. In particular, endotoxins of gram-negative bacteria signal through NF-kB after ligation of their LPS moieties to receptors of the Toll-like receptor (TLR) family. TLR/NFkB– mediated response to bacteria has been a key mechanism through evolution for the protection of multicellular organisms against pathogenic invaders (Maniatis et al, 1995; Janeway et al, 1997)

NF-kB in Acute Lung Injury (ALI)

Acute lung injury (ALI) and its more severe manifestation, acute respiratory distress syndrome (ARDS), are characterized by acute inflammation that affects the function of the gas exchange surface of the lung.

The disorder affects all age groups, and has an incidence of approximately 200,000 cases per year in the United States and a mortality of around 35% (Hudson et al, 2005).

NF-κB activation has been implicated as an important factor in humans with acute respiratory distress syndrome (ARDS), which is characterized by neutrophilic lung inflammation and diffuse alveolar damage, and can result from systemic inflammation. Schwartz et al (Janeway et al, 1997; Hudson et al, 2005; Abraham et al, 2013), reported that NF-κB is activated in alveolar macrophages from patients with ARDS to a significantly higher degree than in alveolar macrophages from critically ill patients with other diseases. In addition, NF-κB activation may be important in the pathogenesis of sepsis (Figure 1).

In other study by Bohrer et al (Nawroth et al, 2007) showed that in peripheral blood monocytes of patients with sepsis, NF-κB activation correlates with mortality. Specifically, all patients in that study who died with sepsis had increased NF-κB activation (greater than twice baseline) in the first 6 d, whereas all patients who survived had NF-κB activation that remained less than twice the baseline value at each time point during the 14-d study period.

Figure 1. NF-kB signaling and lung injury

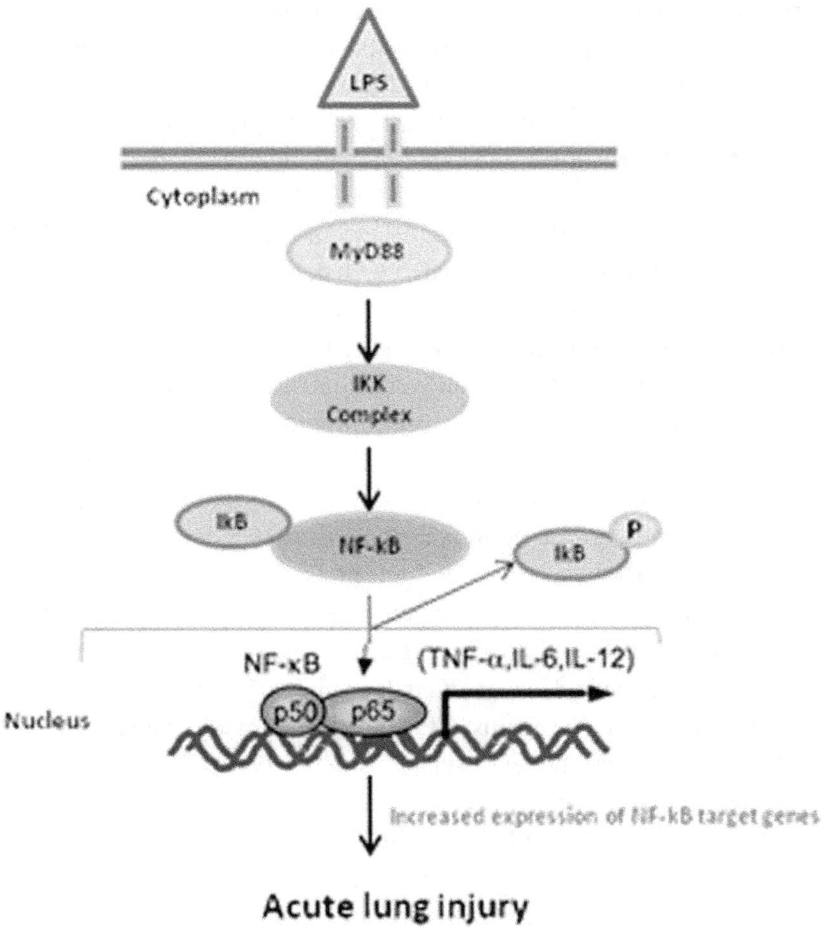

Using a transgenic mice model in which the lueciferase promoter gene was placed under the control of NF-kB dependent promoter. In 2002 Blackwell et al (Blackwell et al, 2000, page 1095-1101), demonstrated increase NF-kB activity in the lung of the mice injected with LPS.

In many mice models, inhibitions of NF-kB activations by varieties of pharmacological inhibitors confirmed the protection against LPS induced ALI. In 2000, Ross SD et al (Ross & Kron et al, 2000) demonstrated that NF-kB is rapidly activated and is associated with poor pulmonary graft function in transplant reperfusion injury, and targeting of NF-kB may be a promising therapy to reduce this injury and improve lung function.

The expression of pro-inflammatory cytokines is rapidly increased in experimental models of the acute respiratory distress syndrome (ARDS), in patients at risk for ARDS, and in patients with established ARDS. Because multiple cytokines are present in bronchoalveolar lavage fluid, a common, proximal activation mechanism may operate in these setting. Clinical studies also suggest a role of NF-kB in path physiology of ALI.

To test the hypothesis that activation of one or more of these nuclear transcriptional regulatory factors might provide a common mechanism for the simultaneous expression of multiple cytokine genes in the setting of ARDS. Schwartz et al (Schwartz et al, 1996, page1285-1292), measured activation of these factors in alveolar macrophages from patients with ARDS and from controls. These experiments demonstrated increased in vivo activation of the nuclear transcriptional regulatory factor NF-kB (but not NF-IL6, cyclic adenosine monophosphate responsive element binding protein, activating protein-1, or serum protein-1) in alveolar macrophages from patients with ARDS. Because binding sequences for NF-kB are present in the enhancer/promoter sequences of multiple proinflammatory cytokines, activation of NF-kB may contribute to the increased expression of multiple cytokines in the lung in the setting of establishedARDS.

In 2000 Moin p et al (Moine et al, 2000, page 85-91), demonstrated the increased NF-kB activation in alveolar macrophages of patients with ALI compared with control. In this study they examined cytoplasmic and nuclear NF-kB counter regulatory mechanisms, involving IkB proteins, in alveolar macrophages obtained from 7 control patients without lung injury and 11 patients with established ARDS. Cytoplasmic levels of the NF-kB subunits p50, p65, and c-Rel were significantly decreased in alveolar macrophages from patients with ARDS, consistent with enhanced migration of liberated NF-kB dimers from the cytoplasm to the nucleus. Cytoplasmic and nuclear levels of IkB-alpha were not significantly altered in alveolar macrophages from patients with established ARDS, compared with controls. In contrast, nuclear levels of Bcl-3 were significantly decreased in patients with ARDS compared with controls ($P = 0.02$). No IkB-gamma, IkB-beta, or p105 proteins were detected in the cytoplasm of alveolar macrophages from control patients or patients with ARDS. The presence of activated NF-kB in alveolar macrophages from patients with established ARDS implies the presence of an ongoing stimulus for NF-kB activation.

In (2005), Matsuda et al (Matsuda, Hattori &Gando et al, 2005) evaluate the effects of "decoy" `cis'-acting oligonucleotides (ODN) directed against NF-κB on inflammatory gene expression and pulmonary function in a cecal-ligation puncture model of sepsis. To test whether functional inactivation of NF-κB could suppress endotoxin-induced lung injury. The authors found that intravenous injection of ODN significantly reduced the increase of NF-κB activity during sepsis, as indicated by electromobility shift analysis. Moreover, NF-κB decoy markedly reduced the expression levels of iNOS, COX-2, histamine H1-receptor, platelet-activating factor receptor, and bradykinin B1 and B2 receptors in the septic lung tissue. It is noteworthy that animals treated with NF-κB ODN displayed an improved outcome with a significant reduction in sepsis-induced lung injury compared with control animals or animals treated with scrambled ODN.

In 2012, study by Xiaojun et al (Xiaojun et al,2012, Pages 209–216) Investigate the protective effect of kaempferol (Kae), a naturally occurring flavonoid compound, on ALI and explore its possible mechanisms and results suggest that Kae exhibits a protective effect on LPS-induced ALI via suppression of MAPKs and NF-κB signaling pathways, which may involve the inhibition of tissue oxidative injury and pulmonary inflammatory process. Kae treatment attenuated pulmonary edema of mice with ALI after LPS challenge, as it markedly decreased the lung W/D ratio of lung samples, protein concentration and the amounts of inflammatory cells in BALF. Similarly, LPS mediated overproduction of proinflammatory cytokines in BALF, including TNF-α, IL-1β and IL-6, was strongly reduced by Kae. In addition, Western blot analysis indicated that the activation of MAPKs and NF-κB signaling pathways stimulated by LPS was significantly blocked by Kae.

In 2014 another important observation by Tirupatthi e al (Tiruppathi et al, 2014, page 239–247) described the potential role of A20 protein (well know NF-Kb inhibitor) to protection against LPS induced ALI by suppressing the NF-kB activation. In these studies, they found that the transcription repressor DREAM (downstream regulatory element antagonist modulator) bound to the promoter of the gene encoding A20 to repress expression of this deubiquitinase that suppresses inflammatory NF-κB signaling. DREAM-deficient mice displayed persistent and unchecked A20 expression in response to endotoxin. DREAM functioned by transcriptionally repressing A20 through binding to downstream regulatory elements (DREs). In contrast, binding of the transcription factor USF1 to the DRE-associated E-box domain in the gene encoding A20 activated its expression in response to inflammatory stimuli. Targeting of DREAM to induce USF1-mediated A20 expression is therefore a potential anti-inflammatory strategy for the treatment of diseases associated with unconstrained NF-κB activity, such as acute lung injury.

The basis of the above findings, it is concluded that NF-κB is playing the crucial role in lung disease as elevated NF-Kb activity is present in the lungs of patients with acute respiratory distress syndrome (ARDS) and experimental models of acute lung injury. Activation of NF-κB contributes to the increased expression of immunoregulatory cytokines and other pro-inflammatory mediators in the lungs.

NF-kB in Cardiovascular Disease

Nuclear factor-kappaB (NF-kappaB) regulates many genes involved in vascular physiopathology through the regulation of several genes, including cytokines, adhesion proteins, NO synthase, and angiotensinogen, as well as other products involved in atherosclerosis, inflammation, proliferation, and immune response (Barnes et al, 1997, page 1066-1071).NFκB primarily resides inactive in the cytoplasm by association with IκB. Its activation can be triggered by a variety of stimuli that ultimately lead to phosphorylation, ubiquitination and degradation of IκB, releasing NFκB dimers to nuclear translocation, where NFκB dependent transcription of a large and diverse array of target genes can be initiated and various physiological and pathological processes modulated (Figure 2).

In 1997, Study by Egido et al (Egido et al,1997, page 1532-1541) has described the elevated tissue specific NF-κB activity in an experimental model of atherosclerosis, correlated with increased macrophage infiltration and monocyte chemoattractant protein-1 (MCP-1) expression, which is diminished by angiotensin-converting enzyme (ACE) inhibition. Atherosclerotic vessels exhibited an increase in NF-κB–like activity, and p50 and p65 NF-κB subunits were identified as components of this activity.

Figure 2. TLR4 mediated NF-kB signaling in cardiac and immune cells

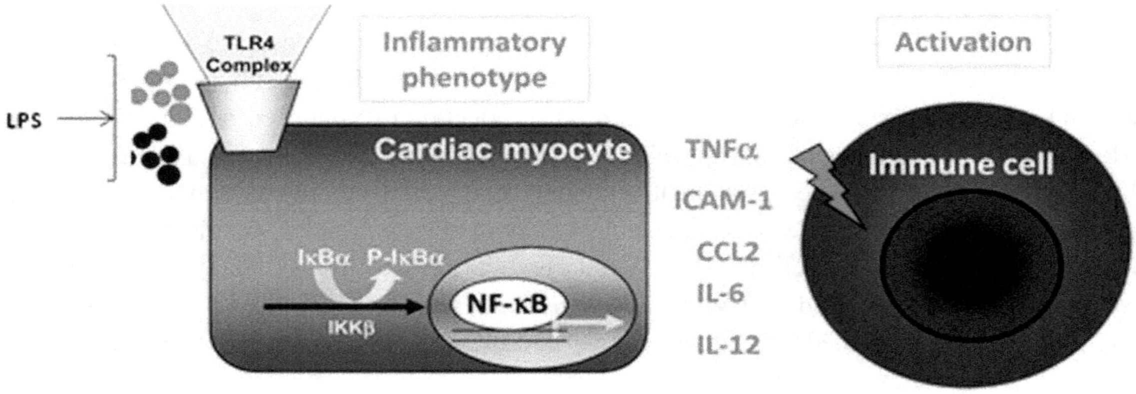

Several years ago, activated NF-κB was demonstrated in human atherosclerotic lesions by Brand et al (Brand et al, 1996, page 715-22) This study demonstrates the presence of activated NF-kappa B in human atherosclerotic tissue for the first time. Atherosclerosis, characterized by features of chronic inflammation and proliferative processes, may be a paradigm for the involvement of NF-kappaB/Rel in chronic inflammatory disease.

Endothelial dysfunction is a well established response to cardiovascular risk factors and development of atherosclerosis.(Deanfield et al, 2007, page 1285-1295) Endothelial dysfunction is involved in lesion formation by the promotion of both the early and late mechanisms of atherosclerosis including up-regulation of adhesion molecules, increased chemokine secretion and leukocyte adherence, increased cell permeability, enhanced low-density lipoprotein oxidation, platelet activation, cytokine elaboration, and vascular smooth muscle cell proliferation and migration(Fei Fang et al, 2013). Endothelial cells at sites of inflammatory responses express a variety of genes that are under the control of nuclear factor NF-kappa B (Deanfield et al, 1994).

In 2008, Gareus, et al (Gareus, 2008, page 372-83) addressed the function of NF-kappa B signaling in vascular endothelial cells in the pathogenesis of atherosclerosis *in vivo*. Endothelium-restricted inhibition of NF-kappa B activation, achieved by ablation of NEMO/IKK gamma or expression of dominant-negative I kappa B alpha specifically in endothelial cells, resulted in strongly reduced atherosclerotic plaque formation in ApoE(-/-) mice fed with a cholesterol-rich diet. Inhibition of NF-kappaB abrogated adhesion molecule induction in endothelial cells, impaired macrophage recruitment to atherosclerotic plaques, and reduced expression of cytokines and chemokines in the aorta. Thus, endothelial NF-kappaB signaling orchestrates proinflammatory gene expression at the arterial wall and promotes the pathogenesis of several cardiovascular diseases, such as atherosclerosis and hypertension (Gareus, 2008, page 372-83).

Using an antibody specifically recognizing activated phosphorylated p65, NF-κB activation was shown in smooth muscle cells, macrophages, and endothelial cells. Moreover, hypercholesterolemia was shown to induce activated NF-κB in the vessel wall in a pig model for atherosclerosis (Lerman et al, 2000). Using mice, Hajra et al showed that there was a colocalization of regions prone to develop atherosclerosis and increased levels of components of the NF-κB system, also indicative for a role of NF-κB in atherosclerosis (Cybulsky et al, 2000).

Innate immunity is the first line of defense against invading pathogens. A family of Toll-like receptors (TLRs) acts as primary sensors that detect a wide variety of microbial components and elicit innate immune responses. All TLR signaling pathways culminate in activation of the transcription factor nuclear factor-kappaB (NF-kappaB), which controls the expression of an array of inflammatory cytokine genes. TLRs, however, are not only expressed on macrophages but also on the other cells commonly found in the arterial wall (Seneviratne, Sivagurunathan & Monaco, 2007)

There is increasing evidence to support the involvement of TLRs, mainly TLR2 and TLR4, in the initiation, progression, and instability of atherosclerotic lesions, leading to plaque rupture (Kristina et al, 2002; Tobias et al, 2009; Bijani et al 2012), as well as their involvement in other cardiovascular diseases (Arditi et al, 2001).

TLR4 over expression has been reported in human and mouse atherosclerotic lesions, mainly in macrophages and endothelial cells (ECs) within the lesion, at different stages of atherogenesis (Pasterkamp et al 2004; Kleijn et al 2004). TLR4 has been shown to be important in the process of expansive arterial remodeling and in matrix breakdown; the latter process involves cell migration and leads to higher expression levels of matrix metalloproteinases (MMPs), mainly MMP-2 and MMP-9, which are involved in extracellular matrix (ECM) degradation (Kleijn et al 2004).

Up-regulation of inflammatory responses is considered a driving force of atherosclerotic lesion development. One key regulator of inflammation is the A20 (also called TNF-α-induced protein 3 or Tnfaip3) gene, which is responsible for NF-κB termination and maps to an atherosclerosis susceptibility locus revealed by quantitative trait locus-mapping studies at mouse proximal chromosome 10.

In 2007 study by Wolfrum et al (Wolfrum 2007, page 18601-18606), examined the role of A20 in atherosclerotic lesion development. At the aortic root lesion size was found to be increased in C57BL/6 (BG) apolipoprotein E-deficient ($ApoE^{-/-}$) mice haploinsufficient for A20, compared with B6 $ApoE^{-/-}$ controls that expressed A20 normally (60% in males and 23% in females; $P < 0.001$ and $P < 0.05$, respectively). The increase in lesions in the A20 haplo insufficient mice correlated with increased expression of pro-atherosclerotic NF-κB target genes, such as vascular cell adhesion molecule 1, intercellular adhesion molecule 1, and macrophage-colony-stimulating factor, and elevated plasma levels of NF-κB-driven cytokines by the basis of above finding it suggest that A20 diminishes atherosclerosis by decreasing NF-κB activity, thereby modulating the pro-inflammatory state associated with lesion development.

The better understanding of the role of NF-kB signaling will lead to the identification of therapeutic targets that down regulate pro-inflammatory and pro-thrombotic responses in atherosclerotic. While blockade of NF-kB could be beneficial in atherosclerosis and other cardio-vascular disease, there are obvious questions regarding the appropriate balance between efficacy and safety levels of NF-kB activity is critical for immune and inflammatory responses and maintenance of homeostasis.

FUTURE PROSPECTS

Despite the reduction in the mortality rate caused by ALI and Cardio-vascular diseases still remains an important serious problem all over the world. Investigational and collaborative efforts directed toward understanding how the overall cellular signaling network translates NF-B activation into the regulation of specific subsets of NF-kB -dependent genes will lead to a mechanistic understanding of how NF-kB mediates diverse and paradoxical biological effects and both animal and clinical studies will provide the necessary insight for improving the detection and treatment of ALI and cardiovascular diseases.

REFERENCES

Anusha, N. (2007, November). Seneviratne, Bawani Sivagurunathan, Claudia Monaco.Toll-like receptors and macrophage activation in atherosclerosis. *Trends in Molecular Medicine*, *13*(11), 460–469. PMID:18029230

Baeuerle, P. A. (1998). IkB–NF-kB Structures: At the interface of inflammation control. *Cell*, *95*, 729–731. doi:10.1016/S0092-8674(00)81694-3 PMID:9865689

Baldwin, A. S. Jr. (1996). The NF-kB and IkB proteins: New discoveries and insights. *Annual Review of Immunology*, *14*(1), 649–681. doi:10.1146/annurev.immunol.14.1.649 PMID:8717528

Bijani, F. M. (2012). Toll-like receptor signaling pathways in cardiovascular diseases: Challenges and opportunities. *International Reviews of Immunology*, *31*(5), 379–395. doi:10.3109/08830185.2012.706761 PMID:23083347

Brand, K., Page, S., Rogler, G., Bartsch, A., Brandl, R., Knuechel, R., & Neumeier, D. et al. (1996, April1). Activated transcription factor nuclear factor-kappa B is present in the atherosclerotic lesion. *The Journal of Clinical Investigation*, *97*(7), 1715–1722. doi:10.1172/JCI118598 PMID:8601637

Chen, X., Yang, X., Liu, T., Guan, M., Feng, X., Dong, W., & Sun, Z. et al. (2012, October). Xiaojun Chen Kaempferol regulates MAPKs and NF-κB signaling pathways to attenuate LPS-induced acute lung injury in mice. *International Immunopharmacology*, *14*(2), 209–216. doi:10.1016/j.intimp.2012.07.007 PMID:22835426

Collins, T., Read, M. A., Neish, A. S., Whitley, M. Z., Thanos, D., & Maniatis, T. (1995). Transcriptional regulation of endothelial cell adhesion molecules: NF-kappa-B and cytokine-inducible enhancers. *The FASEB Journal*, *9*, 899–909. PMID:7542214

Deanfield, J. E. et al.. (2007). Contemporary Reviews in Cardiovascular Medicine Endothelial Function and Dysfunction Testing and Clinical Relevance. *Circulation*, *115*, 1285–1295. PMID:17353456

Edfeldt, K. (2002, March12). Expression of Toll-Like Receptors in Human Atherosclerotic Lesions: A Possible Pathway for Plaque Activation.Circulation. *Journal of the American Heart Association Issue*, *105*(10), 1158–116.

Egido, J. et al.. (1997). Angiotensin-Converting Enzyme Inhibition Prevents Arterial Nuclear Factor-κB Activation, Monocyte Chemoattractant Protein-1 Expression, and Macrophage Infiltration in a Rabbit Model of Early Accelerated Atherosclerosis. *Circulation*, *95*(6), 1532–1541. doi:10.1161/01.CIR.95.6.1532 PMID:9118522

Fang, F., Chen, D., Yu, L., Dai, X., Yang, Y., Tian, W., & Xu, Y. et al. (2013). Proinflammatory Stimuli Engage Brahma Related Gene 1 and Brahma in Endothelial Injury. *Circulation Research*, *113*(8), 986–996. doi:10.1161/CIRCRESAHA.113.301296 PMID:23963727

Gareus, R., Kotsaki, E., Xanthoulea, S., van der Made, I., Gijbels, M. J. J., Kardakaris, R., & Pasparakis, M. et al. (2008, November). Endothelial cell-specific NF-kappaB inhibition protects mice from atherosclerosis. *Cell Metabolism*, *8*(5), 372–383. doi:10.1016/j.cmet.2008.08.016 PMID:19046569

Hajra, L., Evans, A. I., Chen, M., Hyduk, S. J., Collins, T., & Cybulsky, M. I. (2000). The NF-kappa B signal transduction pathway in aortic endothelial cells is primed for activation in regions predisposed to atherosclerotic lesion formation. *Proceedings of the National Academy of Sciences of the United States of America*, *97*(16), 9052–9057. doi:10.1073/pnas.97.16.9052 PMID:10922059

Hayden, M. S., & Ghosh, S. (2004). Signaling to NF-kB. *Genes & Development*, *18*(18), 2195–2224. doi:10.1101/gad.1228704 PMID:15371334

Hollestelle, S. C., De Vries, M. R., Van Keulen, J. K., Schoneveld, A. H., Vink, A., Strijder, C. F., & De Kleijn, D. P. et al. (2004). Toll-like receptor 4 is involved in outward arterial remodeling. *Circulation*, *109*(3), 393–398. doi:10.1161/01.CIR.0000109140.51366.72 PMID:14699006

Karin, M., & Ben-Neriah, Y. (2000). Phosphorylation meets ubiquitination: The control of NF-kB activity. *Annual Review of Immunology*, *18*(1), 621–663. doi:10.1146/annurev.immunol.18.1.621 PMID:10837071

Linda, K. (2009). Curtiss and Peter S. Tobias.Emerging role of Toll-like receptors in atherosclerosis. *Journal of Lipid Research*, *50*(Supplement), S340–S345. PMID:18980945

Matsuda, N., Hattori, Y., Jesmin, S., & Gando, S. (2005). Nuclear factor-κB decoy oligodeoxynucleotides prevent acute lung injury in mice with cecal ligation and puncture-induced sepsis. *Molecular Pharmacology*, *67*(4), 1018–1025. doi:10.1124/mol.104.005926 PMID:15576632

Medzhitov, R., & Janeway, C. A. Jr. (1997). Innate immunity: The virtues of a nonclonal system of recognition. *Cell*, *91*(3), 295–298. doi:10.1016/S0092-8674(00)80412-2 PMID:9363937

Moine, P., McIntyre, R., Schwartz, M. D., Kaneko, D., Shenkar, R., Tulzo, Y. L., & Abraham, E. et al. (2000, February). NF-kappaB regulatory mechanisms in alveolar macrophages from patients with acute respiratory distress syndrome. *Shock (Augusta, Ga.)*, *13*(2), 85–91. doi:10.1097/00024382-200013020-00001 PMID:10670837

Morgan, M. J., & Liu, Z. (2011, January). Crosstalk of reactive oxygen species and NF-κB signaling. *Cell Research*, *21*(1), 103–115. doi:10.1038/cr.2010.178 PMID:21187859

Oeckinghaus & Ghosh. (2009, October). The NF-κB Family of Transcription Factors and Its Regulation. *Cold Spring Harbor Perspectives in Biology*, *1*(4), a000034. PMID:20066092

Pasterkamp, G., Van Keulen, J. K., & De Kleijn, D. P. (2004). Role of Toll-like receptor 4 in the initiation and progression of atherosclerotic disease. *European Journal of Clinical Investigation*, *34*(5), 328–334. doi:10.1111/j.1365-2362.2004.01338.x PMID:15147329

Peter, J. (1997). Barnes.Nuclear Factor-κB — A Pivotal Transcription Factor in Chronic Inflammatory Diseases. *The New England Journal of Medicine*, *336*(15), 1066–1071. doi:10.1056/NEJM199704103361506 PMID:9091804

Ross, S. D., & Kron, I. L. (2000, September). Attenuation of lung reperfusion injury after transplantation using an inhibitor of nuclear factor-kappaB. *American Journal of Physiology. Lung Cellular and Molecular Physiology*, *279*(3), L528–L536. PMID:10956628

Rubenfeld, G. D., Caldwell, E., Peabody, E., Weaver, J., Martin, D. P., Neff, M., & Hudson, L. D. et al. (2005). Incidence and outcomes of acute lung injury. *The New England Journal of Medicine*, *353*(16), 1685–1693. doi:10.1056/NEJMoa050333 PMID:16236739

Schwartz, M. D., Moore, E. E., Moore, F. A., Shenkar, R., Moine, P., Haenel, J. B., & Abraham, E. (2013). Nuclear factor-κB is activated in alveolar macrophages from patients with acute respiratory distress syndrome. *Critical Care Medicine*. PMID:8706481

Sorensen, K. E., Celermajer, D. S., Georgakopoulos, D., Hatcher, G., Betteridge, D. J., & Deanfield, J. E. (1994, January). Impairment of endothelium-dependent dilation is an early event in children with familial hypercholesterolemia and is related to the lipoprotein(a) level. *The Journal of Clinical Investigation*, *93*(1), 50–55. doi:10.1172/JCI116983 PMID:8282821

Teresa, A. (2007). Hopkins, Noriyuki Ouchi, Rei Shibata, Kenneth Walsh.Adiponectin actions in the cardiovascular system. *Cardiovascular Research*, 11–18.

Tiruppathi, C., Soni, D., Wang, D.-M., Xue, J., Singh, V., Thippegowda, P. B., & Malik, A. B. et al. (2014). The transcription factor DREAM represses the deubiquitinase A20 and mediates inflammation. c.tiruppathi. *Nature Immunology*, *15*(3), 239–247. doi:10.1038/ni.2823 PMID:24487321

Tiruppathi, C., Soni, D., Wang, D.-M., Xue, J., Singh, V., Thippegowda, P. B., & Malik, A. B. et al. (2014). The transcription factor DREAM represses the deubiquitinase A20 and mediates inflammation. *Nature Immunology*, *15*(3), 239–247. doi:10.1038/ni.2823 PMID:24487321

Van der Heiden, K., & Cuhlmann, S. (2010). Luong le A, Zakkar M, Evans PC.Role of nuclear factor kappaB in cardiovascular health and disease. *Clinical Science (London, England)*, *118*(10), 593–605. doi:10.1042/CS20090557

Vink, A., de Kleijn, D. P., & Pasterkamp, G. (2004). Functional role for toll-like receptors in atherosclerosis and arterial remodeling. *Current Opinion in Lipidology*, *15*(5), 515–521. doi:10.1097/00041433-200410000-00004 PMID:15361786

Wilson, S. H., Caplice, N. M., Simari, R. D., Holmes, D. R. Jr, Carlson, P. J., & Lerman, A. (2000). Activated nuclear factor-kappaB is present in the coronary vasculature in experimental hypercholesterolemia. *Atherosclerosis*, *148*(1), 23–30. doi:10.1016/S0021-9150(99)00211-7 PMID:10580167

Wolfrum, S., Teupser, D., Tan, M., Chen, K. Y., & Breslow, J. L. (2007). The protective effect of A20 on atherosclerosis in apolipoprotein E-deficient mice is associated with reduced expression of NF-κB target gene. *Proceedings of the National Academy of Sciences of the United States of America*, *104*(47), 18601–18606. doi:10.1073/pnas.0709011104 PMID:18006655

Xu, X. H., Shah, P. K., Faure, E., Equils, O., Thomas, L., Fishbein, M. C., & Arditi, M. et al. (2001). Toll-like receptor-4 is expressed by macrophages in murine and human lipid-rich atherosclerotic plaques and upregulated by oxidized LDL. *Circulation*, *104*(25), 3103–3108. doi:10.1161/hc5001.100631 PMID:11748108

Chapter 4
Store-Operated Calcium Entry Channels:
Potential Role in Cardiac Function

Diptiman D. Bose
Western New England University, USA

ABSTRACT

Store-operated Ca^{2+} entry (SOCE) channels mediate Ca^{2+} influx from the extracellular milieu into the cytosol to regulate a myriad of cellular functions. The Ca^{2+}-release activated Ca^{2+} current has been well characterized in non-excitable cells such as immune cells. However, the role of SOCE proteins in cardiomyocytes and cardiac function has only been recently investigated. The localized endoplasmic reticulum protein, stromal interaction molecule (STIM) and plasma membrane Ca^{2+} channels, ORAI form the minimal functional unit of SOCE. The documentation of STIM and Orai expression in cardiomyocytes has raised questions regarding their role in cardiac function. Recent evidence supports the central role of STIM and Orai in gene transcription and, subsequent phenotypic changes associated with cardiac remodeling and hypertrophy. The purpose of this chapter is to provide an overview of our current understanding of SOCE proteins and, to explore their contributions to cardiovascular function and role in cardiac disorders.

INTRODUCTION

Calcium's role as a ubiquitous intracellular messenger is demonstrated by its central role in a wide range of cellular functions from cell growth, proliferation, function and even cell death. In order to elicit to cellular response, a cell recruits various pumps, exchangers and channels to regulate the concentration of Ca^{2+} (Berridge, Bootman, & Roderick, 2003; Prakriya & Lewis, 2015; J. W. Putney, 2011). The endoplasmic reticulum/sarcoplasmic reticulum (ER/SR) act as an intracellular storage of Ca^{2+}, while plasma membrane (PM) channels regulate gating of Ca^{2+} from the extracellular space. Store operated Ca^{2+} entry (SOCE), is a major mechanism representing Ca^{2+} entry in many excitable and non-excitable cells. Since the first characterization of SOCE through electrophysiology, the two major components of the SOCE

DOI: 10.4018/978-1-5225-2092-4.ch004

process were identified; the ER/SR Ca^{2+} sensor, stromal interaction molecule (STIM) and, the plasma membrane (PM) localized Orai protein as the store-operated channels (Fahrner, Derler, Jardin, & Romanin, 2013; J. W. Putney, 2011; Shaw & Feske, 2012). Upon depletion of inositol-1, 4, 5-trisphosphate (IP_3) or Ryanodine (RyR)-sensitive ER/SR stores, localized ER sensor STIM directly couples with PM Orai channels mediating Ca^{2+} influx. Since the depletion of ER/SR Ca^{2+} is the trigger for PM Ca^{2+} entry, this pathway was appropriately named "store operated Ca^{2+} entry". SOCE-mediated Ca^{2+} entry not only allows for refilling of the ER/SR stores but also helps maintain Ca^{2+} homeostasis. The sustained entry of Ca^{2+} also serves other purposes such as activation of secretion, modulation of enzyme activation, and initiation of transcriptional signaling (J. W. Putney, 2011). Since SOCE-mediated Ca^{2+} influx is involved in vital cellular processes, it is not surprising that aberrant SOCE function has been implicated in many disease states including immunodeficiency, acute pancreatitis, Alzheimer's disease, Duchenne muscular dystrophy and cardiac hypertrophy (Karlstad, Sun, & Singh, 2012; J. W. Putney, 2011)

Since its discovery, the SOCE phenomenon has been well characterized in non-excitable immune cells (Prakriya & Lewis, 2015; Shaw & Feske, 2012). Soon after, SOCE-induced Ca^{2+} influx was shown to play a critical role in excitable cell such as neurons, skeletal muscle cells, and cardiomyocytes (Hartmann et al., 2014; Liu, Xin, Benson, Allen, & Ju, 2015; Majewski & Kuznicki, 2015; Stiber et al., 2008; Tojyo, Morita, Nezu, & Tanimura, 2014). Several studies have demonstrated the expression of STIM and Orai in adult cardiomyoctes, ventricular myocardium, and the sinoatrial node (Wolkowicz et al., 2011; Zhu-Mauldin, Marsh, Zou, Marchase, & Chatham, 2012). In fact, strong evidence suggests that the STIM1 and Orai play a key role in the progression of cardiac hypertrophy. Recent investigations have shown the increased expression of STIM1 in a hypertrophic response (Collins, Zhu-Mauldin, Marchase, & Chatham, 2013). With advances in molecular techniques and transgenic models, studies have provided insight into the role of Orai and transient receptor potential (TRP) channels in the etiology of several cardiovascular diseases (Yue et al., 2015). The goal of this chapter is to provide an overview of our current understanding of molecular regulation of SOCE and highlight the role of STIM1/Orai-1-mediated SOCE in cardiomyocyte function and pathology.

STORE OPERATED CALCIUM ENTRY

The ligation of agonists such as growth factors, neurohormonal stimuli, and inflammatory mediators to G-protein coupled receptors or receptor tyrosine kinases initiates the activation of phospholipase (PLC) enzymes. PLC hydrolyzes phosphatidylinositol 4, 5 bisphosphate into diacylglycerol and inositol 1, 4, 5-trisphosphate (IP_3). IP_3 binds to the IP_3 receptor (IP_3R) on the ER/SR, triggering Ca^{2+} release into the cytosol and mobilizing an increase in cytosolic Ca^{2+} ($[Ca^{2+}]_i$) (Berridge et al., 2003; Oh-hora & Rao, 2008). The increase in $[Ca^{2+}]_i$ can fuel activation of localized events such as calcium-induced Ca^{2+} release via the Ryanodine receptors (RyRs) or even induce downstream transcriptional events (Bers, 2008; J. W. Putney, 2011). The discovery of IP_3 led to our understanding that the consequence of IP_3 production was a transient increase in $[Ca^{2+}]_i$, followed by a sustained influx of Ca^{2+} from the extracellular space. While the increase in $[Ca^{2+}]_i$ was identified as a product of IP_3 activating the IP_3R in the ER/SR, the mechanism underlying Ca^{2+} influx remained unclear (Berridge, 1993). Several studies suggested that a PM-Ca^{2+} pathway was responsible for directly reloading the ER/SR stores. The idea of SOCE, initially described as "capacitative Ca^{2+} entry (CCE)", first described by Putney, reflected these conclusions. This model suggested that Ca^{2+} from extracellular space directly loaded the ER (the "capacitor") (J.

W. Putney, Jr., 1986). This hypothesis was later revised as studies indicated that Ca^{2+} first entered the cytoplasm rather the ER/SR stores and the ER/SR Ca^{2+} release was sufficient signal to induce Ca^{2+} influx. Thus, the CCE model was renamed SOCE to show that Ca^{2+} store depletion activated Ca^{2+} entry into the cytosol mediated by PM Ca^{2+} channels (J. W. Putney, 2011; J. W. Putney, Jr., 1990). In order to regulate cellular processes, it is essential for a cell to maintain steady level of Ca^{2+} in the ER and the cytosol. SOCE functions to help replenish the ER/SR Ca^{2+} stores, while the sustained Ca^{2+} entry allows for downstream activation of various cellular processes. This process allows SOCE to play a pivotal role in a wide range of physiological functions such as cell proliferation, cell motility, exocytosis, inflammation, exocytosis, gene transcription and apoptosis (Berridge et al., 2003; Majewski & Kuznicki, 2015; J. W. Putney, 2011). The identification of SOCE machinery, which included STIM as the ER Ca^{2+} sensor and Orai as the SOC subunit, represent major advances in our understanding of molecular mechanisms regulating SOCE.

Stromal Interaction Molecule (STIM)

The mammalian STIM (stromal interaction molecule) family comprises of two proteins: STIM1 and STIM2. STIM proteins were first discovered while screening for stromal cell transmembrane and secreted proteins that promote cell survival and/or proliferation of pre-B lymphocytes (Oritani & Kincade, 1996). Screening of *Drosophila S2* cells identified STIM dsRNA as a potent inhibitor of SOCE-mediated Ca^{2+} influx (Roos et al., 2005). This study also showed that knockdown of STIM1 in Jurkat T-cells and HEK293 cells suppressed Ca^{2+} influx. Independent investigation on siRNA screen for SOCE inhibition by Meyer and colleagues, also identified STIM1 and STIM2 as potential targets for SOCE inhibition (Liou et al., 2005).

Subsequent studies have shown that STIM protein function as the Ca^{2+} sensor from localized areas in the ER in resting state (Shen, Frieden, & Demaurex, 2011; Shim, Tirado-Lee, & Prakriya, 2015). However, fluorescently labeled STIM1 redistributed into puncta near the PM upon ER-mediated Ca^{2+} release (Liou et al., 2005). Studies on structural organization of STIM1 showed a transmembrane protein with an NH_2 terminal comprising of an EF-hand domain (cEF), a non-Ca^{2+} binding hidden EF-hand domain (hEF), and a sterile alpha motif domain (SAM) (Stathopulos, Li, Plevin, Ames, & Ikura, 2006) (Figure 1). Overexpression of STIM1 proteins with cEF mutations showed increased formation of puncta and SOCE-mediated Ca^{2+} influx (Liou et al., 2005; Spassova et al., 2006). These studies confirmed that Ca^{2+} only binds to the STIM1 cEF domain. The cytoplasmic side of STIM proteins comprises of the STIM1-Orai activating region (SOAR) (Yuan et al., 2009). Depletion of ER/SR Ca^{2+}, results in release of Ca^{2+} from the cEF domain, exposing the SOAR domains. This enhances STIM1 oligomerization into multivalent interactions, which localizes STIM1 to the ER/SR-PM junction. The juxtaposition allows for tight interaction with Orai channels leading to further Ca^{2+} influx (Figure 2) (Covington, Wu, & Lewis, 2010; Park et al., 2009).

Many factors have been shown to regulate STIM function. STIM1 phosphorylation has been known to decrease SOCE-mediated Ca^{2+} influx. Phosphorylation of S486 and S668 in particular, has been shown to inhibit the translocation of STIM1 to the ER-PM junctions (Smyth et al., 2009). Phosphorylation of S575, 608, and 621 by ERK1/2 was found to be necessary for STIM-Orai1 coupling leading to SOCE-mediated Ca^{2+} influx induced by thapsigargin (Pozo-Guisado et al., 2010). Additionally, STIM1 is also thought to be sensitive to various modes of redox modulation. The *S*-glutathionylation of STIM1 Cys-56 caused a decrease in ER-Ca^{2+} sensitivity of the EF-hand. Interestingly, oxidation of STIM1 mediated Ca^{2+}

influx in the presence of replete stores, leading to mitochondrial dysfunction and cell death (Hawkins et al., 2010). The mechanisms underlying the dissociation of STIM1/Orai interaction is not completely understood. An ER localized protein, SOCE-associated regulatory factor, SARAF, binds to both STIM1 and STIM2, and translocates to the ER-PM junction following ER store depletion. It has been postulated that SARAF may facilitate STIM1 dissociation from the PM, thus negatively regulating SOCE function (Palty, Raveh, Kaminsky, Meller, & Reuveny, 2012).

Although much is known about the role of STIM1, the function of STIM2 in regulating Ca^{2+} influx remains unclear. The Ca^{2+} dissociation constant (K_d) is about 2-fold higher than that of STIM1. STIM2 was shown to be a more sensitive senor for detecting ER Ca^{2+} levels, since small change in ER luminal Ca^{2+} levels resulted in STIM2 activation (Shim et al., 2015). In fact, STIM2 has been suggested as a feedback tool to maintain a tight control on basal cytosolic and ER Ca^{2+} levels (Brandman, Liou, Park, & Meyer, 2007). Studies have also shown that STIM2 activation yields slower activation of the CRAC current (Stathopulos, Zheng, & Ikura, 2009). Upregulation of STIM2 protein has been shown to occur in patients with idiopathic pulmonary arterial hypertension (IPAH). Additionally, siRNA mediated knockdown of STIM2 decreased Ca^{2+} influx and proliferation in the IPAH affected cells, whereas the STIM2 knockout had no effect on control pulmonary arterial smooth muscle cells (PASMC) (Song, Makino, & Yuan, 2011). More recent evidence has pointed to the involvement of STIM2 and Orai1 in the phenotypic transition of pulmonary smooth muscle cells from a contractile state to the more proliferative state. The enhancement of Ca^{2+} influx resulting from STIM2/Orai1 upregulation is thought to contribute to PASMC proliferation (Fernandez et al., 2015). Since the discovery of STIM, we have gained significant insights into the function and regulation of STIM in non-excitable cells. However, additional studies investigating whether similar or different mechanisms govern STIM regulation in excitable cells such as cardiomyocytes are lacking, and are needed to fill to the knowledge gaps.

ORAI

Electrophysiological recordings conducted in mast cells identified a Ca^{2+} selective current activated in whole cell recordings by agents such as ionomycin, IP_3 and EGTA. This was named the Ca^{2+}-release-activated Ca^{2+} (CRAC) channel (Hoth & Penner, 1992). CRAC channels were activated by pharmacological agents that deplete the free ER/SR Ca^{2+} rather than changes in $[Ca^{2+}]_i$. The CRAC channel is extremely Ca^{2+} selective with a Ca^{2+}:Na^+ permeability ratio of >1000 (Hoth, 1995). The unitary Ca^{2+} conductance is between 10-35fS and, they have a strong inward-rectifying current voltage (I-V) relationship (Prakriya & Lewis, 2006). Additionally, the CRAC channels lacked voltage dependent activation and were insensitive to common voltage-dependent Ca^{2+} channel inhibitors. However, these channels were sensitive to inhibition by lanthanides, 2-aminoethoxydiphenyl borate (2-APB) and SKF96365 (Aussel, Marhaba, Pelassy, & Breittmayer, 1996; Goto et al., 2010; Kozak, Kerschbaum, & Cahalan, 2002). These properties taken together made CRAC channels the prototypical SOC and the primary target to decipher the molecular identity of SOCE channels.

The discovery of STIM1 protein led to the hunt for the CRAC channel gene using various screening techniques. The investigations originated from the understanding that defective CRAC channel function was the underlying cause of severe combined immunodeficiency (SCID)(Feske, Giltnane, Dolmetsch, Staudt, & Rao, 2001; Partiseti et al., 1994). The mutation was localized to a region of chromosome 12 covering ~74 genes. Genome-wide RNAi screen in S2 cells led to the identification of the homolog in the region of human chromosome 2. This region expressed a surface protein with four transmembrane domains; the protein was named Orai1 (Feske et al., 2006). These investigations along with independent siRNA screen led to the identification of three Orai homologs in the human genome named Orai1, 2 and 3 (Zhang et al., 2006). Ectopically expressed wild-type Orai1 was able to restore SOCE in T-cells isolated from SCID patients. SCID patients were also found to be homozygous for a single missense mutation in Orai1 that led to dysfunctional SOCE-mediated Ca^{2+} influx in these patients (Feske et al., 2006). While STIM1 was established as the Ca^{2+} sensor for SOCE, functional links with endogenous CRAC channels led to the acceptance of Orai1 as the component of CRAC channel pore (Prakriya & Lewis, 2015).

The Orai family of protein is made up of three isoforms; the founding member Orai1, and two highly conserved homologs Orai2 and Orai3. The molecular mechanism regulating Orai1 activity and its functional role has been studied and characterized in great detail. The physiological role of Orai2 and Orai3 are less defined in comparison to Orai1. Orai1 channels are made up of four transmembrane domains and conduct Ca^{2+} ions with selectivity 1000 times more than that of Na^+ (Fahrner et al., 2013; Hoth & Penner, 1992). The permeability of monovalent cations are inhibited in the presence of Ca^{2+}. Under resting conditions, Orai channels can exist as homodimer or homotetramer, while during activation of SOCE they form hexamers (Hou, Pedi, Diver, & Long, 2012). The activation of Orai is dependent on rate of Ca^{2+} depletion and translocation of STIM and Orai to the ER/SR junctions (Figure 3). Orai1 channels displayed both fast and slow Ca^{2+}-dependent inactivation (Lis et al., 2007). As observed with STIM regulation, phosphorylation is also thought to regulate Orai activity. PKC-mediated phosphorylation of Orai1 inhibits SOCE mediated Ca^{2+} influx. The inhibition is thought to occur in a Ca^{2+}-dependent manner (Kawasaki, Ueyama, Lange, Feske, & Saito, 2010). PKC phosphorylation was also found to regulate SOCE-mediated Ca^{2+} influx in primary human myotubes suffering from Duchenne muscular dystrophy (Harisseh, Chatelier, Magaud, Deliot, & Constantin, 2013). Studies have shown that both Orai2 and Orai3 are activated by store depletion and that these channels are more selective for Ca^{2+} over Na^{+}. As observed with endogenous CRAC channel current, both Orai 2 and 3 displayed inwardly rectifying current-voltage relationship (DeHaven, Smyth, Boyles, & Putney, 2007; Potier & Trebak, 2008). Orai 2 and Orai 3 show fast inactivation; Orai 3 displayed much faster inactivation in comparison to Orai2 (Lis et al., 2007). Pharmacological inhibitor of 2-APB was shown to inhibit Orai2, but was insensitive to Orai3 mediated Ca2+ entry. This suggests that in the presence of STIM1, Orai3 may function in a store-depletion-independent manner (Zhang et al., 2008).

Transient Receptor Potential (TRP) Channels

Before the identification of Orai as SOC channels, transient receptor potential channels (TRP) were considered as a potential SOC candidate. The *trp* gene family is divided into six subfamilies consisting of canonical TRP (TRPC), vanilloid TRP (TRPV), melastatin TRP (TRPM), ankyrin TRP (TRPA), polycystic TRP (TRPP) and mucolipin TRP (TRPML) groups. Most TRP channels are Ca^{2+} permeable nonselective cation channels that are activated by various non-voltage-dependent stimuli. TRP channels can sense thermal, mechanical, chemical and intracellular stimuli. Among the TRP family, the TRPCs were thought to be the putative SOCE channels. One of the earliest studies on TRPC1 showed that the channel exhibits store-dependent activation and, hence was identified as the putative SOC channel (Zitt et al., 1996). Subsequently other TRPCs, such as TRPC3, TRPC4 and TRPC7 were also identified as possible candidates for SOC channels (Cheng, Ong, Liu, & Ambudkar, 2013; Zagranichnaya, Wu, & Villereal, 2005). Soon, TRPC expression was also documented in the cardiovascular system. For instance, the presence of TRPC isoforms, TRPC1 and TRPC3-7, was shown in the whole heart (Watanabe, Murakami, Ohba, Takahashi, & Ito, 2008). Although, TRPC5 was not expressed in the SA nodal cells, all other members of the TRPC family were detected (Ju et al., 2007). However, TRPC5 has been shown to have an increased expression levels in heart failure patients (Bush et al., 2006). TRPC6 mediated Ca^{2+} entry has been recorded in cardiomyocytes and, the vascular system such as rodent aorta (Watanabe et al., 2008). A complex picture of TRPC channel characteristics as SOC is emerging and whether TRPCs are potential SOC channels is debatable. A complete discussion on TRP channels and their biophysical characteristics is beyond the scope of this chapter. However, this chapter will focus the discussion on expression patterns of TRPCs in the cardiovascular system and, their role in the development of cardiac hypertrophy (discussed in the next section).

ROLE OF SOCE IN THE HEART

Regulation of cardiac function is dependent on carefully orchestrated spatio-temporal modulation of cytosolic Ca^{2+}. In cardiomyocytes, membrane depolarization mediates opening of voltage-gated Ca^{2+} channels, leading to excitation-contraction coupling (EC) coupling. The voltage-gated Ca^{2+} channels engage with the SR localized RyR2 receptors to induce Ca^{2+} induced Ca^{2+}-release. The product of this interaction mobilizes Ca^{2+} from the SR into the cytosol, leading to activation of actin-myosin cross-bridge cycling (Bers, 2002). Given that the voltage-gated Ca^{2+} entry is the predominant Ca^{2+} influx pathway in cardiomyocytes, one might question what functional role the SOCE-mediated Ca^{2+} influx can play in cardiac function.

Recent studies however, have demonstrated the presence of the SOCE machinery in cardiomyocytes, and highlighted their contribution in maintaining normal cardiac function. Studies conducted in neonatal and embryonic cardiomyocytes, have shown that ER/SR Ca^{2+} store-depletion yielded a sustained Ca^{2+} influx that was sensitive to inhibition by SOCE inhibitors, such as Lanthanium (La^{3+}) and Zinc, but not by the voltage-gated channel inhibitors, Nifedipine and Verapamil (Hunton, Zou, Pang, & Marchase, 2004; Uehara, Yasukochi, Imanaga, Nishi, & Takeshima, 2002). Interestingly, SOCE activity in the embryonic and neonatal cardiomyocytes was more prominent than in comparison to the adult cardiomyocytes. This indicated that SOCE activity was developmentally regulated in the heart (Pan, Brotto, & Ma, 2014). The presence of Orai and STIM1 has been demonstrated in immortalized mouse atrial cardiomyocyte cell line, HL-1. Additionally, Orai1 knockdown in HL-1 cells attenuated SOCE-mediated Ca^{2+} entry, and lowered baseline Ca^{2+} levels (Touchberry et al., 2011). Voelkers et al. showed that neonatal rat ventricular cardiomyocytes not only express STIM1 and Orai1, but that these proteins play an important role in regulating store Ca^{2+} levels and cardiomyocyte growth (Voelkers et al., 2010). Cardiac contractions are initiated by spontaneous firing of pacemaker cells in the sinoatrial node (SAN) of the heart. Cardiac pacemaker tissue has also been shown to express Orai1, STIM1 and STIM2. In isolated single mouse sinoatrial node cells, Orai1 was predominantly shown to be distributed in the sarcolemma, whereas STIM1 had a more diffused expression (Liu et al., 2015). In addition to SAN and neonatal cardiomyocytes, the presence of Orai and STIM expression was also demonstrated in rat ventricular myocardium. In the same study, Orai1 and Orai3 were shown to initiate of arrhythmias in atrial and ventricular myocytes, linking SOCE proteins to aberrant electrophysiological activity leading to arrhythmias. (Wolkowicz et al., 2011). The Cardiac c-kit^{+} progenitor cells also express STIM1, Orai and TRPC1 proteins. Downregulation of TRPC1, STIM1 and Orai1 were shown to decrease proliferation and migration of human cardiac c-kit$^+$ cells. A knockdown of SOCE proteins resulted in decreased expression of factors regulating cell cycle and migration such as cyclin D1, cyclin E and *p*-Akt, thus demonstrating the role of SOCE in myocardial repair and regeneration (Che et al., 2015). These studies provide strong evidence that STIM, Orai and TRPCs contribute in regulating Ca^{2+} homeostasis in the heart in normal physiology and in the setting of several cardiovascular diseases.

SOCE and Cardiac Hypertrophy

Congestive heart failure is a condition characterized by the heart's inability to maintain sufficient blood supply to the body's tissue. This decrease in perfusion results in an increase in ventricular wall thickness. Cardiac hypertrophy is characterized by cardiomyocyte enlargement, reorganization of sarcomere assembly and, activation of hypertrophic genes. Hypertrophic growth occurs as an adaptive growth response to various triggers such as hypertension, myocardial infarction, and valvular defects (Ruhle & Trebak, 2013). Dysfunctional Ca^{2+} homeostasis has been known to be one of the major factors contributing to the development of cardiac hypertrophy. A sustained increase in $[Ca^{2+}]_i$ causes activation of the calcineurin/Nuclear factor of activated T cells (NFAT) pathway; one of signaling pathways implicated in the progression of hypertrophy. Ca^{2+}calmodulin-activated serine/threonine phosphatase, calcineurin dephosphorylates the NFAT; resulting in nuclear translocation of NFAT. The interaction of NFAT with other transcription promoters such as, GATA and AP-1 results in the activation of prohypertrophic gene expression (Figure 4) (Zarain-Herzberg, Fragoso-Medina, & Estrada-Aviles, 2011).

TRPC channels, long thought to be the SOCE channel, have been shown to play an essential role in the development of cardiac hypertrophy. When activated by G_q-linked receptors (such as AngII or endothelin-1 receptors) or catacholaminergic receptors, TRPC mediated Ca^{2+} entry activates calcineurin, resulting in the activation and nuclear translocation of NFAT; thus inducing hypertropic gene expression. Using mouse or rat-based pressure-overload models and molecular techniques, several labs have demonstrated the role of TRP in cardiac hypertrophy. For instance, activation by agonists such as angiotensin II (AngII), phenylephrine, and endothelin-1 led to the upregulation of TRPC1, TRPC3, and TRPC7 expression (Brenner & Dolmetsch, 2007; Ohba et al., 2007). TRP3 and TRP6 were shown to be essential for the development of AngII-induced hypertrophy (Onohara et al., 2006). TRPC3-overexpressing mice models showed increased calcineurin/NFAT activation and AngII-induced hypertrophy (Nakayama, Wilkin, Bodi, & Molkentin, 2006). In addition, phosphorylation of TRPC3 and TRPC6 by protein kinase G (PKG) resulted in inhibition of channel activity, negatively regulated calcineurin/NFAT activation and, led to antihypertrophic effects of natriuretic peptides-Guanylyl Cyclase-A (GC-A). The overexpression of TRPC6 in GC-A knockdown mice increases cardiac hypertrophy, while the inhibition of TRPC6 activity by PKG phosphorylation was also shown to contribute towards the antihypertrophic effects of natriuretic peptide GC-A signaling pathway (Kinoshita et al., 2010; Yue, Zhang, Xie, Jiang, & Yue, 2013). Interestingly, the calcineurin/NFAT pathway causes upregulation of TRPC1, TRPC3 and TRPC6; thus this positive feedback mechanism contributes to the development of long-term hypertrophy and cardiac remodeling (Kuwahara et al., 2006; Ohba et al., 2007).

The discovery of STIM and Orai as mediators of SOCE prompted investigations into their role in SOCE-induced cardiac hypertrophy. In neonatal rat cardiomyocytes, activation of SOCE by agonist such as AngII and endothelin-1 enhanced SOCE, NFAT nuclear translocation and the development of hypertrophy (Hunton et al., 2002; Ohba et al., 2009). The SOCE mediated Ca^{2+} entry and NFAT translocation were inhibited by non-selective inhibitor of SOCE, SKF96365. However, MEK1-induced hypertrophy was demonstrated to be independent of NFAT localization and, was unaffected by SKF96365 (Hunton et al., 2002). The knockdown of STIM1 inhibited the upregulation of TRPC1 and the development of hypertrophic response induced by AngII, phenylephrine and endothelin-1(Ohba et al., 2009). STIM1 knockdown was shown to decrease diastolic Ca^{2+} levels and caffeine-induced Ca^{2+} release from the SR in rat neonatal cardiomyocytes. Interestingly, Orai1 knockdown not only attenuated SOCE mediated Ca^{2+} entry, but also decreased the cardiomyocyte cell size, atrial natriuretic peptide (ANP) and brain-type natriuretic peptide (BNP) anp and bnp levels and significantly decreased calcineurin-NFAT signaling activity Phenylephrine mediated hypertrophic growth was inhibited by STIM1 and Orai1 knockdown. While expression of Orai2 and STIM2 was not detectable in rat neonatal cardiomyocytes, knock down of Orai1 and STIM1 resulted in an increase in Orai2 and STIM2 expression (Volkers et al., 2012). STIM1-dependent Ca^{2+} entry was nominal in adult cardiomyocyte, but it significantly increases in adults animals with cardiac hypertrophy. Additionally, STIM1 knockdown diminished hypertrophic growth in elevated in pressure-overload hearts, thus protecting the heart from compensated cardiac hypertrophy (Hulot et al., 2011). Recent evidence has demonstrated that an Orai3-dependent increase in Ca^{2+} influx may also play a role in the development of hypertrophied cardiomyocytes. Expression of Orai1 and Orai3 were detected in normal and hypertrophied cardiomyocytes, however Orai2 was not detectable. More importantly, the knockdown of Orai3 inhibited Ca^{2+} entry and prevented development of abdominal aortic banding induced cardiomyocyte hypertrophy. The increase in Orai3-mediated Ca^{2+} influx was attributed to the interaction between Orai3/Orai1 and STIM1 in the hypertrophied cardiomyocytes (Saliba et al., 2015).

These studies provide strong evidence that the players involved in SOCE-mediated Ca^{2+} influx play a key role in the development of cardiac hypertrophy. Although these studies have highlighted the role of STIM, Orai and TRPC in cardiac hypertrophy, there are gaps are in our current understanding of the mechanisms underlying the development of hypertrophy. Therefore, additional studies are clearly necessary to decipher the role of these proteins in a hypertrophic response.

Cardiac Reperfusion Injury

The characteristic features of myocardial ischemic/reperfusion (I-R) injury include oxidative stress and an increase in $[Ca^{2+}]_i$ leading to lethal Ca^{2+} overload. A decrease in mitochondrial ATP production accompanied by decrease in pH causes activation of Na^+/H^+ exchanger and reversal of Na^+-Ca^{2+} exchanger (NCX) function, subsequently leading to increase in Ca^{2+} overload. The rise in $[Ca^{2+}]_i$ is attributed to NCX reversal, but L-type Ca^{2+} channels and T-type Ca^{2+} channels are also thought to contribute to Ca^{2+} overload associated by IR (Mozaffari, Liu, Abebe, & Baban, 2013). Recently, evidence has beginning to emerge hinting at the possible role of SOCE in IR-associated Ca^{2+} overload. The Orai-STIM complex was shown to operate by a pH-dependent mechanism, wherein hypoxia resulted in STIM1 junctional accumulation. This suggested that hypoxia, in disease states like IR, could trigger activation of SOCE-mediated Ca^{2+} influx. The study also revealed that acidification led to uncoupling of the Orai-STIM1 complex, thereby providing a mechanism to protect the cells from a Ca^{2+} overload under hypoxic conditions (Mancarella et al., 2011). Several studies have shown that pharmacological inhibitors of SOCE protect the heart against I/R Ca^{2+} overload, indicating a potential role of SOCE. Ca^{2+} overload induced in cardiac microvascular endothelial cells was attenuated by pharmacological inhibitors of SOCE such as 2-APB and gadolinium (Gd^{3+}) (Peters & Piper, 2007). The volatile anesthetic sevoflurane, shown to protect the heart from myocardial injury, inhibited SOCE-mediated Ca^{2+} influx and Ca^{2+} overload in mouse ventricular myocytes (Kojima, Kitagawa, Omatsu-Kanbe, Matsuura, & Nosaka, 2012). Glucosamine has been known to protect the heart against Ca^{2+} overload and I-R injury. The application of glucosamine resulted in inhibiting the SOCE response in neonatal cardiomyocytes (Nagy, Champattanachai, Marchase, & Chatham, 2006; Zhu-Mauldin et al., 2012). Overexpression of TRPC3 in transgenic mouse model increased calpain activation and apoptosis; both of which were attenuated by treatment with SOCE inhibitor, SKF96363 (Shan, Marchase, & Chatham, 2008). These studies have suggested the possible involvement of SOCE-mediated Ca^{2+} influx in I-R injury, however direct evidence linking the two processes is missing.

CONCLUSION

In recent years, research aimed at deciphering the molecular mechanisms governing SOCE-mediated Ca^{2+} influx has helped us understand the physiological functions of SOCE. Communication between depleted ER stores and PM channels is necessary for proper Ca^{2+} influx and further intracellular Ca^{2+} homeostasis. Studies have shown that direct coupling between ER sensor STIM and, SOC channel Orai is necessary for such communication. Although the SOCE pathway was thought to exist in non-excitable cells, recent evidence has demonstrated the presence of various STIM/Orai in cardiomyocytes. More importantly these studies have revealed that STIM1 plays a prominent role in regulating SOCE. Indeed modulation of STIM1 and STIM2 function consequently lead to the development of pathological conditions effecting cardiovascular function. This is especially true in the context of cardiac hypertrophy. STIM1 function in particular, has been linked to the activation of downstream calcineurin-NFAT pathway, driving transcriptional factors that consequently induce hypertrophic signaling (Figure 4). The presence of SOC channels Orai and TRPCs has also been demonstrated in cardiomyocytes however, their role in pathogenesis of diseases is not fully understood. Given the diversity of TRPC channel genes, more cell-specific or tissue-specific information is required to elucidate their role in disease progression. While deficit in Orai function does not result in cardiac phenotype, patients with mutations in Orai develop myopathies such as Duchenne disease, which can later cause cardiomyopathy. Several studies have concluded that Orai channels play a role in the development of cardiac hypertrophy. Additionally, use of SOCE channel inhibitors have been shown to ameliorate I-R injury. Although there is an interest in exploring Orai channels as therapeutic targets to treat diseases such as cardiac hypertrophy and ischemia, the lack of specific channel blockers has been an impediment. The ubiquitous expression and prominent role of SOCE proteins in the immune function necessitates the development of cell-specific delivery systems for the treatment of cardiovascular diseases. Understanding the STIM/Orai structural organization as well as factors regulating SOC function will hopefully aid in the development of novel therapeutic strategies for the treatment of cardiovascular diseases.

ACKNOWLEDGMENT

The author wishes to thank Dr. Clinton Mathias, Assistant Professor at WNEU, College of Pharmacy for his valuable input in reviewing the chapter. The author also acknowledges the contribution of Matthew Murphy, Pharm D student and Dr. Abhishek Deshpande, Assistant Professor of Medicine at Cleveland Clinic Lerner College of Medicine at Case Western Reserve University for assisting in the preparation of this chapter.

REFERENCES

Aussel, C., Marhaba, R., Pelassy, C., & Breittmayer, J. P. (1996). Submicromolar La3+ concentrations block the calcium release-activated channel, and impair CD69 and CD25 expression in CD3- or thapsigargin-activated Jurkat cells. *The Biochemical Journal*, *313*(Pt 3), 909–913. doi:10.1042/bj3130909 PMID:8611174

Berridge, M. J. (1993). Inositol trisphosphate and calcium signalling. *Nature*, *361*(6410), 315–325. doi:10.1038/361315a0 PMID:8381210

Berridge, M. J., Bootman, M. D., & Roderick, H. L. (2003). Calcium signalling: Dynamics, homeostasis and remodelling. *Nature Reviews. Molecular Cell Biology*, *4*(7), 517–529. doi:10.1038/nrm1155 PMID:12838335

Bers, D. M. (2002). Cardiac excitation-contraction coupling. *Nature*, *415*(6868), 198–205. doi:10.1038/415198a PMID:11805843

Bers, D. M. (2008). Calcium cycling and signaling in cardiac myocytes. *Annual Review of Physiology*, *70*(1), 23–49. doi:10.1146/annurev.physiol.70.113006.100455 PMID:17988210

Brandman, O., Liou, J., Park, W. S., & Meyer, T. (2007). STIM2 is a feedback regulator that stabilizes basal cytosolic and endoplasmic reticulum Ca2+ levels. *Cell*, *131*(7), 1327–1339. doi:10.1016/j.cell.2007.11.039 PMID:18160041

Brenner, J. S., & Dolmetsch, R. E. (2007). TrpC3 regulates hypertrophy-associated gene expression without affecting myocyte beating or cell size. *PLoS ONE*, *2*(8), e802. doi:10.1371/journal.pone.0000802 PMID:17726532

Bush, E. W., Hood, D. B., Papst, P. J., Chapo, J. A., Minobe, W., Bristow, M. R., & McKinsey, T. A. et al. (2006). Canonical transient receptor potential channels promote cardiomyocyte hypertrophy through activation of calcineurin signaling. *The Journal of Biological Chemistry*, *281*(44), 33487–33496. doi:10.1074/jbc.M605536200 PMID:16950785

Che, H., Li, G., Sun, H. Y., Xiao, G. S., Wang, Y., & Li, G. R. (2015). Roles of store-operated Ca2+ channels in regulating cell cycling and migration of human cardiac c-kit+ progenitor cells. *American Journal of Physiology. Heart and Circulatory Physiology*, *309*(10), H1772–H1781. PMID:26453325

Cheng, K. T., Ong, H. L., Liu, X., & Ambudkar, I. S. (2013). Contribution and regulation of TRPC channels in store-operated Ca2+ entry. *Curr Top Membr*, *71*, 149–179. doi:10.1016/B978-0-12-407870-3.00007-X PMID:23890115

Collins, H. E., Zhu-Mauldin, X., Marchase, R. B., & Chatham, J. C. (2013). STIM1/Orai1-mediated SOCE: Current perspectives and potential roles in cardiac function and pathology. *American Journal of Physiology. Heart and Circulatory Physiology*, *305*(4), H446–H458. doi:10.1152/ajpheart.00104.2013 PMID:23792674

Covington, E. D., Wu, M. M., & Lewis, R. S. (2010). Essential role for the CRAC activation domain in store-dependent oligomerization of STIM1. *Molecular Biology of the Cell*, *21*(11), 1897–1907. doi:10.1091/mbc.E10-02-0145 PMID:20375143

DeHaven, W. I., Smyth, J. T., Boyles, R. R., & Putney, J. W. Jr. (2007). Calcium inhibition and calcium potentiation of Orai1, Orai2, and Orai3 calcium release-activated calcium channels. *The Journal of Biological Chemistry*, *282*(24), 17548–17556. doi:10.1074/jbc.M611374200 PMID:17452328

Fahrner, M., Derler, I., Jardin, I., & Romanin, C. (2013). The STIM1/Orai signaling machinery. *Channels (Austin, Tex.)*, *7*(5), 330–343. doi:10.4161/chan.26742 PMID:24107921

Fernandez, R. A., Wan, J., Song, S., Smith, K. A., Gu, Y., Tauseef, M., & Yuan, J. X.-J. et al. (2015). Upregulated expression of STIM2, TRPC6, and Orai2 contributes to the transition of pulmonary arterial smooth muscle cells from a contractile to proliferative phenotype. *American Journal of Physiology. Cell Physiology*, *308*(8), C581–C593. doi:10.1152/ajpcell.00202.2014 PMID:25673771

Feske, S., Giltnane, J., Dolmetsch, R., Staudt, L. M., & Rao, A. (2001). Gene regulation mediated by calcium signals in T lymphocytes. *Nature Immunology*, *2*(4), 316–324. doi:10.1038/86318 PMID:11276202

Feske, S., Gwack, Y., Prakriya, M., Srikanth, S., Puppel, S. H., Tanasa, B., & Rao, A. et al. (2006). A mutation in Orai1 causes immune deficiency by abrogating CRAC channel function. *Nature*, *441*(7090), 179–185. doi:10.1038/nature04702 PMID:16582901

Goto, J., Suzuki, A. Z., Ozaki, S., Matsumoto, N., Nakamura, T., Ebisui, E., & Mikoshiba, K. et al. (2010). Two novel 2-aminoethyl diphenylborinate (2-APB) analogues differentially activate and inhibit store-operated Ca(2+) entry via STIM proteins. *Cell Calcium*, *47*(1), 1–10. doi:10.1016/j.ceca.2009.10.004 PMID:19945161

Harisseh, R., Chatelier, A., Magaud, C., Deliot, N., & Constantin, B. (2013). Involvement of TRPV2 and SOCE in calcium influx disorder in DMD primary human myotubes with a specific contribution of alpha1-syntrophin and PLC/PKC in SOCE regulation. *American Journal of Physiology. Cell Physiology*, *304*(9), C881–C894. doi:10.1152/ajpcell.00182.2012 PMID:23426965

Hartmann, J., Karl, R. M., Alexander, R. P., Adelsberger, H., Brill, M. S., Ruhlmann, C., & Konnerth, A. et al. (2014). STIM1 controls neuronal Ca(2)(+) signaling, mGluR1-dependent synaptic transmission, and cerebellar motor behavior. *Neuron*, *82*(3), 635–644. doi:10.1016/j.neuron.2014.03.027 PMID:24811382

Hawkins, B. J., Irrinki, K. M., Mallilankaraman, K., Lien, Y. C., Wang, Y., Bhanumathy, C. D., & Madesh, M. et al. (2010). S-glutathionylation activates STIM1 and alters mitochondrial homeostasis. *The Journal of Cell Biology*, *190*(3), 391–405. doi:10.1083/jcb.201004152 PMID:20679432

Hoth, M. (1995). Calcium and barium permeation through calcium release-activated calcium (CRAC) channels. *Pflugers Archiv*, *430*(3), 315–322. doi:10.1007/BF00373905 PMID:7491254

Hoth, M., & Penner, R. (1992). Depletion of intracellular calcium stores activates a calcium current in mast cells. *Nature*, *355*(6358), 353–356. doi:10.1038/355353a0 PMID:1309940

Hou, X., Pedi, L., Diver, M. M., & Long, S. B. (2012). Crystal structure of the calcium release-activated calcium channel Orai. *Science*, *338*(6112), 1308–1313. doi:10.1126/science.1228757 PMID:23180775

Hulot, J. S., Fauconnier, J., Ramanujam, D., Chaanine, A., Aubart, F., Sassi, Y., & Engelhardt, S. et al. (2011). Critical role for stromal interaction molecule 1 in cardiac hypertrophy. *Circulation*, *124*(7), 796–805. doi:10.1161/CIRCULATIONAHA.111.031229 PMID:21810664

Hunton, D. L., Lucchesi, P. A., Pang, Y., Cheng, X., Dellltalia, L. J., & Marchase, R. B. (2002). Capacitative calcium entry contributes to nuclear factor of activated T-cells nuclear translocation and hypertrophy in cardiomyocytes. *The Journal of Biological Chemistry*, *277*(16), 14266–14273. doi:10.1074/jbc.M107167200 PMID:11827959

Hunton, D. L., Zou, L., Pang, Y., & Marchase, R. B. (2004). Adult rat cardiomyocytes exhibit capacitative calcium entry. *American Journal of Physiology. Heart and Circulatory Physiology*, *286*(3), H1124–H1132. doi:10.1152/ajpheart.00162.2003 PMID:14630640

Ju, Y. K., Chu, Y., Chaulet, H., Lai, D., Gervasio, O. L., Graham, R. M., & Allen, D. G. et al. (2007). Store-operated Ca2+ influx and expression of TRPC genes in mouse sinoatrial node. *Circulation Research*, *100*(11), 1605–1614. doi:10.1161/CIRCRESAHA.107.152181 PMID:17478725

Karlstad, J., Sun, Y., & Singh, B. B. (2012). Ca(2+) signaling: An outlook on the characterization of Ca(2+) channels and their importance in cellular functions. *Advances in Experimental Medicine and Biology*, *740*, 143–157. doi:10.1007/978-94-007-2888-2_6 PMID:22453941

Kawasaki, T., Ueyama, T., Lange, I., Feske, S., & Saito, N. (2010). Protein kinase C-induced phosphorylation of Orai1 regulates the intracellular Ca2+ level via the store-operated Ca2+ channel. *The Journal of Biological Chemistry*, *285*(33), 25720–25730. doi:10.1074/jbc.M109.022996 PMID:20534587

Kinoshita, H., Kuwahara, K., Nishida, M., Jian, Z., Rong, X., Kiyonaka, S., & Nakao, K. et al. (2010). Inhibition of TRPC6 channel activity contributes to the antihypertrophic effects of natriuretic peptides-guanylyl cyclase-A signaling in the heart. *Circulation Research*, *106*(12), 1849–1860. doi:10.1161/CIRCRESAHA.109.208314 PMID:20448219

Kojima, A., Kitagawa, H., Omatsu-Kanbe, M., Matsuura, H., & Nosaka, S. (2012). Presence of store-operated Ca2+ entry in C57BL/6J mouse ventricular myocytes and its suppression by sevoflurane. *British Journal of Anaesthesia*, *109*(3), 352–360. doi:10.1093/bja/aes212 PMID:22777657

Kozak, J. A., Kerschbaum, H. H., & Cahalan, M. D. (2002). Distinct properties of CRAC and MIC channels in RBL cells. *The Journal of General Physiology*, *120*(2), 221–235. doi:10.1085/jgp.20028601 PMID:12149283

Kuwahara, K., Wang, Y., McAnally, J., Richardson, J. A., Bassel-Duby, R., Hill, J. A., & Olson, E. N. (2006). TRPC6 fulfills a calcineurin signaling circuit during pathologic cardiac remodeling. *The Journal of Clinical Investigation*, *116*(12), 3114–3126. doi:10.1172/JCI27702 PMID:17099778

Liou, J., Kim, M. L., Heo, W. D., Jones, J. T., Myers, J. W., & Ferrell, J. E. Jr et al.. (2005). STIM is a Ca2+ sensor essential for Ca2+-store-depletion-triggered Ca2+ influx. *Current Biology*, *15*(13), 1235–1241. doi:10.1016/j.cub.2005.05.055 PMID:16005298

Lis, A., Peinelt, C., Beck, A., Parvez, S., Monteilh-Zoller, M., Fleig, A., & Penner, R. (2007). CRACM1, CRACM2, and CRACM3 are store-operated Ca2+ channels with distinct functional properties. *Current Biology*, *17*(9), 794–800. doi:10.1016/j.cub.2007.03.065 PMID:17442569

Liu, J., Xin, L., Benson, V. L., Allen, D. G., & Ju, Y. K. (2015). Store-operated calcium entry and the localization of STIM1 and Orai1 proteins in isolated mouse sinoatrial node cells. *Frontiers in Physics*, *6*, 69. PMID:25806000

Majewski, L., & Kuznicki, J. (2015). SOCE in neurons: Signaling or just refilling? *Biochimica et Biophysica Acta*, *1853*(9), 1940–1952. doi:10.1016/j.bbamcr.2015.01.019 PMID:25646572

Mancarella, S., Wang, Y., Deng, X., Landesberg, G., Scalia, R., Panettieri, R. A., & Gill, D. L. et al. (2011). Hypoxia-induced acidosis uncouples the STIM-Orai calcium signaling complex. *The Journal of Biological Chemistry*, *286*(52), 44788–44798. doi:10.1074/jbc.M111.303081 PMID:22084246

Mozaffari, M. S., Liu, J. Y., Abebe, W., & Baban, B. (2013). Mechanisms of load dependency of myocardial ischemia reperfusion injury. *Am J Cardiovasc Dis*, *3*(4), 180–196. PMID:24224132

Nagy, T., Champattanachai, V., Marchase, R. B., & Chatham, J. C. (2006). Glucosamine inhibits angiotensin II-induced cytoplasmic Ca2+ elevation in neonatal cardiomyocytes via protein-associated O-linked N-acetylglucosamine. *American Journal of Physiology. Cell Physiology*, *290*(1), C57–C65. doi:10.1152/ajpcell.00263.2005 PMID:16107505

Nakayama, H., Wilkin, B. J., Bodi, I., & Molkentin, J. D. (2006). Calcineurin-dependent cardiomyopathy is activated by TRPC in the adult mouse heart. *The FASEB Journal*, *20*(10), 1660–1670. doi:10.1096/fj.05-5560com PMID:16873889

Oh-hora, M., & Rao, A. (2008). Calcium signaling in lymphocytes. *Current Opinion in Immunology*, *20*(3), 250–258. doi:10.1016/j.coi.2008.04.004 PMID:18515054

Ohba, T., Watanabe, H., Murakami, M., Sato, T., Ono, K., & Ito, H. (2009). Essential role of STIM1 in the development of cardiomyocyte hypertrophy. *Biochemical and Biophysical Research Communications*, *389*(1), 172–176. doi:10.1016/j.bbrc.2009.08.117 PMID:19715666

Ohba, T., Watanabe, H., Murakami, M., Takahashi, Y., Iino, K., Kuromitsu, S., & Ito, H. et al. (2007). Upregulation of TRPC1 in the development of cardiac hypertrophy. *Journal of Molecular and Cellular Cardiology*, *42*(3), 498–507. doi:10.1016/j.yjmcc.2006.10.020 PMID:17174323

Onohara, N., Nishida, M., Inoue, R., Kobayashi, H., Sumimoto, H., Sato, Y., & Kurose, H. et al. (2006). TRPC3 and TRPC6 are essential for angiotensin II-induced cardiac hypertrophy. *The EMBO Journal*, *25*(22), 5305–5316. doi:10.1038/sj.emboj.7601417 PMID:17082763

Oritani, K., & Kincade, P. W. (1996). Identification of stromal cell products that interact with pre-B cells. *The Journal of Cell Biology*, *134*(3), 771–782. doi:10.1083/jcb.134.3.771 PMID:8707854

Palty, R., Raveh, A., Kaminsky, I., Meller, R., & Reuveny, E. (2012). SARAF inactivates the store operated calcium entry machinery to prevent excess calcium refilling. *Cell*, *149*(2), 425–438. doi:10.1016/j.cell.2012.01.055 PMID:22464749

Pan, Z., Brotto, M., & Ma, J. (2014). Store-operated Ca2+ entry in muscle physiology and diseases. *BMB Rep*, *47*(2), 69–79. doi:10.5483/BMBRep.2014.47.2.015 PMID:24411466

Park, C. Y., Hoover, P. J., Mullins, F. M., Bachhawat, P., Covington, E. D., Raunser, S., & Lewis, R. S. et al. (2009). STIM1 clusters and activates CRAC channels via direct binding of a cytosolic domain to Orai1. *Cell*, *136*(5), 876–890. doi:10.1016/j.cell.2009.02.014 PMID:19249086

Partiseti, M., Le Deist, F., Hivroz, C., Fischer, A., Korn, H., & Choquet, D. (1994). The calcium current activated by T cell receptor and store depletion in human lymphocytes is absent in a primary immunodeficiency. *The Journal of Biological Chemistry*, *269*(51), 32327–32335. PMID:7798233

Peters, S. C., & Piper, H. M. (2007). Reoxygenation-induced Ca2+ rise is mediated via Ca2+ influx and Ca2+ release from the endoplasmic reticulum in cardiac endothelial cells. *Cardiovascular Research*, *73*(1), 164–171. doi:10.1016/j.cardiores.2006.09.015 PMID:17097624

Potier, M., & Trebak, M. (2008). New developments in the signaling mechanisms of the store-operated calcium entry pathway. *Pflugers Archiv*, *457*(2), 405–415. doi:10.1007/s00424-008-0533-2 PMID:18536932

Pozo-Guisado, E., Campbell, D. G., Deak, M., Alvarez-Barrientos, A., Morrice, N. A., Alvarez, I. S., & Martin-Romero, F. J. et al. (2010). Phosphorylation of STIM1 at ERK1/2 target sites modulates store-operated calcium entry. *Journal of Cell Science*, *123*(Pt 18), 3084–3093. doi:10.1242/jcs.067215 PMID:20736304

Prakriya, M., & Lewis, R. S. (2006). Regulation of CRAC channel activity by recruitment of silent channels to a high open-probability gating mode. *The Journal of General Physiology*, *128*(3), 373–386. doi:10.1085/jgp.200609588 PMID:16940559

Prakriya, M., & Lewis, R. S. (2015). Store-Operated Calcium Channels. *Physiological Reviews*, *95*(4), 1383–1436. doi:10.1152/physrev.00020.2014 PMID:26400989

Putney, J. W. Jr. (1986). A model for receptor-regulated calcium entry. *Cell Calcium*, *7*(1), 1–12. doi:10.1016/0143-4160(86)90026-6 PMID:2420465

Putney, J. W. Jr. (1990). Capacitative calcium entry revisited. *Cell Calcium*, *11*(10), 611–624. doi:10.1016/0143-4160(90)90016-N PMID:1965707

Putney, J. W. (2011). The physiological function of store-operated calcium entry. *Neurochemical Research*, *36*(7), 1157–1165. doi:10.1007/s11064-010-0383-0 PMID:21234676

Roos, J., DiGregorio, P. J., Yeromin, A. V., Ohlsen, K., Lioudyno, M., Zhang, S., & Stauderman, K. A. et al. (2005). STIM1, an essential and conserved component of store-operated Ca2+ channel function. *The Journal of Cell Biology*, *169*(3), 435–445. doi:10.1083/jcb.200502019 PMID:15866891

Ruhle, B., & Trebak, M. (2013). Emerging roles for native Orai Ca2+ channels in cardiovascular disease. *Curr Top Membr*, *71*, 209–235. doi:10.1016/B978-0-12-407870-3.00009-3 PMID:23890117

Saliba, Y., Keck, M., Marchand, A., Atassi, F., Ouille, A., Cazorla, O., & Lompre, A.-M. et al. (2015). Emergence of Orai3 activity during cardiac hypertrophy. *Cardiovascular Research*, *105*(3), 248–259. doi:10.1093/cvr/cvu207 PMID:25213556

Shan, D., Marchase, R. B., & Chatham, J. C. (2008). Overexpression of TRPC3 increases apoptosis but not necrosis in response to ischemia-reperfusion in adult mouse cardiomyocytes. *American Journal of Physiology. Cell Physiology*, *294*(3), C833–C841. doi:10.1152/ajpcell.00313.2007 PMID:18184877

Shaw, P. J., & Feske, S. (2012). Physiological and pathophysiological functions of SOCE in the immune system. *Frontiers in Bioscience (Elite Edition)*, *4*(6), 2253–2268. doi:10.2741/e540 PMID:22202035

Shen, W. W., Frieden, M., & Demaurex, N. (2011). Local cytosolic Ca2+ elevations are required for stromal interaction molecule 1 (STIM1) de-oligomerization and termination of store-operated Ca2+ entry. *The Journal of Biological Chemistry*, *286*(42), 36448–36459. doi:10.1074/jbc.M111.269415 PMID:21880734

Shim, A. H., Tirado-Lee, L., & Prakriya, M. (2015). Structural and functional mechanisms of CRAC channel regulation. *Journal of Molecular Biology*, *427*(1), 77–93. doi:10.1016/j.jmb.2014.09.021 PMID:25284754

Smyth, J. T., Petranka, J. G., Boyles, R. R., DeHaven, W. I., Fukushima, M., Johnson, K. L., & Putney, J. W. Jr et al.. (2009). Phosphorylation of STIM1 underlies suppression of store-operated calcium entry during mitosis. *Nature Cell Biology*, *11*(12), 1465–1472. doi:10.1038/ncb1995 PMID:19881501

Song, M. Y., Makino, A., & Yuan, J. X. (2011). STIM2 Contributes to Enhanced Store-operated Ca Entry in Pulmonary Artery Smooth Muscle Cells from Patients with Idiopathic Pulmonary Arterial Hypertension. *Pulm Circ*, *1*(1), 84–94. doi:10.4103/2045-8932.78106 PMID:21709766

Spassova, M. A., Soboloff, J., He, L. P., Xu, W., Dziadek, M. A., & Gill, D. L. (2006). STIM1 has a plasma membrane role in the activation of store-operated Ca(2+) channels. *Proceedings of the National Academy of Sciences of the United States of America*, *103*(11), 4040–4045. doi:10.1073/pnas.0510050103 PMID:16537481

Stathopulos, P. B., Li, G. Y., Plevin, M. J., Ames, J. B., & Ikura, M. (2006). Stored Ca2+ depletion-induced oligomerization of stromal interaction molecule 1 (STIM1) via the EF-SAM region: An initiation mechanism for capacitive Ca2+ entry. *The Journal of Biological Chemistry*, *281*(47), 35855–35862. doi:10.1074/jbc.M608247200 PMID:17020874

Stathopulos, P. B., Zheng, L., & Ikura, M. (2009). Stromal interaction molecule (STIM) 1 and STIM2 calcium sensing regions exhibit distinct unfolding and oligomerization kinetics. *The Journal of Biological Chemistry*, *284*(2), 728–732. doi:10.1074/jbc.C800178200 PMID:19019825

Stiber, J., Hawkins, A., Zhang, Z. S., Wang, S., Burch, J., Graham, V., & Rosenberg, P. et al. (2008). STIM1 signalling controls store-operated calcium entry required for development and contractile function in skeletal muscle. *Nature Cell Biology*, *10*(6), 688–697. doi:10.1038/ncb1731 PMID:18488020

Tojyo, Y., Morita, T., Nezu, A., & Tanimura, A. (2014). Key components of store-operated Ca2+ entry in non-excitable cells. *Journal of Pharmacological Sciences*, *125*(4), 340–346. doi:10.1254/jphs.14R06CP PMID:25030742

Touchberry, C. D., Elmore, C. J., Nguyen, T. M., Andresen, J. J., Zhao, X., Orange, M., & Wacker, M. J. et al. (2011). Store-operated calcium entry is present in HL-1 cardiomyocytes and contributes to resting calcium. *Biochemical and Biophysical Research Communications*, *416*(1-2), 45–50. doi:10.1016/j.bbrc.2011.10.133 PMID:22079292

Uehara, A., Yasukochi, M., Imanaga, I., Nishi, M., & Takeshima, H. (2002). Store-operated Ca2+ entry uncoupled with ryanodine receptor and junctional membrane complex in heart muscle cells. *Cell Calcium*, *31*(2), 89–96. doi:10.1054/ceca.2001.0257 PMID:11969249

Voelkers, M., Salz, M., Herzog, N., Frank, D., Dolatabadi, N., Frey, N., & Most, P. et al. (2010). Orai1 and Stim1 regulate normal and hypertrophic growth in cardiomyocytes. *Journal of Molecular and Cellular Cardiology*, *48*(6), 1329–1334. doi:10.1016/j.yjmcc.2010.01.020 PMID:20138887

Volkers, M., Dolatabadi, N., Gude, N., Most, P., Sussman, M. A., & Hassel, D. (2012). Orai1 deficiency leads to heart failure and skeletal myopathy in zebrafish. *Journal of Cell Science*, *125*(Pt 2), 287–294. doi:10.1242/jcs.090464 PMID:22302996

Watanabe, H., Murakami, M., Ohba, T., Takahashi, Y., & Ito, H. (2008). TRP channel and cardiovascular disease. *Pharmacology & Therapeutics*, *118*(3), 337–351. doi:10.1016/j.pharmthera.2008.03.008 PMID:18508125

Wolkowicz, P. E., Huang, J., Umeda, P. K., Sharifov, O. F., Tabengwa, E., Halloran, B. A., & Grenett, H. E. et al. (2011). Pharmacological evidence for Orai channel activation as a source of cardiac abnormal automaticity. *European Journal of Pharmacology*, *668*(1-2), 208–216. doi:10.1016/j.ejphar.2011.06.025 PMID:21745466

Yuan, J. P., Zeng, W., Dorwart, M. R., Choi, Y. J., Worley, P. F., & Muallem, S. (2009). SOAR and the polybasic STIM1 domains gate and regulate Orai channels. *Nature Cell Biology*, *11*(3), 337–343. doi:10.1038/ncb1842 PMID:19182790

Yue, Z., Xie, J., Yu, A. S., Stock, J., Du, J., & Yue, L. (2015). Role of TRP channels in the cardiovascular system. *American Journal of Physiology. Heart and Circulatory Physiology*, *308*(3), H157–H182. doi:10.1152/ajpheart.00457.2014 PMID:25416190

Yue, Z., Zhang, Y., Xie, J., Jiang, J., & Yue, L. (2013). Transient receptor potential (TRP) channels and cardiac fibrosis. *Current Topics in Medicinal Chemistry*, *13*(3), 270–282. doi:10.2174/1568026611313030005 PMID:23432060

Zagranichnaya, T. K., Wu, X., & Villereal, M. L. (2005). Endogenous TRPC1, TRPC3, and TRPC7 proteins combine to form native store-operated channels in HEK-293 cells. *The Journal of Biological Chemistry*, *280*(33), 29559–29569. doi:10.1074/jbc.M505842200 PMID:15972814

Zarain-Herzberg, A., Fragoso-Medina, J., & Estrada-Aviles, R. (2011). Calcium-regulated transcriptional pathways in the normal and pathologic heart. *IUBMB Life*, *63*(10), 847–855. doi:10.1002/iub.545 PMID:21901815

Zhang, S. L., Kozak, J. A., Jiang, W., Yeromin, A. V., Chen, J., Yu, Y., & Cahalan, M. D. et al. (2008). Store-dependent and -independent modes regulating Ca2+ release-activated Ca2+ channel activity of human Orai1 and Orai3. *The Journal of Biological Chemistry*, *283*(25), 17662–17671. doi:10.1074/jbc.M801536200 PMID:18420579

Zhang, S. L., Yeromin, A. V., Zhang, X. H., Yu, Y., Safrina, O., Penna, A., & Cahalan, M. D. et al. (2006). Genome-wide RNAi screen of Ca(2+) influx identifies genes that regulate Ca(2+) release-activated Ca(2+) channel activity. *Proceedings of the National Academy of Sciences of the United States of America*, *103*(24), 9357–9362. doi:10.1073/pnas.0603161103 PMID:16751269

Zhu-Mauldin, X., Marsh, S. A., Zou, L., Marchase, R. B., & Chatham, J. C. (2012). Modification of STIM1 by O-linked N-acetylglucosamine (O-GlcNAc) attenuates store-operated calcium entry in neonatal cardiomyocytes. *The Journal of Biological Chemistry*, *287*(46), 39094–39106. doi:10.1074/jbc.M112.383778 PMID:22992728

Zitt, C., Zobel, A., Obukhov, A. G., Harteneck, C., Kalkbrenner, F., Luckhoff, A., & Schultz, G. (1996). Cloning and functional expression of a human Ca2+-permeable cation channel activated by calcium store depletion. *Neuron*, *16*(6), 1189–1196. doi:10.1016/S0896-6273(00)80145-2 PMID:8663995

KEY TERMS AND DEFINITIONS

Cardiac Hypertrophy: Cardiac hypertrophy is the thickening of the myocardium in response to various stimuli such as hypertension, myocardial injury and valvular defects. The disease is characterized by cardiomyocyte enlargement, reorganization of sarcomere assembly and activation of hypertrophic genes.

Orai Channels: Orai are calcium selective plasma membrane ion channels activated in response to intracellular store depletion. Depletion of Ca^{2+} stores, triggers colocalization of Orai and ER sensors STIM; leading to STIM-Orai coupling, which mediates Ca^{2+} entry.

Store Operated Calcium Entry: Store operated calcium entry is the process by which Ca^{2+} influx across the plasma membrane occurs in response to intracellular store depletion in the endoplasmic reticulum/sarcoplasmic reticulum.

Stromal Interaction Molecule (STIM): STIM is an ER-localized single transmembrane protein, which acts a sensor for depleted Ca^{2+} stores. Store depletion causes oligomerization and translocation of STIM to colocalize with plasma membrane store operated channels mediating Ca^{2+} influx.

APPENDIX

Figure 1. Comparison of STIM domain structures: STIM1 and 2 include an N-terminus EF-hand, a sterile a motif (SAM), followed by a transmembrane (TM) domain. The C-terminus comprises of a three coiled-coil domains, a STIM-Orai activating region (SOAR) and a lysine-rich domain (K). STIM1 and STIM2 are identical except that the STIM2 has a longer tail consisting of proline/histidine-rich (PM) domain. STIM1 contains a proline/serine rich domain (PS).

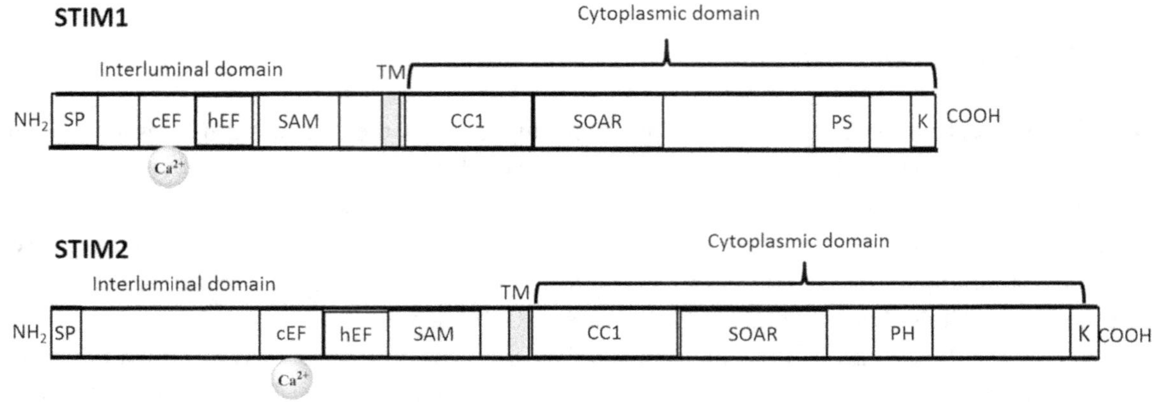

Figure 2. Mechanism of Ca^{2+} influx: Depletion of Endoplasmic reticulum/sarcoplasmic reticulum (ER/SR) Ca^{2+} stores results in dissociation of Ca^{2+} from the EF terminal of STIM, causing the STIM oligomerization, and translocation of STIM to the ER-PM junction. Store depletion also results in the co-localization of Orai at the ER-PM junction. The coupling of STIM to Orai leads to the opening of Orai channels, and elicits localized Ca^{2+} entry.

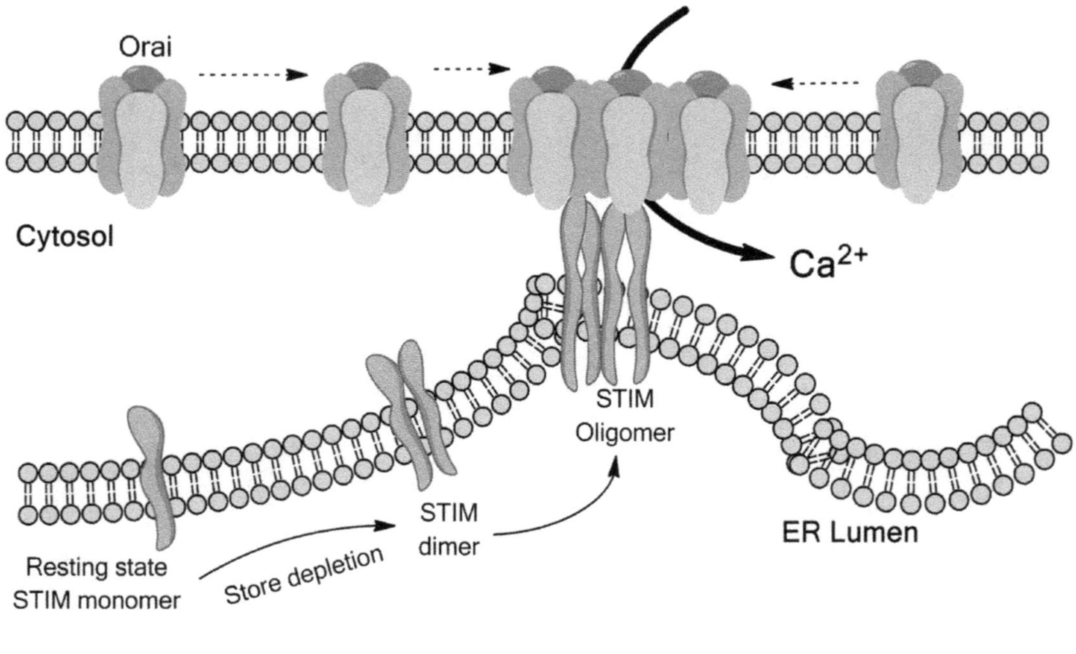

Figure 3. Structural topology of Orai1: Orai channels contain 4 transmembrane domains. The black lines depict the mutations effecting ion selectivity. The dashed black line shows the region of gain of function mutation. The gray region region marked CC depicts the region of STIM binding to the Orai-COOH termini.

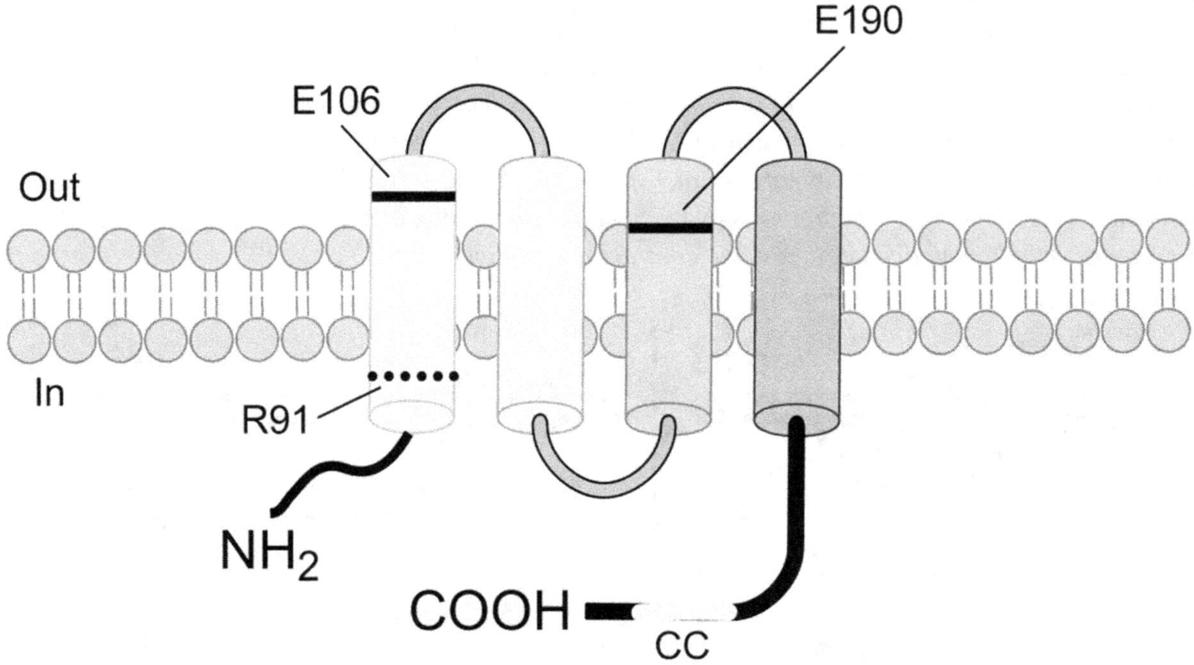

Figure 4. SOCE-dependent activation of cardiac gene expression. Machinery required for SOCE in cardiomyocytes, STIM, Orai and TRPC co-exist in cardiomyocytes. Activation of G_q-coupled receptors by agonists such as angiotensin II, endothelin-1 and phenylephrine activates membrane bound phospholipase C (PLC). PLC hydrolysis phophatidylinositol to inositol 1,4,5-trisphosphate (IP_3). IP_3 diffuses across the cytosol to bind to IP_3 receptors (IP_3R) mobilizing the release of Ca^{2+} into the cytosol. Ca^{2+} subsequently causes more Ca^{2+} release via the Ryanodine receptor (RyR), resulting in ER/SR Ca^{2+} depletion. The depletion of ER/SR stores is sensed by STIM. STIM proteins oligomerizes, and couples to plasma membrane Orai, resulting in pore opening and Ca^{2+} entry. The sustained entry of Ca^{2+} induces downstream pathways such as calcineurin/Nuclear factor of activated T cells (NFAT), triggering the transcriptional pathways resulting in cardiac hypertrophy. The Ca^{2+} increase could cause disruption of mitochondrial membrane potential or activate calpain, culminating in activation of apoptotic pathways leading to myofilament disintegration and contractile dysfunctions.

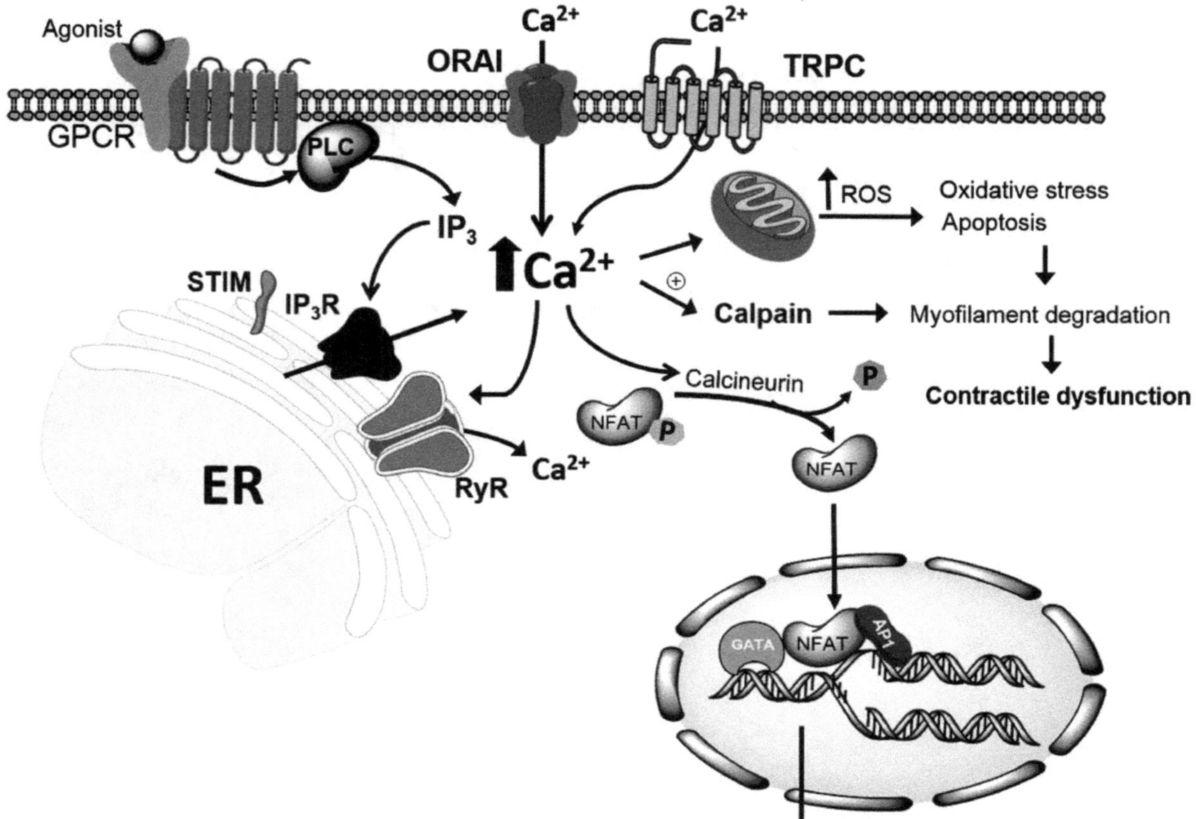

Chapter 5
Examining the Effect of Mitochondrial Fission and Fusion Events on the Heart:
Role of the Mitochondria in Heart Disease

Ashim Malhotra
Pacific University, USA

Shivani Soni
California State University, Fullerton, USA & Chapman University, USA & Alabama State University, USA

ABSTRACT

Mitochondria constitute an integral structural and functional part of the cardiac muscle. The heart muscle relies on the mitochondrial production of fatty acids and ATP as sources of energy during different stages of human growth and development. New mitochondria are created from existing ones by a process called mitochondrial biogenesis which involves both fusion and fission events controlled by a bevy of proteins such as Drp1, OPA1, Mfn1, and Mfn2. In this chapter, we examine the role of these mitochondrial fission and fusion proteins in regulating various heart diseases, particularly, reperfusion injury, dilated cardiomyopathy, and heart failure. It is our intent to examine whether any of these proteins may serve as future candidates for cardiovascular therapy.

INTRODUCTION

Introduction to Heart Disease

Heart disease is a major contributor to morbidity and mortality in the developed world, and particularly in the United States. According to the Centers for Disease Control, 1 in 4 people, about 610,000 individuals, die annually due to heart disease. This loss of life is accompanied by a huge economic burden,

DOI: 10.4018/978-1-5225-2092-4.ch005

especially due to hospitalization and loss of productivity for the even greater numbers of surviving individuals who live with heart disease and require lifelong care and services. Thus, understanding the molecular mechanisms of the normal physiology and pathology of the heart will foster the development of newer pharmacological interventions by identifying novel therapeutic targets for this devastating disease. Thus, exploring new ideas and therapeutic approaches to dealing with cardiovascular diseases constitute an urgent need.

Cardiovascular diseases may manifest in a variety of forms. The most common cardiovascular disease is Ischemic Heart Disease (IHD) that is also known by a variety of other names such as Coronary Artery Disease (CAD) or Acute Coronary Syndrome (ACS). This disease develops due to hypoxia of cardiac muscle when the blood flow to the heart is interrupted, most commonly due to atherosclerosis of the coronary blood vessels. IHD leads to the death of the myocardium and may lead to Sudden Cardiac Death of individuals. However, IHD may also induce arrhythmias. Contradictorily, surgical intervention such as angioplasty to remove the blood vessel clot has been shown to suddenly restore the myocardial oxygen supply and may lead to reperfusion injury.

Other examples of heart disease include those that develop as a consequence of structural damage to the heart or as a result of the compensatory adjustments that the heart undergoes to overcome heart failure. Heart failure is the inability of the heart to meet the oxygen demands of the body. To compensate for this deficiency, the heart undergoes structural modification over time such as the dilation of the ventricles, or an increase in the cell size or cell cumber of cardiomyocytes. These structural changes result in cardiomyopathy, which may be due to different causes ranging from alcohol abuse to genetic causes. These are only some examples of heart disease discussed in this chapter.

Need for Mitochondrial Research in Heart Disease

Mitochondria are essential for cell function as they serve as sources of energy by allowing the production of ATP in the Electron Transport Chain; they are important for the production of fatty acids in the β oxidation process; regulate apoptosis; orchestrate phospholipid production, and modulate a variety of biochemical and cellular processes. In fact in the mammalian heart muscle, even the spatial arrangement of mitochondria is integral to the architecture of the muscle, since they are arranged in a "crystal-like" pattern, intertwined with myofilaments. These observations emphasize the central role played by the mitochondria in the development and function of the heart muscle.

Interestingly, mitochondria are not static organelles. In fact, they undergo cytoplasmic streaming in most cells, except cardiomyocytes, and also undergo fusion and fission. The latter two processes account for the creation of new mitochondria in cells. Thus, it is reasonable to assume that changes in mitochondrial ultrastructure or function or changes in mitochondrial number, or in the regulation of fission or fusion events may lead to overall changes in the heart muscle.

Thus, it is essential to explore the role of mitochondrial defects, deficiencies, and mutations in mitochondrial proteins in the development and exacerbation of heart disease. Not only will this provide a deeper understanding of the molecular processes involved in etiology and pathological progression of heart disease, this strategy may also identify novel therapeutic targets for heart disease.

MITOCHONDRIAL BIOGENESIS

Interestingly, most of the mitochondria at birth are derived from the female oocyte, since the human sperm cell has very little cytoplasm and minimal if any, mitochondrial contribution to the zygote – a phenomenon commonly known as cytoplasmic inheritance. Thus, if there are abnormalities in maternal mitochondrial structure or function, these may be inherited by the offspring. To understand this better, it is important to consider the role that both nuclear and mitochondrial genes play in the biogenesis of new mitochondria.

Mitochondrial biogenesis is a complex process involving high-fidelity generation of 1) membrane components such as phospholipids, lipids, cholesterol, and lipid-rafts required for the generation of the mitochondrial outer and inner membranes; 2) mitochondrial proteins, such as the respiratory complex constituents, or other proteins involved in phospholipid synthesis or in heme synthesis, or the urea cycle or multiple other biochemical processes regulated by the mitochondria; and, 3) the adequate and timely generation of the protein machinery responsible for trafficking, transporting, and integrating mitochondrial proteins into the mitochondrial membranes or inner mitochondrial space or the mitoplast following their translation in the cytoplasm. In other words, for the daughter mitochondria to have proper structure and viability, multiple complex biochemical processes must occur in a synchronized or step-wise, but orchestrated fashion. Failure at any one step in this process may result in mitochondrial abnormalities. In fact, it is possible to classify mitochondrial aberrations by the specific process which is altered or affected during mitochondrial biogenesis. Next, we will discuss mitochondrial biogenesis in the context of mitochondrial fission and fusion. Following that we will examine the relevance of mitochondrial fission and fusion to the normal heart and in heart disease.

THE ROLE OF MITOCHONDRIAL FISSION PROTEINS IN MITOCHONDRIAL BIOGENESIS

Research to understand the molecular regulation of mitochondrial dynamics got a tremendous boost two decades ago with the discovery of the first protein that was shown to regulate the process of mitochondrial fusion in budding yeast (Hales and Fuller, 1997). It was a year later that the first mammalian protein required for mitochondrial fission was identified as the Dynamin related protein (Drp1) (Smirinova, 2001; Yoon, 1998). Since those early years, although a lot has been gleaned about the steps in the process for mitochondrial fusion and fission, only a few more molecular players, at least in human tissues, have been identified. This leaves a lot unknown about the actual process of mitochondrial fusion and fission in human organs. Not only will this knowledge serve to improve our understanding of the regulation of mitochondrial biogenesis in health and illness, but it may also help in identifying therapeutic targets that reside within the mitochondria which can be pharmacologically manipulated to overcome the structural or functional aberration due to deficient mitochondria.

The first possibility of developing mitochondrial disease occurs due to abnormalities during the formation of mitochondrial membranes, or more precisely during the fission or fusion of mitochondria. Importantly, at the cellular level, mitochondria are not static organelles. Instead, they undergo dynamic changes in number, morphology, size, and turnover in every tissue. Most cells retain the ability to upregulate mitochondrial biogenesis in response to physiological stress. This is important due to the central role that mitochondria play in energetics. Mitochondria are involved in the production of ATP through substrate phosphorylation and as such house the mitochondrial respiratory complex proteins which are required for electron transport and the production of ATP. Thus, mitochondria are of prime functional importance in organs with a strong oxygen demand such as the brain, heart, and the liver. Physiological stressors increase oxygen demand and induce mitochondrial biogenesis. This may be evidenced by an increase in mitochondrial fission and an upregulation of proteins that regulate it.

The process of mitochondrial fission has been hypothesized to occur in steps requiring multiple protein factors. It has been suggested that an initial step is a constriction of the mitochondria at specific sites, followed by the recruitment of the fission-regulating Drp1 protein to the mitochondrial outer membrane. Following this event, there appears to be a recruitment and assembly of a protein complex that will allow fission to occur, the fission event itself, and the eventual disassembly of the scission complex (Liesa, 2009).

MITOCHONDRIAL FISSION PROTEINS IN HUMANS

Over the past decade, a few proteins have been discovered that are thought to be involved in mitochondrial fission in human tissues. In addition to the Drp-1 protein, other examples include the human mitochondrial fission protein 1 (hFis1), mitochondrial fission factor, mitochondrial dynamics proteins of two different molecular weights (MiD49 and MiD51).

The Drp-1 Fission Protein

The helical protein Drp1 was discovered in 1998, and shown to be a GTPase which integrates into the mitochondrial outer membrane and causes the scission process to be completed, resulting in mitochondrial fission. Interestingly, Drp1 is usually located in the cytoplasm of the cell, from where it translocates to the mitochondria, binding to many protein receptors. In fact, Fis1, MiD49, and MiD51 may act as receptors for Drp1 and have been shown to mediate mitochondrial fission downstream of Drp1 translocation to the mitochondria. Smirnova et al. (Smirnova, 2001) showed that in mammalian cells, Drp1 was arranged in a spiral formation and was recruited to and aggregated at mitochondrial sites where the scission event would occur, suggesting its direct relevance for mitochondrial fission. Importantly, using an expression system to overexpress a mutant and non-functional dominant negative form of Drp1, the authors also presented strong evidence that the Drp1 protein was only involved in regulating dynamics of the mitochondria, but not that of any other organelle in the COS-7 cells they employed in their study.

Smirnova's seminal work on the function of one of the fission proteins was subsequently enriched in later years by the work of a number of investigators who expanded this research by investigated the effect of non-functional Drp1 on a number of mitochondrial functional parameters. At the present time, not is the Drp1 protein known to be recruited to the mitochondria to regulate mitochondrial fission and overall mitochondrial number and morphology, it is also implicated in the control of Reactive Oxidative Species (ROS) production, oxygen consumption, reduced coupled respiration, and regulating the rate of ATP synthesis in the mitochondria (Benard, 2007). In particular, Benard et al. demonstrated that the expression of a non-functional, dominant negative form of Drp1in HeLa cells resulted in a number of changes to mitochondrial morphology, network, and function. Dominant negative Drp1 was shown to cause 1) a shift from the reticular and highly interconnected mitochondrial network arrangement within the cells, 2) enhanced mitochondrial membrane fluidity, and, 3) significantly diminished potential for ATP production through the OXPHOS pathway.

Using the endocrine, insulin-producing pancreatic β cells, Twig et al. (Twig, 2008) demonstrated that the inhibition of mitochondrial fission by the expression of a dominant negative form of Drp1 resulted in an inhibition of mitochondrial autophagy. Further, their work showed that these mitochondria were impaired in respiratory capability, while also accumulating carbonylated-amino acid containing oxidized proteins that suggested an overall decrease in mitochondrial oxygen consumption and function. Thus, Drp1 was shown to be important not only for mitochondrial morphology by controlling mitochondrial fission, but also for regulating mitochondrial function in β cells. The authors also provided evidence to link autophagy-based removal of damaged mitochondria following defective fission events in these cells.

However, the effects of interrupting mitochondrial fission may be different in different tissues. Although mitochondrial fission has largely been studied in non-cardiac systems, some researchers have recently investigated its role in the maintenance of healthy heart cells. Thus, to understand the physiological relevance of mitochondrial fission and the regulation of mitochondrial dynamics, particularly in the context of the heart, multiple investigators have used an approach similar to the one described above, namely of expressing the non-functional, dominant negative form of the Drp1 protein.

An important example of this approach comes from the work of Ong et al. who studied the effect of mutation of the mitochondrial fission protein Drp1 in the context of ischemia-reperfusion injury to the heart (Ong, 2010). Ischemia-reperfusion injury to the myocardium most commonly occurs as a consequence of acute coronary syndrome (ACS). In ACS, there is a progressive and chronic decrease in the supply of oxygen to the heart tissue, due to complications such as atherosclerosis or atheroma of the blood vessels supplying blood to the heart. Surgical manipulation to restore blood supply results in a sudden upsurge of oxygen-rich blood, and counter-intuitively leads to myocardial damage. This is the most common cause of ischemia-reperfusion injury and eventually for the development of heart failure.

Drp1 and Heart Disease: Ischemia Reperfusion Injury

To investigate the role of mitochondrial fission in heart disease, particularly in the context of ischemia-reperfusion injury and heart failure, Ong et al. expressed the dominant negative form of the Drp1 protein in the cardiac-derived HL cell line. Subsequently, they induced ischemia in these cells and measured various mitochondrial parameters. The expression of dominant negative Drp1 in HL cells, increased the percentage of cells containing elongated mitochondria (63±6%, versus 46±6% in control: n=80 cells per group; $P<0.05$), decreased mitochondrial permeability transition pore sensitivity (by 2.4±0.3-fold; n=80 cells per group; $P<0.05$), and reduced cell death after simulated ischemia/reperfusion injury (12.1±2.9% versus 41.8±4.1% in control: n=320 cells per group; $P<0.05$). These findings led the authors to conclude that inhibiting mitochondrial fission resulted in cardioprotection following ischemia-reperfusion injury (Ong, 2010).

Interestingly, Ong's work was followed by the publication of three independent papers in 2013, all of which emphasize the potential of targeting the Drp1 protein to achieve cardioprotection in various models of heart disease.

In an alternative approach to only expressing the dominant negative form of Drp1 as attempted by Ong et al., the authors Din et al. (Din, 2013) investigated the effect of phosphorylation of Drp1 on the regulation of mitochondrial fission in the context of ischemia-reperfusion injury. Their work provided important insight into the use of some pharmacological agents that can inhibit the phosphorylation of

Drp1 as potential future drugs that can protect the heart from the biochemical effects if ischemic damage. Their work was based on the observation that phosphorylation of Drp1 at serine 637 prevents the translocation of Drp1 from the cytosol to the mitochondria, in a manner similar to the inhibition of translocation of the dominant negative mutant form of the protein. This suggested that post-translational protein modification mechanisms like phosphorylation events may also play a central role in regulating mitochondrial fission events. Based on this, Din et al. studied the effect of phosphorylation of Drp1 on mitochondrial integrity, reticular mitochondrial morphology, mitochondrial fission, and cell viability using both transgenic hearts and neonatal rat cardiomyocytes. Specifically, the authors demonstrated that a serine-threonine protein kinase called Pim-1 was responsible for the phosphorylation of Drp1 at serine 637. They accomplished this by isolating the hearts from transgenic mice that overexpressed the Pim-1 protein, followed by measuring the phosphorylated Pim-1 protein by Western blot of the whole heart homogenates and comparing its expression between normal and Pim-1 overexpressing transgenic hearts. The reported that Pim-1 overexpression resulted in a 2.7 fold increase in the phosphorylation of Drp1 compared to control hearts. Interestingly, the increase in phosphorylation was matched by a reciprocal decrease in the translocation of Drp1 to the mitochondria. The authors also mentioned that "consistent with these findings, adenoviral-induced Pim-1 neonatal rat cardiomyocytes retained a reticular mitochondrial phenotype after simulated ischemia and decreased Drp1 mitochondrial sequestration". The authors concluded that Pim-1 activity resulted in phosphorylation and inhibition of translocation of Drp1 to the mitochondria in response to ischemia-reperfusion injury and prevented mitochondrial fission and fragmentation while allowing the mitochondria to maintain a reticular arrangement in these cells. Thus this work identified Pim-1 as a potential therapeutic target to achieve cardioprotection by inhibiting mitochondrial fission.

Another line of evidence of the direct involvement and central importance of Drp1 in mediating cardiac-specific effects at the physiological level also came in the same year as the work by Din et al. cited above. Gao et al. employed a pharmacological strategy to inhibit Drp1, by utilizing the non-competitive dynamin protein GTPase inhibitor drug called dynasore. Similar to the models cited thus far, these authors studied the effect of inhibition of Drp1 in the context of a reperfusion ischemia injury model as an etiological mechanism in the development of heart failure. Briefly, Gao et al. induced global ischemia for 3o minutes, followed by 1 hour of reperfusion and utilized Langendorff perfused mouse hearts. They pre-treated a group of mice with 1 μM dynasore and measured Left Ventricular End Diastolic Pressure (LVEDP). The authors reported that dynasore pre-treatment before the induction of ischemia-reperfusion prevented the ischemia-reperfusion-mediated elevation in LVEDP. They also observed that dynasore prevented mitochondrial fragmentation and increased the survival and viability of the heart cells, and correlated their findings to the preservation of ATP levels and of mitochondrial morphology in these heart cells. Importantly, this work provided evidence that pharmacological inhibition of Drp1 was a viable strategy for achieving cardioprotection and needs further exploration (Gao, 2013).

Finally, also in the year 2013, Disatnik et al. synthesized a novel Drp1 inhibitor. Specifically, this molecule inhibited the protein interaction of Drp1 with another mitochondrial fission protein called Fis-1. Employing the strategy of rational drug design, Disatnik et al. synthesized a molecule which they named P110. This molecule was designed to disrupt the protein interaction of Drp1 and Fis-1, which was achieved by first identifying the homologous sequence between Drp1 and Fis-1 which would be the most likely site of protein interaction, and then synthesizing a compound that would specifically bind this amino acid sequence. It was the particular intent of the authors to achieve a high degree of specificity of inhibition, such that only Drp1 and Fis-1 interaction would be disrupted by P110, while the drug was designed to spare Drp1's interaction with other proteins regulating mitochondrial dynamics such as mitofusin 1 and mitofusin 2. To investigate the whether P110 would prevent mitochondrial fission and elicit cardioprotection, the authors employed three separate model systems of ischemia-reperfusion injury, namely 1) primary rat cultured cardiac myocytes, 2) an *ex vivo* rat heart model, and, 3) an *in vivo* rat model of myocardial infarction. The authors demonstrated that Drp1 translocated to the mitochondria following the induction of reperfusion ischemic injury, but that this was prevented by the drug P110. Further, "compared with control treatment, P110 (1 μmol/L) decreased infarct size by 28±2% and increased ATP levels by 70+1% after injury relative to control in the *ex vivo* model. Intraperitoneal injection of P110 (0.5 mg/Kg) at the onset of reperfusion in an *in vivo* model resulted in improved mitochondrial oxygen consumption by 68% when measured 3 weeks after ischemic injury, improved cardiac fractional shortening by 35%, reduced mitochondrial H_2O_2 uncoupling state by 70%, and improved overall mitochondrial functions" (Disatnik, 2013). Taken together, the authors were able to demonstrate the successful creation of a specific Drp1 inhibitor that has the potential of pharmacological use in the prevention of mitochondrial fission and fragmentation following ischemia-reperfusion injury.

Conclusion: Mitochondrial Fission Proteins in Ischemic Heart Disease

In summary, the work of Simirnova et al., Din et al., Gao et al., and Disatnik et al. emphasize the central role of mitochondrial dynamics, specifically mitochondrial fission events in regulating the etiology and progression of ischemia-reperfusion injury in the larger context of Acute Coronary Syndrome and heart failure. Further, the field seems to be moving in the direction of creating pharmacological inhibitors that can interfere with the specific function of mitochondrial fission proteins such as Drp1 to effectuate cardioprotection and longer survival of patients suffering from ACS and heart failure, making these novel inhibitors potential cardiac drugs of the future.

Mitochondrial Fission Proteins and Dilated Cardiomyopathy

Further direct evidence for the critical role of Drp1 in regulating mitochondrial and cellular energetics comes from a study conducted by Ashrafian et al. In an attempt to characterize and study a large-scale mutation screen obtained through mutagenesis by treating with *N*-ethyl-*N*-nitrosourea, the authors identified a mouse phenotype known as "Python" which resulted in an inherited dilated cardiomyopathy. Upon analysis, it was found that this particular phenotype was the result of a mutation in the Drp1 gene, which resulted in the C452F mutation which was shown to result in protein modification of Drp1 such that it altered this protein's ability to interact with other proteins in the mitochondria. The eventual biochemical outcome of this was a significant decrease in the levels of ATP, a reduction in the expression of important mitochondrial enzymes such as complex IV and succinate dehydrogenase, and structural aberrations of the mitochondria leading to the development of "abnormal" mitochondria. These observations led the authors to speculate that the reduction in mitochondrial ATP production and the changes in mitochondrial structure and appearance resulted in the dilated cardiomyopathy. Interestingly, homozygosity for this mutation resulted in lethality, suggesting the critical role of Drp1 in the regulation of mitochondrial energetics, morphology, function and by extension the normal physiology of the murine heart. This work provided an important link connecting mitochondrial dynamics to the molecular basis of heart disease (Ashrafian, 2010).

Following this initial report, Cahill et al. (Cahill, 2014) conducted a detailed biochemical analysis of the effect of the C452F Drp1 mutation on mitochondrial dynamics which was published in 2015. In this follow-up study, the authors closely examined the consequence of this mutation on the function and assembly of Drp1 in murine cardiac mitochondria. Importantly, they discovered that this mutation caused an increase in the GTPase activity of Drp1. Further, the C452F mutant Drp1 protein also exhibited abnormalities of assembly and oligomerization in the mitochondrial membrane. The latter was concluded from the observation that compared to their effect on the control non-mutant form of Drp1, even high concentration salt or nucleotide solutions were unable to induce disassembly of the mutant oligomerized protein, suggesting a mutation-induced defect in protein interaction resulting in abnormality in self-aggregation and oligomerization in the mitochondrial membrane. This, in turn, suggested the inability of the C452F Drp1 mutant to integrate into the mitochondrial membranes properly, leading to deficiencies in mitochondrial fission. To test this hypothesis, the authors induced the same mutation in mouse embryonic fibroblasts and analyzed the effect of the mutant Drp1 on mitochondrial morphology, and specifically on mitochondrial fission. They found defects in mitochondrial morphology in the mutant Drp1 mouse embryonic fibroblasts and were further able to demonstrate that in the mutant cells, the removal of damaged and abnormal mitochondria by the process of autophagy (or more appropriately, mitophagy) was impaired. The authors also demonstrated that Drp1 mutation not only caused a defect in mitochondrial morphology in the mouse embryonic fibroblast model system but also caused mitochondrial functional defects related to energy production. This was similar to their study conducted in 2010 and further confirmed that expression of mutant Drp1 was sufficient to produce energy deficiency, changes in mitochondrial morphology, and inhibition of mitophagy in the context of heart cells. Lastly, the authors showed that a partial rescue in terms of restoration of mitochondrial tissue health could be obtained by a long-term feeding of the Drp1 mutant mouse on a low protein diet, which enhanced the autophagy-related removal of damaged mitochondria. The eventual pathological development of dilated cardiomyopathy included a generalized sterile inflammation of the heart.

Conclusion: Mitochondrial Fission Proteins and Dilated Cardiomyopathy

In summary, these two instances of work provided evidence that the C452F mutation of Drp1 results in a monogenic dilated cardiomyopathy due to defects of protein oligomerization and integration in the mitochondrial membranes, resulting in ATP deficit, and accumulation of faulty mitochondria. The overall impact of these studies is to highlight the possibility of exploring Drp1 as a novel therapeutic target in the treatment of heart disease, including heart failure and cardiomyopathy.

MITOCHONDRIAL FUSION PROTEINS AND MITOCHONDRIAL BIOGENESIS

Mitochondrial biogenesis and regeneration require the coordinated and timely initiation of a number of cellular processes. It is important to realize that following mitosis, mitochondria in the new daughter cells do not originate by de novo synthesis, but are derived from previously existing mitochondria in the parent cells. This is relevant because, given the fact of generation from pre-existing mitochondria, new mitochondria can only be created by two processes: division of older mitochondria to produce smaller and fragmented mitochondria or the fusion of existing mitochondria to create newer and larger mitochondria. The molecular aspects of mitochondrial fission events, including the prominent proteins required for this process and their impact on cardiac physiology and pathology, have been discussed in detail above. We will now focus on the regulation of mitochondrial dynamics by mitochondrial fusion events and the role of mitochondrial fusion in the physiology and pathology of cardiovascular disease. We will conclude this section by exploring potential therapeutic strategies based on mitochondrial fusion proteins that may be employed to treat cardiovascular disease in the future.

In addition to contributing to the birthing process for creating new mitochondria, mitochondrial fusion is an important event that may occur in different tissues at different time points depending on the microenvironment. Thus, it is feasible to expect mitochondrial fusion in the absence of mitosis and in response to specific stimuli or drugs. In general, mitochondrial fusion in the human system usually results in the creation of longer mitochondria. This is considered a break from the other possible mitochondrial morphologies generally found in cells, namely 1) the existence of mitochondria as a network, closely linked to the endoplasmic reticulum; 2) the presence of numerous smaller condensed mitochondria; and, 3) the presence of elongated mitochondria. Of course, special mitochondrial arrangements are found in specialized tissue and cells within humans, and are also found in other species, most notably the giant fused Nebenkern mitochondria found in the fruit fly *Drosophila* sperm cells. In fact, we have learned a lot about the molecular process of mitochondrial fusion from studying the molecular events that generate the specialized mitochondria in species such *Drosophila*. In human cells, multiple investigators have reported the apparent flexibility of mitochondrial arrangement which can morph and transiently shift from the reticular form to the more commonly known condensed variant. In fact, in some cells, mitochondrial morphology and fission and fusion events are considered to also contribute to the cytoplasmic circulation of the mitochondria. It is, however, important to emphasize that mitochondrial arrangement and morphology in cardiac tissue is dramatically different from that in other tissues.

Mitochondrial Fusion in the Context of Cardiac Muscle Architecture

In the heart, as indeed in skeletal muscle, mitochondria have a very well defined spatial and topographical orientation. In these muscles, mitochondria are distributed in between the myofibrils of actin and myosin within each myofiber (or muscle cell). In fact, investigators have reported that in the rat skeletal muscle, the mitochondrial arrangement is so precise and periodic that it appears "crystal-like" or like beads on a necklace, especially upon analyzing live myofibers obtained from the muscle (Vendelin, 2005). It has been speculated that this may be particularly relevant in enabling the molecular cross-talk between these mitochondria and in maintaining regular muscle physiology. In fact, it was demonstrated that such a special spatial arrangement made it possible for all adjoining mitochondria in cardiac cells to depolarize by controlling the production of ROS, where ROS produced by the initiating mitochondria may drive ROS changes in the adjacent mitochondria (Zorov, 2000; Brady, 2004). Given such a special arrangement of mitochondria within the skeletal and cardiac muscle, it is reasonable to assume that both mitochondrial fusion and fission events will appear different and may work differently in muscle cells as compared to cells of other tissues. Thus, one must reference mitochondrial fission and fusion in the cardiac tissue as a specialized case of these events elsewhere.

MITOCHONDRIAL FUSION PROTEINS

Researchers have identified three main proteins thus far that participate in initiating and contribute to mitochondrial fusion events. These are the two mitochondrial fusion proteins named mitofusin 1 and 2 (Mfn1 and 2), and the optic atrophy factor 1 (OPA1) proteins. Just as there is a complex multi-step process for mitochondrial fission, mitochondrial fusion, though somewhat simpler, also involves site-specific reactions proceeding in a sequential manner. As is well documented, mitochondria have distinct suborganellar compartments that vary greatly in the content and distribution of enzymes and carry out distinct metabolic process. Essentially, mitochondria have a Mitochondrial Outer Membrane (MOM) and a mitochondrial inner membrane (MIM). The MIM is thrown into folds known as cristae but comes in contact with the MOM at specialized contact sites. Such an architecture creates two distinct functional compartments in the mitochondria, namely, 1) an inner membrane space which exists between the MOM and the outer surface of the MIM, and, 2) a mitoplast compartment which is entirely enclosed by the MIM. Thus, when considering events such as mitochondrial fusion, it is important to recognize the inherent complexity of such a process. For mitochondrial fusion to be effective, it is essential that contents of the newly created mitochondria following the fusion event must be equally distributed within the new mitochondria and so should be "well mixed".

It is, therefore, interesting to note that each protein listed above plays very specific roles in the fusion of the mitochondria. Mfn 1 and 2 are associated with fusion of the MOM, while OPA1 has been shown to mediate the MIM.

The story of the discovery of the mitofusin proteins begins in 1997, strangely enough, with the fruit fly testes. In the fruit fly, sperm cell production occurs in stages. In the early stages, within the developing sperm cells, Electron Microscopy shows the presence of a nucleus, accompanied by one giant, fused mitochondrion. Upon closer examination, the mitochondrion has the appearance of multiple layers, like the skin of an onion. In their seminal work, Hales and Fuller noted that mutations in the gene responsible for coding for the protein that results in this special mitochondrial arrangement resulted in fusion defects and fragmented mitochondria. Since the protein coded for the mitochondria to take on the appearance of layers of onion skin, the protein, and the gene, were named fuzzy onions (fzo). The authors demonstrated that in the absence of this gene, the mitochondrial fusion defects that occurred ultimately led to a failure of spermatogenesis in the fruit fly, and the production of sterile flies. Using sequence analysis and prediction software available at that time, the authors also speculated that the *Fzo* gene encoded a membrane bound GTPase. They were additionally able to demonstrate that mutation in the Fzo gene, while allowing proper translocation of the fzo protein to the mitochondria, resulted in fragmented mitochondria (Hales and Fuller, 1997)

Santel and Fuller identified the first mammalian homologs of the *Drosophila* Fzo gene and called them mitofusins, Mfn1 and Mfn2. They demonstrated that expressing these proteins using transient transfections in human fibroblast cell lines caused the mitochondria to fuse together in these cells. Further, the authors also identified a transmembrane domain within the sequence of the Mfn2 protein and showed that upon interaction with hydrophobic regions of the mitochondrial membrane, it was able to integrate the protein, suggesting the mitochondrial translocation and integration of Mfn2 (Santel & Fuller, 2001).

The importance of mitofusins was realized when it was discovered that mitochondrial fusion is a tightly regulated process and all the required steps must be completed for the proper generation of fused mitochondria. For instance, to ensure cell and mitochondrial viability, it is not enough for the just the MOM of the interacting mitochondria to fuse as a consequence of mitofusin activity. The MIM and the matrix must also fuse and result in the homogenous distribution of mitochondrial content, including of mitochondrial DNA. Thus, when the MIM was prevented from fusing, the resultant mitochondria did not mix their contents well, leading to dysfunction.

MITOFUSINS AND HEART DISEASE

Mitofusin proteins are essential in regulating mitochondrial morphology and dynamics. Interestingly, the role of mitofusins is not restricted to the time of embryonic development of the heart but continues into the adult organism. This is interesting because it provides evidence that heart cell mitochondria are not "static" as once thought, but undergo dynamic changes, alternating between reticular and condensed morphologies throughout life. In fact, although heart cells have restricted cytoplasmic streaming or local movement of mitochondria when compared to isotropic cells from other tissues, these proteins still play an important role in allowing tubular formation and regulating other morphological changes to the mitochondria, some of which may be important for exchanging mitochondrial content.

In addition, upon birth, there are other notable changes that occur in heart cells, perhaps the most relevant of which is the shift in cellular metabolism and energetics. Prior to birth, in the prenatal heart, the primary source of energy is glucose and anaerobic respiration; however, in the first few days of the postnatal period, this shifts substantially to the utilization of fatty acids as the source of energy. This shift in the source of fuel is also accompanied by changes in the mitochondrial morphology.

We will separately examine the role of mitofusins in the developing and adult heart.

Mitofusins and Embryonic Development

To examine the role of Mfn1 and Mfn2 during embryonic development, Chen et al. (Chen, 2003) generated knock-out mice where either Mfn1 or Mfn2 was genetically ablated. Mice heterozygous for either Mfn1 or Mfn2 were able to survive, while homozygous deletion of either gene resulted in lethality. Further, the authors reported that while ablation of either isoform was lethal to the mice, there were differences in the time point and the type of cells where these deletions showed maximum effect. For example, while depleting the Mfn2 gene resulted in abnormalities of the placental trophoblast "giant cells", deleting Mfn1 did not have any apparent effects on these cells. In terms of time, they reported that homozygous mutant embryos died earlier than their heterozygous counterparts, and displayed greater developmental delay. Depleting Mfn1 produced normal frequencies of live mutant embryos till embryonic day 10.5, while ablation of Mfn2 generated normal frequencies of live mutant embryos till embryonic day 9.5. Using the 10.5-day embryos, the authors derived and established an embryonic fibroblast cell line from normal and Mfn1 and Mfn2 knockout mice to examine the specific effects of Mfn1 or Mfn1 depletion on mitochondrial morphology compared to control. They showed a dramatic shift in mitochondrial morphology from the more than 90% tubular arrangement of mitochondria in normal mouse embryonic fibroblasts to the presence of fragmented mitochondria in Mfn1 and Mfn2 knock-outs. Further, the majority of the mitochondria in the knockouts appeared to be spherical. These observations record a major change in mitochondrial morphology and arrangement from a more "tubular" to a more spherical appearance. The authors used time-lapse microscopy to illustrate that fusion events were affected by the loss of either Mfn1 or Mfn2, while mitochondrial DNA content was not much affected, though mitochondrial mobility was altered. To demonstrate that all these changes occurred due to the depletion of the mitofusins, the authors performed a rescue experiment, where restoring mitofusin function also restored mitochondrial morphology to the reticular formation. Chen and colleagues concluded that "mitochondrial fusion is essential for embryonic development, and by enabling cooperation between mitochondria, has protective effects on the mitochondrial population".

Papanicolaou et al. (Papanicolaou, 2011) ablated the Mfn2 gene in mice and studied the effect on the heart and on mitochondrial dynamics in isolated heart cells from these mice. They reported that similar to the finding by Chen et al. (Chen, 2003), mitochondria in the Mfn2 ablated mice heart cells appeared fragmented. Further, an examination of the hearts from these mice indicated a cardiac enlargement, but not ventricular dilatation, while there was an increase in the left ventricular mass in Mfn2 deleted mice. In general, the authors noted that depletion of Mfn2 resulted in "modest myocyte hypertrophy accompanied by mild deterioration of left ventricular function". The modest increase in hypertrophy caused an increase in the "heart weight/body weight" ratio. Moreover, Mfn2 depletion did not change the activities of various mitochondrial enzymes such as citrate synthase, isocitrate dehydrogenase, or medium-chain acyl-CoA dehydrogenase (MCAD).

But perhaps their most significant finding was the difference in the function of Mfn2 discovered by analyzing and comparing mitochondrial permeability transition in neonatal and adult heart cardiomyocyte lacking this gene. In the adult heart cardiomyocyte, Mfn2 depletion protected against the formation of the mitochondrial permeability transition pore and thus prevented the consequent mitochondrial compromise. Thus, it seemed that when Mfn2 protein was present in adult heart cardiomyocyte, it mediated mitochondrial permeability in response to calcium-induced stress. This conclusion was based on the observation that in Mfn2 depleted heart cells, twice the amount of Ca^{2+} was required to induce mitochondrial permeability transition when compared to the Mfn2 wild-type cells. However, Mfn2 ablation resulted in the opposite effect of destabilizing the mitochondria in neonatal cardiomyocytes. The authors interpreted this apparent contradiction in mitochondrial response to Mfn2 deletion by suggesting that mitochondrial dynamics, morphology, and structure and its regulation were substantially different between the adult and the neonatal heart. The authors summarized their findings by reporting that Mfn2 was required to suppress mitochondria from undergoing excessive growth in cardiomyocytes.

I feel that the fact that Mfn2 has distinct and diametrically opposite roles in regulating mitochondrial permeability transition pore in response to Ca^{2+}-induced stress is a significant finding that may have far-reaching consequences when considering drug treatment. This is because it explains the molecular differences between the adult and the neonatal heart. Further, since mitochondria are important sources of ATP and regulators of apoptosis, among other very important biochemical functions, subtle molecular differences like these can affect the cardiotoxicity of drugs, especially in the neonate.

Mitofusins and the Adult Heart

In a subsequent study, Papanicolaou et al. examined the role of the Mfn1 protein in regulating mitochondrial dynamics in the heart. Their results for the role of Mfn1 were diametrically opposite to those for Mfn2. Using cardiocyte-restricted Mfn1 knock-outs, the authors reported that Mfn1 protected against "shrinkage/fragmentation" of the mitochondria. This work began by deleting Mfn1 specifically in cardiac myocytes in mice and examining the effect of this ablation on mice hearts. Interestingly, the authors reported that Mfn1 lacking mice hearts appeared to be smaller than normal hearts, but were structurally and functionally sound. This was determined by the use of noninvasive echocardiography. The parameters measured included heart rate, cardiac mass, diastolic and systolic left ventricular volumes, ejection fractions, cardiac output, fractional shortening of the sarcomere, and peak aortic outflow and none showed any significant differences between the Mfn1 knockout mice when compared to the Mfn wild-type. These data led the authors to conclude that ablation of Mfn1 did not directly affect the systolic and diastolic or pump function of the heart.

However, upon analysis of the adult cardiac myocytes isolated from Mfn1 ablated mice for mitochondrial assessment, the cells showed smaller and spherical mitochondria when compared to cardiac myocytes isolated from Mfn1 wild-type cells. Although the authors noted a lack of overall change in mitochondrial mass, they did observe that Mfn1 ablation seemed to alter the overall morphology of the adult cardiac myocyte mitochondria from a reticular formation to the spherical form. Interestingly, this was accompanied by specific changes in the expression of Electron Transport Chain proteins involved in ATP generation.

However, the most significant effect of the deletion of the Mfn1 gene was reported to be protection from ROS damage. This manifested as a delayed depolarization of the mitochondrial membrane potential in Mfn1 lacking isolated adult cardiac myocytes when compared to the Mfn1 containing control cells. The authors reasoned that since the loss of the mitochondrial membrane potential or "depolarization" of the mitochondria leads to the development of the mitochondrial permeability transition pore, it was plausible to expect that delayed depolarization would have a pro-survival effect. They tested this idea by comparing ROS induction initiated by exposure to hydrogen peroxide in isolated Mfn1-lacking or wild-type murine cardiac myocytes, followed by an assessment of cell viability by the trypan-blue staining method. They reported a significant decrease in cell viability in Mfn1 wild-type cells, while the Mfn1 ablated cells seemed to tolerate ROS better and resisted cell death (Papanicolaou, 2012).

Thus far, it seemed that knocking out either Mfn1 or Mfn2 affected mitochondrial biogenesis, development, and morphology in mice hearts or mice heart cells. However, it was not clear whether Mfn1 and Mfn2 shared some functions in common between them. Papanicolaou et al. designed a system to study the effect of depleting both Mfn1 and Mfn2 simultaneously and specifically only in heart cells. They used an inducible Cre-based animal model approach where administration of raloxifene could induce ablation of both genes. Using this model, the authors reported that there appeared to be some redundancy between Mfn1 and Mfn2, and especially the pathways they affected. This was true because although during the pre-natal period mice seemed to normal mitochondria, following birth, and with increasing number of post-natal days, mitochondria progressively became fragmented in response to Mfn1 and Mfn2 depletion. The authors speculated that mitochondrial fragmentation was a physiological compensatory response that resulted in an increase in mitochondrial number, perhaps as a means of cardiac muscle adaptation to the lack of the mitofusin proteins. However, as this state of mitochondrial fragmentation persisted, especially past post-natal day 7, and the numbers of mitochondria remained persistently expanded, all Mfn1 and Mfn2 lacking mice developed cardiomyopathy and died by postnatal day 16.

With particular reference to the structure and function of the heart, the authors observed that in normal, Mfn1 and Mfn2 wild-type hearts, there was an increase in the mRNA levels of Mfn1 and Mfn2 following birth, up to post-natal day 7. This increase in Mfn1 and Mfn2 seemed to be necessary for the regulation of the morphological and functional viability of heart cells as they transition from a "pre-birth" to an after-birth stage. Other authors had previously speculated on the need for such a change, based on the difference in cellular metabolism and energetics between adult and embryonic cardiac cells, as mentioned above. However, in the current animal model, since both Mfn1 and Mfn2 were ablated, the authors used this system to investigate the effect of this molecular change on the structure and development of the heart. They reported the development of a severe dilated cardiomyopathy in the knock-out mice compared to controls by post-natal day 7. Further, heart function was assessed by measuring heart rate, fractional sarcomere shortening, left ventricular volume, and ventricular wall thickness. All parameters showed significant changes between the mitofusin knockout animals compared to wild-type controls. Thus, for instance, there was a significant reduction in the fractional shortening of the sarcomere, and in the heart rate, followed by an increase in the left ventricular volume and in left ventricular wall thickness in the mitofusin knockout animals by post-natal day 7.

The authors further investigated the structural basis for the observed physiological defects and development of severe dilated cardiomyopathy. Using electron microscopy to analyze the arrangement and ultrastructural appearance of cardiac muscle cells, the authors found significant changes in both the number and shape of the mitochondria, as well as their packing and arrangement when comparing the mitofusin knock-outs to the wild-type cells. In particular, heart cells lacking mitofusins developed spherical mitochondria as mentioned above. But additionally, instead of being arranged in parallel with the actin and myosin filaments as they would under the wild-type conditions, in the mitofusin knock-out cells, the mitochondria were packed in between the myofilaments, resulting in a slight increase in the volume of the muscle cell. Not only was the internal arrangement of the mitochondria different, these mitochondria also appeared to have multiple structural deformations such as the presence of "finger-like" protrusions that were absent from the mitofusin wild-type samples.

Finally, the authors also compared the expression pattern of mitofusins in cardiac myocytes in perinatal mice to that of the protein Peroxisome proliferator-activated receptor gamma coactivator (PGC-1α). They reasoned that this was due to the fact that PGC-1α was known to participate in mitochondrial biogenesis, especially in the context of a reduction in cellular ATP levels. Since there was a decrease in ATP in mitofusin knock-out cardiac myocytes, and also a similarity in the expression pattern of PGC-1α and Mfn1 and Mfn2 in perinatal cardiac myocytes, the authors speculated that PGC-1α and mitofusins could be temporally regulated. To support this claim, they measured changes in mRNA by quantitative RT-PCR, in cardiac cells from post-natal day 0, 3, and 7. The authors reported that no significant changes were found on postnatal days 0 and 3 between mitofusin knock-out and wild-type cardiac myocytes in PGC-1α, Tfam, and Nrf-1, the latter two being transcriptional factors regulating mitochondrial biogenesis. However, interestingly, all three were suppressed on pot-natal day 7. This suggested that mitofusins also regulate mitochondrial biogenesis in the perinatal period in cardiac myocytes.

The Mitochondrial Fusion Protein: OPA1

The optic atrophy 1 protein (OPA1) is essential for the fusion of mitochondria. Just as the mitofusins promote the fusion of the mitochondrial outer membranes, OPA1 promotes the fusion of the inner membranes of the mitochondria. Fusion of the inner membranes is an important event that allows proper mixing of mitochondrial contents, including mitochondrial DNA (mtDNA). The absence of OPA1 prevents mtDNA and mitochondrial content mixing. In fact, it has been reported that in addition to facilitating mixing of mtDNA, OPA1 is actually also required for mtDNA replication. siRNA directed against alternative splice variants of OPA1, and specifically at the exon 4, and demonstrated a decrease in a hydrophobic, 10 kDa peptide generated from this sequence. The absence of this peptide coincided with faulty replication of mtDNA. This led the authors to conclude that OPA1 was directly involved in regulating the replication of mtDNA.

OPA1 is a member of the dynamin-related protein family. The dynamin-related protein family differs from dynamin-related proteins in lacking a proline-rich and a pleckstrin domain. However, both protein families retain the GTPase, a central coiled-coil region, and GTPase effector domains, a dynamin central region, and a C-terminal coiled-coil region. These proteins also contain a highly alkaline domain towards the N-terminal region which is required for mitochondrial targeting. OPA1 was first identified by Nagase et al. in 1998 (Nagase, 1998), but was identified as a regulator of mitochondrial DNA in yeast. Further, significant characterization of this protein as a mitochondrial protein came from the work of Delettre et al. and Olichon et al (Delettre, 2001; Olichon, 2003). Both groups identified the specific exons within the coding region of human OPA1. Collectively, they found that OPA had 8 alternative splice variants in humans and that all the splice variants shared a basic N-terminal domain that targeted the proteins to the mitochondria. Their work also suggested that these alternative splice variants differed in the absence or the presence of the domains encoded by exons 4, 4b and 5b. In summary, their work suggested that there were important domains within the protein structure that regulated its function.

To further explore the role of the domains in the OPA1 protein, various workers introduced mutations in these domains and investigated the effect of these mutations on mitochondrial function and energetics. Interestingly, none of the mutations reported thus far have resulted in a negation of mitochondrial function. The only time an effect was observed in mitochondrial function was when OPA1 was depleted using siRNA technology in mouse embryonic fibroblast cells by Chen et al. These authors demonstrated that ablating the OPA1 resulted in growth and mitochondrial defects. In particular, in the absence of OPA1 mitochondrial respiration was considerably suppressed. Restoration of OPA1 also restored mitochondrial respiration. This experiment suggested that OPA1 was required not only for mitochondrial fusion, and replication of mtDNA but also for the healthy biochemical functioning of the mitochondria (Chen, 2005).

Kasahara et al. (Kasahara, 2013) reported that along with other fusion proteins such as the mitofusins, OPA1 was essential for cardiocyte development during the process of embryogenesis and organogenesis. These authors demonstrated that OPA1 mediated mitochondrial fusion was required for the regulation of a complex molecular pathway which ultimately controlled the signal transduction protein called Notch-1. They reached this conclusion by gene-trapping OPA1 in mouse embryonic stem cells and observing the effects of this on cardiocyte development. They noticed that restricting the function of OPA1 also resulted in impaired cardiocyte development, and damaged signaling involving calcium-calcineurin and the transcription factors tumor growth factor beta (Tgf-β) and serum response factor (SRF), among others. Thus, OPA1 was required for the adequate functioning of a complex and interconnected signal transduction pathway required for cardiocyte development and growth.

OPA1 is reduced in heart failure and in cardiomyopathy. Chen et al. employed two models of heart failure to investigate the effect of OPA1 on mitochondrial fusion and on heart health and function. The authors use an explanted failing human heart which was removed during surgical transplantation. They also employed a high coronary ligation rat model of heart failure. In the latter model, heart failure resulted in the suppression of the OPA1 protein. In rats, OPA1 is known to have 5 alternative splice variants, and reductions in protein expression were noted across all 5 variants. Curiously, this model did not show a decrease in Mfn1 or Mfn2. This decrease in OPA1 in this rat model was mimicked by its decrease in the failing human hearts, which was found to be statistically significant. However, measurement of mRNA levels by RT-PCR showed no difference in OPA1 mRNA between normal and failing hearts, either in the rat model or in failing human hearts. The authors interpreted this to suggest that OPA1 was post-transcriptionally regulated. Further, reduction in OPA1 protein levels was accompanied by changes in mitochondrial morphology. In particular, upon examination by electron microscopy, failing hearts, whether in the rat model or human, showed an increase in fragmented mitochondria and cristae defects. Further analysis by immunogold labeling demonstrated a reduction in OPA1 localization to the mitochondria in the heart failure models. The decrease in OPA1 was also accompanied by an increase in apoptosis, especially in the externalization of cytochrome c from the mitochondria to the cytoplasm, which is recognized as the hallmark and irreversible signal for apoptosis. In fact, the apoptotic effects of the absence of OPA1 could be exaggerated by the application of ischemia to these cells. This confirmed that OPA1 was important for protection against apoptosis (Chen, 2009).

Piquereau et al. (Piquereau, 2012) used a heterogeneous mouse model and reduced the function of OPA1 to 50% in these mice. They investigated the effect of reduced OPA1 on a number of cardiac parameters but found that not only did the mice survive, but most of the cardiac functions were not significantly different from controls. But they reported three important changes. First, they found that even with a 50% reduction in OPA1, there was a disruption of mitochondrial morphology from a reticular to a more spherical, condensed, and fragmented formation. They also found that accompanying this morphological change, was the altered levels of adenosine dinucleotide phosphate (ADP), which they interpreted to be the first evidence for a link between mitochondrial morphology and cellular energetics. Finally, they also measured the formation of the mitochondrial permeability transition pore in response to calcium uptake by the mitochondria in cells lacking OPA1 and compared these to the wild-type control cells. They reported that "the mitochondrial permeability transition pore opening in isolated permeabilized cardiomyocytes and in isolated mitochondria was significantly less sensitive to mitochondrial calcium accumulation". Additionally, they discovered that six weeks following transversal aortic constriction, hearts that were heterogeneous for OPA1, demonstrated hypertrophy "almost two-fold higher ($P< 0.01$) than in wild-type mice with altered ejection fraction (decrease in 43 vs. 22% in $Opa1^{+/+}$ mice, $P< 0.05$)". The authors concluded that decreased expression of OPA1 was of consequence in maintaining mitochondrial morphology and energy transfer between organelles. They further concluded that OPA1 may play a vital role in the response of the heart to hemodynamic changes and may be a significant player in the regulation of cardiac physiology by controlling the response of cardiac mitochondria to calcium.

FUTURE RESEARCH DIRECTIONS AND CONCLUSION

Understanding the role of mitochondrial fission and fusion proteins in different heart diseases, using both cellular and animal models, will provide insight into the molecular mechanisms responsible for its development and progression. We have primarily discussed the role of Mfn1, Mfn2, OPA1, and Drp1 in selected heart disease such as ischemia reperfusion, dilated cardiomyopathy, and heart failure. For future studies, the role of these proteins in other heart diseases must also be explored. It is also important to identify existing drugs that can modulate the expression of these proteins, and hence, indirectly affect the health outcomes in patients. Development of gene therapy, gene editing and their combination with nanotechnology will provide the tools for timely pharmacological intervention if heart disease is identified, allowing the potential delivery of personalized medicine to the patient.

REFERENCES

Ashrafian, H., Docherty, L., Leo, V., Towlson, C., Neilan, M., Steeples, V., & Dear, T. N. et al. (2010). A mutation in the mitochondrial fission gene Dnm1l leads to cardiomyopathy. *PLOS Genetics*, *6*(6), e1001000. doi:10.1371/journal.pgen.1001000 PMID:20585624

Benard, G., Bellance, N., James, D., Parrone, P., Fernandez, H., Letellier, T., & Rossignol, R. (2007). Mitochondrial bioenergetics and structural network organization. *Journal of Cell Science*, *120*(Pt 5), 838–848. doi:10.1242/jcs.03381 PMID:17298981

Brady, N. R., Elmore, S. P., van Beek, J. J., Krab, K., Courtoy, P. J., Hue, L., & Westerhoff, H. V. (2004). Coordinated behavior of mitochondria in both space and time: A reactive oxygen species-activated wave of mitochondrial depolarization. *Biophysical Journal*, *87*(3), 2022–2034. doi:10.1529/biophysj.103.035097 PMID:15345578

Cahill, T. J., Leo, V., Kelly, M., Stockenhuber, A., Kennedy, N. W., Bao, L., & Ashrafian, H. et al. (2015). Resistance of dynamin-related protein 1 oligomers to disassembly impairs mitophagy, resulting in myocardial inflammation and heart failure. *The Journal of Biological Chemistry*, *290*(43), 25907–25919. doi:10.1074/jbc.M115.665695 PMID:26370078

Chen, H., Chomyn, A., & Chan, D. C. (2005). Disruption of fusion results in mitochondrial heterogeneity and dysfunction. *The Journal of Biological Chemistry*, *280*(28), 26185–26192. doi:10.1074/jbc.M503062200 PMID:15899901

Chen, H., Detmer, S. A., Ewald, A. J., Griffin, E. E., Fraser, S. E., & Chan, D. C. (2003). Mitofusins Mfn1 and Mfn2 coordinately regulate mitochondrial fusion and are essential for embryonic development. *The Journal of Cell Biology*, *160*(2), 189–200. doi:10.1083/jcb.200211046 PMID:12527753

Chen, L., Gong, Q., Stice, J. P., & Knowlton, A. A. (2009). Mitochondrial OPA1, apoptosis, and heart failure. *Cardiovascular Research*, *84*(1), 91–99. doi:10.1093/cvr/cvp181 PMID:19493956

Delettre, C., Griffoin, J.-M., Kaplan, J., Dollfus, H., Lorenz, B., Faivre, L., & Hamel, C. P. et al. (2001). Mutation spectrum and splicing variants in the OPA1 gene. *Human Genetics*, *109*(6), 584–591. doi:10.1007/s00439-001-0633-y PMID:11810270

Din, S., Mason, M., Völkers, M., Johnson, B., Cottage, C. T., Wang, Z., & Sussman, M. A. et al. (2013). Pim-1 preserves mitochondrial morphology by inhibiting dynamin-related protein 1 translocation. *Proceedings of the National Academy of Sciences of the United States of America*, *110*(15), 5969–5974. doi:10.1073/pnas.1213294110 PMID:23530233

Disatnik, M., Ferreira, J. C. B., Campos, J. C., Gomes, K. S., Dourado, P. M. M., Qi, X., & Mochly-Rosen, D. (2013). Acute inhibition of excessive mitochondrial fission after myocardial infarction prevents long-term cardiac dysfunction. *Journal of the American Heart Association: Cardiovascular and Cerebrovascular Disease*, *2*(5), e000461. doi:10.1161/JAHA.113.000461 PMID:24103571

Gao, D., Zhang, L., Dhillon, R., Hong. T. T., Shaw, R. M., Zhu, J. (2013). Dynasore protects mitochondria and improves cardiac lusitropy in Langendorff perfused mouse heart. *PLoS One, 15*(4), e60967.

Hales, K. G., & Fuller, M. T. (1997). Developmentally regulated mitochondrial fusion mediated by a conserved, novel, predicted GTPase. *Cell*, *90*(1), 121–129. doi:10.1016/S0092-8674(00)80319-0 PMID:9230308

Kasahara, A., Cipolat, S., Chen, Y., Dorn, G. W. II, & Scorrano, L. (2013). Mitochondrial fusion directs cardiomyocyte differentiation via calcineurin and Notch signaling. *Science*, *342*(6159), 734–737. doi:10.1126/science.1241359 PMID:24091702

Liesa, M., Palacin, M., & Zorzano, A. (2009). Mitochondrial dynamics in mammalian health and disease. *Physiological Reviews*, *89*(3), 799–845. doi:10.1152/physrev.00030.2008 PMID:19584314

Nagase, T., Ishikawa, K., Miyajima, N., Tanaka, A., Kotani, H., & Nomura, N. et al.. (1998). Prediction of the coding sequences of unidentified human genes. IX. The complete sequences of 100 new cDNA clones from brain which can code for large proteins *in vitro*. *DNA Research*, *5*(1), 31–39. doi:10.1093/dnares/5.1.31 PMID:9628581

Olichon, A., Baricault, L., Gas, N., Guillou, E., Valette, A., & Belenguer, P. et al.. (2003). Loss of OPA1 perturbates the mitochondrial inner membrane structure and integrity, leading to cytochrome c release and apoptosis. *The Journal of Biological Chemistry*, *278*(10), 7743–7746. doi:10.1074/jbc.C200677200 PMID:12509422

Ong, S., Subrayan, S., Lim, S. Y., Yellon, D. M., Davidson, S. M., & Hausenloy, D. J. (2010). Inhibiting mitochondrial fission protects the heart against ischemia/reperfusion injury. *Circulation*, *121*(18), 2012–2022. doi:10.1161/CIRCULATIONAHA.109.906610 PMID:20421521

Papanicolaou, K. N., Khairallah, R. J., Ngoh, G. A., Chikando, A., Luptak, I., & O'Shea, K. M. et al.. (2011). Mitofusin-2 maintains mitochondrial structure and contributes to stress-induced permeability transition in cardiac myocytes. *Molecular and Cellular Biology*, *6*(130), 9–28. PMID:21245373

Papanicolaou, K. N., Kikuchi, R., Ngoh, G. A., Coughlan, K. A., Dominguez, I., Stanley, W. C., & Walsh, K. (2012). Mitofusins 1 and 2 are Essential for Postnatal Metabolic Remodeling in Heart. *Circulation Research*, *111*(8), 1012–1026. doi:10.1161/CIRCRESAHA.112.274142 PMID:22904094

Papanicolaou, K. N., Ngoh, G. A., Dabkowski, E. R., OConnell, K. A., Ribeiro, R. F. Jr, Stanley, W. C., & Walsh, K. (2012). Cardiomyocyte deletion of mitofusin-1 leads to mitochondrial fragmentation and improves tolerance to ROS-induced mitochondrial dysfunction and cell death. *American Journal of Physiology. Heart and Circulatory Physiology*, *302*(1), H167–H179. doi:10.1152/ajpheart.00833.2011 PMID:22037195

Piquereau, J., Caffin, F., Novotova, M., Prola, A., Garnier, A., Mateo, P., & Joubert, F. et al. (2012). Down-regulation of OPA1 alters mouse mitochondrial morphology, PTP function, and cardiac adaptation to pressure overload. *Cardiovascular Research*, *94*(3), 408–417. doi:10.1093/cvr/cvs117 PMID:22406748

Santel, A., & Fuller, M. T. (2001). Control of mitochondrial morphology by a human mitofusin. *Journal of Cell Science*, *114*(Pt 5), 867–874. PMID:11181170

Smirnova, E., Griparic, L., Shurland, D. L., & van der Bliek, A. M. (2001). Dynamin-related protein Drp1 is required for mitochondrial division in mammalian cells. *Molecular Biology of the Cell*, *12*(8), 2245–2256. doi:10.1091/mbc.12.8.2245 PMID:11514614

Smirnova, E., Shurland, D. L., Ryazantsev, S. N., & van der Bliek, A. M. (1998). A human dynamin-related protein controls the distribution of mitochondria. *The Journal of Cell Biology*, *143*(2), 351–358. doi:10.1083/jcb.143.2.351 PMID:9786947

Twig, G., Elorza, A., Molina, A. J. A., Mohamed, H., Wikstrom, J. D., Walzer, G., & Shirihai, O. S. et al. (2008). Fission and selective fusion govern mitochondrial segregation and elimination by autophagy. *The EMBO Journal*, *27*(2), 433–446. doi:10.1038/sj.emboj.7601963 PMID:18200046

Vendelin, M., Béraud, N., Guerrero, K., Andrienko, T., Kuznetsov, A. V., & Olivares, J. et al.. (2005). Mitochondrial regular arrangement in muscle cells: A crystal-like pattern. *American Journal of Physiology. Cell Physiology, 288*(3), C757–C767. doi:10.1152/ajpcell.00281.2004 PMID:15496480

Yoon, Y., Pitts, K. R., Dahan, S., & McNiven, M. A. (1998). A novel dynamin-like protein associates with cytoplasmic vesicles and tubules of the endoplasmic reticulum in mammalian cells. *The Journal of Cell Biology, 140*(4), 779–793. doi:10.1083/jcb.140.4.779 PMID:9472031

Zorov, D. B., Filburn, C. R., Klotz, L. O., Zweier, J. L., & Sollott, S. J. (2000). Reactive oxygen species (ROS)-induced ROS release: A new phenomenon accompanying induction of the mitochondrial permeability transition in cardiac myocytes. *The Journal of Experimental Medicine, 192*(7), 1001–1014. doi:10.1084/jem.192.7.1001 PMID:11015441

ADDITIONAL READING

An, H. J., Cho, G., Lee, J. O., Paik, S. G., Kim, Y. S., & Lee, H. (2013). Higd-1a interacts with Opa1 and is required for the morphological and functional integrity of mitochondria. *Proceedings of the National Academy of Sciences of the United States of America, 110*(32), 13014–13019. doi:10.1073/pnas.1307170110 PMID:23878241

Ashrafian, H., Docherty, L., Leo, V., Towlson, C., Neilan, M., Steeples, V., & Dear, T. N. et al. (2010). A mutation in the mitochondrial fission gene Dnm1l leads to cardiomyopathy. *PLOS Genetics, 6*(6), e1001000. doi:10.1371/journal.pgen.1001000 PMID:20585624

Baughman, J. M., Perocchi, F., Girgis, H. S., Plovanich, M., Belcher-Timme, C. A., Sancak, Y., & Mootha, V. K. et al. (2011). Integrative genomics identifies MCU as an essential component of the mitochondrial calcium uniporter. *Nature, 476*(7360), 341–345. doi:10.1038/nature10234 PMID:21685886

Cereghetti, G. M., Stangherlin, A., Martins de Brito, O., Chang, C. R., Blackstone, C., & Bernardi, P. et al.. (2008). Dephosphorylation by calcineurin regulates translocation of Drp1 to mitochondria. *Proceedings of the National Academy of Sciences of the United States of America, 105*(41), 15803–15808. doi:10.1073/pnas.0808249105 PMID:18838687

Cerqua, C., Anesti, V., Pyakurel, A., Liu, D., Naon, D., Wiche, G., & Scorrano, L. et al. (2010). Trichoplein/mitostatin regulates endoplasmic reticulum-mitochondria juxtaposition. *EMBO Reports, 11*(11), 854–860. doi:10.1038/embor.2010.151 PMID:20930847

Chalmers, S., Saunter, C., Wilson, C., Coats, P., Girkin, J. M., & McCarron, J. G. (2012). Mitochondrial motility and vascular smooth muscle proliferation. *Arteriosclerosis, Thrombosis, and Vascular Biology, 32*(12), 3000–3011. doi:10.1161/ATVBAHA.112.255174 PMID:23104850

Chang, C. R., & Blackstone, C. (2007). Cyclic AMP-dependent protein kinase phosphorylation of Drp1 regulates its GTPase activity and mitochondrial morphology. *The Journal of Biological Chemistry, 282*(30), 21583–21587. doi:10.1074/jbc.C700083200 PMID:17553808

Chen, H., Chomyn, A., & Chan, D. C. (2005). Disruption of fusion results in mitochondrial heterogeneity and dysfunction. *The Journal of Biological Chemistry*, *280*(28), 26185–26192. doi:10.1074/jbc.M503062200 PMID:15899901

Chen, H., Detmer, S. A., Ewald, A. J., Griffin, E. E., Fraser, S. E., & Chan, D. C. (2003). Mitofusins MFN1 and Mfn2 coordinately regulate mitochondrial fusion and are essential for embryonic development. *The Journal of Biological Chemistry*, *160*, 189–200. PMID:12527753

Chen, L., Liu, T., Tran, A., Lu, X., Tomilov, A. A., Davies, V., & Knowlton, A. A. et al. (2012a). OPA1 mutation and late-onset cardiomyopathy: Mitochondrial dysfunction and mtDNA instability. *Journal of the American Heart Association*, *1*(5), 3012–3024. doi:10.1161/JAHA.112.003012 PMID:23316298

de Brito, O. M., & Scorrano, L. (2008). Mitofusin 2 tethers endoplasmic reticulum to mitochondria. *Nature*, *456*(7222), 605–610. doi:10.1038/nature07534 PMID:19052620

Hall, A. R., Burke, N., Dongworth, R. K., & Hausenloy, D. J. (2014). Mitochondrial fusion and fission proteins: Novel therapeutic targets for combating cardiovascular disease. *British Journal of Pharmacology*, *171*(8), 1890–1906. doi:10.1111/bph.12516 PMID:24328763

KEY TERMS AND DEFINITIONS

Dilated Cardiomyopathy: Expansion of the ventricles of the heart to compensate for the inability of the heart muscle to meet the oxygen demands of the body during heart failure.

Ischemia-Reperfusion Injury: The surgical or pharmacological restoration of oxygen supply to the myocardium by removing the clot in the coronary vessels results in damage to the heart muscle.

Mitochondrial Biogenesis: The process by which new mitochondria are created.

Mitochondrial Fission Proteins: Proteins that control the division of the mitochondria. The more common mitochondrial fission protein that has been identified in humans is the dynamin-related protein, Drp1. Fission proceeds in steps which start with a constriction at the "scission" site at the mitochondrial membranes.

Mitochondrial Fission: The act of division or splitting of a mitochondrion to form smaller, fragmented mitochondria. This allows for changes in mitochondrial morphology from the reticular to the spherical and condensed form.

Mitochondrial Fusion Proteins: Proteins that regulate the merger of two or more mitochondria. These proteins mediate the fusion of both the outer and inner mitochondrial membrane and allow the mixing of mitochondrial content, including mitochondrial DNA. In humans, the most common mitochondrial fusion proteins are the mitofusins, Mfn1 and Mfn2, which regulate the fusion of the outer mitochondrial membranes, and the optic atrophy protein, OPA1, which mediates the fusion of the inner mitochondrial membranes.

Mitochondrial Fusion: The act of merger of two or more mitochondria. This allows for the formation of "longer", tube-like mitochondria and allows proper mixing of mitochondrial content, including that of mitochondrial DNA.

Chapter 6
Cardiac Remodeling Under Hyperoxic Conditions:
Hyperoxia and Heart Diseases

Siva Kumar Panguluri
University of South Florida, USA

ABSTRACT

Cardiovascular complications and arrhythmias account for high mortality in cardiopulmonary patients in intensive care unites (ICU) and critical care unites. Patients in ICU are often administered with 100% oxygen for treatment with many diseases. According to American Heart Association (AHA), more than 2200 deaths related to cardiac failure are reported every day with an average of 1 in every 39 seconds. Cardiomyopathy is also reported in many diseased conditions including acute lung injury, diabetes, obesity, hypertension, and cancer. Recent studies indicate that hyperoxia induces cardiac injury due to dysfunctional lung and compromised pulmonary functioning. The exact mechanism of cardiovascular complications in ICU/ critical care remains unknown. This review will discuss the effect of hyeproxia on cardiac remodeling with more emphasis on ventricular and electrical remodeling. Understanding the exact mechanism of hyperoxia induced cardiomyopathy is not only important to understand the disease development and progression but also open new avenues for targeted therapy.

INTRODUCTION

Administration of 100% oxygen (O_2) is widely used intervention in critically ill patients at Critical care or Intensive Care Units (ICU). Although O_2 administration is supported by many guidelines for the patients with various medical emergencies (Anderson et al., 2007; Dickstein et al., 2008; O'Driscoll et al., 2008), the clinical implication of hyperoxia remain an important subject of debate (Altemeier & Sinclair, 2007). Recent studies indicate that hyperoxia induces cardiac injury due to dysfunctional lung and compromised pulmonary functioning (Visser, Walther, Laghmani el, Laarse, & Wagenaar, 2010). As pulmonary and cardiovascular systems are known to be in cooperative regulation, changes in cardiovascular systems may influence pulmonary function and vice versa (Howden et al., 2012b). Further-

DOI: 10.4018/978-1-5225-2092-4.ch006

more, smoke inhalation induced lung injury has been shown to have cardiovascular changes in previous study (Demling, Lalonde, Youn, & Picard, 1995) and continuous exposure of rabbits to hyperoxia for 72h caused elevated heart rate and low blood pressure (Sventek & Zambraski, 1988) indicating a close regulation between cardiovascular and pulmonary systems. More recent studies exploring the functional implications of hyperoxia from a cardiovascular stand point identify functional changes in heart rate and heart rate variability and linked it to polymorphisms and candidate gene loci (Howden et al., 2012b). Although the damage caused by delivering 100% oxygen treatment is to the lung and pulmonary system, patients supplemented with 96% of oxygen (hyperoxic), causes accumulation of lung fluid leading to pulmonary dysfunction causing oxidative stress in the heart. Additionally, many clinical reports indicating that hyperoxia was independently associated with increased in-hospital mortality in ICU following resuscitation from cardiac arrest, stroke, and traumatic brain injury (Damiani et al., 2014; Helmerhorst et al., 2014; Kilgannon et al., 2010; Nelskyla, Parr, & Skrifvars, 2013; Rincon, Kang, Maltenfort, et al., 2014; Rincon, Kang, Vibbert, et al., 2014).

Hyperoxia and Lung Injury

Administration of supraphysiological concentrations of oxygen as a mechanical ventilation is often a standard practice to treat newborns, older children, and adults with various diseases and surgeries (Andrea Porzionato et al., 2015). Nevertheless, there were also concerns that breathing pure O_2 might cause irreparable harm and death, which became a prominent clinical concern with the emergence of ICU in 1960s (Kallet & Matthay, 2013). Hyperoxia can cause lung cell injury and death due to accumulation of extremely toxic reactive oxygen species (ROS) (Xu, Guthrie, Mabry, Sack, & Truog, 2006). Induction of extensive inflammatory response and damage to the alveolar-capillarity barrier, which can lead to impaired gas exchange and pulmonary edema are the characteristics of hyperoxia induced lung injury. These characteristics are known to be accompanied by injury and apoptotic or necrotic death of pulmonary cells (Mantell & Lee, 2000; Petrache et al., 1999). Hyperoxia can also induce acute and chronic lung diseases such as acute inflammatory lung injury and bronchopulmonary dysplasia (BPD) under prolonged exposure (Andrea Porzionato et al., 2015).

Generation of ROS including superoxide anions, hydrogen peroxide, hydroxyl radicals, and hypochlorous acid by activated NADPH oxidase, which in turn injure pulmonary cells via lipid peroxidation, protein sulfhydryl oxidation, enzyme inactivation, DNA damage, and depletion of cellular reducing agents (Figure 1) are some of the events that occur in acute inflammatory lung injury (Cacciuttolo, Trinh, Lumpkin, & Rao, 1993; X. Zhang et al., 2003). This can also induce endothelial and epithelial cells to stress responses, and modulation of cell growth, inflammation, and/or death (Lee & Choi, 2003).

The most common chronic lung disease of prematurity is BPD, which results in impaired alveolar growth and a dysmorphic vascular architecture (Thébaud & Abman, 2007). Hyperoxia or high oxygen concentrations are directly correlated to BPD and most of the animal models of BPD involve hyperoxic exposure. Disruption of postnatal alveolar development leading to smaller numbers of enlarged and simplified alveoli, thick septa, and an increase in alveolar macrophages are some of the pathophysiological effects for BPD (Balasubramaniam, Mervis, Maxey, Markham, & Abman, 2007; Dauger et al., 2003; Grisafi et al., 2013; Grisafi et al., 2012; A. Porzionato et al., 2012; A. Porzionato et al., 2013). Changes in microvascular development and thickening of the medial muscle layer of arteries, pulmonary hypertension, increase in number of lung mast cells, which eventually accumulate around the vessels are also reported in experimental models of BPD (Brock & Giulio, 2006; Grisafi et al., 2013; Grisafi et

Figure 1. Schematic diagram showing the events of hyperoxia induced acute inflammatory lung injury

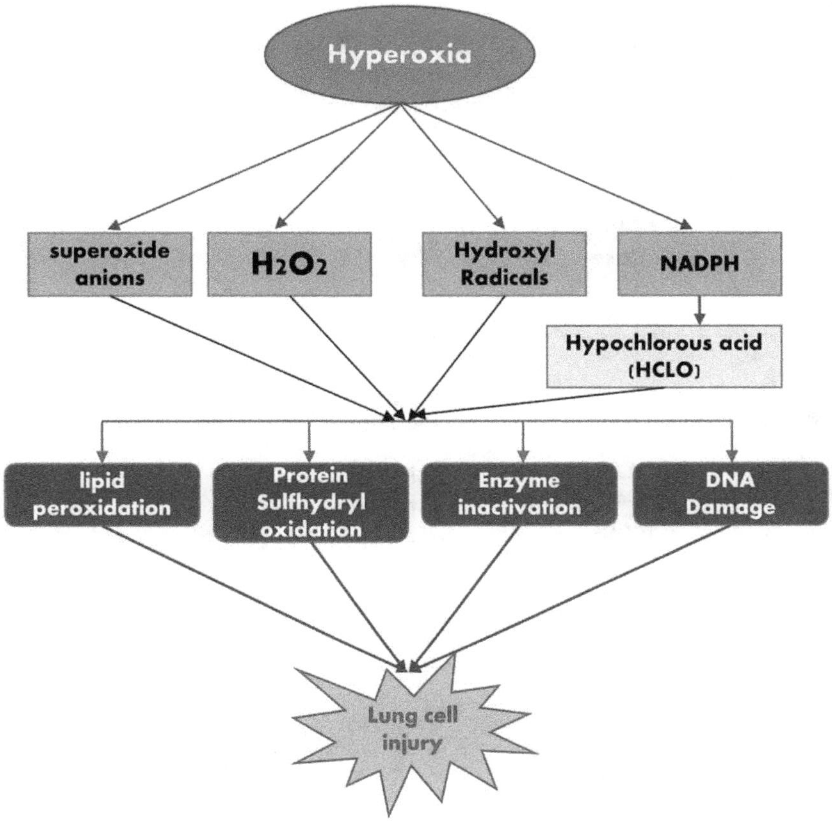

al., 2012; Jones, 1984; Koppel, Han, Cox, Tanswell, & Rabinovitch, 1994; A. Porzionato et al., 2012; A. Porzionato et al., 2013).

Hyperoxia induced lung damage is known to activate many different cascades of intracellular signaling pathways, in particular, protein kinases such as mitogen-activated protein kinases (MAPKs). Extracellular signal-regulated kinase 1 and 2 (ERK 1/2), c-jun N-terminal kinase (JNK family), p38 kinase, and ERK5 are the four well known mammalian MAPK cascades (Plotnikov, Zehorai, Procaccia, & Seger, 2011) and these cascades can be activated by various extracellular stimuli, such as hyperoxia (Figure 2), which in turn control a wide range of cellular processes including cell growth, proliferation, differentiation, motility, stress responses, survival, and apoptosis (Lee & Choi, 2003; Plotnikov et al., 2011; Son et al., 2011; Zaher, Miller, Morrow, Javdan, & Mantell, 2007).

Hyperoxia and Cardiovascular Complications in Neonates

Although the effect of hyperoxia inducing pulmonary diseases is well known, its effects on other organs in both neonates and adults have only been under investigation more recently. Children born at premature condition or undergoing cardiopulmonary bypass (CPB) or extracorporeal membrane oxygenation (ECMO) require to be admitted to critical care units and are often exposed to high oxygen levels (Hyperoxia) during their stay (Allen, Barth, & Ilbawi, 2001; Aoshima et al., 1988; Rosenberg & Cook, 1991;

Figure 2. Hyperoxia induced lung damage via activation of MAPK cascade

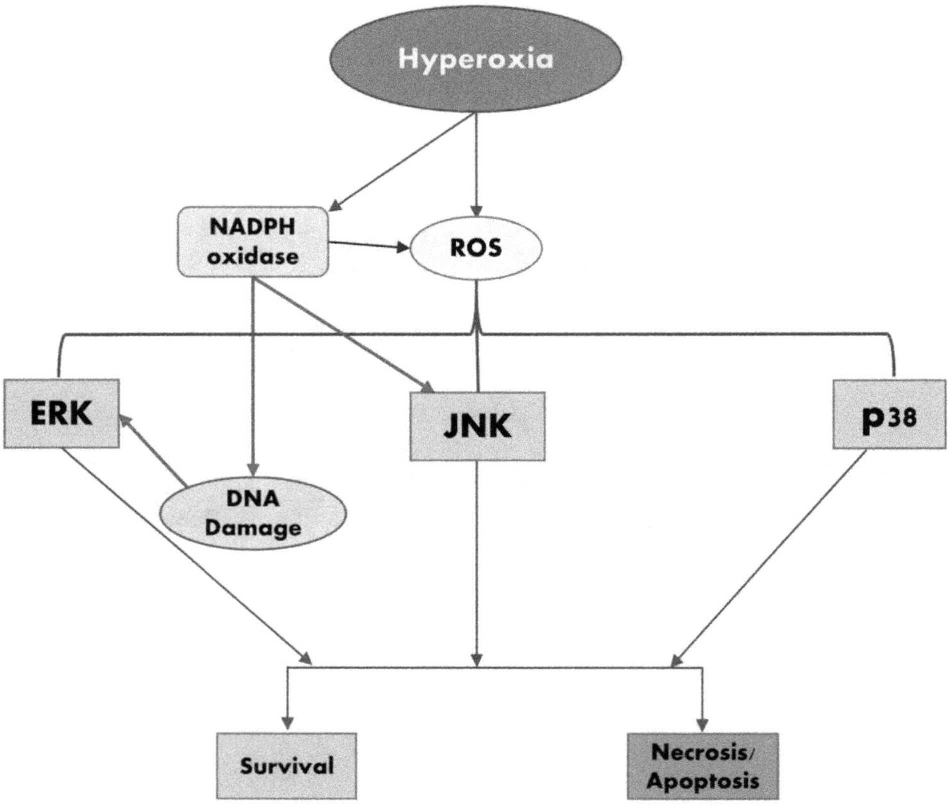

Wittnich, Torrance, & Carlyle, 2000). In order to identify whether the hyperoxia alone can compromise myocardial function and hemodynamic changes in newborn, Bandali et al. (2004) subjected Yorkshire piglets to either 5h of normoxia or hyperoxia, and myocardial function and hemodynamic assessments were recorded hourly (Bandali, Belanger, & Wittnich, 2004). Left ventricular (LV) biopsies were taken to measure the activity of antioxidant enzymes such as superoxide dismutase (SOD), glutathione peroxidase (GPx), and catalase (CAT) in this study. They also measured malondialdehyde (MDA) and 4-hydroxynonenal (4-HNE) as an indicators of oxygen free radical-mediated membrane injury. In this study they found that hyperoxia significantly reduced cardiac contractile function along with reduction of systolic blood pressure and mean atrial blood pressure. Significant reduction of SOD and GPx enzyme activities were observed in LV of these hyperoxia treated piglets, whereas significant elevation of MDA and 4-HNE, indicating the possibility of hyperoxia triggering oxygen free radical-mediated membrane injury in these newborn hearts together with an inability to upregulate its antioxidant enzyme defenses while impairing myocardial function and hemodynamics.

In a separate study to investigate whether the vascular function and blood pressure are altered in adult rats exposed to hyperoxic conditions as neonates also reported similar observation (Yzydorczyk et al., 2008). In this study the both male and female newborn rat pups were kept with their mother in hyperoxia (80% O_2) or room air from days 3 to 10 postnatal. Blood pressure was measured from weeks 7 to 15 and rats were euthanized to measure vascular reactivity, oxidative stress, microvascular density, and nephron counts. This study showed that neonatal hyperoxia leads in the adult rat to elevated blood pressure. Vascular dysfunction, microvascular rarefactions, and reduced nephron counts in both genders.

Hyperoxia and Cardiovascular Complications in Adults

Administration of 100% oxygen in patients treated with acute cardiac dysfunction is a common practice. Although this is done to enhance oxygenation to the tissue, supplementation of oxygen at 15 L/min through a nonrebreather mask for 1h has been shown to not only reduce heart rate and cardiac index (CI) but also increase systemic vascular resistance (SVR) and mean arterial pressure in healthy volunteers (Waring et al., 2003). Also hyperoxia treatment has been shown to reduce stroke volume in healthy volunteers (Thomson, Drummond, Waring, Webb, & Maxwell, 2006). Similarly other studies also confirmed the effect of hyperoxia on hemodynamic changes along with other cardiac functions including cardiac output, stroke volume, and left ventricular end diastolic pressure in both healthy subjects and patients with congestive cardiac failure (Haque et al., 1996; Mak, Azevedo, Liu, & Newton, 2001). Many other studies also reported that hyperoxia treatment affect coronary vascular blood flow (Farquhar et al., 2009; Ganz, Donoso, Marcus, & Swan, 1972; McNulty et al., 2005; McNulty et al., 2007).

Inflammation and oxidative stress are two well studies mechanisms taking a crucial role in the effects of hyperoxia. Cardiopulmonary bypass induces biomaterial-dependent and independent systemic inflammation (Spoelstra-de Man, Smit, Oudemans-van Straaten, & Smulders, 2015). The first one happens when blood touches artificial surfaces and changes the hemodynamic state like a continuous blood flow pattern during bypass (Elahi, Yii, & Matata, 2008); the second one appears during anesthesia; surgical trauma; cardioplegia; ischemia-reperfusion; release of endotoxin; transfusion; and changes in body temperature (Oudemans-van Straaten et al., 1996; Spoelstra-de Man et al., 2015). Altogether these influence a series of humoral and cell-mediated inflammatory responses including the activation of cytokines, adhesion molecules, arachidonic acid metabolites, endothelins, platelet-activating factors (Elahi et al., 2008), the complement system (Spoelstra-de Man et al., 2015), increase of total white blood cell count and number of circulating neutrophils.

In vivo studies with healthy rodents also reported an increase in oxidative stress and inflammation. For example a study on healthy mice exposed to 100% oxygen showed increased cellular infiltration of the lungs, secretion of the pro-inflammatory cytokines like tumor necrosis factor-α (TNF-a) and interleukin (IL-6) (Nagato et al., 2012). Likewise studies involving different septic models (lipopolysaccharide-induced lung inflammation or a caecal ligation and puncture sepsis model) where hyperoxia was induced elevated inflammatory and oxidative stress response (Rodriguez-Gonzalez et al., 2014; Waisman et al., 2012), organ inflammation and mortality (Thiel et al., 2005). There are also studies showing treatment 100% oxygen along with pretreatment of a ROS scavenger (e.g. Vitamin C or N-acetylcysteine) reduces serum levels of pro-inflammatory cytokines. This is the case on a zymosan-stimulated mice model in which serum levels of TNF-alpha, IL-6, and high-mobility group box 1 decreased, it also increased serum anti-inflammatory cytokine (IL-10), and upregulated tissue antioxidant enzymes such as superoxide dismutase, catalase, and glutathione peroxidase (Hou et al., 2010; Waisman et al., 2003; Young, 2012).

Ventricular Remodeling in Hyperoxia Induced Hearts

Hyperoxia or high oxygen concentrations are directly correlated to bronchopulmonary dysplasia (BPD), a common complication of prematurity, affecting approximately one-third of extremely low birth weight infants (Fanaroff et al., 1995; Walsh et al., 2006). Also many studies have reported that approximately 25-35% of infants with moderate to severe BPD develop other complications such as pulmonary hypertension, right ventricular hypertrophy (RVH), and right ventricle (RV) failure (An et al., 2010; Baker, Abman, & Mourani, 2014; Check et al., 2013; Khemani et al., 2007). The pathophysiological consequences of BPD are increase in pulmonary vascular resistance (PVR), which in turn increase afterload and strain on right ventricle. This increasing pressure load on right ventricle will further increase ventricular thickness, initially as a compensatory mechanism, but eventually can lead to RV dilation and failure (Bogaard, Abe, Vonk Noordegraaf, & Voelkel, 2009; Gien, Seedorf, Balasubramaniam, Markham, & Abman, 2007; Stenmark & Abman, 2005; Tsai & Kass, 2009).

Previous studies on mice exposed to neonatal hyperoxia induces alterations in cardiac structure and function leading to cardiac failure in adulthood (Velten et al., 2011). In this study the mice exposed to neonatal hyperoxia showed significantly lower LV wet weights and LV to body weight ratio compared to normoxia controls. Myosin filaments in the heart are composed of α and β subunits. In rodent hearts the myosin heavy chain-α (MHCα) levels predominates the expression of MHCβ levels in healthy cardiac tissue. MHCα has the highest ATPase activity and contractile velocity, whereas MHCβ has lowest contractile capability (Gustafson, Bahl, Markham, Roeske, & Morkin, 1987). Under pathological condition of cardiac remodeling and experimental heart failure, MHCβ levels predominates MHCα (Dillmann, 2010). Therefore, a decrease in MHCα/MHCβ ratio is used as a marker of cardiac hypertrophy (Hui et al., 2006). But in this study, where mice were exposed to neonatal hyperoxia showed increased MHCα expressions compared to MHCβ. Nevertheless, there are no reports on effect of hyperoxia in adult mice hearts until 2013, where we have shown for the first time that adult mice when exposed to hyperoxia conditions for 3 days significantly increase heart wet weight as well as heart weight to tibia length ratio when compared to its normoxia controls (Panguluri, Tur, Fukumoto, et al., 2013). In this study we also showed that both MHCα and MHCβ mRNA as well as protein levels were significantly elevated in hyperoxia treated mice hearts compared to its normoxia controls, suggesting that adult mice respond differently to hyperoxia conditions than the neonates. These findings are further evident by the increased LV wall thickness and overall cross sectional area in hyperoxia treated mice heart (cryostat sections treated with H&E staining) in our study compared with the normoxia controls.

As we know that structural remodeling will obviously influence the cardiac output and other hemodynamic changes, similar to other studies, hyperoxia exposed adult hearts in our study also showed significant reduction of heart rate, cardiac output (Bak, Sjoberg, Rousseau, Steinvall, & Janerot-Sjoberg, 2007; Gole et al., 2011; Howden et al., 2012a; Lund et al., 1999; Panguluri, Tur, Fukumoto, et al., 2013; Rousseau, Bak, Janerot-Sjoberg, & Sjoberg, 2005). The hyperoxia exposed neonates also showed cardiac dysfunction with significant increase in LV end systolic diameter and decreased fractional shortening (FS) (Velten et al., 2011). Taken together, all these studies clearly reported that hyperoxia can induce cardiac structural remodeling, which in turn cause cardiac dysfunction and heart failure via hemodynamic changes and cardiac output.

Electrical Remodeling in Hyperoxia Induced Hearts

Electric remodeling is one of the major characteristic of many cardiomyopathies (Costantini et al., 2005b; Nishiyama et al., 2001; Petkova-Kirova et al., 2006), which in turn leading to left ventricular hypertrophy and heart failure. Potassium channels and its auxiliary subunits such as potassium channel interacting protein-2 (KChIP2) are abundantly expressed in the heart (Brunet et al., 2004; Costantini et al., 2005b;

Teutsch et al., 2007). Of all the potassium channels Kv4.2 and Kv1.5 are responsive to oxygen changes (Perez-Garcia, Lopez-Lopez, & Gonzalez, 1999; Weir, Lopez-Barneo, Buckler, & Archer, 2005). Potassium channels are known to regulate the shape and duration of the action potential, which in turn governs the function of the heart. The outward potassium currents regulate the membrane potential and the action potential duration. Among the various members of potassium channel family (Kv1-12), the Kv4.2 (Voltage gate potassium channel: Kv4.2) is the major ion channel that helps the heart maintain the repolarization reserve.

Mechanical and electrophysiological dysfunctions in heart failure are often observed with reduction of Kv4.2 expressions and increased Kv1.4 expressions (Nishiyama et al., 2001; Qin et al., 2001). Qin et al. (Qin et al., 2001) in their study with streptozotocin (STZ) injected type I diabetic rats showed a significant reduction of Kv4.2, 4.3 and 2.1 transcript as well as protein levels in left ventricle. In another study, the STZ-induced diabetic rats showed a significant reduction of both Kv4.2 mRNA and protein levels and increased Kv1.4 transcripts and protein levels, but no significant change in Kv4.3 expression in ventricle (Nishiyama et al., 2001). They also showed an increase in MHC7 and reduced levels of MHC6 in diabetic rats. Similarly, our laboratory also showed that Kv4.2 and Kv1.5 expressions levels are significantly reduced in diabetic mice (db/db) hearts compared to their wild type controls (Panguluri, Tur, Chapalamadugu, et al., 2013). Although there are no reports on effect of hyperoxia on Kv channel expressions in adult hearts, for the first time our laboratory showed that Kv4.2 and Kv1.5 transcripts as well as protein expression are significantly reduced in hyperoxia treated mice hearts compared to normoxia controls, but no significant change in Kv1.4 at both transcriptional as well as translational levels (Chapalamadugu, Panguluri, Bennett, Kolliputi, & Tipparaju, 2015; Panguluri, Tur, Fukumoto, et al., 2013). In contrast to previous studies, we found a significant increase in transcripts of Kv2.1 and 4.3, which may be a compensatory mechanism for the loss of Kv4.2 expression in these hearts as both Kv4.2 and 4.3 are the molecular co-relates regulating transient outward currents (Ito_{fast}).

In addition to Kv4.2, the slowly inactivating potassium channel, Kv1.5 is also an important determinant of action potential duration in the ventricular myocytes (Fiset, Clark, Larsen, & Giles, 1997; Scheuermann-Freestone et al., 2003), the decreased expression of which is expected to reduce the cardiac repolarization reserve. Previous studies demonstrate that both Kv4.2 and Kv1.5 are sensitive to oxygen levels (Perez-Garcia et al., 1999; Pozeg, 2003), and altered expression and/or activity of these channels and Kvβ subunits (Fiset, Clark, Larsen, et al., 1997; Scheuermann-Freestone et al., 2003; Tipparaju et al., 2012a) modulate repolarization reserves. Due to down-regulation of Kv4.2 in hyperoxia treated hearts, our laboratory also investigated the expression of Kv1.5 gene in both hyperoxia treated as well as diabetic (db/db) mice hearts and showed that Kv1.5 is significantly down-regulated in these two conditions (Chapalamadugu et al., 2015; Panguluri, Tur, Chapalamadugu, et al., 2013).

Transcriptional factors plays a major role in regulating gene expressions in many cellular pathways, especially during pathological conditions. As we know that Kv channel regulation occur in many cardiomyopathies including hyperoxic conditions, our laboratory investigated the expression and activity of transcriptional factors that can regulate oxygen sensitive Kv4.2 and Kv1.5 including homeobox transcriptional factor Iroquois protein 5 (Irx5), nuclear factor kappa B (NFκB), GATA, Myocyte enhancer factor-2 (Mef2), C-terminal binding protein (CtBP), and SiRT1. Additionally Kv channel-interacting proteins (KChIP), which is a chaperon that binds to Kv4.2 and 4.3 was also investigated. Among all the isoforms, KChIP2 is most abundant and highly express in heart tissue and decreased levels of this chaperon has been previously reported in hypertrophy and heart failure (Kuo et al., 2001; Radicke et al., 2006). Recent studies by Jin et al. (Jin et al., 2010), showed that gene transfer of KChIP2 in neonatal cardiomyocytes increased Kv4.2 and 4.3 protein expressions and *in vivo* transfer of this gene in adult rats significantly reduced the left ventricular hypertrophy. As expected, down-regulation of Kv4.2 expression was also in line with the down-regulation of its interacting protein KChIP2 in diabetic mice (db/db) hearts compared to their wild type controls (Panguluri, Tur, Chapalamadugu, et al., 2013). Similarly, our laboratory also reported a significant down-regulation of KChIP2 mRNA as well as protein levels in hyperoxia treated hearts (Panguluri, Tur, Fukumoto, et al., 2013).

Homeobox transcriptional factor Iroquois protein 5 (Irx5), which is known to regulate Kv4.2 is reported to be differentially expressed in a gradient across the left ventricle of heart (Costantini et al., 2005a; Rosati, Grau, & McKinnon, 2006). Costantini et al. (Costantini et al., 2005a) also showed that Irx5 inhibit the activity of Kv4.2 promoter in dose-dependent manner with the association of a cardiac-specific corepressor, mBop. Our laboratory also investigated the expression of Kv4.2 repressor, Irx5 in both diabetic (db/db) and hyperoxia treated mice hearts and showed a significant increase in expression of irx5 in these hearts (Panguluri, Tur, Chapalamadugu, et al., 2013; Panguluri, Tur, Fukumoto, et al., 2013).

GATA4 and GATA6 are other important transcriptional factors, expression of which resembles Kv4.2 expression in heart and is known to be important in cardiac development and function (Laverriere et al., 1994). Recent investigation by Jia et al. (Jia & Takimoto, 2003) showed that GATA4 produce larger increase in Kv4.2 expression via its promoter than GATA6. Earlier reports also suggest that activation of GATA4 is associated with cardiac hypertrophy (Liang et al., 2001), and GATA4 also activate MHC-α promoter (Lu et al., 1999). These findings were further confirmed by investigations in our laboratory, which showed a significantly down-regulation of GATA4 and GATA6 in diabetic (db/db) hearts, but only GATA4 in hyperoxia treated hearts compared to their controls (Panguluri, Tur, Chapalamadugu, et al., 2013; Panguluri, Tur, Fukumoto, et al., 2013). This suggests a difference in molecular mechanism(s) of Kv channel regulation in hyperoxia treated hearts compared to diabetic hearts, although both these conditions share some similarity in pathophysiology.

Myocyte enhancer factor-2 (Mef2) is a transcriptional factor that regulate majority of muscle-specific genes (Amat et al., 2009; Black & Olson, 1998; Wei et al., 2008). This gene was also reported to have an important role in regulation of cardiac hypertrophy (Q. Lin, Schwarz, Bucana, & N. Olson, 1997; Streicher, Ren, Herschman, & Wang, 2010; Tessier & Storey, 2012). Due to its important role in cardiac hypertrophy and muscle cell differentiation, our laboratory examine the expression levels of this transcriptional factor and found that it is significant down-regulated in both hyperoxia treated mice hearts as well as diabetic (db/db) mice hearts (Panguluri, Tur, Chapalamadugu, et al., 2013; Panguluri, Tur, Fukumoto, et al., 2013).

Increasing expressions of nuclear factor kappa B (NFκB) is reported in cardiac hypertrophy and heart diseases (Gupta et al., 2008; Gupta, Young, & Sen, 2005; Higuchi et al., 2002; Purcell et al., 2001; Wong, Fukuchi, Melnyk, Rodger, & Giaid, 1998). In one study, activation of NFκB decreasing KChIP2 expressions and thereby $I_{to,f}$ and inhibition of its activity increased both (Panama et al., 2011). This was further supported by reports from our laboratory in which both diabetic (db/db) as well as hyperoxia treated mice hearts showed a significant increased expression and/or activity of NFκB. The down-regulation of Mef2c in these studies also correlate with the increasing expression and activity of NFκB, which inhibits the function of Mef2c (Kumar, Lin, SenBanerjee, & Jain, 2005). As the existing reports suggests that TNF-α induction in myocytes, increased both expression and activity of NFκB (Bhatnagar et al., 2010) and possibility of TNF-α in regulating Kv4.2 and KChIP2 gene expression levels (Kawada et al., 2006), our laboratory examined the intracellular concentrations of TNF-α in both hyperoxia treated and diabetic (db/db) micea hearts and found that the Kv4.2 and KChIP regulation in both cases are independent of TNF-α (Panguluri, Tur, Chapalamadugu, et al., 2013; Panguluri, Tur, Fukumoto, et al., 2013).

Alteration of various cellular signaling mechanisms such as oxidative stress is known to be associated with cardiac hypertrophy (Sawyer et al., 2002). Existing literature reported the disruption of Hif signaling (Heather & Clarke, 2011), and change in redox status of pyridine nucleotides in various diseased conditions (Ceconi et al., 2000; Ido, 2007). The C-terminal binding protein (CtBP) and SiRT1 are two such important regulators initiated during redox imbalance. The C-terminal binding protein (CtBP) is a transcriptional repressor that requires NAD^+ or NADH for its activity (Chinnadurai, 2003). Studies showed that hypoxic conditions increase NADH levels and activation of CtBP, which in turn interact with other transcriptional factor and thereby enhancing transcriptional repression (Chinnadurai, 2003). Another study showed that CtBP interacts with Mef2-interacting transcription repressor (MITR) and class II histone deacetylase (HDAC) and suppress the Mef2c transcriptional activity (C. L. Zhang, McKinsey, Lu, & Olson, 2001). Similarly, SiRT1 is known to be an important transcriptional repressor in cardiovascular and metabolic diseases, which has histone deacetylase activity (Pillarisetti, 2008). In contrast to CtBP, SiRT1 requires NAD^+ for its deacetylation reaction and increase in NADH levels reduces its activity (S. J. Lin, Ford, Haigis, Liszt, & Guarente, 2004). A wide range of cellular processes are regulated by SiRT1 which includes cell survival, apoptosis, cell growth and metabolism, and deacetylation of histones and non-histone proteins(Finkel, Deng, & Mostoslavsky, 2009). Increase in levels of SiRT1 is found in hypertrophied and failing hearts (Li et al., 2009; Vahtola et al., 2008). Studies also showed that the mice defective of SiRT1 exhibit severe developmental defects in the heart and most of them died after birth (Cheng et al., 2003; McBurney et al., 2003). Explorations in our laboratory on hyperoxia mice showed a significant increase in CtBP transcripts (unpublished data), whereas observed a significant reduction in its protein levels of SiRT1in left ventricle of hyperoxia treated mice (Chapalamadugu et al., 2015). In this study we also showed that reduced expression of SiRT1 is correlated with the down-regulation of Kv1.5, where inhibition of SiRT1 expression with Splitomicin (100 μM) significantly reduced Kv1.5 mRNA levels in cardiomyocytes.

Pulmonary and cardiovascular systems are known to be in cooperative regulation, therefore changes in cardiovascular systems influence pulmonary function and vice versa (Howden et al., 2012b). In a previous study continuous exposure of rabbits to hyperoxia for 72h caused changes in heart rate and low blood pressure (Sventek & Zambraski, 1988) indicating a close regulation between cardiovascular and pulmonary systems. We also know that under normal physiology the LV free wall depicts transmural heterogeneity of ionic currents and is important for physiological activity in the heart. Higher density of potassium outward current (I_{to}) is reported on epicardial region of the left ventricular free wall than that in the inside (Antzelevitch et al., 1991; Furukawa, Myerburg, Furukawa, Bassett, & Kimura, 1990; Liu, Gintant, & Antzelevitch, 1993). The ventricular repolarization occurs through this transmural gradient of I_{to} and travel from epicardium to endocardial portion. A large portion of this current is carried by family of Kv4 channels (Fiset, Clark, Shimoni, & Giles, 1997; Johns, Nuss, & Marban, 1997). As discussed above, suppression of Kv4.2 and its auxiliary protein KChIP2 affects I_{to} currents (Kuo et al., 2001; Panama et al., 2011) and transcriptional factors such as Irx5 and NFκB regulated Kv4.2 expressions (Costantini et al., 2005b; He, Jia, & Takimoto, 2009; Panguluri, Tur, Chapalamadugu, et al., 2013; Panguluri, Tur, Fukumoto, et al., 2013). Additionally hyperoxia exposure can cause hemodynamic changes that include bradycardia, decreased stroke volume and cardiac output (How et al., 2006; Panguluri, Tur, Fukumoto, et al., 2013; Seals, Johnson, & Fregosi, 1991). Therefore, our laboratory for the first time investigated if hyperoxia treatment affects electrical activity, repolarization reserve and susceptibility to ischemia reperfusion injury in the mouse heart. For this surface electrocardiogram (ECG) and ventricular monophasic action potentials (MAPs) recordings were utilized. From this study we reported that hyperoxia treatment causes bradyarrhythmia, with a significant bradycardia and multiple episodes of sinus pause (Chapalamadugu et al., 2015). Most importantly, hyperoxia exposure in this study altered QTc and JT interval significantly, which are key components of ECG measurement of repolarization reserve, which further suggests defects in cardiac repolarization reserve in the hyperoxia treated mice hearts (Crow, Hannan, & Folsom, 2003; Yan & Antzelevitch, 1998). At the tissue level, ventricular monophasic action potentials (MAPs) using *ex vivo* perfused hearts showed significant prolongation of action potential duration (APD) measured at different levels of repolarization, confirming repolarization defects in hyperoxia exposed hearts, which is in correlation with ECG data. Existing literature also suggested that the rapid repolarization accomplished by $I_{to,f}$ currents in ventricles supports the high resting heart rate in mice (Nerbonne & Kass, 2005). The slowly inactivating potassium channel, Kv1.5 is also an important determinant of action potential duration in the ventricular myocytes (Fiset, Clark, Larsen, et al., 1997; Scheuermann-Freestone et al., 2003), and decreased expression of Kv1.5 is expected to reduce the cardiac repolarization reserve. Previous studies demonstrate that both Kv4.2 and Kv1.5 are sensitive to oxygen levels (Perez-Garcia et al., 1999; Pozeg, 2003), and altered expression and/or activity of these channels and auxiliary subunits (Fiset, Clark, Larsen, et al., 1997; Scheuermann-Freestone et al., 2003; Tipparaju et al., 2012b) modulate repolarization reserves. Therefore, decreased expression of Kv1.5 (a molecular correlate of $I_{k,slow1}$ currents) in the mouse heart upon hyperoxia exposure further confirms that the repolarization deficits in hyperoxia treated mice hearts may at least in part regulated by these potassium channels (Chapalamadugu et al., 2015).

Kir2.1 is the major potassium channel responsible for maintaining cardiac resting membrane potential. Recent studies showed that miR-1 injected healthy hearts showed arrhythmic response and impaired inward rectifier K^+ current (I_{K1}) (Yang et al., 2007). In this study, the authors also showed that miR-1 targets Kir2.1 and cause arrhythmia. Studies from our laboratory showed that the transcript levels of *kcnj2* (Kir2.1) was significantly elevated in hyperoxia treated hearts (Panguluri, Tur, Fukumoto, et al., 2013), which further confirms the possible role of Kir2.1 in arrhythmic response in hyperoxia treated mice hearts (Chapalamadugu et al., 2015). Elevation of Kir2.1 in this study may be playing an important role by hyperpolarizing the resting membrane potential (RMP), which shortens the action potential duration (APD), and increase the CV. Recent studies by Milstein et al. (Milstein et al., 2012) showed that changes in functional expression of Kir2.1 modulates expression of Scn5a ($Na_V1.5$) and vice versa to alter cardiac excitability. Interestingly, data from our laboratory also showed a significant increase in transcript levels of Scn5a in hyperoxia treated mice hearts, which further confirms their findings (Panguluri, Tur, Fukumoto, et al., 2013).

CONCLUSION

Supplementing O_2 for enhancement of O_2 delivery is an essential process in cardiopulmonary disease management and end stage failure mainly occurring in lung fibrosis and heart failure patients. Pulmonary and cardiovascular systems are known to be in cooperative regulation, therefore changes in cardiovascular systems influence pulmonary function and vice versa. Although many studies have been reported on the effect of hyperoxia treatment in neonates, our laboratory for the first time reported the effect of hyperoxia on ventricular and electrical remodeling in adult mice hearts (Chapalamadugu et al., 2015;

Figure 3. Schematic representation of events occurring with hyperoxia leading to hypertrophy and arrhythmias. Here the lightly colored upwards arrow indicates up-regulation and the darker downwards arrow indicates down-regulation

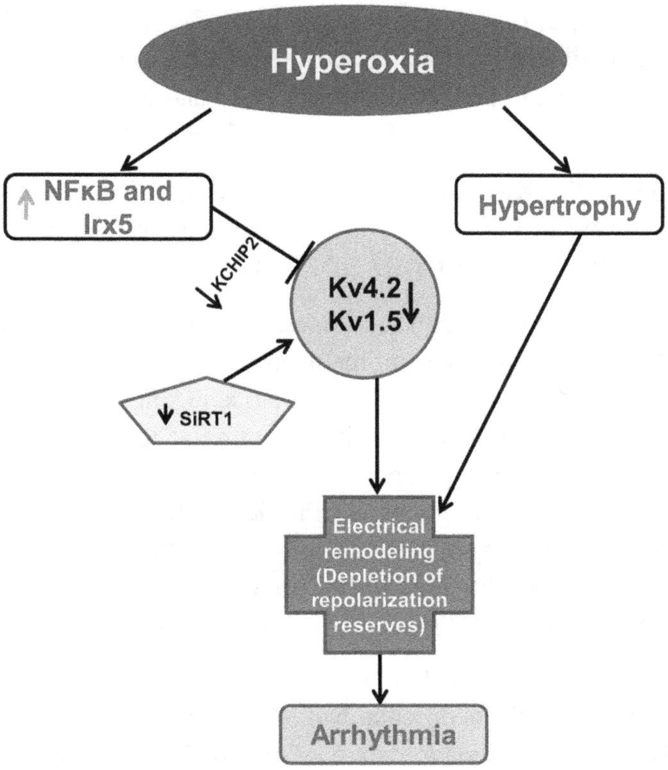

Panguluri, Tur, Fukumoto, et al., 2013). Based on the results obtained from our laboratory, it was evident that hyperoxia exposure for more than 3 days can significantly increase the expression and/or activity of key transcriptional factors such as NFκB and IRx5, which further down-regulates Kv4.2 and its chaperon KChIP2 in ventricles. Additionally, other transcriptional repressors SiRT1 inhibit the expressions of Kv1.5, which is also an important determinant of action potential duration in the ventricular myocytes. Together, the down-regulation of these two important oxygen sensitive Kv channels, further effects the electrical activity and repolarization reserves by prolonged QTc and JT intervals, as well as prolonged action potential durations (APDs). Bradycardia along with the multiple episodes of sinus pause further complicates the hyperoxia induced cardiomyopathy. Cardiac hypertrophy and altered hemodynamics are also added effects of hyperoxia treatment in adult mice hearts. Precisely, exposure of adult mice to hyperoxia for 3 days induces cardiac hypertrophy, ventricular and electrical remodeling by regulation of many key ion channel genes and transcriptional factors (Figure 3).

REFERENCES

Allen, B. S., Barth, M. J., & Ilbawi, M. N. (2001). Pediatric myocardial protection: An overview. *Seminars in Thoracic and Cardiovascular Surgery*, *13*(1), 56–72. doi:10.1053/stcs.2001.22738 PMID:11309728

Altemeier, W. A., & Sinclair, S. E. (2007). Hyperoxia in the intensive care unit: Why more is not always better. *Current Opinion in Critical Care, 13*(1), 73–78. doi:10.1097/MCC.0b013e32801162cb PMID:17198052

Amat, R., Planavila, A., Chen, S. L., Iglesias, R., Giralt, M., & Villarroya, F. (2009). SIRT1 Controls the Transcription of the Peroxisome Proliferator-activated Receptor-γ Co-activator-1α (PGC-1α) Gene in Skeletal Muscle through the PGC-1α Autoregulatory Loop and Interaction with MyoD. *The Journal of Biological Chemistry, 284*(33), 21872–21880. doi:10.1074/jbc.M109.022749 PMID:19553684

An, H. S., Bae, E. J., Kim, G. B., Kwon, B. S., Beak, J. S., Kim, E. K., & Yun, Y. S. et al. (2010). Pulmonary Hypertension in Preterm Infants With Bronchopulmonary Dysplasia. *Korean Circ J, 40*(3), 131–136. doi:10.4070/kcj.2010.40.3.131 PMID:20339498

Anderson, J. L., Adams, C. D., Antman, E. M., Bridges, C. R., Califf, R. M., Casey, D. E. Jr, & Riegel, B. et al. (2007). ACC/AHA 2007 guidelines for the management of patients with unstable angina/non-ST-elevation myocardial infarction: A report of the American College of Cardiology/American Heart Association task force on practice guidelines (writing committee to revise the 2002 guidelines for the management of patients with unstable angina/non-ST-elevation myocardial infarction) developed in collaboration with the American College of Emergency Physicians, the Society for Cardiovascular Angiography and Interventions, and the Society of Thoracic Surgeons endorsed by the American Association of Cardiovascular and Pulmonary Rehabilitation and the Society for Academic Emergency Medicine. *Journal of the American College of Cardiology, 50*(7), e1–e157. doi:10.1016/j.jacc.2007.02.013 PMID:17692738

Antzelevitch, C., Sicouri, S., Litovsky, S. H., Lukas, A., Krishnan, S. C., Di Diego, J. M., & Liu, D. W. et al. (1991). Heterogeneity within the ventricular wall. Electrophysiology and pharmacology of epicardial, endocardial, and M cells. *Circulation Research, 69*(6), 1427–1449. doi:10.1161/01.RES.69.6.1427 PMID:1659499

Aoshima, M., Yokota, M., Shiraishi, Y., Kyoku, I., Kitano, M., Shimada, I., & Mizuhara, S. (1988). Prolonged aortic cross-clamping in early infancy and method of myocardial preservation. *The Journal of Cardiovascular Surgery, 29*(5), 591–595. PMID:3182928

Bak, Z., Sjoberg, F., Rousseau, A., Steinvall, I., & Janerot-Sjoberg, B. (2007). Human cardiovascular dose-response to supplemental oxygen. *Acta Physiologica (Oxford, England), 191*(1), 15–24. doi:10.1111/j.1748-1716.2007.01710.x PMID:17506865

Baker, C. D., Abman, S. H., & Mourani, P. M. (2014). Pulmonary Hypertension in Preterm Infants with Bronchopulmonary Dysplasia. *Pediatric Allergy, Immunology, and Pulmonology, 27*(1), 8–16. doi:10.1089/ped.2013.0323 PMID:24669351

Balasubramaniam, V., Mervis, C. F., Maxey, A. M., Markham, N. E., & Abman, S. H. (2007). Hyperoxia reduces bone marrow, circulating, and lung endothelial progenitor cells in the developing lung: Implications for the pathogenesis of bronchopulmonary dysplasia. *American Journal of Physiology. Lung Cellular and Molecular Physiology, 292*(5), L1073–L1084. doi:10.1152/ajplung.00347.2006 PMID:17209139

Bandali, K. S., Belanger, M. P., & Wittnich, C. (2004). Hyperoxia causes oxygen free radical-mediated membrane injury and alters myocardial function and hemodynamics in the newborn. *American Journal of Physiology. Heart and Circulatory Physiology*, *287*(2), H553–H559. doi:10.1152/ajpheart.00657.2003 PMID:15277198

Bhatnagar, S., Panguluri, S. K., Gupta, S. K., Dahiya, S., Lundy, R. F., & Kumar, A. (2010). Tumor necrosis factor-alpha regulates distinct molecular pathways and gene networks in cultured skeletal muscle cells. *PLoS ONE*, *5*(10), e13262. doi:10.1371/journal.pone.0013262 PMID:20967264

Black, B. L., & Olson, E. N. (1998). Transcriptional control of muscle development by myocyte enhancer factor-2 (mef2) proteins. *Annual Review of Cell and Developmental Biology*, *14*(1), 167–196. doi:10.1146/annurev.cellbio.14.1.167 PMID:9891782

Bogaard, H. J., Abe, K., Vonk Noordegraaf, A., & Voelkel, N. F. (2009). The right ventricle under pressure: Cellular and molecular mechanisms of right-heart failure in pulmonary hypertension. *Chest*, *135*(3), 794–804. doi:10.1378/chest.08-0492 PMID:19265089

Brock, T. G., & Giulio, C. D. (2006). Prolonged Exposure to Hyperoxia Increases Perivascular Mast Cells in Rat Lungs. *The Journal of Histochemistry and Cytochemistry*, *54*(11), 1239–1246. doi:10.1369/jhc.6A7007.2006 PMID:16899761

Brunet, S., Aimond, F., Li, H., Guo, W., Eldstrom, J., Fedida, D., & Nerbonne, J. M. et al. (2004). Heterogeneous expression of repolarizing, voltage-gated K+ currents in adult mouse ventricles. *The Journal of Physiology*, *559*(Pt 1), 103–120. doi:10.1113/jphysiol.2004.063347 PMID:15194740

Cacciuttolo, M. A., Trinh, L., Lumpkin, J. A., & Rao, G. (1993). Hyperoxia induces DNA damage in mammalian cells. *Free Radical Biology & Medicine*, *14*(3), 267–276. doi:10.1016/0891-5849(93)90023-N PMID:8458584

Ceconi, C., Bernocchi, P., Boraso, A., Cargnoni, A., Pepi, P., Curello, S., & Ferrari, R. (2000). New insights on myocardial pyridine nucleotides and thiol redox state in ischemia and reperfusion damage. *Cardiovascular Research*, *47*(3), 586–594. doi:10.1016/S0008-6363(00)00104-8 PMID:10963731

Chapalamadugu, K. C., Panguluri, S. K., Bennett, E. S., Kolliputi, N., & Tipparaju, S. M. (2015). High level of oxygen treatment causes cardiotoxicity with arrhythmias and redox modulation. *Toxicology and Applied Pharmacology*, *282*(1), 100–107. doi:10.1016/j.taap.2014.10.019 PMID:25447406

Check, J., Gotteiner, N., Liu, X., Su, E., Porta, N., Steinhorn, R., & Mestan, K. K. (2013). Fetal growth restriction and pulmonary hypertension in premature infants with bronchopulmonary dysplasia. *Journal of Perinatology*, *33*(7), 553–557. doi:10.1038/jp.2012.164 PMID:23328924

Cheng, H. L., Mostoslavsky, R., Saito, S., Manis, J. P., Gu, Y., Patel, P., & Chua, K. F. et al. (2003). Developmental defects and p53 hyperacetylation in Sir2 homolog (SIRT1)-deficient mice. *Proceedings of the National Academy of Sciences of the United States of America*, *100*(19), 10794–10799. doi:10.1073/pnas.1934713100 PMID:12960381

Chinnadurai, G. (2003). CtBP family proteins: more than transcriptional corepressors. *BioEssays: News and Reviews in Molecular, Cellular and Developmental Biology, 25*(1), 9-12. doi: 10.1002/bies.10212

Costantini, D. L., Arruda, E. P., Agarwal, P., Kim, K. H., Zhu, Y., Zhu, W., & Bruneau, B. G. et al. (2005b). The homeodomain transcription factor Irx5 establishes the mouse cardiac ventricular repolarization gradient. *Cell*, *123*(2), 347–358. doi:10.1016/j.cell.2005.08.004 PMID:16239150

Costantini, D. L., Arruda, E. P., Agarwal, P., Kim, K. H., Zhu, Y. H., Zhu, W., & Bruneau, B. G. et al. (2005a). The homeodomain transcription factor lrx5 establishes the mouse cardiac ventricular repolarization gradient. *Cell*, *123*(2), 347–358. doi:10.1016/j.cell.2005.08.004 PMID:16239150

Crow, R. S., Hannan, P. J., & Folsom, A. R. (2003). Prognostic Significance of Corrected QT and Corrected JT Interval for Incident Coronary Heart Disease in a General Population Sample Stratified by Presence or Absence of Wide QRS Complex: The ARIC Study With 13 Years of Follow-Up. *Circulation*, *108*(16), 1985–1989. doi:10.1161/01.CIR.0000095027.28753.9D PMID:14517173

Damiani, E., Adrario, E., Girardis, M., Romano, R., Pelaia, P., Singer, M., & Donati, A. (2014). Arterial hyperoxia and mortality in critically ill patients: A systematic review and meta-analysis. *Critical Care (London, England)*, *18*(6), 711. doi:10.1186/s13054-014-0711-x PMID:25532567

Dauger, S., Ferkdadji, L., Saumon, G., Vardon, G., Peuchmaur, M., Gaultier, C., & Gallego, J. (2003). Neonatal Exposure to 65% Oxygen Durably Impairs Lung Architecture and Breathing Pattern in Adult Mice*. *Chest*, *123*(2), 530–538. doi:10.1378/chest.123.2.530 PMID:12576377

Demling, R., Lalonde, C., Youn, Y. K., & Picard, L. (1995). Effect of graded increases in smoke inhalation injury on the early systemic response to a body burn. *Critical Care Medicine*, *23*(1), 171–178. doi:10.1097/00003246-199501000-00027 PMID:8001368

Dickstein, K., Cohen-Solal, A., Filippatos, G., McMurray, J. J., Ponikowski, P., Poole-Wilson, P. A., & Tendera, M. et al. (2008). ESC guidelines for the diagnosis and treatment of acute and chronic heart failure 2008: The task force for the diagnosis and treatment of acute and chronic heart failure 2008 of the European Society of Cardiology. Developed in collaboration with the heart failure association of the ESC (HFA) and endorsed by the European Society of Intensive Care Medicine (ESICM). *European Heart Journal*, *29*(19), 2388–2442. doi:10.1093/eurheartj/ehn309 PMID:18799522

Dillmann, W. (2010). Cardiac hypertrophy and thyroid hormone signaling. *Heart Failure Reviews*, *15*(2), 125–132. doi:10.1007/s10741-008-9125-7 PMID:19125327

Elahi, M. M., Yii, M., & Matata, B. M. (2008). Significance of oxidants and inflammatory mediators in blood of patients undergoing cardiac surgery. *J Cardiothorac Vasc Anesth, 22*(3), 455-467. doi: 10.1053/j.jvca.2007.12.022

Fanaroff, A. A., Wright, L. L., Stevenson, D. K., Shankaran, S., Donovan, E. F., Ehrenkranz, R. A., & Verter, J. et al. (1995). Very-low-birth-weight outcomes of the National Institute of Child Health and Human Development Neonatal Research Network, May 1991 through December 1992. *American Journal of Obstetrics and Gynecology*, *173*(5), 1423–1431. doi:10.1016/0002-9378(95)90628-2 PMID:7503180

Farquhar, H., Weatherall, M., Wijesinghe, M., Perrin, K., Ranchord, A., Simmonds, M., & Beasley, R. (2009). Systematic review of studies of the effect of hyperoxia on coronary blood flow. *American Heart Journal*, *158*(3), 371–377. doi:10.1016/j.ahj.2009.05.037 PMID:19699859

Finkel, T., Deng, C. X., & Mostoslavsky, R. (2009). Recent progress in the biology and physiology of sirtuins. *Nature*, *460*(7255), 587–591. doi:10.1038/nature08197 PMID:19641587

Fiset, C., Clark, R. B., Larsen, T. S., & Giles, W. R. (1997). A rapidly activating sustained K+ current modulates repolarization and excitation-contraction coupling in adult mouse ventricle. *The Journal of Physiology*, *504*(Pt 3), 557–563. doi:10.1111/j.1469-7793.1997.557bd.x PMID:9401964

Fiset, C., Clark, R. B., Shimoni, Y., & Giles, W. R. (1997). Shal-type channels contribute to the Ca2+-independent transient outward K+ current in rat ventricle. *The Journal of Physiology*, *500*(Pt 1), 51–64. doi:10.1113/jphysiol.1997.sp021998 PMID:9097932

Furukawa, T., Myerburg, R. J., Furukawa, N., Bassett, A. L., & Kimura, S. (1990). Differences in transient outward currents of feline endocardial and epicardial myocytes. *Circulation Research*, *67*(5), 1287–1291. doi:10.1161/01.RES.67.5.1287 PMID:2225360

Ganz, W., Donoso, R., Marcus, H., & Swan, H. J. (1972). Coronary hemodynamics and myocardial oxygen metabolism during oxygen breathing in patients with and without coronary artery disease. *Circulation*, *45*(4), 763–768. doi:10.1161/01.CIR.45.4.763 PMID:5016013

Gien, J., Seedorf, G. J., Balasubramaniam, V., Markham, N., & Abman, S. H. (2007). Intrauterine pulmonary hypertension impairs angiogenesis in vitro: Role of vascular endothelial growth factor nitric oxide signaling. *American Journal of Respiratory and Critical Care Medicine*, *176*(11), 1146–1153. doi:10.1164/rccm.200705-750OC PMID:17823355

Gole, Y., Gargne, O., Coulange, M., Steinberg, J. G., Bouhaddi, M., Jammes, Y., & Boussuges, A. et al. (2011). Hyperoxia-induced alterations in cardiovascular function and autonomic control during return to normoxic breathing. *European Journal of Applied Physiology*, *111*(6), 937–946. doi:10.1007/s00421-010-1711-4 PMID:21069379

Grisafi, D., Pozzobon, M., Dedja, A., Vanzo, V., Tomanin, R., Porzionato, A., & Zaramella, P. et al. (2013). Human amniotic fluid stem cells protect rat lungs exposed to moderate hyperoxia. *Pediatric Pulmonology*, *48*(11), 1070–1080. doi:10.1002/ppul.22791 PMID:23533160

Grisafi, D., Tassone, E., Dedja, A., Oselladore, B., Masola, V., Guzzardo, V., & Zaramella, P. et al. (2012). L-citrulline Prevents Alveolar and Vascular Derangement in a Rat Model of Moderate Hyperoxia-induced Lung Injury. *Lung*, *190*(4), 419–430. doi:10.1007/s00408-012-9382-z PMID:22430123

Gupta, S., Young, D., Maitra, R. K., Gupta, A., Popovic, Z. B., Yong, S. L., & Sen, S. et al. (2008). Prevention of cardiac hypertrophy and heart failure by silencing of NF-kappaB. *Journal of Molecular Biology*, *375*(3), 637–649. doi:10.1016/j.jmb.2007.10.006 PMID:18037434

Gupta, S., Young, D., & Sen, S. (2005). Inhibition of NF-kappaB induces regression of cardiac hypertrophy, independent of blood pressure control, in spontaneously hypertensive rats. *American Journal of Physiology. Heart and Circulatory Physiology*, *289*(1), H20–H29. doi:10.1152/ajpheart.00082.2005 PMID:15749748

Gustafson, T. A., Bahl, J. J., Markham, B. E., Roeske, W. R., & Morkin, E. (1987). Hormonal regulation of myosin heavy chain and alpha-actin gene expression in cultured fetal rat heart myocytes. *The Journal of Biological Chemistry*, *262*(27), 13316–13322. PMID:2888758

Haque, W. A., Boehmer, J., Clemson, B. S., Leuenberger, U. A., Silber, D. H., & Sinoway, L. I. (1996). Hemodynamic effects of supplemental oxygen administration in congestive heart failure. *Journal of the American College of Cardiology*, *27*(2), 353–357. doi:10.1016/0735-1097(95)00474-2 PMID:8557905

He, W., Jia, Y., & Takimoto, K. (2009). Interaction between transcription factors Iroquois proteins 4 and 5 controls cardiac potassium channel Kv4.2 gene transcription. *Cardiovascular Research*, *81*(1), 64–71. doi:10.1093/cvr/cvn259 PMID:18815185

Heather, L. C., & Clarke, K. (2011). Metabolism, hypoxia and the diabetic heart. *Journal of Molecular and Cellular Cardiology*, *50*(4), 598–605. doi:10.1016/j.yjmcc.2011.01.007 PMID:21262230

Helmerhorst, H., Schultz, M., van der Voort, P., Bosman, R., Juffermans, N., de Jonge, E., & van Westerloo, D. (2014). Self-reported attitudes versus actual practice of oxygen therapy by ICU physicians and nurses. *Annals of Intensive Care*, *4*(1), 23. doi:10.1186/s13613-014-0023-y PMID:25512878

Higuchi, Y., Otsu, K., Nishida, K., Hirotani, S., Nakayama, H., Yamaguchi, O., & Hori, M. et al. (2002). Involvement of reactive oxygen species-mediated NF-kappa B activation in TNF-alpha-induced cardiomyocyte hypertrophy. *Journal of Molecular and Cellular Cardiology*, *34*(2), 233–240. doi:10.1006/jmcc.2001.1505 PMID:11851362

Hou, L., Xie, K., Qin, M., Peng, D., Ma, S., Shang, L., & Xiong, L. et al. (2010). Effects of reactive oxygen species scavenger on the protective action of 100% oxygen treatment against sterile inflammation in mice.[doi]. *Shock (Augusta, Ga.)*, *33*(6), 646–654. doi:10.1097/SHK.0b013e3181c1b5d4 PMID:19789462

How, O. J., Aasum, E., Severson, D. L., Chan, W. Y., Essop, M. F., & Larsen, T. S. (2006). Increased myocardial oxygen consumption reduces cardiac efficiency in diabetic mice. *Diabetes*, *55*(2), 466–473. doi:10.2337/diabetes.55.02.06.db05-1164 PMID:16443782

Howden, R., Cho, H. Y., Miller-DeGraff, L., Walker, C., Clark, J. A., Myers, P. H., & Kleeberger, S. R. et al. (2012a). Cardiac physiologic and genetic predictors of hyperoxia-induced acute lung injury in mice. *American Journal of Respiratory Cell and Molecular Biology*, *46*(4), 470–478. doi:10.1165/rcmb.2011-0204OC PMID:22052878

Howden, R., Cho, H. Y., Miller-DeGraff, L., Walker, C., Clark, J. A., Myers, P. H., & Kleeberger, S. R. et al. (2012b). Cardiac physiologic and genetic predictors of hyperoxia-induced acute lung injury in mice. *American Journal of Respiratory Cell and Molecular Biology*, *46*(4), 470–478. doi:10.1165/rcmb.2011-0204OC PMID:22052878

Hui, H. P., Li, X. Y., Liu, X. H., Sun, S., Lu, X. C., Liu, T., & Yang, W. (2006). Adeno-associated viral gene transfer of SERCA2a improves heart function in chronic congestive heart failure rats. *Zhonghua Xin Xue Guan Bing Za Zhi*, *34*(4), 357–362. PMID:16776934

Ido, Y. (2007). Pyridine nucleotide redox abnormalities in diabetes. *Antioxidants & Redox Signalling*, *9*(7), 931–942. doi:10.1089/ars.2007.1630 PMID:17508915

Jia, Y., & Takimoto, K. (2003). GATA and FOG2 transcription factors differentially regulate the promoter for Kv4.2 K+ channel gene in cardiac myocytes and PC12 cells. *Cardiovascular Research*, *60*(2), 278–287. doi:10.1016/S0008-6363(03)00528-5 PMID:14613857

Jin, H., Hadri, L., Palomeque, J., Morel, C., Karakikes, I., Kaprielian, R., & Lebeche, D. et al. (2010). KChIP2 attenuates cardiac hypertrophy through regulation of Ito and intracellular calcium signaling. *Journal of Molecular and Cellular Cardiology*, *48*(6), 1169–1179. doi:10.1016/j.yjmcc.2009.12.019 PMID:20051248

Johns, D. C., Nuss, H. B., & Marban, E. (1997). Suppression of neuronal and cardiac transient outward currents by viral gene transfer of dominant-negative Kv4.2 constructs. *The Journal of Biological Chemistry*, *272*(50), 31598–31603. doi:10.1074/jbc.272.50.31598 PMID:9395498

Jones, R. H. (1984). Must Enlightened Mystics Be Moral? *Philosophy East & West*, *34*(3), 273–293. doi:10.2307/1398629

Kallet, R. H., & Matthay, M. A. (2013). Hyperoxic Acute Lung Injury. *Respiratory Care*, *58*(1), 123–141. doi:10.4187/respcare.01963 PMID:23271823

Kawada, H., Niwano, S., Niwano, H., Yumoto, Y., Wakisaka, Y., Yuge, M.,... Izumi, T. (2006). Tumor necrosis factor-alpha downregulates the voltage gated outward K+ current in cultured neonatal rat cardiomyocytes: a possible cause of electrical remodeling in diseased hearts. *Circulation Journal: Official Journal of the Japanese Circulation Society, 70*(5), 605-609.

Khemani, E., McElhinney, D. B., Rhein, L., Andrade, O., Lacro, R. V., Thomas, K. C., & Mullen, M. P. (2007). Pulmonary artery hypertension in formerly premature infants with bronchopulmonary dysplasia: Clinical features and outcomes in the surfactant era. *Pediatrics*, *120*(6), 1260–1269. doi:10.1542/peds.2007-0971 PMID:18055675

Kilgannon, J. H., Jones, A. E., Shapiro, N. I., Angelos, M. G., Milcarek, B., & Hunter, K.Emergency Medicine Shock Research Network, Investigators. (2010). Association between arterial hyperoxia following resuscitation from cardiac arrest and in-hospital mortality. *Journal of the American Medical Association*, *303*(21), 2165–2171. doi:10.1001/jama.2010.707 PMID:20516417

Koppel, R., Han, R. N. N., Cox, D., Tanswell, A. K., & Rabinovitch, M. (1994). [alpha]1-Antitrypsin Protects Neonatal Rats from Pulmonary Vascular and Parenchymal Effects of Oxygen Toxicity. *Pediatric Research*, *36*(6), 763–770. doi:10.1203/00006450-199412000-00014 PMID:7898985

Kumar, A., Lin, Z., SenBanerjee, S., & Jain, M. K. (2005). Tumor necrosis factor alpha-mediated reduction of KLF2 is due to inhibition of MEF2 by NF-kappaB and histone deacetylases. *Molecular and Cellular Biology*, *25*(14), 5893–5899. doi:10.1128/MCB.25.14.5893-5903.2005 PMID:15988006

Kuo, H. C., Cheng, C. F., Clark, R. B., Lin, J. J., Lin, J. L., Hoshijima, M., & Chien, K. R. et al. (2001). A defect in the Kv channel-interacting protein 2 (KChIP2) gene leads to a complete loss of I(to) and confers susceptibility to ventricular tachycardia. *Cell*, *107*(6), 801–813. doi:10.1016/S0092-8674(01)00588-8 PMID:11747815

Laverriere, A. C., MacNeill, C., Mueller, C., Poelmann, R. E., Burch, J. B., & Evans, T. (1994). GATA-4/5/6, a subfamily of three transcription factors transcribed in developing heart and gut. *The Journal of Biological Chemistry*, *269*(37), 23177–23184. PMID:8083222

Lee, P. J., & Choi, A. M. K. (2003). Pathways of cell signaling in hyperoxia. *Free Radical Biology & Medicine*, *35*(4), 341–350. doi:10.1016/S0891-5849(03)00279-X PMID:12899937

Li, L., Zhao, L., Yi-Ming, W., Yu, Y. S., Xia, C. Y., Duan, J. L., & Su, D. F. (2009). Sirt1 hyperexpression in SHR heart related to left ventricular hypertrophy. *Canadian Journal of Physiology and Pharmacology, 87*(1), 56–62. doi:10.1139/Y08-099 PMID:19142216

Liang, Q., De Windt, L. J., Witt, S. A., Kimball, T. R., Markham, B. E., & Molkentin, J. D. (2001). The transcription factors GATA4 and GATA6 regulate cardiomyocyte hypertrophy in vitro and in vivo. *The Journal of Biological Chemistry, 276*(32), 30245–30253. doi:10.1074/jbc.M102174200 PMID:11356841

Lin, Q., Schwarz, J., Bucana, C., & Olson, N. (1997). Control of Mouse Cardiac Morphogenesis and Myogenesis by Transcription Factor MEF2C. *Science, 276*(5317), 1404–1407. doi:10.1126/science.276.5317.1404 PMID:9162005

Lin, S. J., Ford, E., Haigis, M., Liszt, G., & Guarente, L. (2004). Calorie restriction extends yeast life span by lowering the level of NADH. *Genes & Development, 18*(1), 12–16. doi:10.1101/gad.1164804 PMID:14724176

Liu, D. W., Gintant, G. A., & Antzelevitch, C. (1993). Ionic bases for electrophysiological distinctions among epicardial, midmyocardial, and endocardial myocytes from the free wall of the canine left ventricle. *Circulation Research, 72*(3), 671–687. doi:10.1161/01.RES.72.3.671 PMID:8431990

Lu, J. R., McKinsey, T. A., Xu, H., Wang, D. Z., Richardson, J. A., & Olson, E. N. (1999). FOG-2, a heart- and brain-enriched cofactor for GATA transcription factors. *Molecular and Cellular Biology, 19*(6), 4495–4502. doi:10.1128/MCB.19.6.4495 PMID:10330188

Lund, V. E., Kentala, E., Scheinin, H., Klossner, J., Helenius, H., Sariola-Heinonen, K., & Jalonen, J. (1999). Heart rate variability in healthy volunteers during normobaric and hyperbaric hyperoxia. *Acta Physiologica Scandinavica, 167*(1), 29–35. doi:10.1046/j.1365-201x.1999.00581.x PMID:10519974

Mak, S., Azevedo, E. R., Liu, P. P., & Newton, G. E. (2001). Effect of hyperoxia on left ventricular function and filling pressures in patients with and without congestive heart failure. *Chest, 120*(2), 467–473. doi:10.1378/chest.120.2.467 PMID:11502645

Mantell, L. L., & Lee, P. J. (2000). Signal transduction pathways in hyperoxia-induced lung cell death. *Molecular Genetics and Metabolism, 71*(1-2), 359–370. doi:10.1006/mgme.2000.3046 PMID:11001828

McBurney, M. W., Yang, X., Jardine, K., Hixon, M., Boekelheide, K., Webb, J. R., & Lemieux, M. et al. (2003). The mammalian SIR2alpha protein has a role in embryogenesis and gametogenesis. *Molecular and Cellular Biology, 23*(1), 38–54. doi:10.1128/MCB.23.1.38-54.2003 PMID:12482959

McNulty, P. H., King, N., Scott, S., Hartman, G., McCann, J., Kozak, M., & Sinoway, L. I. et al. (2005). Effects of supplemental oxygen administration on coronary blood flow in patients undergoing cardiac catheterization. *American Journal of Physiology. Heart and Circulatory Physiology, 288*(3), H1057–H1062. doi:10.1152/ajpheart.00625.2004 PMID:15706043

McNulty, P. H., Robertson, B. J., Tulli, M. A., Hess, J., Harach, L. A., Scott, S., & Sinoway, L. I. (2007). Effect of hyperoxia and vitamin C on coronary blood flow in patients with ischemic heart disease. *J Appl Physiol (1985), 102*(5), 2040-2045. doi: 10.1152/japplphysiol.00595.2006

Milstein, M. L., Musa, H., Balbuena, D. P., Anumonwo, J. M. B., Auerbach, D. S., Furspan, P. B., & Jalife, J. et al. (2012). Dynamic reciprocity of sodium and potassium channel expression in a macromolecular complex controls cardiac excitability and arrhythmia.*Proceedings of the National Academy of Sciences*. doi:10.1073/pnas.1109370109

Nagato, A. C., Bezerra, F. S., Lanzetti, M., Lopes, A. A., Silva, M. A., Porto, L. C., & Valenca, S. S. (2012). Time course of inflammation, oxidative stress and tissue damage induced by hyperoxia in mouse lungs. *International Journal of Experimental Pathology*, *93*(4), 269–278. doi:10.1111/j.1365-2613.2012.00823.x PMID:22804763

Nelskyla, A., Parr, M. J., & Skrifvars, M. B. (2013). Prevalence and factors correlating with hyperoxia exposure following cardiac arrest - an observational single centre study. *Scan J Trauma Resusc Emerg Med*, *21*(1), 35. doi:10.1186/1757-7241-21-35 PMID:23639102

Nerbonne, J. M., & Kass, R. S. (2005). Molecular physiology of cardiac repolarization. *Physiological Reviews*, *85*(4), 1205–1253. doi:10.1152/physrev.00002.2005 PMID:16183911

Nishiyama, A., Ishii, D. N., Backx, P. H., Pulford, B. E., Birks, B. R., & Tamkun, M. M. (2001). Altered K(+) channel gene expression in diabetic rat ventricle: Isoform switching between Kv4.2 and Kv1.4. *American Journal of Physiology. Heart and Circulatory Physiology*, *281*(4), H1800–H1807. PMID:11557574

ODriscoll, R., Davison, A., Elliott, M., Howard, L., Wedzicha, J., Mackway-Jones, K., & Hinshaw, K. et al. (2008). BTS guideline for emergency oxygen use in adult patients. *Thorax*, *63*(Supplement 6), vi1–vi68. doi:10.1136/thx.2008.102947 PMID:18838559

Oudemans-van Straaten, H. M., Jansen, P. G., Hoek, F. J., van Deventer, S. J., Sturk, A., Stoutenbeek, C. P.,... Eysman, L. (1996). Intestinal permeability, circulating endotoxin, and postoperative systemic responses in cardiac surgery patients. *J Cardiothorac Vasc Anesth*, *10*(2), 187-194. doi: S1053-0770(96)80235-7 [pii]

Panama, B. K., Latour-Villamil, D., Farman, G. P., Zhao, D., Bolz, S. S., Kirshenbaum, L. A., & Backx, P. H. (2011). Nuclear factor kappaB downregulates the transient outward potassium current I(to,f) through control of KChIP2 expression. *Circulation Research*, *108*(5), 537–543. doi:10.1161/CIRCRESAHA.110.229112 PMID:21252158

Panguluri, S. K., Tur, J., Chapalamadugu, K. C., Katnik, C., Cuevas, J., & Tipparaju, S. M. (2013). MicroRNA-301a mediated regulation of Kv4.2 in diabetes: Identification of key modulators. *PLoS ONE*, *8*(4), e60545. doi:10.1371/journal.pone.0060545 PMID:23573265

Panguluri, S. K., Tur, J., Fukumoto, J., Deng, W., Sneed, K. B., Kolliputi, N., & Tipparaju, S. M. et al. (2013). Hyperoxia-induced hypertrophy and ion channel remodeling in left ventricle. *American Journal of Physiology. Heart and Circulatory Physiology*, *304*(12), H1651–H1661. doi:10.1152/ajpheart.00474.2012 PMID:23585127

Perez-Garcia, M. T., Lopez-Lopez, J. R., & Gonzalez, C. (1999). Kvbeta1.2 subunit coexpression in HEK293 cells confers O2 sensitivity to kv4.2 but not to Shaker channels. *The Journal of General Physiology*, *113*(6), 897–907. doi:10.1085/jgp.113.6.897 PMID:10352037

Petkova-Kirova, P. S., Gursoy, E., Mehdi, H., McTiernan, C. F., London, B., & Salama, G. (2006). Electrical remodeling of cardiac myocytes from mice with heart failure due to the overexpression of tumor necrosis factor-alpha. *American Journal of Physiology. Heart and Circulatory Physiology*, *290*(5), H2098–H2107. doi:10.1152/ajpheart.00097.2005 PMID:16339842

Petrache, I., Choi, M. E., Otterbein, L. E., Chin, B. Y., Mantell, L. L., Horowitz, S., & Choi, A. M. K. (1999). Mitogen-activated protein kinase pathway mediates hyperoxia-induced apoptosis in cultured macrophage cells. *American Journal of Physiology. Lung Cellular and Molecular Physiology*, *277*(3), L589–L595. PMID:10484467

Pillarisetti, S. (2008). A review of Sirt1 and Sirt1 modulators in cardiovascular and metabolic diseases. *Recent Patents on Cardiovascular Drug Discovery*, *3*(3), 156–164. doi:10.2174/157489008786263989 PMID:18991791

Plotnikov, A., Zehorai, E., Procaccia, S., & Seger, R. (2011). The MAPK cascades: Signaling components, nuclear roles and mechanisms of nuclear translocation. *Biochimica et Biophysica Acta*, *1813*(9), 1619–1633. doi:10.1016/j.bbamcr.2010.12.012 PMID:21167873

Porzionato, A., Sfriso, M. M., Mazzatenta, A., Macchi, V., De Caro, R., & Di Giulio, C. (2015). Effects of hyperoxic exposure on signal transduction pathways in the lung. *Respiratory Physiology & Neurobiology*, *209*, 106–114. doi:10.1016/j.resp.2014.12.002 PMID:25485998

Porzionato, A., Zaramella, P., Macchi, V., Grisafi, D., Salmaso, R., Baraldi, M., & De Caro, R. et al. (2012). Fluoxetine may worsen hyperoxia-induced lung damage in neonatal rats. *Histology and Histopathology*, *27*(12), 1599–1610. PMID:23059890

Porzionato, A., Zaramella, P., Macchi, V., Sarasin, G., Di Giulio, C., Rigon, A., & De Caro, R. et al. (2013). Cyclosporine and hyperoxia-induced lung damage in neonatal rats. *Respiratory Physiology & Neurobiology*, *187*(1), 41–46. doi:10.1016/j.resp.2013.02.018 PMID:23454024

Pozeg, Z. I. (2003). In Vivo Gene Transfer of the O2-Sensitive Potassium Channel Kv1.5 Reduces Pulmonary Hypertension and Restores Hypoxic Pulmonary Vasoconstriction in Chronically Hypoxic Rats. *Circulation*, *107*(15), 2037–2044. doi:10.1161/01.CIR.0000062688.76508.B3 PMID:12695303

Purcell, N. H., Tang, G., Yu, C., Mercurio, F., DiDonato, J. A., & Lin, A. (2001). Activation of NF-kappa B is required for hypertrophic growth of primary rat neonatal ventricular cardiomyocytes. *Proceedings of the National Academy of Sciences of the United States of America*, *98*(12), 6668–6673. doi:10.1073/pnas.111155798 PMID:11381115

Qin, D., Huang, B., Deng, L., El-Adawi, H., Ganguly, K., Sowers, J. R., & El-Sherif, N. (2001). Downregulation of K(+) channel genes expression in type I diabetic cardiomyopathy. *Biochemical and Biophysical Research Communications*, *283*(3), 549–553. doi:10.1006/bbrc.2001.4825 PMID:11341759

Radicke, S., Cotella, D., Graf, E. M., Banse, U., Jost, N., Varro, A., & Wettwer, E. et al. (2006). Functional modulation of the transient outward current Ito by KCNE beta-subunits and regional distribution in human non-failing and failing hearts. *Cardiovascular Research*, *71*(4), 695–703. doi:10.1016/j.cardiores.2006.06.017 PMID:16876774

Rincon, F., Kang, J., Maltenfort, M., Vibbert, M., Urtecho, J., Athar, M. K., & Bell, R. et al. (2014). Association between hyperoxia and mortality after stroke: A multicenter cohort study. *Critical Care Medicine*, *42*(2), 387–396. doi:10.1097/CCM.0b013e3182a27732 PMID:24164953

Rincon, F., Kang, J., Vibbert, M., Urtecho, J., Athar, M. K., & Jallo, J. (2014). Significance of arterial hyperoxia and relationship with case fatality in traumatic brain injury: A multicentre cohort study. *Journal of Neurology, Neurosurgery, and Psychiatry*, *85*(7), 799–805. doi:10.1136/jnnp-2013-305505 PMID:23794718

Rodriguez-Gonzalez, R., Martin-Barrasa, J. L., Ramos-Nuez, A., Canas-Pedrosa, A. M., Martinez-Saavedra, M. T., Garcia-Bello, M. A., & Villar, J. et al. (2014). Multiple system organ response induced by hyperoxia in a clinically relevant animal model of sepsis. *Shock (Augusta, Ga.)*, *42*(2), 148–153. doi:10.1097/SHK.0000000000000189 PMID:24978892

Rosati, B., Grau, F., & McKinnon, D. (2006). Regional variation in rnRNA transcript abundance within the ventricular wall. *Journal of Molecular and Cellular Cardiology*, *40*(2), 295–302. doi:10.1016/j.yjmcc.2005.11.002 PMID:16412459

Rosenberg, E. M., & Cook, L. N. (1991). Electromechanical dissociation in newborns treated with extracorporeal membrane oxygenation: An extreme form of cardiac stun syndrome. *Critical Care Medicine*, *19*(6), 780–784. doi:10.1097/00003246-199106000-00009 PMID:2055055

Rousseau, A., Bak, Z., Janerot-Sjoberg, B., & Sjoberg, F. (2005). Acute hyperoxaemia-induced effects on regional blood flow, oxygen consumption and central circulation in man. *Acta Physiologica Scandinavica*, *183*(3), 231–240. doi:10.1111/j.1365-201X.2005.01405.x PMID:15743383

Sawyer, D. B., Siwik, D. A., Xiao, L., Pimentel, D. R., Singh, K., & Colucci, W. S. (2002). Role of oxidative stress in myocardial hypertrophy and failure. *Journal of Molecular and Cellular Cardiology*, *34*(4), 379–388. doi:10.1006/jmcc.2002.1526 PMID:11991728

Scheuermann-Freestone, M., Madsen, P. L., Manners, D., Blamire, A. M., Buckingham, R. E., Styles, P., & Clarke, K. et al. (2003). Abnormal cardiac and skeletal muscle energy metabolism in patients with type 2 diabetes. *Circulation*, *107*(24), 3040–3046. doi:10.1161/01.CIR.0000072789.89096.10 PMID:12810608

Seals, D. R., Johnson, D. G., & Fregosi, R. F. (1991). Hyperoxia lowers sympathetic activity at rest but not during exercise in humans. *American Journal of Physiology. Regulatory, Integrative and Comparative Physiology*, *260*(5), R873–R878. PMID:2035699

Son, Y., Cheong, Y.-K., Kim, N.-H., Chung, H.-T., Kang, D. G., & Pae, H.-O. (2011). Mitogen-Activated Protein Kinases and Reactive Oxygen Species: How Can ROS Activate MAPK Pathways? *Journal of Signal Transduction*, *792639*. doi:10.1155/2011/792639 PMID:21637379

Spoelstra-de Man, A. M., Smit, B., Oudemans-van Straaten, H. M., & Smulders, Y. M. (2015). Cardiovascular effects of hyperoxia during and after cardiac surgery. *Anaesthesia*, *70*(11), 1307–1319. doi:10.1111/anae.13218 PMID:26348878

Stenmark, K. R., & Abman, S. H. (2005). Lung vascular development: Implications for the pathogenesis of bronchopulmonary dysplasia. *Annual Review of Physiology*, *67*(1), 623–661. doi:10.1146/annurev.physiol.67.040403.102229 PMID:15709973

Streicher, J. M., Ren, S., Herschman, H., & Wang, Y. (2010). MAPK-Activated Protein Kinase-2 in Cardiac Hypertrophy and Cyclooxygenase-2 Regulation in Heart. *Circulation Research*, *106*(8), 1434–1443. doi:10.1161/CIRCRESAHA.109.213199 PMID:20339119

Sventek, J. C., & Zambraski, E. J. (1988). Effects of chronic hyperoxia on the cardiovascular responses to vasoactive compounds in the rabbit. *Aviation, Space, and Environmental Medicine*, *59*(4), 314–320. PMID:3163478

Tessier, S. N., & Storey, K. B. (2012). Myocyte enhancer factor-2 and cardiac muscle gene expression during hibernation in thirteen-lined ground squirrels. *Gene*, *501*(1), 8–16. doi:10.1016/j.gene.2012.04.004 PMID:22513076

Teutsch, C., Kondo, R. P., Dederko, D. A., Chrast, J., Chien, K. R., & Giles, W. R. (2007). Spatial distributions of Kv4 channels and KChip2 isoforms in the murine heart based on laser capture microdissection. *Cardiovascular Research*, *73*(4), 739–749. doi:10.1016/j.cardiores.2006.11.034 PMID:17289005

Thébaud, B., & Abman, S. H. (2007). Bronchopulmonary Dysplasia. *American Journal of Respiratory and Critical Care Medicine*, *175*(10), 978–985. doi:10.1164/rccm.200611-1660PP PMID:17272782

Thiel, M., Chouker, A., Ohta, A., Jackson, E., Caldwell, C., Smith, P.,... Sitkovsky, M. V. (2005). Oxygenation inhibits the physiological tissue-protecting mechanism and thereby exacerbates acute inflammatory lung injury. *PLoS Biol, 3*(6), e174. doi: 10.1371/journal.pbio.0030174

Thomson, A. J., Drummond, G. B., Waring, W. S., Webb, D. J., & Maxwell, S. R. (2006). Effects of short-term isocapnic hyperoxia and hypoxia on cardiovascular function. *J Appl Physiol (1985), 101*(3), 809-816. doi: 10.1152/japplphysiol.01185.2005

Tipparaju, S. M., Li, X. P., Kilfoil, P. J., Xue, B., Uversky, V. N., Bhatnagar, A., & Barski, O. A. (2012a). Interactions between the C-terminus of Kv1.5 and Kvbeta regulate pyridine nucleotide-dependent changes in channel gating. *Pflugers Archiv*, *463*(6), 799–818. doi:10.1007/s00424-012-1093-z PMID:22426702

Tipparaju, S. M., Li, X. P., Kilfoil, P. J., Xue, B., Uversky, V. N., Bhatnagar, A., & Barski, O. A. (2012b). Interactions between the C-terminus of Kv1.5 and Kvbeta regulate pyridine nucleotide-dependent changes in channel gating. *Pflugers Archiv: European journal of physiology, 463*(6), 799-818. doi: 10.1007/s00424-012-1093-z

Tsai, E. J., & Kass, D. A. (2009). Cyclic GMP signaling in cardiovascular pathophysiology and therapeutics. *Pharmacology & Therapeutics*, *122*(3), 216–238. doi:10.1016/j.pharmthera.2009.02.009 PMID:19306895

Vahtola, E., Louhelainen, M., Merasto, S., Martonen, E., Penttinen, S., Aahos, I., & Mervaala, E. et al. (2008). Forkhead class O transcription factor 3a activation and Sirtuin1 overexpression in the hypertrophied myocardium of the diabetic Goto-Kakizaki rat. *Journal of Hypertension*, *26*(2), 334–344. doi:10.1097/HJH.0b013e3282f293c8 PMID:18192848

Velten, M., Hutchinson, K. R., Gorr, M. W., Wold, L. E., Lucchesi, P. A., & Rogers, L. K. (2011). Systemic Maternal Inflammation and Neonatal Hyperoxia Induces Remodeling and Left Ventricular Dysfunction in Mice. *PLoS ONE*, *6*(9), e24544. doi:10.1371/journal.pone.0024544 PMID:21935422

Visser, Y. P., Walther, F. J., Laghmani, E. H., Laarse, A., & Wagenaar, G. T. M. (2010). Apelin attenuates hyperoxic lung and heart injury in neonatal rats. *American Journal of Respiratory and Critical Care Medicine*, *182*(10), 1239–1250. doi:10.1164/rccm.200909-1361OC PMID:20622042

Waisman, D., Brod, V., Rahat, M. A., Amit-Cohen, B. C., Lahat, N., Rimar, D., & Bitterman, H. et al. (2012). Dose-related effects of hyperoxia on the lung inflammatory response in septic rats.[doi]. *Shock (Augusta, Ga.)*, *37*(1), 95–102. doi:10.1097/SHK.0b013e3182356fc3 PMID:21921827

Waisman, D., Brod, V., Wolff, R., Sabo, E., Chernin, M., Weintraub, Z.,... Bitterman, H. (2003). Effects of hyperoxia on local and remote microcirculatory inflammatory response after splanchnic ischemia and reperfusion. *Am J Physiol Heart Circ Physiol, 285*(2), H643-652. doi: 10.1152/ajpheart.00900.2002

Walsh, M. C., Szefler, S., Davis, J., Allen, M., Van Marter, L., Abman, S., & Jobe, A. et al. (2006). Summary proceedings from the bronchopulmonary dysplasia group. *Pediatrics*, *117*(3 Pt 2), S52–S56. doi:10.1542/peds.2005-0620I PMID:16777823

Waring, W. S., Thomson, A. J., Adwani, S. H., Rosseel, A. J., Potter, J. F., Webb, D. J., & Maxwell, S. R. (2003). Cardiovascular effects of acute oxygen administration in healthy adults. *Journal of Cardiovascular Pharmacology*, *42*(2), 245–250. doi:10.1097/00005344-200308000-00014 PMID:12883329

Wei, J. Q., Shehadeh, L. A., Mitrani, J. M., Pessanha, M., Slepak, T. I., Webster, K. A., & Bishopric, N. H. (2008). Quantitative Control of Adaptive Cardiac Hypertrophy by Acetyltransferase p300. *Circulation*, *118*(9), 934–946. doi:10.1161/CIRCULATIONAHA.107.760488 PMID:18697823

Weir, E. K., Lopez-Barneo, J., Buckler, K. J., & Archer, S. L. (2005). Acute oxygen-sensing mechanisms. *The New England Journal of Medicine*, *353*(19), 2042–2055. doi:10.1056/NEJMra050002 PMID:16282179

Wittnich, C., Torrance, S. M., & Carlyle, C. E. (2000). Effects of hyperoxia on neonatal myocardial energy status and response to global ischemia. *The Annals of Thoracic Surgery*, *70*(6), 2125–2131. doi:10.1016/S0003-4975(00)01756-2 PMID:11156132

Wong, S. C., Fukuchi, M., Melnyk, P., Rodger, I., & Giaid, A. (1998). Induction of cyclooxygenase-2 and activation of nuclear factor-kappaB in myocardium of patients with congestive heart failure. *Circulation*, *98*(2), 100–103. doi:10.1161/01.CIR.98.2.100 PMID:9679714

Xu, D., Guthrie, J. R., Mabry, S., Sack, T. M., & Truog, W. E. (2006). Mitochondrial aldehyde dehydrogenase attenuates hyperoxia-induced cell death through activation of ERK/MAPK and PI3K-Akt pathways in lung epithelial cells. *American Journal of Physiology. Lung Cellular and Molecular Physiology*, *291*(5), L966–L975. doi:10.1152/ajplung.00045.2006 PMID:16782756

Yan, G.-X., & Antzelevitch, C. (1998). Cellular Basis for the Normal T Wave and the Electrocardiographic Manifestations of the Long-QT Syndrome. *Circulation*, *98*(18), 1928–1936. doi:10.1161/01.CIR.98.18.1928 PMID:9799215

Yang, B., Lin, H., Xiao, J., Lu, Y., Luo, X., Li, B., & Wang, Z. et al. (2007). The muscle-specific microRNA miR-1 regulates cardiac arrhythmogenic potential by targeting GJA1 and KCNJ2. *Nature Medicine*, *13*(4), 486–491. doi:10.1038/nm1569 PMID:17401374

Young, R. W. (2012). Hyperoxia: A review of the risks and benefits in adult cardiac surgery. *The Journal of Extra-Corporeal Technology*, *44*(4), 241–249. PMID:23441567

Yzydorczyk, C., Comte, B., Cambonie, G., Lavoie, J.-C., Germain, N., & Shun, T. (2008). Neonatal Oxygen Exposure in Rats Leads to Cardiovascular and Renal Alterations in Adulthood. *Hypertension*, *52*(5), 889–895. doi:10.1161/HYPERTENSIONAHA.108.116251 PMID:18852387

Zaher, T. E., Miller, E. J., Morrow, D. M. P., Javdan, M., & Mantell, L. L. (2007). Hyperoxia-induced signal transduction pathways in pulmonary epithelial cells. *Free Radical Biology & Medicine*, *42*(7), 897–908. doi:10.1016/j.freeradbiomed.2007.01.021 PMID:17349918

Zhang, C. L., McKinsey, T. A., Lu, J. R., & Olson, E. N. (2001). Association of COOH-terminal-binding protein (CtBP) and MEF2-interacting transcription repressor (MITR) contributes to transcriptional repression of the MEF2 transcription factor. *The Journal of Biological Chemistry*, *276*(1), 35–39. doi:10.1074/jbc.M007364200 PMID:11022042

Zhang, X., Shan, P., Sasidhar, M., Chupp, G. L., Flavell, R. A., Choi, A. M. K., & Lee, P. J. (2003). Reactive Oxygen Species and Extracellular Signal-Regulated Kinase 1/2 Mitogen-Activated Protein Kinase Mediate Hyperoxia-Induced Cell Death in Lung Epithelium. *American Journal of Respiratory Cell and Molecular Biology*, *28*(3), 305–315. doi:10.1165/rcmb.2002-0156OC PMID:12594056

Chapter 7
Platelet Function Disorders

Zubair A. Karim
The University of Texas at El Paso, USA

Fadi T. Khasawneh
The University of Texas at El Paso, USA

ABSTRACT

Platelets play an important role in thrombosis and hemostasis. Moreover, platelet dysfunction due to congenital and acquired etiologies is also one of the most common causes of bleeding encountered in clinical practice. Mostly, platelet function disorders are deficiencies of glycoprotein mediators of adhesion and aggregation, whereas defects of primary receptors for stimuli include those of the P2Y12 ADP receptor. Studies on inherited defects of (1) secretion for storage organelles (dense and alpha-granules), (2) the platelet cytoskeleton, and (3) the generation of pro-coagulant activity have allowed for the identification of genes directly and/or indirectly controlling specific functional responses. This chapter will review recent advances in the molecular characterization of platelet function defects, the spectrum of clinical manifestations of these disorders and their management.

INTRODUCTION

Abnormality in platelet function causes bleeding in patient which is disturbance in hemostasis. The term hemostasis applies to a myriad of physiological processes that are involved in maintaining vascular integrity and keeping the blood in fluid form. Human platelets are multifunctional anucleated cells that play an important role in hemostasis. Here we will discuss the physiology of platelets in hemostasis and defects in platelet function.

Platelet Structure and Function

Platelets originate from the cytoplasm of bone marrow megakaryocyte (Figure 1).

It lack genomic DNA but contain megakaryocyte-derived mRNA and the translational machinery needed for protein synthesis. Circulating platelets are discoid in shape, which dimensions of approximately 2-4 µm. Their shape and small size enables the platelets to be pushed to the edge of vessels, placing

DOI: 10.4018/978-1-5225-2092-4.ch007

Figure 1. The diagram summarizes the production of platelets from the defragmentation of megakaryocyte

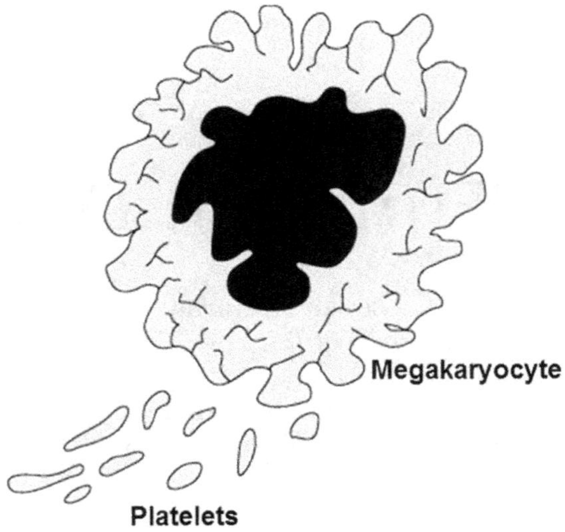

them in the optimum location to constantly survey the integrity of the vasculature. Platelets circulate in a concentration of 150,000-450,000 cells/mL. Of the total body platelets, about 70% stay in the circulation while the remaining 30% are continually but transiently sequestered in the spleen. Platelets remain in circulation for an average of 10 days (Kile, 2014). Most platelets are removed from the circulation by the spleen and liver after senescence, but a constant small fraction is continually removed through involvement in maintenance of vascular integrity (Kile, 2014).

On peripheral blood smears stained with Wright-Giemsa stain, platelets appear as small, granular staining cells with a rough membrane, and are normally present as 3-10 platelets per high-power oil-immersion field (Dunning, 2011). Despite their simple appearance on the peripheral blood smear, platelets have a complex structure (Figure 2). Platelets internal structure has been divided into four zones:

- Peripheral zone,
- Sol-gel zone,
- Organelle zone, and
- Membrane zone.

The peripheral zone includes the outer membranes and closely associated structures. The platelet has a surface-connected system of channels called the open canalicular system (OCS). The walls of the OCS are included in this zone. The OCS provides access to the interior of the platelet to plasma membranes, and an outlet channel for platelet products. The release of platelet products through the OCS after platelet activation is called “the release reaction”.

The membranes of the platelet are rich in platelet receptors, which determine its specific cellular identity. These receptors are constitutively expressed on the platelets and require conformational change during platelet activation to express receptor function. The major classes of receptors and their ligands are shown in Table 1.

The peripheral zone also includes membrane phospholipids (Kowata, 2014). Phospholipids are an important component of coagulation as they provide the surface upon which coagulation protein react.

Figure 2. The diagram summarizes ultrastructural features observed in thin sections of discoid platelets cut in cross-section. Components of the peripheral zone include the exterior coat, and submembrane area containing specialized filaments (SMF) that form the wall of the platelet and line channels of the surface-connected open calnalicular system (OCS). The matrix of the platelet interior is the sol-gel zone containing actin microfilaments, structural filaments, the circumferential band of microtubules, and glycogen. Formed elements embedded in the sol-gel zone include mitochondria, alpha, and dense granules. Collectively they constitute the organelle zone. The membrane systems include the surface-connected open canalicular system and the dense tubular system, which serve as the platelet sarcoplasmic reticulum.

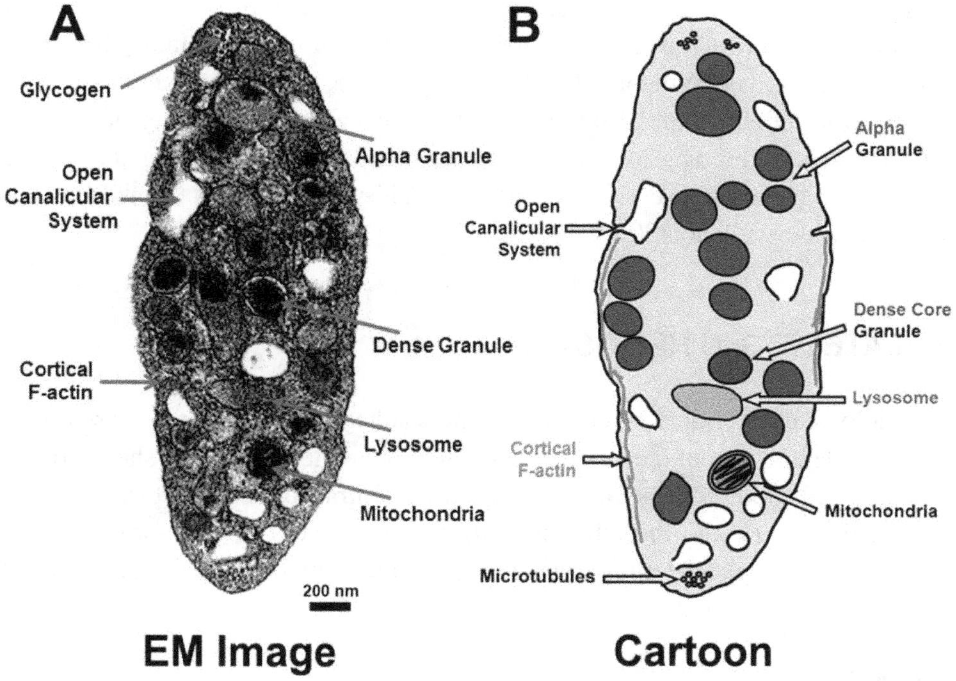

Table 1. Structure and function of glycoprotein receptor

Glycoprotein (GP) Receptor	Structure	Function/Ligand
GPIIb/IIIa	Integrin αIIbβ3	Receptor for fibrinogen, VWF, fibronectin, vitronectin and thrombospondin
GPIa/IIa	Integrin α2β1	Receptor for collagen
GPIb/IX/V	Leucine-rich repeats receptor	Receptor for insoluble VWF
GPVI	Non-integrin receptor, immunoglobulin superfamily receptor	Receptor for collagen

Phospholipids also serve as the initial substrate for platelet enzymatic reactions to produce thromboxane A_2 (TXA_2), an important product of platelet activation and a powerful platelet agonist (substance that causes platelet aggregation). The platelet membrane also has the ability to translate signals from the surface into the internal chemical signals (Pothapragada, 2015).

The sol-gel zone is beneath the peripheral zone and consists of the framework of the platelets, the cytoskeleton (Loftus, 1984). The cytoskeleton forms the support for the maintenance of the platelet's discoid shape as well as the contractile system that allows, upon activation, shape change, pseudopod extension, internal contraction, and release of granule constituents. The cytoskeleton comprises somewhere between 30-50% of the total protein.

The organelle zone consists of the granules and cellular components such as alpha granule, dense granule, lysosomes, mitochondria etc. these organelle serve in the metabolic processes of the platelet and store enzymes and a large variety of other substances critical to platelet function (van Nispen tot Pannerden, 2010). There are two compartments of adenine nucleotides: the storage or secretable pool in dense and alpha granules and the metabolic or cytoplasmic pool.

The dense granules contain non-metabolic adenosine triphosphate (ATP) and adenosine diphosphate (ADP), serotonin, and calcium (Jonnalagadda, 2012). The alpha granules contain adhesive proteins such as fibrinogen, fibronectin, von Willebrand factor V, high molecular weight kininogen, factor XI, and plasminogen activator inhibitor-I are also present in the alpha granule (Jonnalagadda, 2012).

The fourth zone is the membrane zone, which includes the dese tubular system. It is here that calcium, important for triggering contractile events, is concerned. This zone also contains the enzymatic systems are prostaglandins synthesis (Choi, 2010).

ROLE OF PLATELETS IN HEMOSTASIS

In a normal physiological state, platelets circulate without adhering to undisturbed vascular endothelium. Upon disruption of the integrity of the vascular endothelium or alteration in the shear stress of the blood flow, platelets are "activated". Platelet activation plays a central role in both benign and pathological responses to vascular injury and thrombus formation. The process of transformation of inactivated platelets into a well-formed platelet plug occurs along a continuum, but may be divided into three steps: (1) adhesion; (2) aggregation; and (3) secretion.

Platelet Adhesion

Subendothelial components (e.g. collagen, VWF, fibronectin, and laminin) are exposed upon vessel damage (Ed Rainger, 2015). VWF facilitates the initial adhesion via binding to the glycoprotein (GP)Ib/IX/V complex, especially under high shear conditions. These interactions enable platelets to slow down sufficiently so that further binding interactions take place with other receptor-ligand pairs, resulting in static adhesion. In particular, the initial interaction between collagen and GPVI induces a conformational change (activation) in the platelet integrins GPIIb/IIIa and GPIa/IIa. VWF and collagen from strong bonds with GPIIb/IIIa and GPIa/IIa, resepectively, anchoring the platelets in place (Ed Rainger, 2015).

Patients with Bernard-Soulier syndrome and Glanzmann's thrombasthenia have defective platelet adhesion due to decrease or absent expression of the glycoprotein receptors that are involved in platelet adhesion: the GPIb/IX/V and GPIIb/IIIa receptors respectively (Li, 2015; Nurden, 2015).

Platelet Aggregation and Secretion

Platelets undergo morphological changes upon activation. Platelet shape changes from a disc to a spiny sphere with multiple pseudopodial extensions. The platelet membrane becomes rearranged, with exposure of negatively charged phospholipids that facilitate the interaction with coagulation proteins to form the tenase and prothrombin complexes. The content of platelet granules are secreted through the surface-connected canalicular system, ADP, fibrinogen, and factor V appearing on the platelet surface and in the milieu immediately surrounding the platelet (Ren, 2008). PDGF is secreted and leads to smooth muscle proliferation and may initiate atherosclerosis. Platelet factor 3 or tissue factor is also expressed after platelet activation. Small pieces of the platelet are able to bud off to form circulating microparticles. Platelet-agonist interactions result in the production or release of a variety of intracellular messenger molecules that facilitate these reactions.

Biochemical Processes Involved in Platelet Aggregation and Secretion

As platelets are recruited to the area of blood vessel damage, they become activated by a range of agonists including ADP, thrombin, and thromboxanes, which interact with transmembrane receptors. Receptor stimulation results in G protein interactions, which enable activation of enzymes involved in cellular metabolic pathways, in particular, phosphatidylinositol 3-kinase and phospholipase C. Metabolic pathway activation results in the elevation of cytoplasmic calcium and phosphorylation of substrate proteins, which bring about changes in the cytoskeleton, enabling platelet shape change and spreading, release of alpha- and dense-granular contents, stimulation of phospholipase A_2 and liberation of TXA_2, induction of a procoagulant surface, and activation of GPIIb/IIIa receptors. The biochemical details of these reactions are illustrated in Figure 3.

Figure 3. Agonists, receptors and effector systems in platelet activation. The diagram summarizes the molecular and biochemical mechanisms involved in platelet activation.

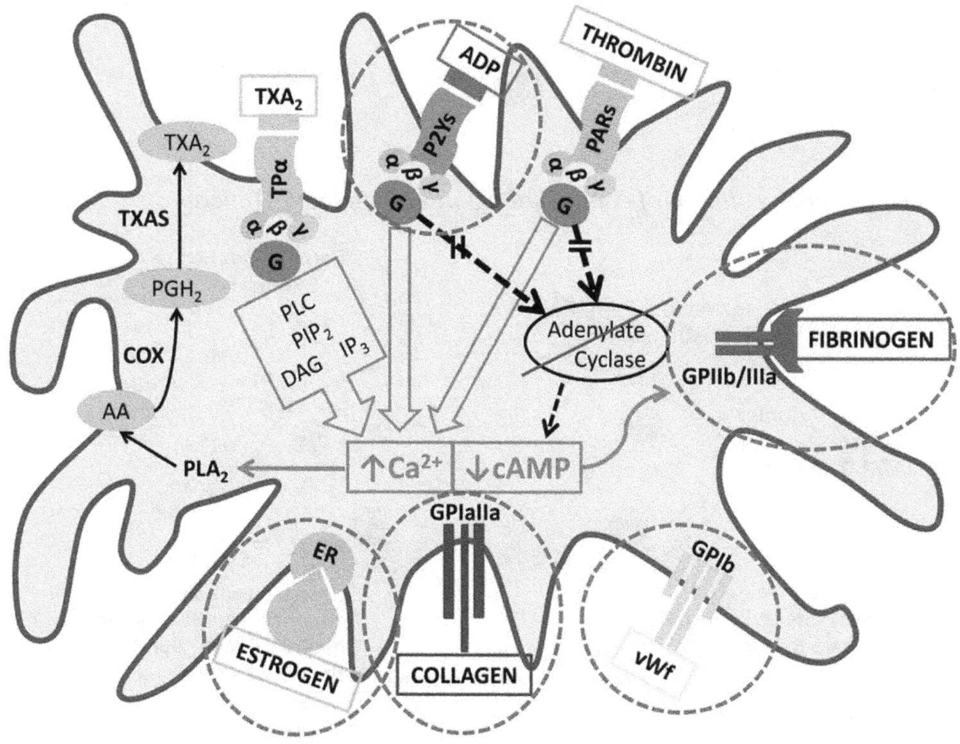

A rare diverse group of disorders of platelet signal transduction have been described, including defects in the agonist receptors for TXA_2, ADP and collagen; the membrane G proteins' and the prostaglandin pathway enzymes cyclooxygenase and TXA_2 synthetase (Figure 4). Disorders of the platelet storage granules are also well described and include dense granule deficiency, alpha granule deficiency, and combined dense and alpha granule deficiency (Figure 5).

Figure 4. Schematic representation of normal platelet response

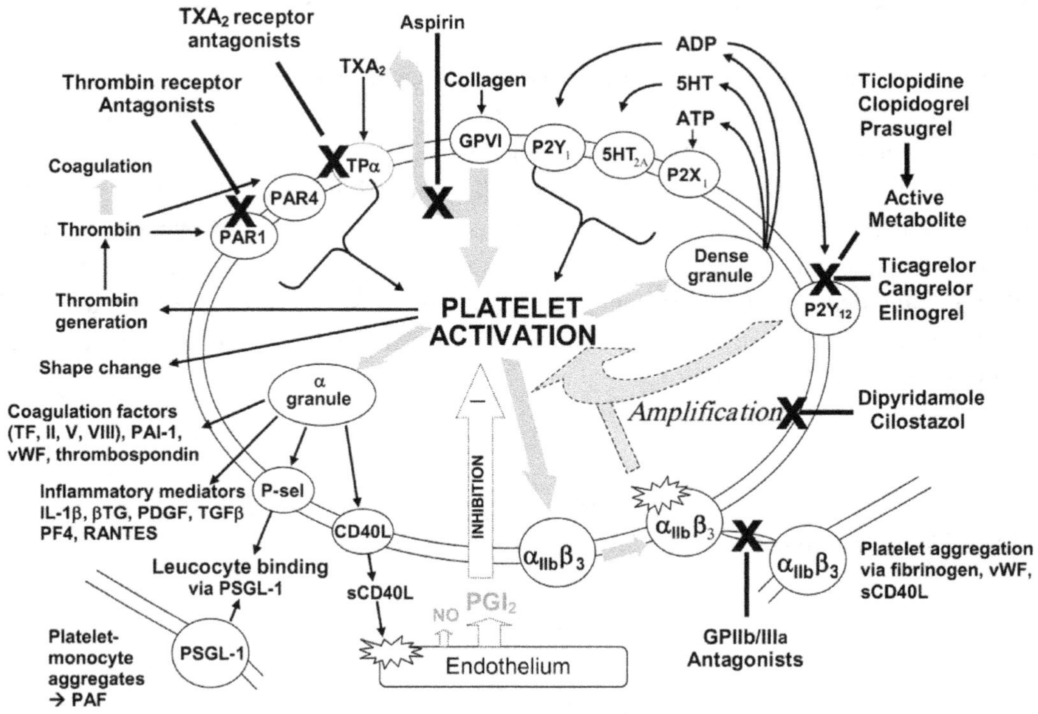

Figure 5. Schematic representation of congenital disorders of platelet function

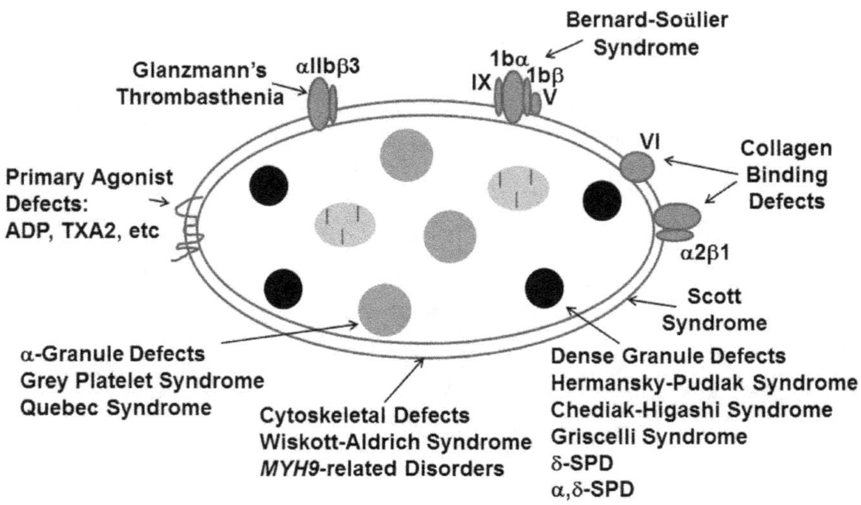

SUMMARY

The contribution of platelets to hemostasis lies in the formation of the primary hemostatic plug, the secretion of important substances for further recruitment of platelets, the provision of a surface for coagulation to proceed, the release of promoters of endothelial repair, and the restoration of normal vessel architecture. Disruption in any of the above described events and biochemical processes may lead to platelet dysfunction, which may be either inherited or acquired.

Specific Disorders of Platelet Function

The following section briefly describes the inherited platelet disorder (Tables 2 and 3).

Table 2. Disorders of adhesion and aggregation due to defects in receptors and defects in signal transduction

Disorder	Inheritance	Structural Defect	Platelet Characteristics	Defect in Platelet Function	Associations	Treatment Options		
						Platelet Transfusion	DDAVP	rFVIIa
Bernard- Soülier Syndrome	AR	GPIb/IX, GPIbα, GPIbβ, GPIX	Giant Platelets	Abnormal adhesion	DiGeorge Velocardio facial Syndrome	Y	Y	?
Glanzmann's Thrombasthenia	AR	GPIIb/IIIa	None	Absent aggregation with physiological agonists, defective clot retraction	↑ bone thickening and ↓ fertility	Y	N	Y
Platelet type VWD	AD	GPIbα	Platelet heterogeneity	Abnormal adhesion: ↓ sensitive to ristocetin	Absence of HMWM	Y	N	?
A2β1 Collagen receptor	?	α2	Normal	Abnormal adhesion: ↓ response to collagen	Modifications in receptor density according to haplotype	Y	Y	?
P_2Y_{12} ADP receptor	AR	P_2Y_{12} ADP receptor	Normal	Abnormal aggregation to ADP	Not known	Y	Y	?
TPα/ Thromboxane A2 receptor		TPα	Normal	Absence of response to TXA2 analogues	Not known	Y	Y	?
Intracellular signaling	?	Phospholipase Cβ	Normal	Variable aggregation and secretion defects on multiple agonists	Not known	Y	Y	?
Cyclooxygenase deficiency	AR	Cyclooxygenase enzyme	Not known	No aggregation with arachidonic acid, ↓ response to collagen and ADP	Not known	Y	Y	?
Scott Syndrome	AR	ATP-binding cassette transporter A1	Normal	↓ procoagulant activity and microparticle release	Defects extend to other cell lines	Y	?	?
Wiskott-Aldrich Syndrome	X-linked	WAS protein mutation	Small size, fewer granules	↓ aggregation and secretion	Eczema, immunodeficiency	Y	?	?

Table 3. Disorders of secretion due to abnormalities of storage granules

Disorder	Inheritance	Structural Defect	Platelet Characteristics	Defect in Platelet Function	Associations	Treatment Options		
						Platelet Transfusion	DDAVP	rFVIIa
Hermansky-Pudlak syndrome	AR	Lysosomal secretion defects	Platelet storage pool defect	↓ aggregation and secretion with collagen	Oculocutaneous albinism, decreased pigmentation	Y	Y	Y
Chediak Higashi syndrome	AR	Mutation of a lysosomal trafficking regulator protein	Decrease in phagocytosis	↓ aggregation and secretion with collagen	Recurrent pyogenic infections, partial albinism and peripheral neuropathy	Y	Y	Y
Gray platelet syndrome	AR or AD	Platelet alpha granule deficiency	Reduction or absence of alpha granules	Abnormal but variable, can be decreased with thrombin, epinephrine and/or collagen	Thrombocytopenia, and abnormally large agranular platelets in peripheral blood smears	Y	?	?
Quebec syndrome	AD	Large amounts of the fibrinolytic enzyme urokinase-type plasminogen activator (u-PA) in platelets	Reduction or absence of alpha granules	Absent aggregation with epinephrine	Unknown	Y	?	?
Paris-Trousseau syndrome	AD	Defective megakaryopoiesis	Giant megakaryocyte granules	Abnormal aggregation and secretion with thrombin, epinephrine, ADP and collagen	Psycomotor retardation, facial and cardiac abnormalities	Y	Y	?
Jacobsen syndrome	AD	Defective megakaryopoiesis	Giant megakaryocyte granules	Abnormal aggregation and secretion with thrombin, epinephrine, ADP and collagen	Psycomotor retardation, facial and cardiac abnormalities	Y	Y	?
Griscelli synderome	AR	Mutations in the genes encoding myosin Va (*MYOSA*), Rab27a (*Rab27a*; a small GTPase),	Rarely bleeding while platelet secretory defects	No secretion with thrombin, collagen and ADP	Myosin Va, Rab27a	Y	?	?
δ storage pool deficiency	AR	Platelet dense granule deficiency	Reduction or absence of dense granules	Absent second wave of aggregation with ADP, epinephrine, ATP:ADP ratio >3	Wiskott-Aldrich syndrome, Thrombocytopenia-absent radius (TAR) syndrome, Ehler-Danlos syndrome	Y	Y	Y
Vacuolar protein sorting-associated protein 33B disorder	AD	Mutations of VPS33B	platelet dysfunction and low granule content with a multisystem disorder featuring renal tubular and other dysfunction	No aggregation with thrombin, collagen and ADP	VPS33B	Y	?	?
Familial haemophagocytic lymphohistiocytosis (FHL)-3	AR	Munc 13-4 mutation	Defects in granule release	No aggregation with thrombin, collagen and ADP	Munc 13-4	Y	?	?
Familial haemophagocytic lymphohistiocytosis (FHL)-4	AR	Syntaxin-11	Defects in granule release	No aggregation with thrombin, collagen and ADP	Syntaxin-11	Y	?	?

continued on following page

Table 3. Continued

Disorder	Inheritance	Structural Defect	Platelet Characteristics	Defect in Platelet Function	Associations	Treatment Options		
						Platelet Transfusion	DDAVP	rFVIIa
Familial haemophagocytic lymphohistiocytosis (FHL)-5	AR	Unc 18-b	Defects in granule release	No aggregation with thrombin, collagen and ADP	Unc 18-b	Y	?	?
MYH9 Disorders								
May-Hegglin syndrome	AD	MYH9, non-muscle myosin heavy chain IIA	Large size	No consistent defect	Neutrophil inclusions	Y	?	?
Fechtner syndrome	AD	MYH9	Large size	No consistent defect	Hereditary nephritis, hearing loss	Y	?	?
Epstein syndrome	AD	MYH9	Large size	Impaired response to collagen	Hereditary nephritis, hearing loss	Y	?	?
Montreal platelet syndrome	AD	Unknown	Large size	Spontaneous agglutination, ↓ response to thrombin	Unknown	Y	?	?

Defects in Platelet Receptors

Glanzmann's Thrombasthenia

Glanzmann's thrombasthenia is a classic inherited platelet disorder; platelets fail to aggregate to all physiological agonists due to absence or decrease of the integrin αIIbβ3 (Binder, 2015). The platelet count, size, shape and life span are normal in this disorder. It is inherited as an autosomal recessive trait: therefore parental history of bleeding is negative. Males and females are equally affected. The bleeding time is invariably prolonged. Clot retraction is poor to absent. Platelet function studies reveal aggregation defects in presence of thrombin (Buitrago, 2015). Adhesion to areas of damaged endothelium is normal but recruitment of further platelets into the primary hemostatic plug is defective. Assessment of integrin αIIbβ3 receptors on the platelet membrane using flow cytometry is possible in reference laboratories (Rubak, 2015). In normal hemostasis, αIIbβ3 on activated platelets binds fibrinogen and other adhesive proteins that link platelets together during aggregation. Other manifestation of Glanzmann's thrombasthenia includes a defective platelet spreading on the nature of the mutation. These manifestations give rise to a variable but sometimes severe bleeding disorder whose treatments with platelet transfusions can be compromised by alloantibody formation (Seligsohn, 2012). Glanzmann's thrombasthenia has been comprehensively dealt with in a series of recent reviews and only essential details will be repeated here (Binder, 2015; Nurden, 2011; Nurden, 2012; Nurden, 2013; Sandrock-Lang, 2015; Sandrock-Lang, 2015; Seligsohn, 2012).

Bernard-Soulier Syndrome

Bernard-Soulier syndrome is a rare syndrome characterized by abnormally large platelets that may also be mildly decreased in number (Savoia, 2014). The bleeding time is markedly prolonged. Platelet aggregation studies reveal that aggregation is defective against thrombin (Andrews, 2013). This abnormality is due to a decrease or absence of GPIb/IX, the VWF receptor. This disorder should be differentiated from VWF, which is due to a defect in the VWF rather than the platelet receptor. Bernard-Soulier syndrome is inherited as an autosomal recessive trait with males and females equally affected (Bragadottir, 2015). Parental history of similar bleeding problems is absent. In contrast, VWF is inherited as an autosomal dominant trait; however, symptoms are variable and therefore parental history is an inadequate guide to excluding this diagnosis. In Bernard-Soulier syndrome, platelet transfusions are used therapeutically; however, as with Glanzmann's thrombasthenia, alloimmunization may occur. There are reports of successful control of bleeding with rFVIIa in patients with Bernard-Soulier syndrome (Ozelo, 2005; Tefre, 2009).

Defects in Granule Content/Storage Pool Deficiencies

Dense granules are storage sites for serotonin, ADP, ATP, and polyphosphate (Jonnalagadda, 2012; Smith, 2014; Smith, 2015). Storage pool disorders are a heterogeneous group of diseases in which there is an abnormality in the ability to store appropriate products within the platelet granules (Masliah-Planchon, 2013). The following represent a few of the recognized storage pool disorders not associated with a systemic disorder.

Grey Platelet Syndrome

Grey platelet syndrome is a disorder characterized by a protein deficiency (e.g. platelet factor 4, β-thromboglobulin, fibrinogen and PDGF) in the alpha granules, both in platelet and megakaryocyte (Gunay-Aygun, 2010). This disorder is a mild to moderate bleeding disorder that can, on occasion, be life-threatening and is characterized by a severe and specific deficiency of α-granules and their contents (Gunay-Aygun, 2010). On the peripheral smear the platelets are grey in color and large. There is consistently impaired aggregation to thrombin in platelet function. Unlike for HPS, platelets from a GPS patient failed to spread when plated on polylysine, collage or fibronectin showing that dense granule and α-granule deficiencies have different effects (Peters, 2012). Electron micrographs shows only vestigial α-granules in platelets. In 2011, it has been shown that mutations in *NBEAL2* (neurobeachin-like 2) in GPS (Albers, 2011; Gunay-Aygun, 2011; Kahr, 2011). GPS is a hetergenous trait whose severity depends on the extent of the α-granule deficiency (Bottega, 2013).

Vacuolar Protein Sorting-Associated Protein 33B Disorder

Mutations of *VPS33B*, which encodes a regulator of soluble N-ethylmaleimide-sensitive factor activating receptor (SNARE)-dependent membrane fusion and of *VIPAS39*, encoding VPS33B-interacting protein, cause the arthrogryposis-renal dysfunction-cholestasis (ARC) syndrome (Smith, 2012). Mostly lethal for young children, ARC associates platelet dysfunction and low granule content with a multisystem disorder featuring renal tubular and other dysfunction. The platelet defect extends to stored and membrane components of α-granules (Urban, 2012).

Quebec Platelet Disorder

Quebec platelet disorder is inherited as an autosomal dominant disorder that is associated with very abnormal aggregation with epinephrine and is unique to French-Canadian families (Blavignac, 2011). There is a defect in alpha granule proteolysis and a deficiency of alpha granule multimerin, a multimeric protein that binds factor V within the granule, thereby leading to a decreased content of platelet factor V and several other proteins (fibrinogen, VWF etc). Thrombocytopenia is sometimes observed and there is a characteristic lack of platelet aggregation response with epinephrine. The genetic basis of this disorder is a tandem duplication of the u-PA gene, *PLAU* (urokinase-type plasminogen activator) (Paterson, 2010).

Hermansky-Pudlak Syndrome

Hermansky-Pudlak syndrome is inherited as an autosomal recessive disorder with associated occulocutaneous albinism. Oculocutaneous albinism is characteristic of HPS as is ceroid-lipofuscin storage in the reticulo-endothelial system while granulomatous colitis, interstitial lung disease and fatal pulmonary fibrosis feature in some subtypes. Defects in nine genes (*HPS1, HPS3-6, DTNBP1, BLOC1S3,* BLOC1S6) cause distinct HPS subtypes in human (Huizing, 2008; Masliah-Planchon, 2013). Interestingly, polyphosphates released from dense granules activate plasma FXII, addition of polyphosphates restored defective clotting in HPS implying that their deficit contributes to the bleeding syndrome (Muller, 2009). Platelet function studies showed an absent secondary wave to ADP, epinephrine, restocetin and abnormal aggregation with collagen.

Chediak-Higashi Syndrome

Chediak-Higashi syndrome is a rare autosomal recessive disorder with large abnormal granules that are apparent in melanocytes, leukocytes, and fibroblasts, but not in platelets. There is a partial occulocutaneous albinism and often recurrent pyogenic infections. The platelet count is normal, with a prolonged bleeding time, decrease dense granule and abnormal platelet aggregation associated with a bleeding tendency, severe immunological defects with life threatening infections and progressive neurological dysfunction (Huizing, 2008). The immunodeficiency leads to the development of a lymphoproliferative syndrome and an accelerated phase in ~85% of patients.

Griscelli Synderome

Patients with Griscelli syndrome have partial albinism and silver hair; different subtypes combine neurological defects and/or severe immunodeficiency with a defective cytotoxic lymphocyte activity. Mutations in the genes encoding myosin Va (*MYOSA*), Rab27a (*Rab27a*; a small GTPase), or melanophilin (*MLPH*) cause 3 subtypes of Griscelli syndrome but rarely bleeding while platelet secretory defects have yet to be described (Masliah-Planchon, 2013).

Familial Haemophagocytic Lymphohistiocytosis

In a new development, defective platelet secretion (dense granule, α-granule and lysosome) in spite of normal granule cargo has been shown in familial haemophagocytic lymphohistiocytosis types 3, 4 and

5, potentially lethal disorders of immune dysregulation caused respectively by defects in Munc 13-4 (*UNC13D*) {Sandrock, 2010 #9}, snytaxin-11 (*STX11*) (Ye, 2012) and Munc18b (*STXBP2*) (Al Hawas, 2012) coding genes. Munc18b appears to be a partner of syntaxin-11 in platelet exocytosis (Al Hawas, 2012; Ye, 2012). This work highlights how platelets may use similar secretory machinery as ctyotoxic T lymphocytes and NK (natural killer) cells.

Wiskott-Aldrich Syndrome

Wiskott-Aldrich syndrome is a rare X-linked recessive disorder caused by a defect in a protein named termed as Wiskott-Aldrich syndrome protein (WASP) (Baldini, 1969). The gene resides on Xp11.12-23, and its expression is limited to cells of hematopoietic lineage. This disease is characterized by thrombocytopenia, with small platelets and immunodeficiency (Grottum, 1969). WAS protein is a key regulator of actin polymerization in hemoatopoietic cells; it is involved in signal transduction with tyrosine phosphorylation sites and adapter protein functins. Patients with this disorder may have bleeding in association with the decreased number as well as abnormal function of the platelets. In some patients a storage pool deficiency has been described (Gunay-Aygun, 2004; Nurden, 2008; White, 1987). Affected patients have a history of recurrent infections and eczema on physical examination. Laboratory abnormalities reveal absent isohemaglutinins. There are associated immunologic defects. Genetic testing has revealed abnormalities in many of these patients. Treatment of acute bleeding is through platelet transfusions. Splenectomy has shown to improve the thrombocytopenia. Bone marrow transplantation should be considered the definitive treatment for these patients (Hongeng, 2001).

Release Defects

This group of patients most likely represent the largest group of platelet function disorders. Release defects may occur due to abnormalities in signal transduction from the membrane, abnormal internal metabolic pathways and abnormal release mechanisms or structures involved in the release reaction (Rendu, 2001; Shapiro, 2000; Huang, 2015). It is clear therefore that release defects are a heterogeneous group of disorders with a wide variety of underlying defects whose mechanisms are not fully elucidated. The final common abnormality within this group of defects is the failure to successfully release granule contents upon platelet activation.

Release defects are associated with a prolonged bleeding time and an abnormal *in vitro* platelet aggregation profile characterized by abnormalities of aggregation in association with ADP, including an absent secondary wave, epinephrine and collagen, which a blunted or absent secondary wave. In more sophisticated studies, there is a measurable defect in ADP release (Rendu, 2001; Shapiro, 2000). There are normal metabolic stores of ADP (those not associated with granule contents). The contents of granules are normal. Many patients with release Defects may be treated with DDAVP (Ghosh, 1993).

Coagulation Factor Defects Affecting Platelet Function

Abnormalities of plasma coagulation factors may lead to defects in platelet function, despite the presence of normal numbers of properly functioning platelets. The most common abnormality in this category is VWD. Absence of plasma and platelet fibrinogen leads to a defect in platelet function, as fibrinogen is important in the platelet-platelet interaction within the primary hemostatic plug. Afibrinogenemia is a rare autosomal recessive defect (de Moerloose, 2013). Both VWD and afibrinogenemia lead to adhesive defects in platelet function: VWD in the platelet vessel interaction, and afibrinogenemia in the platelet-platelet interaction (Azzam, 2012; Eid, 2008; Matsui, 2002).

Von Willebrand Disease

Platelet-type von Willebrand disease (VWD) is an autosomal dominant disease with mild to moderate bleeding and thrombocytopenia with enlarged platelets characterized by spontaneous VWF-binding to GPIbα (Othman, 2011). The defect in VWD resides with the VWF, which plays an important part in platelet function and whose platelet receptor is GPIb/IX. Abnormalities in VWF may lead to mucocutaneous bleeding similar to that seen in platelet function defects. VWD is inherited as an autosomal dominant trait with males and females equally affected (Mitrovic, 2014). The bleeding time may be prolonged. Coagulation factor studies may reveal abnormalities in factor VIII activity, quantitative VWF antigen, VWF activity (commonly measured in the ristocetin cofactor assay), and the structure of the protein itself (usually assessed through multimeric analysis by gel electrophoresis).

Afibrinogenemia

This is a rare autosomal recessive disorder in which there are extremely low or absent levels of fibrinogen. The bleeding time may be prolonged. In some patients there may be an associated decrease in platelet counts as well as an abnormal platelet aggregation profile. The absence or severe deficiency of plasma fibrinogen leads to impaired platelet-platelet interaction (de Moerloose, 2013).

Defects in Platelet Pro-Coagulant Activity

Scott Syndrome

Scott syndrome is a rare inherited disorder caused by defective scrambling of phospholipids on blood cells (Lhermusier, 2011). It manifests by a decreased fibrin formation during shear-dependent adhesion of platelets to subendothelium. When activated Scott platelets are unable to translocate PS to the outer leaflet of the membrane bilayer; factors Va and Xa fail to bind leading to a decreased capacity of platelets to convert prothrombin in thrombin. This lack of thrombin generation is sufficient to induce a bleeding syndrome. The disease is caused by mutations in *ANO6* (anoctamin 6, also known as *TMEM16F*) that encodes transmembrane protein 16F, a Ca^{2+}-activated channel essential for Ca^{2+}-dependent PS exposure (Suzuki, 2010; Yang, 2012).

Miscellaneous Congenital Disorders

There are disorders of platelet function that have been reported to occur in association with connective tissue disorders. These include but are not limited to such disorders as Ehlers-Danlos syndrome, Marfan's syndrome, osteogenesis imperfect, and fragile X syndrome (Brusin, 2008; Cheng, 2015; Gross, 2015; Malfait, 2014). May-Hegglin anomaly is an autosomal dominant disorder characterized by ineffective thrombopoiesis with normal platelet function studies, and abnormal inclusion granules in leukocytes

(Althaus, 2011). Platelet function defects have also been reported to occur in association with Down's syndrome (Boleracki, 2015).

Thrombocytopenia and absent radii syndrome (TAR) is characterized by thrombocytopenia and defects of the radial bone (Idahosa, 2014). Platelet function defects have been reported in TAR syndrome (Bottillo, 2013; Wilson, 2014). Infants with this syndrome may suffer severe and even fatal bleeding in the first year of life, after which the thrombocytopenia gradually improves (Bottillo, 2013; Wilson, 2014). Prophylactic platelet transfusions are recommended in this population of patients. Hereditary autosomal dominant thrombocytopenia resembling idiopathic thrombocytopenic purpura (ITP) has been reported and may be associated with a platelet function defect (Mihalov, 2014). Platelet function defects have also been reported to occur in association with increased serum IgA, nephritis, deafness, and giant platelets (Mihalov, 2014).

Defects in Intracellular Signaling Pathways

Pathologies of signal transduction pathways concern patients with defects of platelet aggregation that affect some stimuli more than others; such disorders may be quite common (Dawood, 2012; Nurden, 2011). Early studies highlighted patients with abnormalities of receptor-linked G-protein signaling, phospholipase C pathways, protein kinase C phosphorylation and Ca^{2+} mobilization; however, as gene sequencing was not available at the time, the genetic defects remains unknown (Rao, 2013). Likewise, patients with purported congenital deficiencies of cyclooxygenase-I, prostagnalding H synthase-I, thromboxane synthase, phospholipase A_2, lipoxygenase, glycogen synthase and ATP metabolism, gp91 phox deficiency associated with impaired isoprostane formation were all the object of initial reports largely based on platelet function testing (Pignatelli, 2011; Rao, 2013). Two examples where specific gene mutations have now been described are (i) thromboxane synthase in Ghosal syndrome (linking defective arachidonic acid-induced platelet aggregation with an increased bone density) (Genevieve, 2008) and (ii) inherited cytosolic phospholipase A2α deficiency associated with impaired eicosanoid biosynthesis, small intestinal ulceration, and platelet dysfunction (Adler, 2008). Signaling defects may directly interfere with platelet activation pathways including αIIbβ3 activation and fibrinogen binding or intervene secondarily by preventing secretion of ADP or formation and release of TXA_2.

A special category of patient with defects in the G-protein cascade involves second messengers or RGS (regulator of G protein signaling) proteins that affect cAMP levels (Alshbool, 2015; Louwette, 2012). RGS are multi-functional GTPase accelerating proteins that enhance GTP hydrolysis by G protein α-subunits and so intervene early in signaling cascades (Alshbool, 2015). The complex-imprinted gene cluster, *GNAS*, regulates Gsα. Direct genetic and epigenetic defects of *GNAS* include both Gsα hypofunction and thrombotic phenotype associated with more generalized hormonal, skeletal defects and sometimes mental retardation (Louwette, 2012; Van Geet, 2009). A paternally inherited 36 bp insertion in the extra-large stimulatory Gsα and stimulates adenylate cyclase and is associated with Gs hyperfunction in platelets, leading to an increased trauma-related bleeding tendency by is also accompanied by neurological problems, growth deficiency and brachydactyly (Van Geet, 2009). Whether Gs defects occur in patients with platelet-specific bleeding disorders is yet unknown.

CONCLUSION

Platelets are essential for primary hemostasis. Platelet function defects comprise a large and heterogeneous group of bleeding disorders that range in severity from mild to severe. Patients may be asymptomatic; however, the majority who are diagnosed present with easy bruising and mucocutaneous bleeding or excessive hemorrhage following injury or surgery. As the complex internal biochemical and signal transduction pathways are further elucidated, and as structural analysis of platelet advances, more of the mechanisms leading to platelet function defects will be understood. Despite our advances in the understanding of the etiology of these defects in function, treatment remains fairly rudimentary. Adjunctive therapies (such as antifibrinolytics, microfibular collagen, fibrin glue, etc.), rFVIIa and platelet transfusions remain the mainstay of therapy available at this time. For platelet function disorders associated with a defect in a plasma coagulation factor such as von Willebrand disease and afibrinogenemia, treatment consists of replacement of the deficient coagulation factor.

REFERENCES

Adler, D. H., Cogan, J. D., Phillips, J. A. III, Schnetz-Boutaud, N., & Milne, G. L. et al.. (2008). Inherited human cPLA(2alpha) deficiency is associated with impaired eicosanoid biosynthesis, small intestinal ulceration, and platelet dysfunction. *The Journal of Clinical Investigation*, *118*, 2121–2131. PMID:18451993

Al Hawas, R., Ren, Q., Ye, S., Karim, Z. A., Filipovich, A. H., & Whiteheart, S. W. (2012). Munc18b/STXBP2 is required for platelet secretion. *Blood*, *120*(12), 2493–2500. doi:10.1182/blood-2012-05-430629 PMID:22791290

Albers, C. A., Cvejic, A., Favier, R., Bouwmans, E. E., Alessi, M. C., Bertone, P., & Ouwehand, W. H. et al. (2011). Exome sequencing identifies NBEAL2 as the causative gene for gray platelet syndrome. *Nature Genetics*, *43*(8), 735–737. doi:10.1038/ng.885 PMID:21765411

Alshbool, F. Z., Karim, Z. A., Vemana, H. P., Conlon, C., Lin, O. A., & Khasawneh, F. T. (2015). The regulator of G-protein signaling 18 regulates platelet aggregation, hemostasis and thrombosis. *Biochemical and Biophysical Research Communications*, *462*(4), 378–382. doi:10.1016/j.bbrc.2015.04.143 PMID:25969426

Althaus, K., Najm, J., & Greinacher, A. (2011). MYH9 related platelet disorders - often unknown and misdiagnosed. *Klinische Padiatrie*, *223*(03), 120–125. doi:10.1055/s-0031-1275664 PMID:21567368

Andrews, R. K., & Berndt, M. C. (2013). Bernard-Soulier syndrome: An update. *Seminars in Thrombosis and Hemostasis*, *39*(06), 656–662. doi:10.1055/s-0033-1353390 PMID:23929303

Azzam HA, Goneim HR, El-Saddik AM, Azmy E, Hassan M, El-Sharawy S. 2012. The condensed MCMDM-1 VWD bleeding questionnaire as a predictor of bleeding disorders in women with unexplained menorrhagia. *Blood Coagulation & Fibrinolysis: An International Journal in Haemostasis and Thrombosis, 23*, 311-5.

Baldini, M. G. (1969). Platelet defect in Wiskott-Aldrich syndrome. *The New England Journal of Medicine, 281*(2), 107. doi:10.1056/NEJM196907102810224 PMID:5784770

Binder, A., & Aledort, L. (2015). Glanzmann's thrombasthenia: meeting the anticoagulation challenge. *Haemophilia: The Official Journal of the World Federation of Hemophilia.*

Blavignac, J., Bunimov, N., Rivard, G. E., & Hayward, C. P. (2011). Quebec platelet disorder: Update on pathogenesis, diagnosis, and treatment. *Seminars in Thrombosis and Hemostasis, 37*(06), 713–720. doi:10.1055/s-0031-1291382 PMID:22102275

Boleracki, M., Farkas, F., Meszely, A., Szikszai, Z., & Sik Lanyi, C. (2015). Developing an Animal Counting Game in Second Life for a Young Adult with Down Syndrome. *Studies in Health Technology and Informatics, 217*, 71–77. PMID:26294455

Bottega, R., Pecci, A., De Candia, E., Pujol-Moix, N., Heller, P. G., Noris, P., & Savoia, A. et al. (2013). Correlation between platelet phenotype and NBEAL2 genotype in patients with congenital thrombocytopenia and alpha-granule deficiency. *Haematologica, 98*(6), 868–874. doi:10.3324/haematol.2012.075861 PMID:23100277

Bottillo, I., Castori, M., De Bernardo, C., Fabbri, R., Grammatico, B., Preziosi, N., & Grammatico, P. et al. (2013). Prenatal diagnosis and post-mortem examination in a fetus with thrombocytopenia-absent radius (TAR) syndrome due to compound heterozygosity for a 1q21.1 microdeletion and a RBM8A hypomorphic allele: A case report. *BMC Research Notes, 6*(1), 376. doi:10.1186/1756-0500-6-376 PMID:24053387

Bragadottir, G., Birgisdottir, E. R., Gudmundsdottir, B. R., Hilmarsdottir, B., Vidarsson, B., Magnusson, M. K., & Onundarson, P. T. et al. (2015). Clinical phenotype in heterozygote and biallelic Bernard-Soulier syndromea case control study. *American Journal of Hematology, 90*(2), 149–155. doi:10.1002/ajh.23891 PMID:25370924

Brusin, J. H. (2008). Osteogenesis imperfecta. *Radiologic Technology, 79*, 535–548, quiz 49–51. PMID:18650529

Buitrago, L., Rendon, A., Liang, Y., Simeoni, I., Negri, A., Filizola, M., & Coller, B. S. et al. (2015). alphaIIbbeta3 variants defined by next-generation sequencing: Predicting variants likely to cause Glanzmann thrombasthenia. *Proceedings of the National Academy of Sciences of the United States of America, 112*(15), E1898–E1907. doi:10.1073/pnas.1422238112 PMID:25827233

Cheng, A., & Owens, D. (2015). Marfan syndrome, inherited aortopathies and exercise: What is the right answer? *Heart (British Cardiac Society), 101*(10), 752–757. doi:10.1136/heartjnl-2014-306440 PMID:25911666

Choi, W., Karim, Z. A., & Whiteheart, S. W. (2010). Protein expression in platelets from six species that differ in their open canalicular system. *Platelets, 21*(3), 167–175. doi:10.3109/09537101003611385 PMID:20196629

Dawood, B. B., Lowe, G. C., Lordkipanidze, M., Bem, D., Daly, M. E., Makris, M., & Watson, S. P. et al. (2012). Evaluation of participants with suspected heritable platelet function disorders including recommendation and validation of a streamlined agonist panel. *Blood*, *120*(25), 5041–5049. doi:10.1182/blood-2012-07-444281 PMID:23002116

de Moerloose, P., Casini, A., & Neerman-Arbez, M. (2013). Congenital fibrinogen disorders: An update. *Seminars in Thrombosis and Hemostasis*, *39*(06), 585–595. doi:10.1055/s-0033-1349222 PMID:23852822

Dunning, K., & Safo, A. O. (2011). The ultimate Wright-Giemsa stain: 60 years in the making. *Biotechnic & Histochemistry*, *86*(2), 69–75. doi:10.3109/10520295.2010.515496 PMID:21395491

Ed Rainger, G., Chimen, M., Harrison, M. J., Yates, C. M., Harrison, P., Watson, S. P., & Nash, G. B. et al. (2015). The role of platelets in the recruitment of leukocytes during vascular disease. *Platelets*, *26*(6), 507–520. doi:10.3109/09537104.2015.1064881 PMID:26196409

Eid, S.S., Kamal, N.R., Shubeilat, T.S., & Wael, A.G. (2008). Inherited bleeding disorders: a 14-year retrospective study. *Clinical Laboratory Science: Journal of the American Society for Medical Technology, 21*, 210-4.

Genevieve, D., Proulle, V., Isidor, B., Bellais, S., Serre, V., Djouadi, F., & Cormier-Daire, V. et al. (2008). Thromboxane synthase mutations in an increased bone density disorder (Ghosal syndrome). *Nature Genetics*, *40*(3), 284–286. doi:10.1038/ng.2007.66 PMID:18264100

Ghosh, S., & Rao, A. K. (1993). Lack of effect of 1-desamino-8-D-arginine vasopressin on direct adhesion of platelets to collagen. *Thrombosis Research*, *70*(5), 417–422. doi:10.1016/0049-3848(93)90083-Z PMID:7690994

Gross, C., Hoffmann, A., Bassell, G. J., & Berry-Kravis, E. M. (2015). Therapeutic Strategies in Fragile X Syndrome: From Bench to Bedside and Back. *Neurotherapeutics; the Journal of the American Society for Experimental NeuroTherapeutics*, *12*(3), 584–608. doi:10.1007/s13311-015-0355-9 PMID:25986746

Grottum, K. A., Hovig, T., Holmsen, H., Abrahamsen, A. F., Jeremic, M., & Seip, M. (1969). Wiskott-Aldrich syndrome: Qualitative platelet defects and short platelet survival. *British Journal of Haematology*, *17*(4), 373–388. doi:10.1111/j.1365-2141.1969.tb01383.x PMID:5346410

Gunay-Aygun, M., Falik-Zaccai, T. C., Vilboux, T., Zivony-Elboum, Y., Gumruk, F., Cetin, M., & Gahl, W. A. et al. (2011). NBEAL2 is mutated in gray platelet syndrome and is required for biogenesis of platelet alpha-granules. *Nature Genetics*, *43*(8), 732–734. doi:10.1038/ng.883 PMID:21765412

Gunay-Aygun, M., Huizing, M., & Gahl, W. A. (2004). Molecular defects that affect platelet dense granules. *Seminars in Thrombosis and Hemostasis*, *30*(5), 537–547. doi:10.1055/s-2004-835674 PMID:15497096

Gunay-Aygun, M., Zivony-Elboum, Y., Gumruk, F., Geiger, D., Cetin, M., Khayat, M., & Falik-Zaccai, T. et al. (2010). Gray platelet syndrome: Natural history of a large patient cohort and locus assignment to chromosome 3p. *Blood*, *116*(23), 4990–5001. doi:10.1182/blood-2010-05-286534 PMID:20709904

Hongeng, S., Benjaponpitak, S., Tardtong, P., Varavithya, W., Chuansumrit, A., et al. (2001). Successful allogeneic peripheral blood stem cell transplantation in Wiskott-Aldrich Syndrome Patients: first report in Thailand. *Asian Pacific Journal of Allergy and Immunology, 19*, 191-5.

Huang, Y., & Whiteheart, S. W. (2015). Platelet secretion paves the way. *Blood*, *126*(4), 433–434. doi:10.1182/blood-2015-05-646687 PMID:26206945

Huizing, M., Helip-Wooley, A., Westbroek, W., Gunay-Aygun, M., & Gahl, W. A. (2008). Disorders of lysosome-related organelle biogenesis: Clinical and molecular genetics. *Annual Review of Genomics and Human Genetics*, *9*(1), 359–386. doi:10.1146/annurev.genom.9.081307.164303 PMID:18544035

Idahosa, C., Berardi, T. R., Shkolnikov, R., & Stoopler, E. T. (2014). Thrombocytopenia absent radius (TAR) syndrome: A case report and review for oral health care providers. *Special Care in Dentistry*, *34*(5), 251–258. doi:10.1111/scd.12060 PMID:25346959

Jonnalagadda, D., Izu, L. T., & Whiteheart, S. W. (2012). Platelet secretion is kinetically heterogeneous in an agonist-responsive manner. *Blood*, *120*(26), 5209–5216. doi:10.1182/blood-2012-07-445080 PMID:23086755

Kahr, W. H., Hinckley, J., Li, L., Schwertz, H., Christensen, H., Rowley, J. W., & Di Paola, J. et al. (2011). Mutations in NBEAL2, encoding a BEACH protein, cause gray platelet syndrome. *Nature Genetics*, *43*(8), 738–740. doi:10.1038/ng.884 PMID:21765413

Kile, B. T. (2014). The role of apoptosis in megakaryocytes and platelets. *British Journal of Haematology*, *165*(2), 217–226. doi:10.1111/bjh.12757 PMID:24467740

Kowata, S., Isogai, S., Murai, K., Ito, S., Tohyama, K., Ema, M., & Ishida, Y. et al. (2014). Platelet demand modulates the type of intravascular protrusion of megakaryocytes in bone marrow. *Thrombosis and Haemostasis*, *112*(4), 743–756. doi:10.1160/TH14-02-0123 PMID:24965909

Lhermusier, T., Chap, H., & Payrastre, B. (2011). Platelet membrane phospholipid asymmetry: From the characterization of a scramblase activity to the identification of an essential protein mutated in Scott syndrome. *Journal of thrombosis and haemostasis. JTH*, *9*, 1883–1891. PMID:21958383

Li, J., Dai, K., Wang, Z., Cao, L., Bai, X., & Ruan, C. (2015). Platelet functional alterations in a Bernard-Soulier syndrome patient with filamin A mutation. *J Hematol Oncol*, *8*(1), 79. doi:10.1186/s13045-015-0171-z PMID:26133172

Loftus, J. C., Choate, J., & Albrecht, R. M. (1984). Platelet activation and cytoskeletal reorganization: High voltage electron microscopic examination of intact and Triton-extracted whole mounts. *The Journal of Cell Biology*, *98*(6), 2019–2025. doi:10.1083/jcb.98.6.2019 PMID:6539337

Louwette, S., Van Geet, C., & Freson, K. (2012). Regulators of G protein signaling: Role in hematopoiesis, megakaryopoiesis and platelet function. *Journal of thrombosis and haemostasis. JTH*, *10*, 2215–2222. PMID:22908964

Malfait, F., & De Paepe, A. (2014). The Ehlers-Danlos syndrome. *Advances in Experimental Medicine and Biology*, *802*, 129–143. doi:10.1007/978-94-007-7893-1_9 PMID:24443025

Masliah-Planchon, J., Darnige, L., & Bellucci, S. (2013). Molecular determinants of platelet delta storage pool deficiencies: An update. *British Journal of Haematology*, *160*(1), 5–11. doi:10.1111/bjh.12064 PMID:23025459

Matsui, H., Sugimoto, M., Mizuno, T., Tsuji, S., & Miyata, S. et al.. (2002). Distinct and concerted functions of von Willebrand factor and fibrinogen in mural thrombus growth under high shear flow. *Blood, 100*(10), 3604–3610. doi:10.1182/blood-2002-02-0508 PMID:12393609

Mihalov, J., & Timarova, G. (2014). A Seeming Paradox: Ischemic Stroke in the Context of Idiopathic Thrombocytopenic Purpura. *Clinical and Applied Thrombosis/Hemostasis*. PMID:25115760

Mitrovic, M., Elezovic, I., Miljic, P., & Suvajdzic, N. (2014). Acquired von Willebrand syndrome in patients with Gaucher disease. *Blood Cells, Molecules & Diseases, 52*(4), 205–207. doi:10.1016/j.bcmd.2013.11.001 PMID:24275154

Muller, F., Mutch, N. J., Schenk, W. A., Smith, S. A., Esterl, L., Spronk, H. M., & Renné, T. et al. (2009). Platelet polyphosphates are proinflammatory and procoagulant mediators in vivo. *Cell, 139*(6), 1143–1156. doi:10.1016/j.cell.2009.11.001 PMID:20005807

Nurden, A., & Nurden, P. (2011). Advances in our understanding of the molecular basis of disorders of platelet function. *Journal of thrombosis and haemostasis. JTH, 9*(Suppl 1), 76–91. PMID:21781244

Nurden, A. T., Fiore, M., Nurden, P., & Pillois, X. (2011). Glanzmann thrombasthenia: A review of ITGA2B and ITGB3 defects with emphasis on variants, phenotypic variability, and mouse models. *Blood, 118*(23), 5996–6005. doi:10.1182/blood-2011-07-365635 PMID:21917754

Nurden, A. T., & Nurden, P. (2015). Inherited disorders of platelet function: Selected updates. *Journal of thrombosis and haemostasis. JTH, 13*(Suppl 1), S2–S9. PMID:26149024

Nurden, A.T., Pillois, X., & Nurden, P. (2012). Understanding the genetic basis of Glanzmann thrombasthenia: implications for treatment. *Expert Review of Hematology, 5*, 487-503.

Nurden, A. T., Pillois, X., & Wilcox, D. A. (2013). Glanzmann thrombasthenia: State of the art and future directions. *Seminars in Thrombosis and Hemostasis, 39*(06), 642–655. doi:10.1055/s-0033-1353393 PMID:23929305

Nurden, P., & Nurden, A. T. (2008). Congenital disorders associated with platelet dysfunctions. *Thrombosis and Haemostasis, 99*, 253–263. PMID:18278172

Othman, M. (2011). Platelet-type von Willebrand disease: A rare, often misdiagnosed and underdiagnosed bleeding disorder. *Seminars in Thrombosis and Hemostasis, 37*(05), 464–469. doi:10.1055/s-0031-1281030 PMID:22102188

Ozelo, M. C., Svirin, P., & Larina, L. (2005). Use of recombinant factor VIIa in the management of severe bleeding episodes in patients with Bernard-Soulier syndrome. *Annals of Hematology, 84*(12), 816–822. doi:10.1007/s00277-005-1080-y PMID:16044315

Paterson, A. D., Rommens, J. M., Bharaj, B., Blavignac, J., Wong, I., Diamandis, M., & Hayward, C. P. M. et al. (2010). Persons with Quebec platelet disorder have a tandem duplication of PLAU, the urokinase plasminogen activator gene. *Blood, 115*(6), 1264–1266. doi:10.1182/blood-2009-07-233965 PMID:20007542

Peters, C. G., Michelson, A. D., & Flaumenhaft, R. (2012). Granule exocytosis is required for platelet spreading: Differential sorting of alpha-granules expressing VAMP-7. *Blood*, *120*(1), 199–206. doi:10.1182/blood-2011-10-389247 PMID:22589474

Pignatelli, P., Carnevale, R., Di Santo, S., Bartimoccia, S., Sanguigni, V., Lenti, L., & Violi, F. et al. (2011). Inherited human gp91phox deficiency is associated with impaired isoprostane formation and platelet dysfunction. *Arteriosclerosis, Thrombosis, and Vascular Biology*, *31*(2), 423–434. doi:10.1161/ATVBAHA.110.217885 PMID:21071703

Pothapragada, S., Zhang, P., Sheriff, J., Livelli, M., Slepian, M. J., Deng, Y., & Bluestein, D. (2015). A phenomenological particle-based platelet model for simulating filopodia formation during early activation. *International Journal for Numerical Methods in Biomedical Engineering*, *31*(3), e02702. doi:10.1002/cnm.2702 PMID:25532469

Rao, A. K. (2013). Inherited platelet function disorders: Overview and disorders of granules, secretion, and signal transduction. *Hematology/Oncology Clinics of North America*, *27*(3), 585–611. doi:10.1016/j.hoc.2013.02.005 PMID:23714313

Ren, Q., Ye, S., & Whiteheart, S. W. (2008). The platelet release reaction: Just when you thought platelet secretion was simple. *Current Opinion in Hematology*, *15*(5), 537–541. doi:10.1097/MOH.0b013e328309ec74 PMID:18695380

Rendu, F., & Brohard-Bohn, B. (2001). The platelet release reaction: Granules constituents, secretion and functions. *Platelets*, *12*(5), 261–273. doi:10.1080/09537100120068170 PMID:11487378

Rubak, P., Nissen, P. H., Kristensen, S. D., & Hvas, A. M. (2015). Investigation of platelet function and platelet disorders using flow cytometry. *Platelets*, 1–9. PMID:25901600

Sandrock, K., Nakamura, L., Vraetz, T., Beutel, K., Ehl, S., & Zieger, B. (2010). Platelet secretion defect in patients with familial hemophagocytic lymphohistiocytosis type 5 (FHL-5). *Blood*, *116*(26), 6148–6150. doi:10.1182/blood-2010-08-302943 PMID:21183701

Sandrock-Lang, K., Oldenburg, J., Wiegering, V., Halimeh, S., Santoso, S., Kurnik, K., & Zieger, B. et al. (2015a). Characterisation of patients with Glanzmann thrombasthenia and identification of 17 novel mutations. *Thrombosis and Haemostasis*, *113*(4), 782–791. doi:10.1160/TH14-05-0479 PMID:25373348

Sandrock-Lang, K., Wentzell, R., Santoso, S., & Zieger, B. (2015b). Inherited platelet disorders. *Hamostaseologie*, 35. PMID:25707719

Savoia, A., Kunishima, S., De Rocco, D., Zieger, B., Rand, M. L., Pujol-Moix, N., & Lanza, F. et al. (2014). Spectrum of the mutations in Bernard-Soulier syndrome. *Human Mutation*, *35*(9), 1033–1045. doi:10.1002/humu.22607 PMID:24934643

Seligsohn, U. (2012). Treatment of inherited platelet disorders. *Haemophilia: The Official Journal of the World Federation of Hemophilia, 18*(S4), 161-5.

Shapiro, A.D. (2000). Platelet function disorders. *Haemophilia: The Official Journal of the World Federation of Hemophilia, 6*(S1), 120-7.

Smith, H., Galmes, R., Gogolina, E., Straatman-Iwanowska, A., Reay, K., Banushi, B., & Gissen, P. et al. (2012). Associations among genotype, clinical phenotype, and intracellular localization of trafficking proteins in ARC syndrome. *Human Mutation*, *33*(12), 1656–1664. doi:10.1002/humu.22155 PMID:22753090

Smith, S. A., & Morrissey, J. H. (2014). Polyphosphate: A new player in the field of hemostasis. *Current Opinion in Hematology*, *21*(5), 388–394. doi:10.1097/MOH.0000000000000069 PMID:25010799

Smith, S. A., & Morrissey, J. H. (2015). 2013 Scientific Sessions Sol Sherry Distinguished Lecture in Thrombosis: Polyphosphate: A Novel Modulator of Hemostasis and Thrombosis. *Arteriosclerosis, Thrombosis, and Vascular Biology.*

Suzuki, J., Umeda, M., Sims, P. J., & Nagata, S. (2010). Calcium-dependent phospholipid scrambling by TMEM16F. *Nature*, *468*(7325), 834–838. doi:10.1038/nature09583 PMID:21107324

Tefre, K.L., Ingerslev, J., & Sorensen, B. (2009). Clinical benefit of recombinant factor VIIa in management of bleeds and surgery in two brothers suffering from the Bernard-Soulier syndrome. *Haemophilia: The Official Journal of the World Federation of Hemophilia, 15*, 281-4.

Urban, D., Li, L., Christensen, H., Pluthero, F. G., Chen, S. Z., Puhacz, M., & Kahr, W. H. A. et al. (2012). The VPS33B-binding protein VPS16B is required in megakaryocyte and platelet alpha-granule biogenesis. *Blood*, *120*(25), 5032–5040. doi:10.1182/blood-2012-05-431205 PMID:23002115

Van Geet, C., Izzi, B., Labarque, V., & Freson, K. (2009). Human platelet pathology related to defects in the G-protein signaling cascade. *Journal of thrombosis and haemostasis. JTH*, *7*(Suppl 1), 282–286. PMID:19630817

White, J. G. (1987). Inherited abnormalities of the platelet membrane and secretory granules. *Human Pathology*, *18*(2), 123–139. doi:10.1016/S0046-8177(87)80331-3 PMID:3542800

Wilson, D. B., Link, D. C., Mason, P. J., & Bessler, M. (2014). Inherited bone marrow failure syndromes in adolescents and young adults. *Annals of Medicine*, *46*(6), 353–363. doi:10.3109/07853890.2014.915579 PMID:24888387

Yang, H., Kim, A., David, T., Palmer, D., Jin, T., Tien, J., & Jan, L. Y. et al. (2012). TMEM16F forms a Ca2+-activated cation channel required for lipid scrambling in platelets during blood coagulation. *Cell*, *151*(1), 111–122. doi:10.1016/j.cell.2012.07.036 PMID:23021219

Ye, S., Karim, Z. A., Al Hawas, R., Pessin, J. E., Filipovich, A. H., & Whiteheart, S. W. (2012). Syntaxin-11, but not syntaxin-2 or syntaxin-4, is required for platelet secretion. *Blood*, *120*(12), 2484–2492. doi:10.1182/blood-2012-05-430603 PMID:22767500

Section 2

Discoveries in Cardiovascular Sciences:

Clinical Perspectives

Chapter 8
Myocardial Infarction:
Disease Mechanisms and Therapeutic Perspectives

Kalyan C. Chapalamadugu
University of South Florida, USA

Rakesh Kukreja
Virginia Commonwealth University, USA

Samhitha Gudla
University of South Florida, USA

Srinivas M. Tipparaju
University of South Florida, USA

ABSTRACT

Myocardial infarction (MI) is a major cardiovascular disease (CVD) and ranks among the leading causes of morbidity and mortality in humans, worldwide. Despite advances in disease prevention and treatment strategies, majority of the developed and developing world's suffer higher disease burden from MI, and incur billions of dollars in healthcare costs (Murray et al., 2015). Global estimates from 2013 show that MI is the major cardiovascular disease (CVD), and that deaths due to MI accounted for nearly half of the 17 million CVD mortalities (GBD, 2013; Mortality and Causes of Death Collaborators, 2015). Within the United States, MI top's the chart of both communicable and non-communicable diseases in terms of health loss that it is estimated to have inflicted in the population (Murray, et al., 2015). It has been estimated that every 2 minutes, three Americans suffer from myocardial infarction (MI), primary cause of MI being coronary blood flow obstruction and myocardial damage. The annual estimates of MI incidence in USA are approximately three quarter million a year while almost two-thirds of these cases represent new attacks (Mozaffarian, et al., 2015). Collectively, MI continues to lead the charts for CVD incidence rates, health loss, mortalities thereby putting enormous strain on healthcare system.

MULTI-ETIOLOGICAL DISORDER

MI primarily arise due to obstruction in the coronary blood flow to one or multiple regions of heart causing subsequent tissue hypoxegenation, metabolic modifications in the myocardium, cell death and decreased contractility. A major condition that leads to this obstruction is coronary artery diseases such as atherosclerosis, which involves plaque build-up (an intimal and/or sub-intimal deposition of lipids,

DOI: 10.4018/978-1-5225-2092-4.ch008

inflammatory cells and fibrous tissue) at the branching portions or in the narrow regions of the larger arteries. While a potential of the plaque to directly block the arterial lumen causing reduced blood flow always exists, atherosclerotic complications primarily arise due to the plaque rupture providing a foci for platelet aggregation and eventual thrombosis in the blood vessels, thereby effectively decreasing or altogether blocking the blood and oxygen supply to the dependent portions of the myocardium (Libby & Theroux, 2005; Naghavi et al., 2003). Plaque rupture leading to MI contributes to almost 70% of the total acute myocardial fatalities (Naghavi, et al., 2003). However, coronary artery diseases and therefore MI is always considered a multi-etiological disease as several factors contribute to atherosclerosis. One retrospective study in a select white male population revealed positive correlations between plaque lesions in aorta or coronary arteries and serum low-density lipoprotein (LDL), total cholesterol, triglycerides, systolic and diastolic blood pressure, and ponderal index (Berenson, Wattigney, Bao, Srinivasan, & Radhakrishnamurthy, 1995). Similar studies in the United Kingdom (Turner et al., 1998) revealed that type-2 diabetes is also a major risk factor for atherosclerosis as not only that hemoglobinA_{1c} and fasting blood glucose levels positively correlate with higher incidence of coronary disease and myocardial infarction, but diabetes can enhance the risk of MI through increasing the predisposition for atherosclerosis to perturbed serum lipid profile (Turner, et al., 1998). Further, life style factors, which include diet, physical activity, smoking, can significantly influence MI incidence (Ambrose & Barua, 2004; Oliveira, Barros, & Lopes, 2009). Epidemiological studies indicate that hypertension is perhaps, one single most risk factor for MI incidence, and estimates suggest that mortality due to coronary heart diseases doubles with every increment of a 20 mm Hg systolic or 10 mm Hg diastolic blood pressure (Cífková, 2008; McAreavey et al., 2016). Hence, conditions that can significantly contribute to hyperlipidemia, inflammation, aberrant vascular tone and hyperglycemia can all contribute to pathogenesis of plaque buildup in the arteries leading to atherosclerosis and associated cardiac complications such as MI.

Pathogenesis of Myocardial Infarction

Heart is one of the high energy demanding contractile tissue, and primarily relies on aerobic metabolism for unabated supply of high energy Adenosine triphosphate (ATP) to meet its energy requirements. Approximately two-third of ATP supply in normal healthy hearts comes through β-oxidation of long chain fatty acids in the mitochondria, while the rest summoned through catabolism of other substrates such as glucose, lactate, ketones and amino acids (Lopaschuk, Ussher, Folmes, Jaswal, & Stanley, 2010). Given that oxygen supply is essential to oxidative metabolism in all cells; it is inevitable that conditions that limit oxygen supply to the tissue would adversely affect the metabolism and energy supply compromising the structural and functional integrity of the heart. Immediate to the onset of ischemia, myocardium switches its reliance on fatty acids for ATP to anaerobic glycolysis, and depending on the severity of ischemia, this shift in metabolism leads to a moderate to severe fall in myocardial ATP and phosphocreatine concentrations and increases in net lactate, NADH, cellular acidosis, which can disrupt the ionic homeostasis in the cell resulting in Ca^{2+} overload. Simultaneously, inhibition of oxidative phosphorylation (OXPHOS) and accumulation of NADH in the mitochondria enhances ROS production. Further deprivation of oxygen and low energy state also affects endoplasmic reticulum leading to UPR and ER stress. These endogenous stress responses combined with energy shortage eventually leads to cell death and infarct formation (Kajstura et al., 1996; Yu et al., 2014). Accumulation of dead cells combined with modified extracellular milieu can signal inflammatory response, which attracts leukocytes to the infarct zone (Frangogiannis, 2008). Establishing blood flow and thereby renewing oxygen and nutrient supply can significantly alleviate infarct size and declined contractile function, however dependent on the timely reperfusion of the affected portions of the heart. Reperfusion rapidly activates OXPHOS and restores intracellular ATP, PH and normalizes lactate levels. Although high oxygen consumption also increases ROS production with potential to damage cell membranes, high Ca2+ accumulation in mitochondria leads to opening of mitochondrial permeability transition pore leading to apoptosis (Frohlich, Meier, White, Yellon, & Hausenloy, 2013; Griffiths & Halestrap, 1995). Further, resumption of blood flow also brings in neutrophils, monocytes and macrophages which release more ROS into the infarct zone can contribute to cell death, ECM remodeling, debris removal and scar formation (Frangogiannis, 2008). Timely reperfusion is recognized as the single most important intervention necessary after an MI event to minimize infarct size, improve cardiac contractility and reduce mortality (Zeymer et al., 2011). Collectively, oxidative stress, reductive stress, ER stress and inflammation represent the major pathological processes that underlie MI (Figure 1).

Oxidative Stress

Reactive oxygen species (ROS) such as superoxide anion ($O2^{-}$), hydroxyl radical ($^{\cdot}OH$) and hydrogen peroxide (H_2O_2) are routinely produced in eukaryotic cells with reported beneficial effects on cell cycle, survival and differentiation. While mitochondrial oxidative phosphorylation (Sena & Chandel, 2012) and NADPH oxidases (NOX) (Lassègue, San Martín, & Griendling, 2012) contribute significantly to intracellular ROS generation, involvement of other systems including xanthine oxidase (Battelli, Polito, Bortolotti, & Bolognesi, 2016), nitric oxide synthase (K. Zhao, Huang, Lu, Zhou, & Wei, 2010) and

Figure 1. Major pathophysiological mechanisms that form the basis for MI and myocardial remodeling

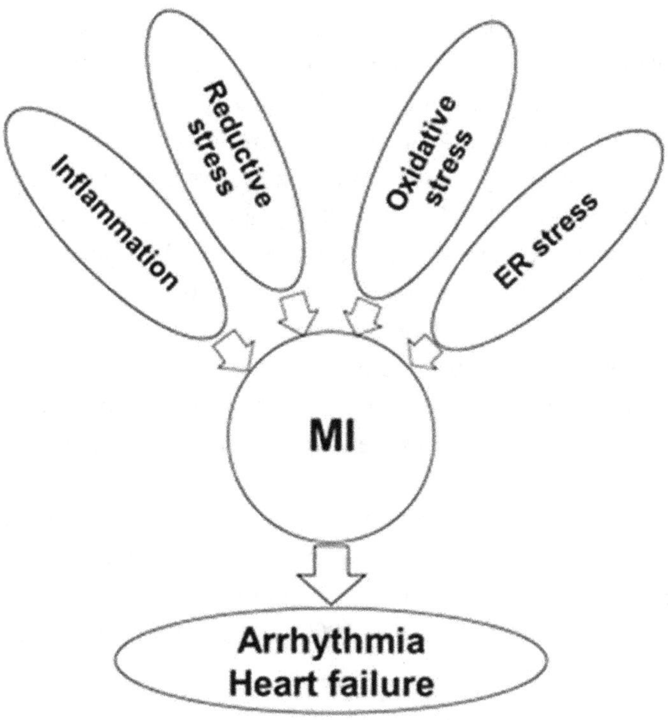

cytochrome P450 (Dostalek et al., 2008) is also well recognized. Extrinsic or intrinsic stressors can significantly enhance ROS production, and the net oxidative state of a cell at any point is determined by the residual ROS in the cell that overcame anti-oxidant defenses driven by enzymatic (superoxide dismutase, catalase, glutathione peroxidase) and non-enzymatic (Vitamin C, β-carotene, Vitamin E, glutaredoxin, thioredoxin, glutathione and peroxiredoxins), scavengers (Birben, Sahiner, Sackesen, Erzurum, & Kalayci, 2012). Because of their ability to readily donate an electron, excessive ROS can oxidize cellular molecules including lipids, proteins and DNA with deleterious consequences on cell growth, survival and function (Birben, et al., 2012).

Oxidative stress has been considered as one of a major pathophysiological basis of MI. Although elevation of ROS production in cardiac cells during hypoxic or anoxic conditions of ischemia are cardiotoxic, damage of ischemic myocardium due to ROS generated during reperfusion appear to be the major cause of adverse post-ischemic remodeling of the heart (Q. Chen, Moghaddas, Hoppel, & Lesnefsky, 2008; H.-L. Lee, Chen, Yeh, Zweier, & Chen, 2012; Zweier, Flaherty, & Weisfeldt, 1987). Studies conducted in dogs showed that reperfusion after a moderate ischemia leads to robust ROS generation that lasts even after 3 hours into reperfusion, with significant effect on the myocardial contractile function (Bolli et al., 1989a, 1989b). Mitochondria is a major source of oxidative stress as elemental oxygen is consumed in electron transfer chain of OXPHOS pathway, and enhanced electron leak due to I/R injury would elevate ROS production. Myocardial I/R injury leads to significant inhibition of complexes I and III, which are mediators of electron transfer chain of the mitochondrial OPXPHOS pathway, thus increasing electron leak and enhanced ROS production (Q. Chen, et al., 2008; H.-L. Lee, et al., 2012; Zhu et al., 2007). Another major source of ROS in cardiac myocytes comes from NADPH oxidase (Nox) (Hoffmeyer et al., 2000; Kuroda et al., 2010), with potential to affect cardiac remodeling and disease pathogenesis in heart. Deletion of Nox1, Nox2 or both has been shown to alleviate myocardial I/R injury in mice, suggesting that mitigating ROS excess through Nox inhibition is cardioprotective (Braunersreuther et al., 2013).

Xanthine oxidase has been extensively studied as a source of ROS in myocardial I/R injury as it also uses oxygen as an end electron acceptor with potential to contribute to cardiac myocyte ROS production during I/R injury. Animal studies have shown that the ischemic cardiac tissue have higher xanthine oxidase activity than its counterpart, Xanthine dehydrogenase that uses NAD+ as end electron acceptor, suggesting that enhanced Xanthine oxidase levels leads to ROS excess and I/R injury (Chambers et al., 1985; Kang et al., 2006). Similarly, dysregulation of β-adrenergic signaling, protein kinase A (Spear et al., 2007) and Cytochrome c Oxidase (Prabu et al., 2006) can each contribute to enhanced mitochondrial ROS excess during ischemia and reperfusion leading to myocardial injury.

Correlative studies have shown that decreased serum concentration of antioxidants such as Vitamin C associate to higher incidence of MI (Gey, Stahelin, & Eichholzer, 1993; Nyyssönen, Parviainen, Salonen, Tuomilehto, & Salonen, 1997). Prospective studies in humans have also shown that myocardial infarction associate to elevated oxidant levels (malondialdehyde) in blood, concurrent to diminished levels of antioxidant defenses measured as decreased superoxide dismutase, glutathione peroxidase and catalase activities as well as lower levels of non-enzymatic antioxidants such as β-carotene ascorbic acid, retinol and α-tocopherol (Hazini et al., 2015). Animal studies further showed that augmentation of antioxidant system through exogenous perfusion can alleviate myocardial I/R injury. Perfusion of ischemic hearts with Vitamin E (Haramaki, Assadnazari, Zimmer, Schepkin, & Packer, 1995), dihydrolipoic acid (Haramaki, et al., 1995), glutathione (Seiler & Starnes, 2000) and ascorbic acid (Tsai et al., 2011) were shown to mitigate myocardial I/R injury.

Reductive Stress

The counterpart of oxidative stress in cells, defined as reductive stress, is primarily determined by the proportion of reducing equivalents of pyridine nucleotides; NADH/NAD, NADPH/NADPH in the intracellular milieu. NAD/NADH partner in OXPHOS and ATP synthesis in the cells, while NADP/NADPH regulates oxidative stress (Circu, Maloney, & Aw, 2011). Both glycolysis and Kreb's cycle generates NADH, which in the mitochondria serves as an electron donor for electron transport chain of OXPHOS system to support ATP synthesis. Additionally, glucose can also enter into polyol pathway when excess or during glycolysis inhibition, which eventually leads to glucose reduction into sorbitol by aldose reductase (AR) and subsequent oxidation by sorbitol dehydrogenase to fructose, and reduction of NAD to NADH (Williamson et al., 1993). On the other hand, NADPH is generated during the first two enzymatic reactions of pentose phosphate pathway; glucose 6-phosphate dehydrogenase (G6-PDH) and 6-phosphogluconate dehydrogenase (6-PGDH), as well as during the substrate catalysis of malic enzyme and isocitrate dehydrogenase (Andrés, Satrústegui, & Machado, 1980). While NADH primarily contributes to OXPHOS, NADPH is used to regenerate the reduced glutathione (GSH) from glutathione disulfide (GSSG) by glutathione reductase, as well as reduce thioredoxin (Trx) by thioredoxin reductase (TrxR) (Birben, et al., 2012). Further, NADPH can also activate Nox leading to elevated ROS production (Circu, et al., 2011; Han et al., 2012). Because the generation of each of these pyridine nucleotide redox pairs is tightly coupled with substrate flux and usage, disruption of metabolic pathways that lead to increased levels of reduced equivalents of nicotinamide nucleotides can induce the reductive stress, and affect the overall redox potential of the cell with profound implications to cell survival and function.

Ischemic myocardium undergoes sever shift in energy substrate utilization as lack of blood flow limits both oxygen as well nutrients. Immediately after the onset of ischemia, glycolytic pathways are upregulated to sustain ATP necessary for cellular function. However, to sustain glycolysis, both NAD and NADH are required, but because of the inhibition of OXPHOS which supplies NAD for the glycolysis to continue, pyruvate which is the end product of glycolysis will instead be converted to lactate by lactate dehydrogenase in the cytoplasm. However, this leads to lactate accumulation, increased PH and accumulation of NADH in the cytosol, increases NADH/NAD ratio and inhibit glycolysis (Solaini & Harris, 2005). It was estimated that NADH/NAD ratio can increase more than 10 fold during ischemia, with potential to inhibit pyruvate oxidation (Salem, Saidel, Stanley, & Cabrera, 2002). As such, several studies have shown that decreasing the reductive stress through decreasing cytosolic NADH/NAD ratio in ischemic myocardium can limit I/R injury. Supplementation of Niacin in perfusion buffer has been shown to significantly decrease lactate/pyruvate ratio, attenuate ATP decline, creatine kinase release and improve lactate efflux in hearts subjected to low-flow ischemia (Trueblood, Ramasamy, Wang, & Schaefer, 2000). Similarly, pharmacological inhibition of aldose-reductase (AR) in the polyol pathway by Zopolrestat was shown to reduce cytosolic reductive stress measured as decreased lactate/pyruvate ratio in the heart subjected to low-flow ischemia and significantly improved high energy phosphate content (Ramasamy, Trueblood, & Schaefer, 1998). Studies have also shown that myocardial I/R injury is associated with decreased NAD levels, leading to elevated NADH/NAD levels, cytosolic reductive stress, and rescuing NAD by genetic or pharmacological means is cardioprotective against I/R injury (Hsu, Oka, Shao, Hariharan, & Sadoshima, 2009; Yamamoto et al., 2014). Further, increased NAD(P)H/NAD(P) has been shown in mouse hearts with Nox suppression, while decreased ratios of the these pairs were observed in Nox4 overexpressing hearts (Yu, et al., 2014), suggesting the redox ratios of these nucleotides is also influenced by Nox enzyme availability and/or activity. Similarly, elevation of mitochondrial NADH/NAD redox stress during ischemia may significantly overwhelm electron transport chain, resulting in excess ROS production (Yu, et al., 2014). Earlier studies have shown that excess NADPH, although a major factor in regenerating anti-oxidant glutathione and thioredoxin levels, can also lead to excess superoxide production in failing myocardium (Gupte et al., 2006). Studies conducted in isolated mitochondria and whole cardiac myocytes showed that reductive stress beyond a certain optimal level is indeed pro-oxidative leading to ROS excess in the cells (Aon, Cortassa, & O'Rourke, 2010).

Endoplasmic Reticulum (ER) Stress

ER is central to synthesis, folding and maturation of proteins in eukaryotic cells. As an intracellular store of ca^{2+} molecules, ER also plays a major role in various cellular processes including, but not limited to; cell cycle, survival, signaling, mobility and contractility. The ability of ER to process proteins is heavily oxygen and glucose dependent, and conditions that limit the supply can lead to accumulation of misfolded or unfolded proteins in the ER lumen, a condition summarized as ER stress (Kaufman, 2002; A. S. Lee, 1992). Cells however, try to correct these perturbations by inhibiting protein synthesis, but increasing the transcription and translation of heat shock proteins (HSPs) and supporting machinery for protein folding and degradation of misfolded proteins. This mechanism also termed as 'unfolded protein response (UPR), involves four major proteins that were identified and extensively characterized as primary mediators of UPR. Localized to the ER membrane, protein kinase-like ER kinase (PERK), inositol-requiring ER-to-nucleus signal kinase 1 (IRE1) and activating transcription factor 6α (ATF6α), stay normally latent due to their binding to glucose regulated protein-78 (Bip/Grp78) on the luminal side (Kaufman, 2002). However, accumulation of unfolded proteins in ER can pull away GPR-78 from these binding partners in the ER membrane relieving the inhibition resulting in UPR activation. Once activated, these proteins can induce transcriptional and posttranslational modulation of specific genes, which leads to inhibition of new protein synthesis, upregulating expression of ER chaperones and proteins involved in ER stress associated degradation (ERAD) (Kaufman, 2002).

Several studies using in vitro and in vivo models have shown UPR is activated in heart during I/R injury. Earlier studies in mice have shown UPR through increased XBP1 and GRP78 expression is upregulated in neonatal ventricular myocytes. Further, the same study showed that ischemia also enhances GRP78 specifically in infarcted myocardial tissue, suggesting that activated transcription factor 6 (ATF6) branch of UPR is elevated in injured myocardium (Thuerauf et al., 2006). Consistently, I/R increases GRP78 and GRP94 expression in heart, and overexpression of ATF6 in the heart, which is upstream of both GRP members, reduced infarct size and cardiomyocyte apoptosis, suggesting that UPR upregulation can be cardioprotective in I/R injury (Martindale et al., 2006). In vitro studies further showed that ischemia but not reoxygenation can increase nuclear translocation of ATF6 promoting GRP78 transcription and UPR upregulation (Doroudgar, Thuerauf, Marcinko, Belmont, & Glembotski, 2009). Studies in cardiac myocytes have also shown that UPR upregulation in I/R injury involves ATF6 dependent upregulation of protein disulfide isomerase associated 6 (PDIA6) gene, which is key to ER protein folding and cytoprotection (Vekich, Belmont, Thuerauf, & Glembotski, 2012). Further the same group have shown that ischemia can upregulate ATF6 and Derlin3, which is an important ERAD protein, both in cardiomyocytes and mouse heart (Belmont et al., 2010). Studies have shown that prolonged injury can increase the severity of ER stress and activate proapoptotic gene networks. Another ER protein involved in UPR is PERK, and activated PERK phosphorylates eukaryotic initiation factor 2-α (eIF2α), but promotes ATF4 expression, which then induces proapoptotic C/EBP homologous protein (CHOP) encoding gene expression (Ma,

Brewer, Alan Diehl, & Hendershot, 2002). Studies in neonatal rat cardiomyocytes showed that while early stages of ischemia upregulates the expression of GRP78, XBP1 and eIF2α phosphorylation inhibiting protein translation, severe ischemia can evoke maladaptive ER stress activating C/EBP homologous protein (CHOP) and caspase -12 activation resulting in cellular apoptosis (Szegezdi et al., 2006). Studies using knockout mice showed that CHOP deletion confers significant protection against myocardial I/R injury as both the extent of infarction and cardiomyocyte apoptosis are attenuated, and the exuberance of ROS that occurs during early reperfusion has been implicated in CHOP upregulation and apoptosis (Miyazaki et al., 2011). ER stress in cardiac myocytes also upregulates a proapoptotic p53-upregulated modulator of apoptosis (PUMA) gene (Nickson, Toth, & Erhardt, 2007), a BCL-2 family member that is a transcriptional target of ATF4/CHOP pair (Galehdar et al., 2010). In vivo studies revealed that I/R injury upregulates PUMA in infarct zone, and deletion of PUMA in cardiomyocytes or in mice rescues myocyte death and preserve contractile function during I/R injury (Toth et al., 2006). Further, low levels of oxidative stress can also elicit ER stress during reperfusion and contribute to myocardial damage (Z. H. Wang, Liu, Wu, Yu, & Yang, 2014). Because of the diverse and critical roles of ER in cell survival and function, ER stress is now recognized as a major pathophysiological regulator in various CVDs including MI.

Inflammation

Inflammation constitutes one of the major pathogenic basis of myocardial remodeling in infarcted heart. Inflammatory responses although are initiated in myocardium during ischemia, changes during reperfusion are profound, and the severity of inflammation appear to be one of major determinants of post MI recovery. Inflammatory responses during I/R injury includes aberrant changes in both vascular endothelium (VE) as well as myocardial cells, and reperfusion phase appear to be a major contributor of VE dysfunction. In cats, VE dependent relaxation of vasculature was significantly decreased to vasoactivator compounds such as acetyl choline (ACh) even with 2.5 minutes of reperfusion, as opposed to 4.5 of ischemia alone (Tsao, Aoki, Lefer, Johnson, & Lefer, 1990; Viehman, Ma, Lefer, & Lefer, 1991), suggesting reperfusion augments VE dysfunction in I/R injury. Although the time of induction depends on the species and duration of reperfusion, within 3 hours into reperfusion, mouse myocardium expresses various chemokines; MIP-1α, MIP-1β, MIP-2, MCP-1, IP-10, CXCR3, cytokines; IL-1β, IL-6, IL-10, TNF-α, LIF, TGFβ1, TGFβ2 and TGFβ3, and adhesion molecules; ICAM-1, selectins and growth factors; M-CSF and SCF (Dewald et al., 2004; Kukielka et al., 1993; Kumar et al., 1997). Further I/R injury also leads to endothelial dysfunction involving decline in vasodilatory ability of vasculature and expression of cytokines, adhesion molecules and chemokines and complement proteins (Singhal, Symons, Boudina, Jaishy, & Shiu, 2010). Neutrophils, which are innate killer cells, reach to the vasculature of the infarct zone, and bind to endothelial cell surfaces, and through interactions between selectins, integrins, cytokines and adhesion molecules, tether to endothelial surface and transmigrate into the perivascular space into the infarcted tissue (Vinten-Johansen, 2004). Upregulated cytokines in the infarct zone can also activate neutrophils, and further enhance the expression of adhesion molecules such as ICAM-1 on cardiac myocytes (Vinten-Johansen, 2004). Neutrophils are rich source of ROS and proteases, which clears the necrotic cell debris and release proinflammatory mediators in the infarcted and surrounding non-infarcted tissue. Further, MI also results in macrophage infiltration into the infarct tissue. While neutrophil infiltration is highest in the first 24 hours of ischemia, monocytes and their successor macrophages descend later into infarcted heart. In murine MI model (Nahrendorf et al., 2007), at least two waves of monocyte infiltration was reported, which include a first wave of Ly-6C^{high} cell population between day 1 to 4 of ischemia, and a second wave of Ly-6C^{lo} population thereafter, and this biphasic recruitment of monocytes into the infarct tissue supports a temporally distinct function of monocytes where Ly-6C^{high} are proinflammatory and scavenge necrotic tissue whereas Ly-6C^{lo} promotes angiogenesis and scar formation.

The fact that inflammation is a necessary process to clear the dead cells and form granulation tissue and heal the injured myocardium, interventions to modulate inflammatory response may minimize tissue injury. Cytokines have attracted the attention in this case as they play a key role in the expression of chemokines, cell adhesion molecules and inflammatory cell recruitment. Tumor necrosis factor alpha (TNFα) is a major cytokine induced in infarcted but not in normal myocardium (Dorge et al., 2002). Genetic ablation studies in mice have shown that TNF receptor type 1 and type 2 double, but not single, deletion, increased apoptotic myocyte cell death and infarct size, suggesting that at least one type of the receptor promotes anti-inflammatory cascade (Kurrelmeyer et al., 2000). Supporting this, inhibition of nuclear translocation of downstream target of TNF, the nuclear factor κB (NFκB) transcription factor, accentuates ischemic injury and infarct size (Misra et al., 2003). Similarly murine studies also have shown that p50 deletion, which is one of the five NFκB subunits, adversely affects post-ischemic left ventricular remodeling and systolic function (Timmers et al., 2009). Contrarily, beneficial effect of TNFα in infarcted hearts was also reported. TNFα deletion in mice reportedly protects against myocardial injury and contractile dysfunction in reperfused ischemic hearts, which was attributed to a potential over expression of this cytokine during reperfusion than ischemia alone (Maekawa et al., 2002). Genetic studies indicate that TNF receptors may be involved as TNF receptor type 1 but not TNF type 2, deletion in mice confers protection against I/R injury (Flaherty et al., 2008). Therefore, inflammation in the setting of MI represents complex pathogenic processes, where same factors such, for example TNFα, can have opposing actions, depending on the phase of injury (ischemia vs. reperfusion).

Interventions to Minimize Post-MI Cardiac Remodeling

Cardiac remodeling and recovery post MI episode depends on various factors, and major ones being the duration of ischemia before restoring perfusion and extent of myocardial tissue that suffered ischemia. Intriguingly, and perhaps justifiably, the major pathological basis of MI: oxidative stress, energy metabolism, reductive stress, ER stress and inflammation, can all adapt and protect or mal-adapt and worsen, with potential to alter the outcome of MI (Blasig, Ebert, Hennig, Pali, & Tosaki, 1990), suggesting that these same mechanisms can be manipulated to minimize the damage and improve the prognosis in MI patients (Figure 2).

In the last 30 years, the concept termed "ischemic conditioning" has received greater attention, and has been advanced as a promising intervention strategy to minimize MI induced damage. Several forms of conditioning strategies have been described in the literature depending on when the conditioning stimulus is applied in relation to timing of a major ischemic event; before vs. after (Ischemic preconditioning; IPC vs. ischemic postconditioning; IPoC) or where the stimulus was applied during ischemia; albeit at a remote site, (remote ischemic pre-conditioning, RIPC).

Earlier studies in animals have shown that preconditioning confers significant cardioprotection against MI. Past studies (Murry, Richard, Reimer, & Jennings, 1990) showed that multiple intermittent ischemia of 5 min durations in coronary circulation in dogs prior to a single continuous 40 minute ischemia can

Figure 2. Changes in metabolic and signaling events in myocardial infarction (MI): NADH-Nicotinamide adenine dinucleotide (oxidized), NADH-Nicotinamide adenine dinucleotide (reduced), ATP-Adenosine triphosphate, AKT/Protein Kinase B, PKC-Protein Kinase C, ERK1/2-Extracellular signal regulated Kinase 1/2, ROS-reactive oxygen Species, EF% ejection fraction and FS% Fractional shortening

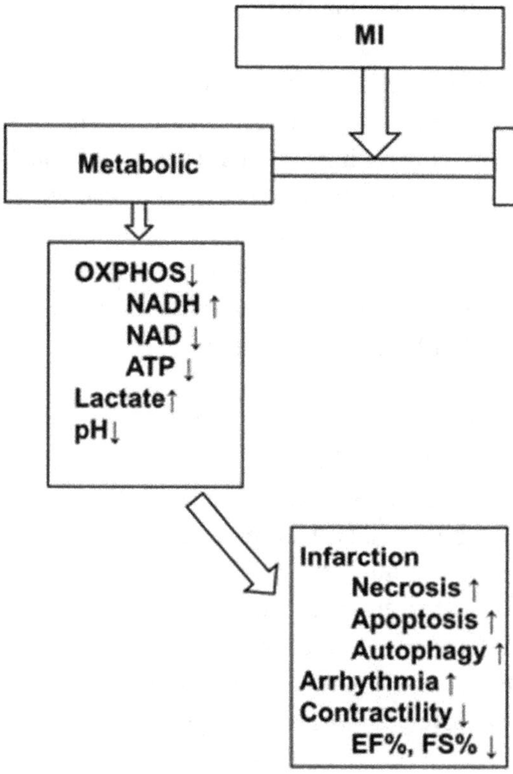

significantly reduce the infarct size, decelerate the fall in ATP levels and alleviate reductive stress associated with catabolites such as lactate. Myocardial damage during I/R is associated with significant increase in ROS and reactive nitrogen species (RNS) levels and decreased mitochondrial oxygen consumption; and preconditioning in mice through applying intermittent ischemic episodes were shown to attenuate ROS and RNS excess levels and promote oxygen consumption, clearly suggesting cardioprotection (Li et al., 2014; X. Zhao et al., 2005; Zhu, et al., 2007). Similarly, pathways involving UPR and ER stress were also investigated as potential mediators of ischemic conditioning, and studies in transgenic mice showed that IPC activates adaptive UPR by ER involving PERK/ATF3/ATF6 signaling pathway, with potential protective effects during early and late stages of I/R remodeling in myocardium (Brooks et al., 2014). Further, several studies have shown that pretreatment with various inflammatory cytokines such as TNF-α, IL-1, IL-1β, LIF at suboptimal doses confer protection of myocardium against I/R injury (Brown et al., 1990; Nelson, Wong, & McCord, 1995; Yamashita et al., 2000).

Both patient data and animal studies indicate that IPoC can also minimize I/R injury. Studies that investigated the effect of IPoC in patients having ST-elevation myocardial infarction (STEMI), and underwent primary percutaneous cutaneous intervention indicate that IPoC can minimize myocardial damage as indicated by reduction in serum markers of cardiac cell death; creatine kinase (CK, CK-MB), cardiac troponin I (cTnI) and improved contractile function, however the infarct sizes are not significantly different (Gao et al., 2015; Khan et al., 2014; L. Wang, Wang, Xu, & Li, 2013). Animal studies also support that IPoC can alleviate I/R injury. IPoC in ex vivo perfused 3 month old mice hearts showed that inducing shorter duration intermittent cycles of ischemia during reperfusion after a major index ischemia can reduce the infarct size, oxidative stress and improve cytoprotective protein expression in heart (Perez et al., 2016). In vivo studies in rats suggest that IPoc induced infarct size reduction also involves decreased superoxide anion production, lipid peroxidation, reduced neutrophil infiltration and cell death (Kin et al., 2004). Further, studies in isolated mitochondria show that IPoC improves the expression of mitochondrial electron transfer chain proteins concomitant to infarct size reduction, however conditional to open mitochondrial K_{ATP} channels, suggesting that IPoC may also improve energy metabolism (Cao et al., 2016). Further, IPoC mediated cardioprotection against I/R injury also involves ER stress attenuation, and studies in rats and rat cardiomyocytes indicate that protection is conferred by inhibiting the proapoptotic gene pathways including downregulation of CHOP, calreticulin, calcineurin, Caspase-12, JNK phosphorylation and increasing p38 MAPK phosphorylation (Y. H. Chen, Wu, Yao, Sun, & Liu, 2011; Liu, Zhang, Sun, & Wu, 2008).

Another mode of myocardial conditioning termed 'remote ischemic preconditioning (RIPC)' was initially reported by Przyklenk et al (1993), where multiple shorter episodes of I/R applied to circumflex coronary artery branches of dog prior to LAD ligation and/or reperfusion resulted in a significant reduction in infarct size, suggesting that the beneficial effects extended beyond the preconditioned vascular bed (Przyklenk, Bauer, Ovize, Kloner, & Whittaker, 1993). Subsequent studies in various animal models have demonstrated that RIPC, even when the preconditioning stimulus was applied to a major vasculature of distant organs; hind limb, intestine, kidney, can also limit the infarct size and confer protection against subsequent myocardial I/R injury (Aon, et al., 2010; Belmont, et al., 2010; Birben, et al., 2012; Braunersreuther, et al., 2013). Several studies investigated the mechanistic basis of RIPC, and concluded that humoral, neural as well as systemic factors may all contribute to myocardial protection (Birben, et al., 2012; Cai, Parajuli, Zheng, & Becker, 2012; Konstantinov et al., 2004; Shimizu et al., 2010). At the signaling level, cardioprotection through RIPC appears to activate prosurvival genetic pathways involving PKC, AKT, ERK1/2 and JNK1, which can converge to suppress proaptotic gene programs resulting in reduction of infarct size (Aon, et al., 2010; Belmont, et al., 2010; Chambers, et al., 1985; Q. Chen, et al., 2008; Cífková, 2008). Additionally, diffusible molecules such as Nitric oxide may be involved in RIPC through alleviating oxidative stress. A recent work (Rassaf et al., 2014) showed that stimulating nitric oxide release by applying shorter cycles of transient ischemia in femoral vascular bed with subsequent reactive hyperemia in mice enhanced plasma and cardiac nitrite levels resulting in elevated NO levels in the heart leading to S-nitrosation of mitochondrial membrane proteins, decreased mitochondrial respiration and reactive oxygen species generation, effectively reducing the infarct size (Rassaf, et al., 2014). Studies conducted in coronary artery bypass grafting patients also indicate that RIPC may activate myocardial antioxidant defenses such as superoxide dismutase, cytochrome C and thioredoxin-1, potentially reducing ischemic injury (Cai, et al., 2012; Yildirim et al., 2016). Further, the beneficial effects of RIPC I/R injury may also involve inflammatory mediators. Microarray studies conducted in circulating leukocytes and neutrophils of humans subjected to non-invasive shorter episodes of I/R revealed decreased proinflammatory gene expression, which suggested that the beneficial effects of RIPC may involve modulation of innate immune system that involves decreased potential of leukocyte and neutrophil adhesion for phagocytosis and exocytosis and production of inflammatory mediators such as cytokine, and chemokines (Konstantinov, et al., 2004; Shimizu, et al., 2010). Studies in mice have further shown that the beneficial effects RIPC may also involve upregulation of both systemic and cardiac anti-inflammatory pathways, as RIPC applied through serial hind limb I/R episodes increased plasma and cardiac IL-10 protein levels, upregulated PI3K/AKT pathway and attenuated I/R injury in a IL-10 dependent manner (Cai, et al., 2012). Given the significance of immune system in myocardial I/R injury, modulation of the inflammatory mediators by RIPC may be cardioprotective. Furthermore, exosomes and microvesicles may also play a role in remote signal transduction in RIPC. Ex vivo studies showed that when these protein, DNA, miRNA rich vesicles that are secreted into cardiac effluents collected from rat hearts subjected to three 5/5min episodes of I/R, when perfused into non-preconditioned recipient hearts that underwent subsequent longer I/R insult, resulted in reducing the infarct size (Giricz et al., 2014).

RIPC is considered one of the most practical to confer cardioprotection through preconditioning in the case of MI, because it can be applied, non-invasively, while patients are in transport or before arrival or in advance of the major procedures such as percutaneous interventions or bypass graft. RIPC is still an active area of research, and although contradictory evidence exists, clinical trials provide some strong evidence of the beneficial effects of RIPC (Table 1).

Table 1. Remote Ischemic Preconditioning (RIPC), clinical trials and outcomes

RIPC Site/Stimulus	Major Intervention	Outcome
Upper arm, three cycles of I/R (5/5 min)	Primary percutaneous intervention surgery in ACS patients	Decreased serum cTnI and decreased ST-segment deviations (Hoole et al., 2009)
Upper arm, four cycles of I/R (5/5 min)	Primary percutaneous intervention surgery in ACS patients	Increased myocardial salvage index (Bøtker et al., 2010)
Upper arm, three cycles of I/R (5/5 min)	Primary percutaneous intervention surgery in ACS patients	Decreased serum cTnT levels (Ahmed et al., 2013)
Upper arm, three cycles of I/R (5/5 min)	Primary percutaneous intervention surgery in ACS patients	No difference in plasma high-sensitivity C-reactive protein, endothelial progenitor cells cell count or serum cTnT (Prasad et al., 2013)
Upper arm, three cycles of I/R (5/5 min)	Coronary artery bypass graft	Decreased perioperative myocardial injury index and serum total troponin levels (Hausenloy et al., 2007)
Common iliac artery, one cycle of I/R (10/10 min)	Abdominal aortic aneurysm repair	Reduced myocardial infarction (Ali et al., 2007)
Upper arm, three cycles of I/R (5/5 min)	Primary percutaneous intervention surgery in ACS patients	Decreased cardiac troponin I, decreased incidence of MI 4a (Luo et al., 2013)
Upper arm, one cycle of I/R (5/5 min)	Primary percutaneous intervention surgery in ACS patients	Decreased cardiac troponin I, decreased incidence of MI 4a (Zografos et al., 2014)
Upper arm, three cycles of I/R (5/5 min)	Coronary artery bypass graft	Short term increase in cardiac contractility, decreased vascular resistance, no change in serum levels of troponin I and creatine kinase-MB. No long term changes detected (24 hours) (Lomivorotov et al., 2012)
Upper arm, four cycles of I/R (5/5 min)	Elective coronary artery bypass graft	No significant change in troponin levels and primary outcomes (Meybohm et al., 2015)

CONCLUSION

MI still represents the major CVD, worldwide. Given that MI is a form of metabolic disease, and complicated by life style factors and other highly prevalent co-morbidities such as diabetes and hypertension, both, the development of new, and improvement of the existing, approaches has to be carried out in order to more effectively decrease the morbidity, mortality and associated health costs of MI.

REFERENCES

Ahmed, R. M., Mohamed, E.-H. A., Ashraf, M., Maithili, S., Nabil, F., Rami, R., & Mohamed, T. I. (2013). Effect of remote ischemic preconditioning on serum troponin T level following elective percutaneous coronary intervention. *Catheterization and Cardiovascular Interventions*, *82*(5), E647–E653. doi:10.1002/ccd.24825 PMID:23404916

Ali, Z. A., Callaghan, C. J., Lim, E., Ali, A. A., Nouraei, S. A., Akthar, A. M., & Gaunt, M. E. et al. (2007). Remote ischemic preconditioning reduces myocardial and renal injury after elective abdominal aortic aneurysm repair: A randomized controlled trial. *Circulation*, *116*(11Suppl), I98–I105. doi:10.1161/circulationaha.106.679167 PMID:17846333

Ambrose, J. A., & Barua, R. S. (2004). The pathophysiology of cigarette smoking and cardiovascular diseaseAn update. *Journal of the American College of Cardiology*, *43*(10), 1731–1737. doi:10.1016/j.jacc.2003.12.047 PMID:15145091

Andrés, A., Satrústegui, J., & Machado, A. (1980). Development of NADPH-producing pathways in rat heart. *The Biochemical Journal*, *186*(3), 799–803. doi:10.1042/bj1860799 PMID:7396838

Aon, M. A., Cortassa, S., & ORourke, B. (2010). Redox-optimized ROS balance: A unifying hypothesis. *Biochimica et Biophysica Acta (BBA) -. Bioenergetics*, *1797*(6–7), 865–877. doi:10.1016/j.bbabio.2010.02.016

Battelli, M. G., Polito, L., Bortolotti, M., & Bolognesi, A. (2016). Xanthine Oxidoreductase-Derived Reactive Species: Physiological and Pathological Effects. *Oxidative Medicine and Cellular Longevity*, *3527579*. doi:10.1155/2016/3527579 PMID:26823950

Belmont, P. J., Chen, W. J., San Pedro, M. N., Thuerauf, D. J., Gellings Lowe, N., Gude, N., & Glembotski, C. C. et al. (2010). Roles for endoplasmic reticulum-associated degradation and the novel endoplasmic reticulum stress response gene Derlin-3 in the ischemic heart. *Circulation Research*, *106*(2), 307–316. doi:10.1161/CIRCRESAHA.109.203901 PMID:19940266

Berenson, G. S., Wattigney, W. A., Bao, W., Srinivasan, S. R., & Radhakrishnamurthy, B. (1995). Rationale to Study the Early Natural History of Heart Disease: The Bogalusa Heart Study. *The American Journal of the Medical Sciences*, *310*, S22–S28. doi:10.1097/00000441-199512000-00005 PMID:7503119

Birben, E., Sahiner, U. M., Sackesen, C., Erzurum, S., & Kalayci, O. (2012). Oxidative Stress and Antioxidant Defense. *The World Allergy Organization Journal*, *5*(1), 9-19. doi: 10.1097/WOX.0b013e3182439613

Blasig, I. E., Ebert, B., Hennig, C., Pali, T., & Tosaki, A. (1990). Inverse relationship between ESR spin trapping of oxyradicals and degree of functional recovery during myocardial reperfusion in isolated working rat heart. *Cardiovascular Research*, *24*(4), 263–270. doi:10.1093/cvr/24.4.263 PMID:2161288

Bolli, R., Jeroudi, M. O., Patel, B. S., DuBose, C. M., Lai, E. K., Roberts, R., & McCay, P. B. (1989a). Direct evidence that oxygen-derived free radicals contribute to postischemic myocardial dysfunction in the intact dog. *Proceedings of the National Academy of Sciences of the United States of America*, *86*(12), 4695–4699. doi:10.1073/pnas.86.12.4695 PMID:2543984

Bolli, R., Jeroudi, M. O., Patel, B. S., DuBose, C. M., Lai, E. K., Roberts, R., & McCay, P. B. (1989b). Direct evidence that oxygen-derived free radicals contribute to postischemic myocardial dysfunction in the intact dog. *Proceedings of the National Academy of Sciences of the United States of America*, *86*(12), 4695–4699. doi:10.1073/pnas.86.12.4695 PMID:2543984

Bøtker, H. E., Kharbanda, R., Schmidt, M. R., Bøttcher, M., Kaltoft, A. K., Terkelsen, C. J., & Nielsen, T. T. et al. (2010). Remote ischaemic conditioning before hospital admission, as a complement to angioplasty, and effect on myocardial salvage in patients with acute myocardial infarction: A randomised trial. *Lancet*, *375*(9716), 727–734. doi:10.1016/S0140-6736(09)62001-8 PMID:20189026

Braunersreuther, V., Montecucco, F., Asrih, M., Pelli, G., Galan, K., Frias, M., & Jaquet, V. et al. (2013). Role of NADPH oxidase isoforms NOX1, NOX2 and NOX4 in myocardial ischemia/reperfusion injury. *Journal of Molecular and Cellular Cardiology*, *64*, 99–107. doi:10.1016/j.yjmcc.2013.09.007 PMID:24051369

Brooks, A. C., Guo, Y., Singh, M., McCracken, J., Xuan, Y. T., Srivastava, S., & Bhatnagar, A. et al. (2014). Endoplasmic reticulum stress-dependent activation of ATF3 mediates the late phase of ischemic preconditioning. *Journal of Molecular and Cellular Cardiology*, *76*, 138–147. doi:10.1016/j.yjmcc.2014.08.011 PMID:25151953

Brown, J. M., White, C. W., Terada, L. S., Grosso, M. A., Shanley, P. F., Mulvin, D. W., & Repine, J. E. et al. (1990). Interleukin 1 pretreatment decreases ischemia/reperfusion injury. *Proceedings of the National Academy of Sciences of the United States of America*, *87*(13), 5026–5030. doi:10.1073/pnas.87.13.5026 PMID:2367521

Cai, Z. P., Parajuli, N., Zheng, X., & Becker, L. (2012). Remote ischemic preconditioning confers late protection against myocardial ischemia-reperfusion injury in mice by upregulating interleukin-10. *Basic Research in Cardiology*, *107*(4), 277–277. doi:10.1007/s00395-012-0277-1 PMID:22752341

Cao, S., Liu, Y., Wang, H., Mao, X., Chen, J., Liu, J.,... Yu, T. (2016). Ischemic postconditioning influences electron transport chain protein turnover in Langendorff-perfused rat hearts. *PeerJ*, *4*, e1706. doi: 10.7717/peerj.1706

Chambers, D. E., Parks, D. A., Patterson, G., Roy, R., McCord, J. M., Yoshida, S., & Downey, J. M. et al. (1985). Xanthine oxidase as a source of free radical damage in myocardial ischemia. *Journal of Molecular and Cellular Cardiology*, *17*(2), 145–152. doi:10.1016/S0022-2828(85)80017-1 PMID:3839024

Chen, Q., Moghaddas, S., Hoppel, C. L., & Lesnefsky, E. J. (2008). Ischemic defects in the electron transport chain increase the production of reactive oxygen species from isolated rat heart mitochondria. *American Journal of Physiology. Cell Physiology*, *294*(2), C460–C466. doi:10.1152/ajpcell.00211.2007 PMID:18077608

Chen, Y. H., Wu, X. D., Yao, S. T., Sun, S., & Liu, X. H. (2011). Calcineurin is involved in cardioprotection induced by ischemic postconditioning through attenuating endoplasmic reticulum stress. *Chinese Medical Journal*, *124*(20), 3334–3340. PMID:22088531

Cífková, R. (2008). Epidemiology and risk of hypertension. *Archives of Medical Science*, *5*(2A), S199–S211.

Circu, M. L., Maloney, R. E., & Aw, T. Y. (2011). Disruption of pyridine nucleotide redox status during oxidative challenge at normal and low-glucose states: Implications for cellular adenosine triphosphate, mitochondrial respiratory activity, and reducing capacity in colon epithelial cells. *Antioxidants & Redox Signalling*, *14*(11), 2151–2162. doi:10.1089/ars.2010.3489 PMID:21083422

Dewald, O., Ren, G., Duerr, G. D., Zoerlein, M., Klemm, C., Gersch, C., & Frangogiannis, N. G. et al. (2004). Of Mice and Dogs: Species-Specific Differences in the Inflammatory Response Following Myocardial Infarction. *American Journal of Pathology*, *164*(2), 665–677. doi:10.1016/S0002-9440(10)63154-9 PMID:14742270

Dorge, H., Schulz, R., Belosjorow, S., Post, H., van de Sand, A., Konietzka, I., & Heusch, G. et al. (2002). Coronary microembolization: The role of TNF-alpha in contractile dysfunction. *Journal of Molecular and Cellular Cardiology*, *34*(1), 51–62. doi:10.1006/jmcc.2001.1489 PMID:11812164

Doroudgar, S., Thuerauf, D. J., Marcinko, M. C., Belmont, P. J., & Glembotski, C. C. (2009). Ischemia Activates the ATF6 Branch of the Endoplasmic Reticulum Stress Response. *The Journal of Biological Chemistry*, *284*(43), 29735–29745. doi:10.1074/jbc.M109.018036 PMID:19622751

Dostalek, M., Hardy, K. D., Milne, G. L., Morrow, J. D., Chen, C., Gonzalez, F. J., & Guengerich, F. P. et al. (2008). Development of Oxidative Stress by Cytochrome P450 Induction in Rodents Is Selective for Barbiturates and Related to Loss of Pyridine Nucleotide-dependent Protective Systems. *The Journal of Biological Chemistry*, *283*(25), 17147–17157. doi:10.1074/jbc.M802447200 PMID:18442974

Flaherty, M. P., Guo, Y., Tiwari, S., Rezazadeh, A., Hunt, G., Sanganalmath, S. K., & Dawn, B. et al. (2008). The role of TNF-α receptors p55 and p75 in acute myocardial ischemia/reperfusion injury and late preconditioning. *Journal of Molecular and Cellular Cardiology*, *45*(6), 735–741. doi:10.1016/j.yjmcc.2008.08.014 PMID:18824172

Frangogiannis, N. G. (2008). The immune system and cardiac repair. *Pharmacological Research*, *58*(2), 88–111. doi:10.1016/j.phrs.2008.06.007 PMID:18620057

Frohlich, G. M., Meier, P., White, S. K., Yellon, D. M., & Hausenloy, D. J. (2013). Myocardial reperfusion injury: Looking beyond primary PCI. *European Heart Journal*, *34*(23), 1714–1722. doi:10.1093/eurheartj/eht090 PMID:23536610

Galehdar, Z., Swan, P., Fuerth, B., Callaghan, S. M., Park, D. S., & Cregan, S. P. (2010). Neuronal apoptosis induced by endoplasmic reticulum stress is regulated by ATF4-CHOP-mediated induction of the Bcl-2 homology 3-only member PUMA. *The Journal of Neuroscience*, *30*(50), 16938–16948. doi:10.1523/JNEUROSCI.1598-10.2010 PMID:21159964

Gao, J., Luo, J., Liu, F., Zheng, Y., Chen, B., Chen, Q., & Yang, Y. (2015). Short-and long-term effects of ischemic postconditioning in STEMI patients: A meta-analysis. *Lipids in Health and Disease*, *14*(1), 147. doi:10.1186/s12944-015-0151-x PMID:26573572

GBD 2013 Mortality and Causes of Death Collaborators. (2015). Global, regional, and national age–sex specific all-cause and cause-specific mortality for 240 causes of death, 1990–2013: a systematic analysis for the Global Burden of Disease Study 2013. *The Lancet, 385*(9963), 117-171. doi: 10.1016/s0140-6736(14)61682-2

Gey, K. F., Stahelin, H. B., & Eichholzer, M. (1993). Poor plasma status of carotene and vitamin C is associated with higher mortality from ischemic heart disease and stroke: Basel Prospective Study. *The Clinical Investigator*, *71*(1), 3–6. doi:10.1007/BF00210955 PMID:8453256

Giricz, Z., Varga, Z. V., Baranyai, T., Sipos, P., Pálóczi, K., Kittel, Á., & Ferdinandy, P. et al. (2014). Cardioprotection by remote ischemic preconditioning of the rat heart is mediated by extracellular vesicles. *Journal of Molecular and Cellular Cardiology*, *68*, 75–78. doi:10.1016/j.yjmcc.2014.01.004 PMID:24440457

Griffiths, E. J., & Halestrap, A. P. (1995). Mitochondrial non-specific pores remain closed during cardiac ischaemia, but open upon reperfusion. *The Biochemical Journal*, *307*(Pt 1), 93–98. doi:10.1042/bj3070093 PMID:7717999

Gupte, S. A., Levine, R. J., Gupte, R. S., Young, M. E., Lionetti, V., Labinskyy, V., & Recchia, F. A. et al. (2006). Glucose-6-phosphate dehydrogenase-derived NADPH fuels superoxide production in the failing heart. *Journal of Molecular and Cellular Cardiology*, *41*(2), 340–349. doi:10.1016/j.yjmcc.2006.05.003 PMID:16828794

Han, C. Y., Umemoto, T., Omer, M., Den Hartigh, L. J., Chiba, T., LeBoeuf, R., & Chait, A. et al. (2012). NADPH Oxidase-derived Reactive Oxygen Species Increases Expression of Monocyte Chemotactic Factor Genes in Cultured Adipocytes. *The Journal of Biological Chemistry*, *287*(13), 10379–10393. doi:10.1074/jbc.M111.304998 PMID:22287546

Haramaki, N., Assadnazari, H., Zimmer, G., Schepkin, V., & Packer, L. (1995). The influence of vitamin E and dihydrolipoic acid on cardiac energy and glutathione status under hypoxia-reoxygenation. *Biochemistry and Molecular Biology International*, *37*(3), 591–597. PMID:8595400

Hausenloy, D. J., Mwamure, P. K., Venugopal, V., Harris, J., Barnard, M., Grundy, E., & Yellon, D. M. et al. (2007). Effect of remote ischaemic preconditioning on myocardial injury in patients undergoing coronary artery bypass graft surgery: A randomised controlled trial. *Lancet*, *370*(9587), 575–579. doi:10.1016/S0140-6736(07)61296-3 PMID:17707752

Hazini, A., Cemek, M., Isildak, I., Alpdagtas, S., Onul, A., Senel, U., & Uyarel, H. et al. (2015). Investigation of ischemia modified albumin, oxidant and antioxidant markers in acute myocardial infarction. *Postepy Kardiol Interwencyjnej*, *11*(4), 298–303. doi:10.5114/pwki.2015.55600 PMID:26677379

Hoffmeyer, M. R., Jones, S. P., Ross, C. R., Sharp, B., Grisham, M. B., Laroux, F. S., & Lefer, D. J. et al. (2000). Myocardial Ischemia/Reperfusion Injury in NADPH Oxidase–Deficient Mice. *Circulation Research*, *87*(9), 812–817. doi:10.1161/01.RES.87.9.812 PMID:11055986

Hoole, S. P., Heck, P. M., Sharples, L., Khan, S. N., Duehmke, R., Densem, C. G., & Dutka, D. P. et al. (2009). Cardiac Remote Ischemic Preconditioning in Coronary Stenting (CRISP Stent) Study: A prospective, randomized control trial. *Circulation*, *119*(6), 820–827. doi:10.1161/CIRCULATIONAHA.108.809723 PMID:19188504

Hsu, C.-P., Oka, S., Shao, D., Hariharan, N., & Sadoshima, J. (2009). Nicotinamide Phosphoribosyltransferase Regulates Cell Survival Through NAD+ Synthesis in Cardiac Myocytes. *Circulation Research*, *105*(5), 481–491. doi:10.1161/CIRCRESAHA.109.203703 PMID:19661458

Kajstura, J., Cheng, W., Reiss, K., Clark, W. A., Sonnenblick, E. H., Krajewski, S., & Anversa, P. et al. (1996). Apoptotic and necrotic myocyte cell deaths are independent contributing variables of infarct size in rats. *Laboratory Investigation*, *74*(1), 86–107. PMID:8569201

Kang, S. M., Lim, S., Song, H., Chang, W., Lee, S., Bae, S. M., & Hwang, K. C. et al. (2006). Allopurinol modulates reactive oxygen species generation and Ca2+ overload in ischemia-reperfused heart and hypoxia-reoxygenated cardiomyocytes. *European Journal of Pharmacology*, *535*(1-3), 212–219. doi:10.1016/j.ejphar.2006.01.013 PMID:16516885

Kaufman, R. J. (2002). Orchestrating the unfolded protein response in health and disease. *The Journal of Clinical Investigation*, *110*(10), 1389–1398. doi:10.1172/JCI0216886 PMID:12438434

Khan, A. R., Binabdulhak, A. A., Alastal, Y., Khan, S., Faricy-Beredo, B. M., Luni, F. K.,... Tinkel, J. (2014). Cardioprotective role of ischemic postconditioning in acute myocardial infarction: a systematic review and meta-analysis. *Am Heart J, 168*(4), 512-521 e514. doi: 10.1016/j.ahj.2014.06.021

Kin, H., Zhao, Z.-Q., Sun, H.-Y., Wang, N.-P., Corvera, J. S., Halkos, M. E., & Vinten-Johansen, J. et al. (2004). Postconditioning attenuates myocardial ischemia–reperfusion injury by inhibiting events in the early minutes of reperfusion. *Cardiovascular Research*, *62*(1), 74–85. doi:10.1016/j.cardiores.2004.01.006 PMID:15023554

Konstantinov, I. E., Arab, S., Kharbanda, R. K., Li, J., Cheung, M. M. H., Cherepanov, V., & Redington, A. N. et al. (2004). The remote ischemic preconditioning stimulus modifies inflammatory gene expression in humans. *Physiological Genomics*, *19*(1), 143–150. doi:10.1152/physiolgenomics.00046.2004 PMID:15304621

Kukielka, G. L., Hawkins, H. K., Michael, L., Manning, A. M., Youker, K., Lane, C., & Anderson, D. C. et al. (1993). Regulation of intercellular adhesion molecule-1 (ICAM-1) in ischemic and reperfused canine myocardium. *The Journal of Clinical Investigation*, *92*(3), 1504–1516. doi:10.1172/JCI116729 PMID:8104198

Kumar, A. G., Ballantyne, C. M., Michael, L. H., Kukielka, G. L., Youker, K. A., Lindsey, M. L., & Entman, M. L. et al. (1997). Induction of Monocyte Chemoattractant Protein-1 in the Small Veins of the Ischemic and Reperfused Canine Myocardium. *Circulation*, *95*(3), 693–700. doi:10.1161/01.CIR.95.3.693 PMID:9024159

Kuroda, J., Ago, T., Matsushima, S., Zhai, P., Schneider, M. D., & Sadoshima, J. (2010). NADPH oxidase 4 (Nox4) is a major source of oxidative stress in the failing heart. *Proceedings of the National Academy of Sciences of the United States of America*, *107*(35), 15565–15570. doi:10.1073/pnas.1002178107 PMID:20713697

Kurrelmeyer, K. M., Michael, L. H., Baumgarten, G., Taffet, G. E., Peschon, J. J., Sivasubramanian, N., & Mann, D. L. et al. (2000). Endogenous tumor necrosis factor protects the adult cardiac myocyte against ischemic-induced apoptosis in a murine model of acute myocardial infarction. *Proceedings of the National Academy of Sciences of the United States of America*, *97*(10), 5456–5461. doi:10.1073/pnas.070036297 PMID:10779546

Lassègue, B., San Martín, A., & Griendling, K. K. (2012). Biochemistry, Physiology, and Pathophysiology of NADPH Oxidases in the Cardiovascular System. *Circulation Research*, *110*(10), 1364–1390. doi:10.1161/CIRCRESAHA.111.243972 PMID:22581922

Lee, A. S. (1992). Mammalian stress response: Induction of the glucose-regulated protein family. *Current Opinion in Cell Biology*, *4*(2), 267–273. doi:10.1016/0955-0674(92)90042-B PMID:1599691

Lee, H.-L., Chen, C.-L., Yeh, S. T., Zweier, J. L., & Chen, Y.-R. (2012). Biphasic modulation of the mitochondrial electron transport chain in myocardial ischemia and reperfusion. *American Journal of Physiology. Heart and Circulatory Physiology*, *302*(7), H1410–H1422. doi:10.1152/ajpheart.00731.2011 PMID:22268109

Li, Y., Cai, M., Cao, L., Qin, X., Zheng, T., Xu, X., & He, G. et al. (2014). Endurance exercise accelerates myocardial tissue oxygenation recovery and reduces ischemia reperfusion injury in mice. *PLoS ONE*, *9*(12), e114205. doi:10.1371/journal.pone.0114205 PMID:25474642

Libby, P., & Theroux, P. (2005). Pathophysiology of Coronary Artery Disease. *Circulation*, *111*(25), 3481–3488. doi:10.1161/CIRCULATIONAHA.105.537878 PMID:15983262

Liu, X. H., Zhang, Z. Y., Sun, S., & Wu, X. D. (2008). Ischemic postconditioning protects myocardium from ischemia/reperfusion injury through attenuating endoplasmic reticulum stress. *Shock (Augusta, Ga.)*, *30*(4), 422–427. doi:10.1097/SHK.0b013e318164ca29 PMID:18323739

Lomivorotov, V. V., Shmyrev, V. A., Nepomnyaschih, V. A., Ponomarev, D. N., Knyazkova, L. G., Lomivorotov, V. N., & Karaskov, A. M. (2012). Remote ischaemic preconditioning does not protect the heart in patients undergoing coronary artery bypass grafting. *Interactive Cardiovascular and Thoracic Surgery*, *15*(1), 18–22. doi:10.1093/icvts/ivs118 PMID:22493101

Lopaschuk, G. D., Ussher, J. R., Folmes, C. D. L., Jaswal, J. S., & Stanley, W. C. (2010). Myocardial Fatty Acid Metabolism in Health and Disease. *Physiological Reviews*, *90*(1), 207–258. doi:10.1152/physrev.00015.2009 PMID:20086077

Luo, S. J., Zhou, Y. J., Shi, D. M., Ge, H. L., Wang, J. L., & Liu, R. F. (2013). Remote ischemic preconditioning reduces myocardial injury in patients undergoing coronary stent implantation. *The Canadian Journal of Cardiology*, *29*(9), 1084–1089. doi:10.1016/j.cjca.2012.11.022 PMID:23414904

Ma, Y., Brewer, J. W., Alan Diehl, J., & Hendershot, L. M. (2002). Two Distinct Stress Signaling Pathways Converge Upon the CHOP Promoter During the Mammalian Unfolded Protein Response. *Journal of Molecular Biology*, *318*(5), 1351–1365. doi:10.1016/S0022-2836(02)00234-6 PMID:12083523

Maekawa, N., Wada, H., Kanda, T., Niwa, T., Yamada, Y., Saito, K., & Seishima, M. et al. (2002). Improved myocardial ischemia/reperfusion injury in mice lacking tumor necrosis factor-α. *Journal of the American College of Cardiology*, *39*(7), 1229–1235. doi:10.1016/S0735-1097(02)01738-2 PMID:11923051

Martindale, J. J., Fernandez, R., Thuerauf, D., Whittaker, R., Gude, N., Sussman, M. A., & Glembotski, C. C. (2006). Endoplasmic Reticulum Stress Gene Induction and Protection From Ischemia/Reperfusion Injury in the Hearts of Transgenic Mice With a Tamoxifen-Regulated Form of ATF6. *Circulation Research*, *98*(9), 1186–1193. doi:10.1161/01.RES.0000220643.65941.8d PMID:16601230

McAreavey, D., Vidal, J. S., Aspelund, T., Eiriksdottir, G., Schelbert, E. B., Kjartansson, O., & Arai, A. E. et al. (2016). Midlife Cardiovascular Risk Factors and Late-Life Unrecognized and Recognized Myocardial Infarction Detect by Cardiac Magnetic Resonance: ICELAND-MI, the AGES-Reykjavik Study. *J Am Heart Assoc*, *5*(2). doi:10.1161/jaha.115.002420 PMID:26873683

Meybohm, P., Bein, B., Brosteanu, O., Cremer, J., Gruenewald, M., Stoppe, C., & Zacharowski, K. et al. (2015). A Multicenter Trial of Remote Ischemic Preconditioning for Heart Surgery. *The New England Journal of Medicine*, *373*(15), 1397–1407. doi:10.1056/NEJMoa1413579 PMID:26436208

Misra, A., Haudek, S. B., Knuefermann, P., Vallejo, J. G., Chen, Z. J., Michael, L. H., & Mann, D. L. et al. (2003). Nuclear Factor-κB Protects the Adult Cardiac Myocyte Against Ischemia-Induced Apoptosis in a Murine Model of Acute Myocardial Infarction. *Circulation*, *108*(25), 3075–3078. doi:10.1161/01.CIR.0000108929.93074.0B PMID:14676146

Miyazaki, Y., Kaikita, K., Endo, M., Horio, E., Miura, M., Tsujita, K., & Oike, Y. et al. (2011). C/EBP Homologous Protein Deficiency Attenuates Myocardial Reperfusion Injury by Inhibiting Myocardial Apoptosis and Inflammation. *Arteriosclerosis, Thrombosis, and Vascular Biology*, *31*(5), 1124–1132. doi:10.1161/ATVBAHA.111.224519 PMID:21330607

Mozaffarian, D., Benjamin, E. J., Go, A. S., Arnett, D. K., Blaha, M. J., Cushman, M., & Turner, M. B. et al. (2015). Heart Disease and Stroke Statistics—2016 Update: A Report From the American Heart Association. *Circulation*. doi:10.1161/CIR.0000000000000152 PMID:26673558

Murray, C. J. L., Barber, R. M., Foreman, K. J., Ozgoren, A. A., Abd-Allah, F., Abera, S. F., & Vos, T. et al. (2015). Global, regional, and national disability-adjusted life years (DALYs) for 306 diseases and injuries and healthy life expectancy (HALE) for 188 countries, 1990–2013: Quantifying the epidemiological transition. *Lancet*, *386*(10009), 2145–2191. doi:10.1016/S0140-6736(15)61340-X PMID:26321261

Murry, C. E., Richard, V. J., Reimer, K. A., & Jennings, R. B. (1990). Ischemic preconditioning slows energy metabolism and delays ultrastructural damage during a sustained ischemic episode. *Circulation Research*, *66*(4), 913–931. doi:10.1161/01.RES.66.4.913 PMID:2317895

Naghavi, M., Libby, P., Falk, E., Casscells, S. W., Litovsky, S., Rumberger, J., & Willerson, J. T. et al. (2003). From Vulnerable Plaque to Vulnerable Patient: A Call for New Definitions and Risk Assessment Strategies: Part I. *Circulation*, *108*(14), 1664–1672. doi:10.1161/01.CIR.0000087480.94275.97 PMID:14530185

Nahrendorf, M., Swirski, F. K., Aikawa, E., Stangenberg, L., Wurdinger, T., Figueiredo, J.-L., & Pittet, M. J. et al. (2007). The healing myocardium sequentially mobilizes two monocyte subsets with divergent and complementary functions. *The Journal of Experimental Medicine*, *204*(12), 3037–3047. doi:10.1084/jem.20070885 PMID:18025128

Nelson, S. K., Wong, G. H. W., & McCord, J. M. (1995). Leukemia inhibitory factor and tumor necrosis factor induce manganese superoxide dismutase and protect rabbit hearts from reperfusion injury. *Journal of Molecular and Cellular Cardiology*, *27*(1), 223–229. doi:10.1016/S0022-2828(08)80021-1 PMID:7760346

Nickson, P., Toth, A., & Erhardt, P. (2007). PUMA is critical for neonatal cardiomyocyte apoptosis induced by endoplasmic reticulum stress. *Cardiovascular Research*, *73*(1), 48–56. doi:10.1016/j.cardiores.2006.10.001 PMID:17107669

Nyyssönen, K., Parviainen, M. T., Salonen, R., Tuomilehto, J., & Salonen, J. T. (1997). Vitamin C deficiency and risk of myocardial infarction: Prospective population study of men from eastern Finland. *BMJ: British Medical Journal*, *314*(7081), 634–638. doi:10.1136/bmj.314.7081.634 PMID:9066474

Oliveira, A., Barros, H., & Lopes, C. (2009). Gender heterogeneity in the association between lifestyles and non-fatal acute myocardial infarction. *Public Health Nutrition*, *12*(10), 1799–1806. doi:10.1017/S1368980008004588 PMID:19161646

Perez, V. V. D. A., Mazo, T., Marchini, T., Caceres, L., Evelson, P., & Gelpi, R. J. (2016). Ischemic postconditioning confers cardioprotection and prevents reduction of Trx-1 in young mice, but not in middle-aged and old mice. *Molecular and Cellular Biochemistry*. doi:10.1007/s11010-016-2677-2

Prabu, S. K., Anandatheerthavarada, H. K., Raza, H., Srinivasan, S., Spear, J. F., & Avadhani, N. G. (2006). Protein Kinase A-mediated Phosphorylation Modulates Cytochrome c Oxidase Function and Augments Hypoxia and Myocardial Ischemia-related Injury. *The Journal of Biological Chemistry*, *281*(4), 2061–2070. doi:10.1074/jbc.M507741200 PMID:16303765

Prasad, A., Gossl, M., Hoyt, J., Lennon, R. J., Polk, L., Simari, R., & Lerman, A. et al. (2013). Remote ischemic preconditioning immediately before percutaneous coronary intervention does not impact myocardial necrosis, inflammatory response, and circulating endothelial progenitor cell counts: A single center randomized sham controlled trial. *Catheterization and Cardiovascular Interventions*, *81*(6), 930–936. doi:10.1002/ccd.24443 PMID:22517646

Przyklenk, K., Bauer, B., Ovize, M., Kloner, R. A., & Whittaker, P. (1993). Regional ischemic preconditioning protects remote virgin myocardium from subsequent sustained coronary occlusion. *Circulation*, *87*(3), 893–899. doi:10.1161/01.CIR.87.3.893 PMID:7680290

Ramasamy, R., Trueblood, N., & Schaefer, S. (1998). Metabolic effects of aldose reductase inhibition during low-flow ischemia and reperfusion. *American Journal of Physiology. Heart and Circulatory Physiology*, *275*(1), H195–H203. PMID:9688914

Rassaf, T., Totzeck, M., Hendgen-Cotta, U. B., Shiva, S., Heusch, G., & Kelm, M. (2014). Circulating Nitrite Contributes to Cardioprotection by Remote Ischemic Preconditioning. *Circulation Research*, *114*(10), 1601–1610. doi:10.1161/CIRCRESAHA.114.303822 PMID:24643960

Salem, J. E., Saidel, G. M., Stanley, W. C., & Cabrera, M. E. (2002). Mechanistic model of myocardial energy metabolism under normal and ischemic conditions. *Annals of Biomedical Engineering*, *30*(2), 202–216. doi:10.1114/1.1454133 PMID:11962772

Seiler, K. S., & Starnes, J. W. (2000). Exogenous GSH protection during hypoxia-reoxygenation of the isolated rat heart: Impact of hypoxia duration. *Free Radical Research*, *32*(1), 41–55. doi:10.1080/10715760000300051 PMID:10625216

Sena, L. A., & Chandel, N. S. (2012). Physiological roles of mitochondrial reactive oxygen species. *Molecular Cell*, *48*(2), 158–167. doi:10.1016/j.molcel.2012.09.025 PMID:23102266

Shimizu, M., Saxena, P., Konstantinov, I. E., Cherepanov, V., Cheung, M. M., Wearden, P., & Redington, A. N. et al. (2010). Remote ischemic preconditioning decreases adhesion and selectively modifies functional responses of human neutrophils. *The Journal of Surgical Research*, *158*(1), 155–161. doi:10.1016/j.jss.2008.08.010 PMID:19540519

Singhal, A. K., Symons, J. D., Boudina, S., Jaishy, B., & Shiu, Y.-T. (2010). Role of Endothelial Cells in Myocardial Ischemia-Reperfusion Injury. *Vascular Disease Prevention*, *7*(1), 1–14. doi:10.2174/1874120701007010001 PMID:25558187

Solaini, G., & Harris, D. A. (2005). Biochemical dysfunction in heart mitochondria exposed to ischaemia and reperfusion. *The Biochemical Journal*, *390*(Pt 2), 377–394. doi:10.1042/BJ20042006 PMID:16108756

Spear, J. F., Prabu, S. K., Galati, D., Raza, H., Anandatheerthavarada, H. K., & Avadhani, N. G. (2007). β1-Adrenoreceptor activation contributes to ischemia-reperfusion damage as well as playing a role in ischemic preconditioning. *American Journal of Physiology. Heart and Circulatory Physiology*, *292*(5), H2459–H2466. doi:10.1152/ajpheart.00459.2006 PMID:17237252

Szegezdi, E., Duffy, A., OMahoney, M. E., Logue, S. E., Mylotte, L. A., OBrien, T., & Samali, A. (2006). ER stress contributes to ischemia-induced cardiomyocyte apoptosis. *Biochemical and Biophysical Research Communications*, *349*(4), 1406–1411. doi:10.1016/j.bbrc.2006.09.009 PMID:16979584

Thuerauf, D. J., Marcinko, M., Gude, N., Rubio, M., Sussman, M. A., & Glembotski, C. C. (2006). Activation of the Unfolded Protein Response in Infarcted Mouse Heart and Hypoxic Cultured Cardiac Myocytes. *Circulation Research*, *99*(3), 275–282. doi:10.1161/01.RES.0000233317.70421.03 PMID:16794188

Timmers, L., van Keulen, J. K., Hoefer, I. E., Meijs, M. F., van Middelaar, B., den Ouden, K., & de Kleijn, D. P. et al. (2009). Targeted deletion of nuclear factor kappaB p50 enhances cardiac remodeling and dysfunction following myocardial infarction. *Circulation Research*, *104*(5), 699–706. doi:10.1161/CIRCRESAHA.108.189746 PMID:19168865

Toth, A., Jeffers, J. R., Nickson, P., Min, J. Y., Morgan, J. P., Zambetti, G. P., & Erhardt, P. (2006). Targeted deletion of Puma attenuates cardiomyocyte death and improves cardiac function during ischemia-reperfusion. *American Journal of Physiology. Heart and Circulatory Physiology*, *291*(1), H52–H60. doi:10.1152/ajpheart.01046.2005 PMID:16399862

Trueblood, N. A., Ramasamy, R., Wang, L. F., & Schaefer, S. (2000). Niacin protects the isolated heart from ischemia-reperfusion injury. *American Journal of Physiology. Heart and Circulatory Physiology*, *279*(2), H764–H771. PMID:10924076

Tsai, M. S., Huang, C. H., Tsai, C. Y., Chen, H. W., Lee, H. C., Cheng, H. J., & Chen, W. J. et al. (2011). Ascorbic acid mitigates the myocardial injury after cardiac arrest and electrical shock. *Intensive Care Medicine*, *37*(12), 2033–2040. doi:10.1007/s00134-011-2362-6 PMID:21953354

Tsao, P. S., Aoki, N., Lefer, D. J., Johnson, G. III, & Lefer, A. M. (1990). Time course of endothelial dysfunction and myocardial injury during myocardial ischemia and reperfusion in the cat. *Circulation*, *82*(4), 1402–1412. doi:10.1161/01.CIR.82.4.1402 PMID:2401073

Turner, R. C., Millns, H., Neil, H. A. W., Stratton, I. M., Manley, S. E., Matthews, D. R., & Holman, R. R. (1998). Risk factors for coronary artery disease in non-insulin dependent diabetes mellitus: United Kingdom prospective diabetes study (UKPDS: 23). *BMJ: British Medical Journal*, *316*(7134), 823–828. doi:10.1136/bmj.316.7134.823 PMID:9549452

Vekich, J. A., Belmont, P. J., Thuerauf, D. J., & Glembotski, C. C. (2012). Protein Disulfide Isomerase-associated 6 is an ATF6-inducible ER Stress Response Protein that Protects Cardiac Myocytes from Ischemia/Reperfusion-mediated Cell Death. *Journal of Molecular and Cellular Cardiology*, *53*(2), 259–267. doi:10.1016/j.yjmcc.2012.05.005 PMID:22609432

Viehman, G. E., Ma, X. L., Lefer, D. J., & Lefer, A. M. (1991). Time course of endothelial dysfunction and myocardial injury during coronary arterial occlusion. *The American Journal of Physiology*, *261*(3 Pt 2), H874–H881. PMID:1653539

Vinten-Johansen, J. (2004). Involvement of neutrophils in the pathogenesis of lethal myocardial reperfusion injury. *Cardiovascular Research*, *61*(3), 481–497. doi:10.1016/j.cardiores.2003.10.011 PMID:14962479

Wang, L., Wang, J., Xu, H., & Li, B. (2013). Postconditioning in patients treated with primary percutaneous coronary intervention: An updated meta-analysis. *Catheterization and Cardiovascular Interventions*, *82*(5), E662–E671. doi:10.1002/ccd.25095 PMID:23804529

Wang, Z. H., Liu, J. L., Wu, L., Yu, Z., & Yang, H. T. (2014). Concentration-dependent wrestling between detrimental and protective effects of H2O2 during myocardial ischemia/reperfusion.[Original Article]. *Cell Death & Disease*, *5*(6), e1297. doi:10.1038/cddis.2014.267 PMID:24946090

Williamson, J. R., Chang, K., Frangos, M., Hasan, K. S., Ido, Y., Kawamura, T., & Tilton, R. G. et al. (1993). Hyperglycemic Pseudohypoxia and Diabetic Complications. *Diabetes*, *42*(6), 801–813. doi:10.2337/diab.42.6.801 PMID:8495803

Yamamoto, T., Byun, J., Zhai, P., Ikeda, Y., Oka, S., & Sadoshima, J. (2014). Nicotinamide mononucleotide, an intermediate of NAD+ synthesis, protects the heart from ischemia and reperfusion. *PLoS ONE*, *9*(6), e98972. doi:10.1371/journal.pone.0098972 PMID:24905194

Yamashita, N., Hoshida, S., Otsu, K., Taniguchi, N., Kuzuya, T., & Hori, M. (2000). The involvement of cytokines in the second window of ischaemic preconditioning. *British Journal of Pharmacology*, *131*(3), 415–422. doi:10.1038/sj.bjp.0703594 PMID:11015290

Yildirim, F., Iskesen, I., Kurdal, A. T., Ozturk, T., Taneli, F., Gozukara, C., & Ozbakkaloglu, A. (2016). Is Attenuation of Oxidative Stress Helpful to Understand the Mechanism of Remote Ischemic Preconditioning in Cardiac Surgery? *Journal of Cardiothoracic and Vascular Anesthesia*, *30*(1), 134–140. doi:10.1053/j.jvca.2015.06.027 PMID:26411813

Yu, Q., Lee, C. F., Wang, W., Karamanlidis, G., Kuroda, J., Matsushima, S., & Tian, R. et al. (2014). Elimination of NADPH Oxidase Activity Promotes Reductive Stress and Sensitizes the Heart to Ischemic Injury. *Journal of the American Heart Association: Cardiovascular and Cerebrovascular Disease*, *3*(1), e000555. doi:10.1161/JAHA.113.000555 PMID:24470522

Zeymer, U., Bauer, T., Gersh, B. J., Zahn, R., Gitt, A., Junger, C., & Senges, J. (2011). Beneficial effect of reperfusion therapy beyond the preservation of left ventricular function in patients with acute ST-segment elevation myocardial infarction. *International Journal of Cardiology*, *146*(2), 177–180. doi:10.1016/j.ijcard.2009.06.034 PMID:19604587

Zhao, K., Huang, Z., Lu, H., Zhou, J., & Wei, T. (2010). Induction of inducible nitric oxide synthase increases the production of reactive oxygen species in RAW264.7 macrophages. *Bioscience Reports*, *30*(4), 233–241. doi:10.1042/BSR20090048 PMID:19673702

Zhao, X., He, G., Chen, Y. R., Pandian, R. P., Kuppusamy, P., & Zweier, J. L. (2005). Endothelium-derived nitric oxide regulates postischemic myocardial oxygenation and oxygen consumption by modulation of mitochondrial electron transport. *Circulation*, *111*(22), 2966–2972. doi:10.1161/CIRCULATIONAHA.104.527226 PMID:15939832

Zhu, X., Liu, B., Zhou, S., Chen, Y. R., Deng, Y., Zweier, J. L., & He, G. (2007). Ischemic preconditioning prevents in vivo hyperoxygenation in postischemic myocardium with preservation of mitochondrial oxygen consumption. *American Journal of Physiology. Heart and Circulatory Physiology*, *293*(3), H1442–H1450. doi:10.1152/ajpheart.00256.2007 PMID:17513495

Zografos, T. A., Katritsis, G. D., Tsiafoutis, I., Bourboulis, N., Katsivas, A., & Katritsis, D. G. (2014). Effect of one-cycle remote ischemic preconditioning to reduce myocardial injury during percutaneous coronary intervention. *The American Journal of Cardiology*, *113*(12), 2013–2017. doi:10.1016/j.amjcard.2014.03.043 PMID:24793669

Zweier, J. L., Flaherty, J. T., & Weisfeldt, M. L. (1987). Direct measurement of free radical generation following reperfusion of ischemic myocardium. *Proceedings of the National Academy of Sciences of the United States of America*, *84*(5), 1404–1407. doi:10.1073/pnas.84.5.1404 PMID:3029779

Chapter 9
Pharmacogenomics and Cardiovascular Disease

Emily K. Dornblaser
University of New England, USA

Craig P. Worby
University of New England, USA

Daniel Alan Brazeau
University of New England, USA

ABSTRACT

Cardiovascular disease is one of the most prevalent disease states in the U.S. and contributes substantially to overall morbidity and mortality. The ability to effectively optimize the treatment of cardiovascular disease has a significant impact on overall disease prevention and treatment. This chapter discusses the relationship between genetic variations and their impact on medications used for the treatment of cardiovascular disorders. Key medications that are susceptible to genetic variation have been identified. The chapter describes the mechanisms by which genetic variation may contribute to altered medication concentrations or effects and briefly reviews the place in therapy for the cardiovascular medications. In addition, this chapter reviews current clinical literature to determine the overall impact these variations may have on clinical outcomes.

INTRODUCTION

The prevalence of cardiovascular disease in the United States is extensive. The American Heart Association estimates that approximately 1 in 3 American adults have at least one cardiovascular condition. Many have multiple conditions. Eighty million Americans are estimated to have hypertension, while 15 million have some form of coronary heart disease. Cardiovascular disease (CVD) encompasses a wide-variety of conditions including hypertension, hyperlipidemia, coronary heart disease, atrial fibrillation and other arrhythmias, and congestive heart failure. CVD accounts for about 30% of all deaths in the United States and is the leading cause of death for both men and women (Mozafarian et al., 2016).

DOI: 10.4018/978-1-5225-2092-4.ch009

Evidence-based therapies of various pharmacologic agents have been shown to reduce morbidity and mortality. Commonly used agents may include beta-blockers, statins, anti-platelets, and anti-coagulants (January et al., 2014; O'Gara et al., 2013; Yancy et al., 2013). The effects of these medications may be profoundly altered by genetic variation among patients in genes responsible for drug metabolism, drug transport or the targets of the drugs themselves. The clinical implications of these genetic variations will be discussed in this chapter.

BACKGROUND

It has been a little over a 15 years since the publication of the initial draft of the human genome (Venter et al. 2001; Lander et al. 2001). Estimates for the final cost to sequence the "first" human genome range from \$500 million to \$1 billion. Since the completion of this first genome sequencing, technologies have undergone two revolutions first with massively parallel sequencing in the 2005 and recently with nanopore sensing technologies that hold out the hope of single molecule sequencing. As these next generation sequencing technologies become readily available, genome sequencing costs has decreased and sequence yields increased exponentially. In large part due to availability of high-throughput sequencing technologies it has become possible to begin to assess and catalogue human genetic variation. In an analysis of sequence data from protein coding regions (exomes) of 60,706 individuals Lek, et al. (2016) have identified over 3,000 genes which are likely loss of function variants; importantly 72% of these identified genes have no established disease phenotype at this time. The ultimate identification and delineating of these variants in human populations are critical to understanding the underlying genetic causes of human disease and drug response.

This revolution in genomic technologies as well as the attendant advances in bioinformatics has led to the appeal for prevention and treatment strategies based upon the individual characteristics of the patient, now referred to as "Precision Medicine".

The recognition that much of the variability among patients in disease severity and treatment response may soon be anticipated (and prevented) with knowledge being acquired in the new fields of genomics, metagenomics (assessment of the patient's microbial community), metabolomics (assessment of the small molecule metabolites in biological systems) and proteomics (assessment of the patient's proteins including enzymes, transporters, receptors) drives the development of precision medicine. Importantly, one of the more successful areas in precision medicine is in pharmacogenetics or pharmacogenomics. The two terms have been used interchangeably and have the ultimate goal of identifying the many underlying genetic factors playing a role in the efficacy or toxicity of all drugs. Pharmacogenetics traditionally considers the action of a single gene in drug response. Pharmacogenomics is the broader term and includes any and all genes and their interactions that may play a role in drug response. Pharmacogenetics/genomics has experienced more success in terms of clinical relevance as compared to success of genomics to predict disease risk because often a single gene will play a large role in drug response and is thus a much more tractable problem (Altman 2011).

For virtually all medications the role of patient variability in drug response either in efficacy, toxicity or adverse reactions is well known. One aspect of patient variability is the incidence of adverse drug reactions (ADR). For example, the Institute of Medicine has estimated that there are ~1.5 million preventable adverse drug reactions in the US each year costing over 3 billion dollars (Aspden et al 2007). This represents a considerable and potentially avoidable burden on the healthcare system. Cardiovascular medications are an all too common cause of ADRs, largely due to warfarin and oral anti-platelets (Budnitz et al 2011). Additionally studies have shown that only 50-75% patients respond beneficially to the first drug administered and this rate is even lower (4%-25%) for the top ten highest-grossing drugs in the US (Schork 2015). For medications to treat cardiac arrhythmias nearly 60% of the drugs first administered provide little or no benefit (Spear et al. 2001). While it is known that much of this variation in patient response is due to factors including age, diet, drug interactions, or non-compliance the concern here is the role of genetic variation in drug response.

In the cardiovascular literature there has been much interest in the role of human genetic variation in drug metabolizing enzymes, drug transporters and drug targets (Myburgh etal 2012; Weeke and Roden 2013; Johnson and Cavallari 2013). Much of what is known in the pharmacogenetics of all drugs, including cardiovascular drugs is compiled, annotated and updated daily in the Pharmacogenomics and Pharmacogenetics Knowledge Base (PharmGKB, http://www.pharmgkb.org/). PharmGKB is an integrated database providing clinical, pharmacokinetic, pharmacodynamic, genotypic, and molecular function data for human genetic polymorphisms and drugs (Klein et al. 2001; Altman et al. 2003). The stated objective PharmGKB is to "aid researchers in understanding how genetic variation among individuals contributes to differences in reactions to drugs". The data within PharmGKB includes:

1. Annotation of genetic variants that play a role in gene-drug-disease relationships.
2. Excellent summaries of important "pharmacogenes" – genes involved in drug response.
3. FDA drug labels that include pharmacogenomic information.
4. Drug metabolism and transport pathways with links to relevant genes.
5. Clinical annotations summarizing the role of human genetic variation in altering clinical endpoints that aid in determining medical practice or policy.
6. Publish pharmacogenomic drug dosing guidelines through the Clinical Pharmacogenetics Implementation Consortium (CPIC).

Most importantly for practitioners the Clinical Pharmacogenetics Implementation Consortium (CPIC) has developed guidelines to assist health care providers with available genetic test results as they apply to the prescribing of medication (Relling and Klein, 2011). The guidelines have been organized around either genes or medications and assigned a CPIC level (A-D) based on whether there are prescribing recommendations based on the evidence (Consortium). The PharmGKB level of evidence scale provides a graded approach to currently published literature with the highest level (1A) reflecting a medical society endorsed guideline ("Clinical Annotation Levels of Evidence"). Importantly, these guidelines are intended to help clinicians understand how to use test results rather than whether the tests should be conducted or not. Table 1 details all cardiovascular medications that have CPIC guidelines as well as the level of evidence associated with each and whether there are actionable dosing recommendations. Medications that are routinely used for cardiovascular disease that have significant levels of evidence or actionable dosing recommendations are reviewed in this chapter including antiplatelet medications, lipid lowering agents, anticoagulants and beta-blockers.

Table 1. Cardiovascular medications with annotated pharmacogenetic indications based upon the Clinical Pharmacogenetics Implementation Consortium (CPIC) and the Pharmcogenomics Knowledgebase (PharmGKB)

	Drugs	Indication	Genes	CPIC Level	PharmGKB Level of Evidence	PGx on FDA Label
1	Acenocoumarol	Anticoagulant	*CYP4F2*	B	2B	
2	Aspirin	Antiplatelet	*LTC4S*	D	2B	
3	Atorvastatin	Statin	*COQ2*	D	2B	
4	Carvedilol	Beta Blocker	*CYP2D6*	C	3	Actionable PGx
5	Clopidogrel	Antiplatelet	*CYP2C19*	A	1A	Genetic testing recommended
			CES1	C/D	2B	
6	Digoxin	Anti-arrythmic	*ABCB1*	C/D	2A	
7	Flecainide	Anti-arrythmic	*CYP2D6*	C	2A	
8	HMG COA Reductase Inhibitors	Statin	*HMGCR*	D	2A	
9	Isosorbide Dinitrate	Vasodilator	*NAT1*	D		
			NAT2	D		Informative PGx
10	Metoprolol	Beta Blocker	*CYP2D6*	C	3	Informative PGx
11	Phenprocoumon	Anticoagulant	*CYP4F2*	B	2A	
12	Propafenone	Anti-arrythmic	*CYP2D6*	C	2A	Actionable PGx
13	Propranolol	Beta Blocker	*CYP2D6*	C	4	Informative PGx
14	Rosuvastatin	Statin	*ABCG2*	D	2B	
			COQ2	D	2B	
15	Simvastatin	Statin	*SLCO1B1*	A	1A	
16	Warfarin	Anticoagulant	*CYP2C9*	A	1A	Actionable PGx
			VKORC1	A	1A	Actionable PGx
			CYP4F2	B	1B	
			CALU	D	2B	
			GGCX	D	3	

PHARMACOGENETICS OF CARDIOVASCULAR DRUGS

The impact of pharmacogenetic variation typically manifests in either a change in the pharmacokinetic profile of a medication or the pharmacodynamic effect of a medication. Pharmacokinetics refers to the process by which a drug moves through the body, often described by absorption, distribution, metabolism, and elimination (ADME). A pharmacogenomic alteration to liver enzyme systems (ex. CYP) may result in an increase or a decrease in the metabolism of a medication thus causing the drug to be either cleared faster or slower by the body respectively. Pharmacodynamics refers to the effect a medication has on the body. Genetic variations in target receptor complexes or intracellular signaling pathways may increase or decrease the effect of the medication.

Antiplatelet Medications (Clopidogrel, Prasugrel, Ticagrelor, Asprin)

- **Mechanism of Action:** Clopidogrel, prasugrel, and ticagrelor are all inhibitors of platelet $P2Y_{12}$ receptors. Clopidogrel and prasugrel inhibit irreversibly while ticagrelor inhibiton is reversible. In normal functioning platelets, ADP binds to $P2Y_{12}$ receptors to reduce cyclic AMP. Cyclic AMP itself inhibits platelet activation; therefore, decreasing cAMP through the $P2Y_{12}$ receptor promotes activation. Clopidogrel blocks the $P2Y_{12}$ receptor, increasing cAMP, and ultimately inhibiting platelet activation. Only clopidogrel has been seen to be profoundly effected by genomic variations (Weitz, 2011).
- **Place in Therapy:** Clopidogrel is frequently used for secondary prevention of stroke, acute coronary syndrome, and prevention of stent thrombosis after percutaneous coronary intervention. Clopidogrel has demonstrated efficacy in reducing rates of stroke, myocardial infarction, and death (Weitz, 2011).
- **Genetic Variations Present:** Clopidogrel is a prodrug that requires transformation in the liver via CYP2C19 to its active form. Variants in the genes encoding CYP2C19 can affect metabolism. The presence of the *CYP2C19*2* loss of function variant can cause marked reductions in platelet aggregation (Hulot et al., 2006). In addition to *CYP2C19*2* there are other alleles (*2-*8) segregating in patient populations that also result in reduced function. There is even one allele *CYP2C19*17* that results in increased enzyme activity and potentially increased platelet inhibition (Scott, et al 2013).
- **Implications:** In January 2009, in response to reports that clopidogrel effectiveness may be reduced in some patients, the FDA initiated an investigation into the genetic factors and other drugs that may influence its effectiveness ("Early Communication about an Ongoing Safety Review of clopidogrel bisulfate (marketed as Plavix)" January 26, 2009).("Early Communication about an Ongoing Safety Review of clopidogrel bisulfate (marketed as Plavix)" January 26, 2009). In a follow-up communication that November, the FDA recommended against the co-administration of clopidogrel with omeprazole, a CYP2C19 inhibitor. In March 2010, the FDA issued a safety warning that poor metabolizers of clopidogrel may not receive the full benefit of the medication ("FDA Drug Safety Communication: Reduced effectiveness of Plavix (clopidogrel) in patients who are poor metabolizers of the drug" March 12, 2010). This recommendation was based on a pharmacokinetic study of 40 healthy subjects that demonstrated higher doses of clopidogrel in PMs would achieve greater anti-platelet response. However, the study was not intended to assess clinical outcomes; therefore definitive recommendations could not be made ("FDA Drug Safety Communication: Reduced effectiveness of Plavix (clopidogrel) in patients who are poor metabolizers of the drug., " March 12, 2010). Since the FDA warning, extensive research has been conducted on the implications of CYP2C19 polymorphisms on clinical outcomes and the need for genetic testing. Genotype testing prior to initiation of clopidogrel has proven to be controversial. Clinical Pharmacogenetics Implementation Consortium (CPIC) recommended in its 2013 guidelines that consideration be given to genetic testing if the results may alter treatment (Scott et al., 2013). The American Heart Association (AHA) recommends against routine genetic testing as no RCT to date has demonstrated improved outcomes (Levine et al., 2016). A meta-analysis of 32 studies dating from 2008-2011 published in 2011 found no difference in clinical outcomes with clopidogrel use between CYP2C19 genotypes. The increase in cardiovascular events effects

seen in individual studies was attributed to significant small study bias in that larger studies trended toward no difference in clinical outcomes (Holmes, Perel, Shah, Hingorani, & Casas, 2011). Recently, Doll et al. published a genetic sub-study of the TRILOGY ACS trial evaluating the effects of CYP2C19 of clopidogrel or prasugrel in medically managed patients with acute coronary syndrome on a composite primary endpoint of cardiovascular death, myocardial infarction, or stroke. Patients were classified as either extensive metabolizers (EM) or reduced metabolizers (RM). While there was a trend to toward decreased events in EMs, no statistically significant difference was found between EMs and RMs for either medication. The authors concluded that genotype testing was not supported by their findings; however, the sub-study included very few patients with 2 non-functioning alleles (Doll et al., 2016). CYP2C19 may be more important in patients undergoing PCI (Wallentin et al., 2010; Mega et al., 2010). As a result of this, the AHA suggests use of prasugrel or ticagrelor over clopidogrel in patients indicated for dual-antiplatelet therapy who have undergone coronary stenting (Levine et al., 2016).

Lipid-Lowering Drugs (Atorvastatin, Rosuvastatin, Simvastatin, HGM Co-A Reductase Inhibitors)

- **Mechanism of Action:** The drug class commonly referred to as 'statins' are classified as HMG-CoA Reductase inhibitors. These medications inhibit the formation of mevalonate, a precursor to LDL cholesterol, and result in lower in vivo synthesis of LDL. The body responds with an up-regulation of LDL receptors increasing catabolism of circulating LDL and increasing the liver's extraction of circulating LDL precursors. The net result is a lowering of circulating LDL cholesterol levels and is one of the primary reasons these medications are utilized for many primary and secondary disease prevention strategies (Malloy & Kane, 2015).
- **Place in Therapy:** The statin medications are primarily used for the treatment and prevention of atherosclerotic cardiovascular disease (acute coronary syndromes, history of myocardial infarction, stable or unstable angina, stroke, transient ischemic attack or peripheral artery disease) and the intensity of therapy should be determined based on the 10-year ASCVD risk score of the patient and their baseline LDL-C levels (Stone et al., 2014).
- **Genetic Variations Present:** In 2008, the SEARCH collaborative group published the results of a genome wide association study to identify any major single-nucleotide polymorphism (SNP) that may be associated with the common statin side effect of myopathy. The study revealed a non-synonymous rs4149056 SNP on the SLC01B1 gene that was associated with statin metabolism ($r^2=0.97$). It is postulated that alterations in this gene result in a lower uptake of the statin mediation into hepatocytes resulting in higher circulating blood concentrations of the medication. Each copy of the C allele present represented an odds ratio for myopathy of 4.5 (95% CI: 2.6-7.7) and of 16.9 (95% CI: 4.7-61.1) for CC alleles compared to TT homozygotes (Link et al., 2008). Similar results were found with a gene-dose effect in an additional genome wide study published within a year of the SEARCH trial (Voora et al., 2009).
- **Implications:** In response to the SEARCH trial results, the FDA updated the prescribing guidelines for simvastatin and no longer recommend initiating therapy at doses of 80 mg of simvastatin a day ("FDA Drug Safety Communication: New restrictions, contraindications, and dose limitations for Zocor (simvastatin) to reduce risk of muscle injury," 2011). The recently published ACC/

AHA guidelines on the treatment of cholesterol identify the impact of pharmacogenetic testing as an area of future clinical consideration (Stone et al., 2014). In 2014, the Clinical Pharmacogenetics Implementation Consortium published an update to their 2012 guideline on simvastatin-induced myopathy. The consortium strongly recommends prescribing a lower dose of simvastatin or an alternative statin in patients with intermediate or low function phenotypes (Ramsey et al., 2014). The translation of genetic testing to clinical prescribing patterns has been minimal, in part because the intensity of statin dosing is the focus of clinical prescribing guidelines and has been associated with better patient outcomes. Although empiric reductions in dosing due to genetic profiling may prevent adverse events patients may not realize the clinical benefits from a lower dose of the medication. Genetic testing may have a role in guiding the selection of the initial medication rather than the initial dose as a means of reducing harm yet ensuring the benefit of the medication is realized.

Anti-Coagulants (Warfarin)

- **Warfarin Mechanism of Action:** Warfarin is an anticoagulant medication that elicits response through inhibition of the vitamin K reduction pathway. The reduced form of vitamin K is responsible for carboxylation and activation of clotting factors. Thus the enzyme vitamin K epoxide reductase (VKOR) is responsible for the reduction of vitamin K; it's inhibition by warfarin results in a depletion of active clotting factors resulting in systemic anticoagulation (Weitz, 2011).
- **Place in Therapy:** Warfarin therapy has traditionally been the basis for nearly all anticoagulation indications including treatment of venous thromboembolism and pulmonary embolism (VTE/PE), stroke prevention in patients with Atrial Fibrillation (AFib), secondary stroke prevention and anticoagulation for valvular disease. However, novel oral anticoagulants (NOACs)- medications that do not require routine monitoring and have fewer drug interactions- are beginning to show superiority over warfarin therapy (Guyatt, Akl, Crowther, Gutterman, & Schuünemann, 2012). In 2012, the CHEST Anticoagulation guidelines recommended dabigatran over warfarin therapy for the secondary prevention of stroke in patients with AFib (You et al., 2012). In 2016, the CHEST guidelines for VTE/PE treatment were updated and now recommend any of the NOAC medications over warfarin therapy (Kearon et al., 2016). Genetic Variations Present: The CYP 2C9 enzyme is primarily responsible for the metabolism of warfarin in the liver. Two major *CYP2C9* variants *2 and *3 have been identified as having a significant impact on the overall dosing requirements for warfarin therapy due to their impact on its metabolism. The CYP enzyme variability is responsible for a pharmacokinetic effect on drug levels and patients with either variant have been found to require larger doses of warfarin (Whirl-Carrillo et al., 2012).A genetic variation in the gene responsible for VKOR enzyme activity, the *VKORC1* gene, results in a pharmacodynamic effect on the medication's activity. (Thorn) The c.-1639G>A or c.1173C>T SNP's present in the regulatory regions of VKORC1 contribute to the variability in warfarin dosing for patient populations. Presence of the c.1639A allele results in an increased sensitivity to the effects of warfarin and therefore requires lower doses of the medications. The genotypes c.1639AA, AG, GG (or 1173TT, CT, CC) correlate to high, medium and low sensitivity to the medication (Johnson & Callavari).
- **Implications:** As the evidence for better outcomes with novel oral anticoagulants builds, the use of warfarin therapy will likely to decrease over time. In the 2012 CHEST guidelines, the routine use of pharmacogenetic testing for guiding the initiation of warfarin dosing was not recommended

with a strong level of evidence, that is Grade 1B (Guyatt et al., 2012). Although there is potential benefit for using genomic testing to determine warfarin dosing, the movement away from clinical use of the medication is likely to limit further studies on dosing based on genomics. It would be likely that without further studies clinical guidelines such as CHEST will not reverse their position on its utility for routine use.

β-blockers (Carvedilol, Metoprolol, Propanolol)

- **Mechanism of Action:** Beta-blockers function by binding to beta-adrenergic receptors to competitively reduce binding of catecholamines and beta-agonists (Robertson & Biaggioni, 2015). Most agents in the class such as metoprolol and carvedilol are pure antagonists; however, some like pindolol and acebutalol act as partial agonists (Robertson & Biaggioni, 2015; Westfall & Westfall, 2011). Beta-blockers decrease heart rate, blood pressure, and myocardial oxygen consumption.
- **Place in Therapy:** Beta-blockers are used to treat a variety of diseases such as hypertension, ischemic heart disease, and atrial fibrillation. Beta-blockers are also guideline-directed therapy to reduce morbidity and mortality from myocardial infarctions and heart failure (O'Gara et al., 2013; Yancy et al., 2013).
- **Genetic Variations:** Metoprolol is extensively metabolized hepatically through CYP2D6, thus variability in the CYP2D6 genotype can lead to dramatic differences in serum concentrations between patients. Poor metabolizers can exhibit serum concentrations three to ten times extensive metabolizers (Robertson & Biaggioni, 2015). CYP2D6 is responsible for up to 60% of the metabolism of oral metoprolol (Lennard et al., 1982).
- **Implications:** CYP2D6 polymorphisms have demonstrated increased concentrations of metoprolol in poor metabolizers (Ismail & Teh, 2006; Sharp et al., 2009). A study of 52 patients demonstrated that patients with 0 to 1 functional alleles had higher serum concentrations, 6.3 times ($p = 0.016$) and 3.2 times ($p = 0.006$) respectively, than patients with 2 fully functional alleles. The study did not find a difference in HR, SBP, or DBP between any group; however, too few patients were enrolled in the 0 functional allele group to draw conclusions (Sharp et al., 2009). The clinical implications of CYP2D6 variations on the effects of metoprolol may exist over a range of outcomes. One recent trial (2014), prospectively evaluated the effects of CYP2D6 polymorphisms in patients receiving oral metoprolol at doses titrated to 100 mg twice daily. 218 patients were classified as poor metabolizers (PM), intermediate metabolizers (IM), extensive metabolizers (EM), and ultra-rapid metabolizers (UM). There was no statistically significant difference seen in the mean daily dose of metoprolol, change in systolic and diastolic blood pressure in each group, or side effects. However, the investigators did find a greater reduction in heart rate in PMs and IMs (-16.6 ± 6.9 and -18.6 ± 5.1) compared to EMs and UMs (-11.4 ± 6.6 and -11.2 ± 8.2, $p = 0.0001$; Hamadeh et al., 2014). As metoprolol dose is titrated to clinical effect, there is no role for pharmacogenomics in determining the dose at this time. While carvedilol is also metabolized through CYP2D6, no pharmacodynamics differences on HR, BP, or adverse effects have been noted (Baudhuin et al., 2010; Sehrt, Meineke, Tzvetkov, Gultepe, & Brockmoller, 2011).

FUTURE RESEARCH DIRECTIONS AND CONCLUSION

There is now substantial pharmacogenetic evidence that could be applied to help guide patient therapy. In one recent review of cardiovascular drugs and pharmacogenomics the authors looked at 289 studies involving cardiovascular drugs and genetics (Kitsios and Kent 2012). The authors identified 289 cardiovascular studies assessing the role of pharmacogenetics in patient response. These studies identified 220 unique genetic polymorphisms in genes involved in drug metabolism, transport and drug action. Of these 9% (19) were confirmed by the authors stringent criteria to have significant associations. However, none of the 19 gene/drug associations have yet to be recommended for use in clinical practice. The authors note that this lack of clinical impact is often due to the fact that genetic testing is never likely to be more accurate in predicting patient response that direct phenotypic measures (INR for examples in warfarin dosing). In a similar study Kaufman et al. reviewed 884 drug/genetic studies involving 51 cardiovascular medications and found evidence of associations strong enough to support clinical alerts for 92 polymorphisms affecting 23 medications (Kaufman et al. 2015). They note that the lack of randomized clinical trials (RCT) has hampered the incorporation of guidelines based upon genetic tests. Such RCTs while foundational to evidence-based medicine are difficult in pharmacogenetic assessments given the cost, time and limited scope of any one allele in patient populations. Lesko et al. suggests that requirement of RCTs to demonstrate clinical utility "represents an unrealistically high evidentiary standard" (Lesko, et al. 2010). Rather RCTs along with a combination of prospective clinical trials and observational studies are needed to hasten the translation of pharmacogenetic research to medical practice (Lesko, et al. 2010). It has been argued that the standard to employ pharmacogenetic information in making clinical decisions should not be superiority to current practice. Given the ever decreasing cost of genotyping and the generally low risk of modifying therapy based upon pharmacogenetics the use of this information should be an important component of any multi-faceted decision making process guiding therapy (Altman 2011).

REFERENCES

Altman, R. B. (2011). Pharmacogenomics: Noninferiority Is Sufficient for Initial Implementation. *Clinical Pharmacology and Therapeutics*, *89*(3), 248–350. doi:10.1038/clpt.2010.310 PMID:21326263

Aspden, P., Wolcott, J., Bootman, J. L., & Cronenwett, L. R. (Eds.). (2007). Committee on Identifying and Preventing Medication Errors. Board on Health Care Services; Institute of Medicine. Preventing Medication Errors. Washington, DC: National Academies Press.

Baudhuin, L. M., Miller, W. L., Train, L., Bryant, S., Hartman, K. A., Phelps, M., & Jaffe, A. S. et al. (2010). Relation of ADRB1, CYP2D6, and UGT1A1 polymorphisms with dose of, and response to, carvedilol or metoprolol therapy in patients with chronic heart failure. *The American Journal of Cardiology*, *106*(3), 402–408. doi:10.1016/j.amjcard.2010.03.041 PMID:20643254

Budnitz, D. S., Lovegrove, M. C., Shehab, N., & Richards, C. L. (2011). Emergency Hospitalizations for Adverse Drug Events in Older Americans. *The New England Journal of Medicine*, *365*(21), 2002–2012. doi:10.1056/NEJMsa1103053 PMID:22111719

Clinical Annotation Levels of Evidence. (n.d.). Retrieved from https://www.pharmgkb.org/page/clinAnnLevels

Consortium, C. P. I. Prioritization of Genes/Drugs. (n.d.). Retrieved from https://cpicpgx.org/prioritization/-cpicLevels

Doll, J. A., Neely, M. L., Roe, M. T., Armstrong, P. W., White, H. D., Prabhakaran, D., & Fox, K. A. et al. (2016). Impact of CYP2C19 Metabolizer Status on Patients With ACS Treated With Prasugrel Versus Clopidogrel. *Journal of the American College of Cardiology*, *67*(8), 936–947. doi:10.1016/j.jacc.2015.12.036 PMID:26916483

Early Communication about an Ongoing Safety Review of clopidogrel bisulfate (marketed as Plavix). (2009). Retrieved from http://www.fda.gov/Drugs/DrugSafety/PostmarketDrugSafetyInformationforPatientsandProviders/DrugSafetyInformationforHeathcareProfessionals/ucm079520.htm

FDA Drug Safety Communication. Reduced effectiveness of Plavix (clopidogrel) in patients who are poor metabolizers of the drug. (2010). Retrieved from http://www.fda.gov/Drugs/DrugSafety/PostmarketDrugSafetyInformationforPatientsandProviders/ucm203888.htm

FDA Drug Safety Communication. New restrictions, contraindications, and dose limitations for Zocor (simvastatin) to reduce risk of muscle injury. (2011). Retrieved from http://www.fda.gov/Drugs/DrugSafety/ucm256581.htm

Guyatt, G. H., Akl, E. A., Crowther, M., Gutterman, D. D., & Schuünemann, H. J. (2012). Executive summary: Antithrombotic therapy and prevention of thrombosis, 9th ed: american college of chest physicians evidence-based clinical practice guidelines. Chest, 141(2), 7S-47S. doi:10.1378/chest.1412S3

Hamadeh, I. S., Langaee, T. Y., Dwivedi, R., Garcia, S., Burkley, B. M., Skaar, T. C., & Johnson, J. A. et al. (2014). Impact of CYP2D6 polymorphisms on clinical efficacy and tolerability of metoprolol tartrate. *Clinical Pharmacology and Therapeutics*, *96*(2), 175–181. doi:10.1038/clpt.2014.62 PMID:24637943

Holmes, M. V., Perel, P., Shah, T., Hingorani, A. D., & Casas, J. P. (2011). CYP2C19 genotype, clopidogrel metabolism, platelet function, and cardiovascular events: A systematic review and meta-analysis. *Journal of the American Medical Association*, *306*(24), 2704–2714. doi:10.1001/jama.2011.1880 PMID:22203539

Hulot, J. S., Bura, A., Villard, E., Azizi, M., Remones, V., Goyenvalle, C., & Gaussem, P. et al. (2006). Cytochrome P450 2C19 loss-of-function polymorphism is a major determinant of clopidogrel responsiveness in healthy subjects. *Blood*, *108*(7), 2244–2247. doi:10.1182/blood-2006-04-013052 PMID:16772608

Ismail, R., & Teh, L. K. (2006). The relevance of CYP2D6 genetic polymorphism on chronic metoprolol therapy in cardiovascular patients. *Journal of Clinical Pharmacy and Therapeutics*, *31*(1), 99–109. doi:10.1111/j.1365-2710.2006.00699.x PMID:16476126

January, C. T., Wann, L. S., Alpert, J. S., Calkins, H., Cigarroa, J. E., Cleveland, J. C. Jr, & Yancy, C. W. et al. (2014). 2014 AHA/ACC/HRS guideline for the management of patients with atrial fibrillation: A report of the American College of Cardiology/American Heart Association Task Force on practice guidelines and the Heart Rhythm Society. *Circulation*, *130*(23), e199–e267. doi:10.1161/CIR.0000000000000041 PMID:24682347

Johnson, J. A., & Cavallari, L. H. (2013). Pharmacogenetics and Cardiovascular Disease—Implications for Personalized Medicine. *Pharmacological Reviews*, *65*(3), 987–1009. doi:10.1124/pr.112.007252 PMID:23686351

Kaufman, A. L., Spitz, J., Jacobs, M., Sorrentino, M., Yuen, S., Danahey, K., & ODonnell, P. H. (2015). Evidence for Clinical Implementation of Pharmacogenomics in Cardiac Drugs. *Mayo Clinic Proceedings*, *90*(6), 716–729. doi:10.1016/j.mayocp.2015.03.016 PMID:26046407

Kearon, C., Akl, E. A., Ornelas, J., Blaivas, A., Jimenez, D., Bounameaux, H., & Moores, L. et al. (2016). Antithrombotic therapy for vte disease: Chest guideline and expert panel report. *Chest*, *149*(2), 315–352. doi:10.1016/j.chest.2015.11.026 PMID:26867832

Kitsios, G. D., & Kent, D. M. (2012). Personalised medicine: Not just in our genes. *BMJ (Clinical Research Ed.)*, *344*, e2161. PMID:22491484

Klein, T. E., Chang, J. T., Cho, M. K., Easton, K. L., Fergerson, R., Hewett, M., & Altman, R. B. et al. (2001). Integrating Genotype and Phenotype Information: An Overview of the PharmGKB Project. *The Pharmacogenomics Journal*, *1*(3), 167–170. doi:10.1038/sj.tpj.6500035 PMID:11908751

Lek, M., Karczewski, K. J., Minikel, E. V., Samocha, K. E., Banks, E., Fennell, T., & MacArthur, D. G. et al. (2016). Analysis of protein-coding genetic variation in 60,706 humans. *Nature*, *536*(7616), 285–291. doi:10.1038/nature19057 PMID:27535533

Lennard, M. S., Silas, J. H., Freestone, S., Ramsay, L. E., Tucker, G. T., & Woods, H. F. (1982). Oxidation phenotypea major determinant of metoprolol metabolism and response. *The New England Journal of Medicine*, *307*(25), 1558–1560. doi:10.1056/NEJM198212163072505 PMID:7144837

Lesko, L. J., Zineh, I., & Huang, S.-M. (2010). What Is Clinical Utility and Why Should We Care? *Clinical Pharmacology and Therapeutics*, *88*(6), 729–733. doi:10.1038/clpt.2010.229 PMID:21081937

Levine, G. N., Bates, E. R., Bittl, J. A., Brindis, R. G., Fihn, S. D., Fleisher, L. A., & Smith, S. C. Jr et al.. (2016). 2016 ACC/AHA Guideline Focused Update on Duration of Dual Antiplatelet Therapy in Patients With Coronary Artery Disease: A Report of the American College of Cardiology/American Heart Association Task Force on Clinical Practice Guidelines. *Journal of the American College of Cardiology*, *68*(10), 1082–1115. doi:10.1016/j.jacc.2016.03.513 PMID:27036918

Link, E., Parish, S., Armitage, J., Bowman, L., Heath, S., Matsuda, F., & Collins, R. et al. (2008). SLCO1B1 variants and statin-induced myopathya genomewide study. *The New England Journal of Medicine*, *359*(8), 789–799. doi:10.1056/NEJMoa0801936 PMID:18650507

Malloy, M., & Kane, J. (2015). Agents used in dyslipidemia. In B. Katzung & A. Trevor (Eds.), Basic & Clinical Pharmacology. New York, NY: McGraw-Hill.

Mega, J. L., Close, S. L., Wiviott, S. D., Shen, L., Walker, J. R., Simon, T., & Sabatine, M. S. et al. (2010). Genetic variants in ABCB1 and CYP2C19 and cardiovascular outcomes after treatment with clopidogrel and prasugrel in the TRITON-TIMI 38 trial: A pharmacogenetic analysis. *Lancet*, *376*(9749), 1312–1319. doi:10.1016/S0140-6736(10)61273-1 PMID:20801494

Mozaffarian, D., Benjamin, E. J., Go, A. S., Arnett, D. K., Blaha, M. J., Cushman, M., & Turner, M. B. et al. (2016). Heart Disease and Stroke Statistics-2016 Update: A Report From the American Heart Association. *Circulation*, *133*(4), e38–e360. doi:10.1161/CIR.0000000000000350 PMID:26673558

Myburgh, R., Hochfeld, W. E., Dodgen, T. M., Ker, J., & Pepper, M. S. (2012). Cardiovascular pharmacogenetics. *Pharmacology & Therapeutics*, *133*(3), 280–290. doi:10.1016/j.pharmthera.2011.11.002 PMID:22123178

OGara, P. T., Kushner, F. G., Ascheim, D. D., Casey, D. E. Jr, Chung, M. K., de Lemos, J. A., & Zhao, D. X. et al. (2013). 2013 ACCF/AHA guideline for the management of ST-elevation myocardial infarction: executive summary: a report of the American College of Cardiology Foundation/American Heart Association Task Force on Practice Guidelines: developed in collaboration with the American College of Emergency Physicians and Society for Cardiovascular Angiography and Interventions. *Catheterization and Cardiovascular Interventions*, *82*(1), E1–E27. doi:10.1002/ccd.24776 PMID:23299937

Ramsey, L. B., Johnson, S. G., Caudle, K. E., Haidar, C. E., Voora, D., Wilke, R. A., & Niemi, M. et al. (2014). The clinical pharmacogenetics implementation consortium guideline for SLCO1B1 and simvastatin-induced myopathy: 2014 update. *Clinical Pharmacology and Therapeutics*, *96*(4), 423–428. doi:10.1038/clpt.2014.125 PMID:24918167

Relling, M. V., & Klein, T. E. (2011). CPIC: Clinical Pharmacogenetics Implementation Consortium of the Pharmacogenomics Research Network. *Clinical Pharmacology and Therapeutics*, *89*(3), 464–467. doi:10.1038/clpt.2010.279 PMID:21270786

Robertson, D., & Biaggioni, I. (2015). Adrenoceptor Antagonist Drugs. In B. Katzung & A. Trevor (Eds.), Basic & Clinical Pharmacology. New York, NY: McGraw-Hill.

Schork, N. J. (2015). Personalized medicine: Time for one-person trials. *Nature*, *520*(7549), 609–611. doi:10.1038/520609a PMID:25925459

Scott, S. A., Sangkuhl, K., Stein, C. M., Hulot, J. S., Mega, J. L., Roden, D. M., & Shuldiner, A. R. et al. (2013). Clinical Pharmacogenetics Implementation Consortium guidelines for CYP2C19 genotype and clopidogrel therapy: 2013 update. *Clinical Pharmacology and Therapeutics*, *94*(3), 317–323. doi:10.1038/clpt.2013.105 PMID:23698643

Sehrt, D., Meineke, I., Tzvetkov, M., Gultepe, S., & Brockmoller, J. (2011). Carvedilol pharmacokinetics and pharmacodynamics in relation to CYP2D6 and ADRB pharmacogenetics. *Pharmacogenomics*, *12*(6), 783–795. doi:10.2217/pgs.11.20 PMID:21599570

Sharp, C. F., Gardiner, S. J., Jensen, B. P., Roberts, R. L., Troughton, R. W., Lainchbury, J. G., & Begg, E. J. (2009). CYP2D6 genotype and its relationship with metoprolol dose, concentrations and effect in patients with systolic heart failure. *The Pharmacogenomics Journal*, *9*(3), 175–184. doi:10.1038/tpj.2009.9 PMID:19365402

Spear, B. B., Heath-Chiozzi, M., & Huff, J. (2001). Clinical application of pharmacogenetics. *Trends in Molecular Medicine*, *7*(5), 201–204. doi:10.1016/S1471-4914(01)01986-4 PMID:11325631

Stone, N. J., Robinson, J. G., Lichtenstein, A. H., Bairey Merz, C. N., Blum, C. B., Eckel, R. H., & Wilson, P. et al. (2014). 2013 ACC/AHA guideline on the treatment of blood cholesterol to reduce atherosclerotic cardiovascular risk in adults: A report of the American College of Cardiology/American Heart Association Task Force on Practice Guidelines. *Journal of the American College of Cardiology*, *63*(2525 Pt B), 2889–2934. doi:10.1016/j.jacc.2013.11.002 PMID:24239923

Voora, D., Shah, S. H., Spasojevic, I., Ali, S., Reed, C. R., Salisbury, B. A., & Ginsburg, G. S. (2009). The SLCO1B1*5 genetic variant is associated with statin-induced side effects. *Journal of the American College of Cardiology*, *54*(17), 1609–1616. doi:10.1016/j.jacc.2009.04.053 PMID:19833260

Wallentin, L., James, S., Storey, R. F., Armstrong, M., Barratt, B. J., Horrow, J., & Becker, R. C. et al. (2010). Effect of CYP2C19 and ABCB1 single nucleotide polymorphisms on outcomes of treatment with ticagrelor versus clopidogrel for acute coronary syndromes: A genetic substudy of the PLATO trial. *Lancet*, *376*(9749), 1320–1328. doi:10.1016/S0140-6736(10)61274-3 PMID:20801498

Weeke, P., & Roden, D. M. (2013). Pharmacogenomics and Cardiovascular Disease. *Current Cardiology Reports*, *15*(7), 376. doi:10.1007/s11886-013-0376-0 PMID:23689943

Weitz, J. (2011). Blood Coagulation and Anticoagulant, Fibrinolytic, and Antiplatelet Drugs. In L. Brunton, B. Chabner, & B. Knollmann (Eds.), Goodman & Gilman's: The Pharmacologic Basis of Therapeutics. New York, NY: McGraw-Hill.

Westfall, T., & Westfall, D. (2011). Adrenergic Agonists and Antagonists. In L. Brunton, B. Chabner, & B. Knollmann (Eds.), Goodman & Gilman's: The Pharmacologic Basis of Therapeutics. New York, NY: McGraw-Hill

Whirl-Carrillo, M., McDonagh, E., Hbert, J., Gong, L., Snghkul, K., Thron, C., & Klein, T. E. et al. (2012). Pharmacogenomics Knowledge for Personalized Medicine. *Clinical Pharmacology and Therapeutics*, *92*(4), 414–417. doi:10.1038/clpt.2012.96 PMID:22992668

Yancy, C. W., Jessup, M., Bozkurt, B., Butler, J., Casey, D. E. Jr, Drazner, M. H., & Wilkoff, B. L. et al. (2013). 2013 ACCF/AHA guideline for the management of heart failure: A report of the American College of Cardiology Foundation/American Heart Association Task Force on Practice Guidelines. *Journal of the American College of Cardiology*, *62*(16), e147–e239. doi:10.1016/j.jacc.2013.05.019 PMID:23747642

You, J. J., Singer, D. E., Howard, P. A., Lane, D. A., Eckman, M. H., Fang, M. C., & Lip, G. Y. H. (2012). Antithrombotic therapy for atrial fibrillation: Antithrombotic therapy and prevention of thrombosis, 9th ed: American college of chest physicians evidence-based clinical practice guidelines. Chest, 141(2), e531S-e575S. doi:10.1378/chest.11-2304

KEY TERMS AND DEFINITIONS

CPIC Levels: A or B Prescribing action recommended, alternative therapies or dosing are highly likely to be effective and safe. C: No prescribing action recommended, alternatives are unclear, but testing is common. D: No prescribing action recommended, alternatives are unclear or evidence is weak; testing is rare or nonexistent.

Genome: The genome of an organism encompasses all the genetic material in the cell. In humans this would include the 3 billion bases pairs contained in the chromosomes in the nucleus and the approximately 16,000 base pairs of the mitochondria.

Genotype: The underlying genetic constitution of an individual usually in relation to a specific trait.

Mechanism of Action: The mechanism by which a medication alters physiology to elicit a response. Mechanisms of action are often described by the manner in which a drug binds to a target receptor (agonist/antagonist). It may be described by enzymatic activity or intracellular action.

Pharmacodynamics: The effect of a drug on a body. The pharmacodynamics of a medication is dependent on the mechanism of action of the medication.

Pharmacogenetics: The study of the role of genetic variation in determining individual drug response. Generally, pharmacogenetics has been limited to the effects of one or a few genes.

Pharmacogenomics: The study of the genome-wide role of human variation in drug response. Pharmacogenomics is a broader term and includes pharmacogenetic effects. Pharmacogenomics also includes the application of genomic technologies in drug discovery, disposition and function.

Pharmacokinetics: The process by which a drug is absorbed, distributed, metabolized and eliminated after it enters the body. Pharmacokinetics describes how a medication moves through the body and therefore impacts the overall concentration, location, and duration of a medication and its effects.

PharmaGKB Level of Evidence: 1A/1B: High, CPIC guideline or known clinical implementation. 2A/2B: Moderate, variant-drug combination with moderate evidence of an association. 3: Low, Annotation for a variant-drug combination based on a single significant (not yet replicated) or annotation for a variant-drug combination evaluated in multiple studies but lacking clear evidence of an association. 4: Annotation based on a case report, non-significant study or in vitro, molecular or functional assay evidence only.

Phenotype: The observable outcome of the interaction of an individual's genes and environmental factors.

Polymorphic: A gene or locus is polymorphic if there are differences among individuals in its DNA sequence or length. Generally, the specific difference must have a frequency of 5% in the population to be considered polymorphic.

Chapter 10
Advances in the Diagnosis and Treatment of Infective Endocarditis

R. Brigg Turner
Pacific University School of Pharmacy, USA

Jacqueline Schwartz
Pacific University School of Pharmacy, USA

ABSTRACT

Infective endocarditis is a relatively uncommon infectious disease that leads to substantial mortality and morbidity. This disease primarily involves bacterial infection of the heart valves. Diagnosis is contingent upon excellent physical examination and radiological and microbiological evidence. While failure to identify the causative microorganism does not preclude the diagnosis of infective endocarditis, management is more difficult. Recent advances have improved the etiological identification and allowed for shorter time to optimal antibiotic therapy. Advances in treatment have focused on therapies to combat drug-resistant microorganisms as well as mitigate adverse events. While new therapies are available, there exists a paucity of clinical evidence and further studies are required.

INTRODUCTION

While cardiovascular infections are relatively uncommon, they carry substantial morbidity and mortality and consume substantial healthcare resources. Three distinct clinical syndromes have been previously described and account for the vast majority of serious infections of the heart: endocarditis, myocarditis, and pericarditis. A variety of infectious pathogens including viruses, bacteria, and fungi are responsible for these syndromes. Rapid diagnosis, identification of etiologic pathogen, and receipt of optimal therapy are necessary to reduce mortality and prevent substantial morbidity.

Infective endocarditis refers to infection of the inner lining of the heart, specifically the valves of the heart. Now considered the fourth most common serious infection leading to mortality, infective endo-

DOI: 10.4018/978-1-5225-2092-4.ch010

carditis has an incidence of only 3-7 cases per 100,000 person-years (Baddour, 2015; Mylonakis, 2001). However, it has been estimated to be responsible for a loss of 1.6 million healthy years globally (Murray, 2012). In this chapter, we explore the epidemiology, pathophysiology, etiology, and diagnosis, with a particular emphasis on treatment advances for the most common infectious pathogens. The objectives of this chapter are to give the reader a comprehensive overview of this disease and an in depth discussion on treatment by discussing evidence-based recommendations and controversies.

EPIDEMIOLOGY AND PATHOPHYSIOLOGY

Two major guidelines have been published regarding the diagnosis and treatment of infective endocarditis; the United States (US) guideline was recently updated in 2015 (Baddour, 2015) as was the European Society of Cardiology guidelines (Habib, 2015). While infection of any part of the inner lining heart would be included in this syndrome, the heart valves have a higher probability of becoming infected (Fowler, 2015).

During the 20th century, the median age of patients with infective endocarditis has gradually increased from less than 30 years to the current estimated median of 50 years of age (Fowler, 2015; Murdoch, 2009). Of note, males more commonly become infected, particularly later in life. This has not always been the case but may be due to a number of factors including the decline in rheumatic fever, the aging population, and immunosenescence (Fowler, 2015).

Of alarming concern is the advent of healthcare-associated infective endocarditis. This new classification is likely due to increased incidence of surgical interventions, insertion of prosthetic material, and duration of indwelling catheters. This increase easily prompts anxiety in light of the rise of widespread antibiotic resistance and the proliferation of pandrug-resistant microorganisms (Spellberg, 2008; Spellberg 2013).

A vast majority of infective endocarditis is localized to either the aortic or mitral valve (left-sided endocarditis). Infection on the tricuspid and pulmonary valves (right-sided endocarditis) occurs infrequently. Of interest, the incidence of aortic valve endocarditis with involvement of other valves has increased substantially from 5% of cases in 1938 to 38% in the year 2000 (Murdoch, 2009). Right sided endocarditis is estimated to account for only 10% of all cases (Moss, 2003). The hypotheses for this difference in location of infection are three-fold: 1). blood on the left-side of the heart has a higher oxygen content which is more conducive to bacterial growth; 2). higher pressures on the left side of the heart may create higher turbulence which leads to higher probability of endothelial damage; 3). congenital and acquired abnormalities of heart structures are more common on the left side (Frontera, 2000). Rheumatic heart disease, once the most common cause of defect leading to infective endocarditis, has reduced in incidence in developed countries to less than 5% of infective endocarditis cases (Murdoch, 2009). Major congenital heart defects are known to predispose to infective endocarditis; however, minor defects are also major risk factors. One of the most common of these defects is a bicuspid aortic valve which was shown in one study to be a contributing factor in 16% of native valve endocarditis cases (Tribouilloy, 2010). This defect is particularly prevalent in elderly males with most patients unaware of the defect until the time of infective endocarditis diagnosis (Lamas, 2000). Other defects include degenerative lesions present in the elderly (Fowler, 2015).

Other factors associated with infection include mechanical heart valves, healthcare contact as mentioned previously, and injection drug use. While the majority of patients have left-sided endocarditis because of the aforementioned reasons, it is estimated that 75% of injection drug users with endocarditis have right-sided endocarditis (Frontera, 2000). Injection drug users often reconstitute illicit drugs for injection with nonsterile fluid, including tap water and saliva, which have high numbers of bacterial organisms. In addition, injection drug users do not routinely perform aseptic technique when injecting, thereby increasing the chance of inoculating the bloodstream with skin flora. If the bloodstream is inoculated during this process, a substantial bacterial load will be introduced to the right-side of the heart.

A distinction is made between infection occurring on native valves and those on prosthetic valves (mechanical or bioprosthetic) valves. The presence of a prosthetic valve is a risk factor for the development of infective endocarditis and the incidence has been increasing. In a study published in 2009, prosthetic valve endocarditis accounted for approximately 20% of cases (Murdoch, 2009). Approximately 90,000 prosthetic valves are implanted in the United States and the incidence of prosthetic valve endocarditis is approximately 0.5% per patient-year. This infection carries an extremely high mortality of 30-50% (Pibarot, 2009).

Multiple factors must be chronologically present for the development of infective endocarditis. First, alteration and subsequent damage of the valve endothelium must be present. In patients with native valves, this is typically caused by high blood turbulence and alterations in blood flow that can be caused by congenital defects, regurgitation, valvular stenosis, and multiple other conditions. The presence of a prosthetic valve qualifies as an alteration of the valve endothelium. Endothelial damage leads to recruitment and attachment of fibrin, platelets, fibronectin, and other factors developing into nonbacterial thrombotic endocarditis (e.g. a blood clot on the valve that is sterile). Second, bacteria must be present in the bloodstream, adhere to the thrombotic lesion, and invade this thrombosis leading to infection. Certain bacteria appear to have a predisposition for adhering and infecting these sterile thrombotic lesions. Once infected, these thrombotic lesions are colloquially referred to as vegetations. While most bacteremias are transient and cleared readily by the intact immune system, microorganisms within a vegetation are, to some degree, protected from the immune system. The vegetation provides an excellent location for bacterial growth, expansion, and subsequent invasion of the surrounding tissue, which finally leads to infective endocarditis. The presence of a large vegetation (> 10 mm in diameter) can, in turn, result in hemodynamic instability, further disturbances in blood flow, and embolic phenomenon (Baddour, 2015). Fortunately, the incidence of embolic events has decreased from an estimated 70 to 95% in the pre-antibiotic era to 15-35% currently (Fowler, 2015). Further damage to the valve and surrounding tissue can occur, particularly with infection caused by *Staphylococcus aureus*. In addition, over activation of the immune system can often result in immune complex deposition which is responsible for Roth spots and Osler's nodes.

The necessity of predisposing endothelial damage was illustrated in animal models. In animals with undamaged heart valves, injection of high inoculums of bacteria did not result in infective endocarditis. In contrast, damage to the valve lining followed by injection of bacteria resulted in rapid development of infective endocarditis (Durack, 1972; Durack, 1972). Transient bacteremia is caused when a mucosal surface colonized with bacteria is traumatized leading to the potential for bacterial entry into the bloodstream. Most bacteremias of this origin are present for only 15 to 30 minutes prior to being eradicated by the intact immune system. Transient bacteremias are most closely related to dental, upper airway, gastrointestinal, urologic, and obstetric/gynecologic procedures (Fowler, 2015).

SIGNS, SYMPTOMS, AND DIAGNOSIS

In a large cohort study, the most common signs and symptoms of infective endocarditis were fever (96%), heart murmur (85%), hematuria (26%), embolic phenomenon (17%), splenomegaly (11%), splinter hemorrhages (8%), Janeway lesions (5%), conjunctival hemorrhage (5%), Osler's nodes (3%), and Roth's spots (2%) (Murdoch, 2009). Symptomatology of infective endocarditis is differentiated into acute cases, presenting within days, and subacute cases, presenting within weeks to months. Particularly in subacute cases, generalized signs of chronic illness are often present and include anorexia, night sweats, low-grade fevers, weight loss, chronic fatigue, and diffuse weakness. Pulmonary compromise can be seen in those with right-sided endocarditis due to embolic events. In those with left-sided endocarditis, embolic events can occur in any organ system leading to some difficulty in diagnosis and often misdiagnosis.

Anemia is very common in patients with subacute infective endocarditis but is uncommon in those with acute presentations; the opposite is true for leukocytosis, as those with subacute infection often have normal leukocyte counts. Non-specific signs of infection also include elevated erythrocyte sedimentation rate and C-reactive protein. Patients will often present with abnormal urinalysis with proteinuria, hematuria, and renal casts present. Despite the potential usefulness of these laboratory values, blood cultures and echocardiography are the most useful diagnostic tools available.

In a prospective study of infective endocarditis, 89% of patients had positive blood cultures (Murdoch, 2009). The most common reasons for culture-negative infective endocarditis include inadequate blood culture volume collected, prior antibiotic administration, and fastidious microorganisms, including cell wall deficient bacteria, *Brucella species, Legionella species, Bartonella species, Tropheryma whipplei*, fungi, mycobacteria, and nutritionally variant streptococci (Baron, 2005). The HACEK organisms (*Haemophilus* species, *Aggregatibacter actinomycetemcomitans*, *Cardiobacterium hominis*, *Eikenella corrodens*, and *Kingella kingae*) were historically thought to be the most common cause of culture negative endocarditis. Currently, HACEK organisms are easily isolated due to improvements in blood culture media and automated blood culture systems (Petti, 2006). Cases of culture-negative infective endocarditis can be difficult to manage as tailoring and optimizing antibiotic regimens is extremely difficult without knowledge of the offending pathogen. Since the source of infection is the vegetation, bacteremia is constant but colony counts are typically low. Collection of appropriate cultures may limit culture-negative endocarditis to approximately 5% of cases (Von Reyn, 1981). In these few cases, additional diagnostic laboratories may be useful (Fowler, 2015). These include serological tests, histopathology and direct immunofluorescence of resected vegetations, and polymerase-chain reaction.

Recent advances in microbiological techniques may decrease the time to identification of the causative pathogen. Two of these techniques are matrix-assisted laser desorption/ionization time of flight (MALDI-TOF) mass spectroscopy and whole genome sequencing. MALDI-TOF is a technique that ionizes bacteria and analyzes the resultant protein composition via mass spectroscopy. It has recently received wide acceptance into clinical laboratories and has been useful in decreasing time to identification of bacteria from clinical cultures; in addition, it has the ability to differentiate bacterial species that were previously difficult to differentiate using traditional techniques commonly employed in clinical laboratories (Huang, 2013; Perez, 2014). While it may aid in precision of organism identification, it is unlikely to decrease the incidence of culture-negative endocarditis as it currently must be performed on bacterial colonies that have grown on culture media. Instead of the proteomics utilized in MALDI-TOF, whole genome sequencing is a technique that rapidly sequences bacterial DNA. It has also been proposed as a method to decrease time to bacterial identification and enhance the precision of identification; however, similar to MALDI-TOF, it is unlikely to decrease the incidence of culture-negative endocarditis. Whole genome sequencing is currently in the experimental phase and has not yet been widely introduced into clinical laboratories (Kwong, 2015). Both of these techniques will enhance bacterial species identification which will further inform clinical practice by allowing for delineation of specific risk factors and advanced treatment options for specific organisms.

Echocardiography is performed in two ways: transthoracic (TTE) and transesophageal (TEE). While TEEs are more invasive requiring the ultrasound transducer to be introduced into the esophagus for visualization, it results in much higher sensitivity at detecting vegetations (Erbel, 1988). As TTE is noninvasive, the recent updates to the guidelines recommend this test in all patients suspected of infective endocarditis. If TTE is negative, then a TEE is recommended. The benefit of TEE appears to be in detection of small vegetations (Erbel, 1988).

Suspicion of endocarditis is reliant upon the clinician's recognition of signs and symptoms consist with this disease. Criteria for diagnosis (first introduced in 1982) were updated in 2000 and are called the modified Duke's criteria (Baddour, 2015). While these criteria can be a useful aid, clinical identification and judgment is the keystone of diagnosis.

ETIOLOGY

The most common bacterial etiologies are described in Table 1 (see Appendix). In intravenous drug users, etiological distribution is altered and is listed in Table 2 (see Appendix). Empiric antimicrobial therapy should be tailored to the most likely pathogens causing infections based upon the clinical presentation, patient specific risk factors, and any clinical laboratory results. Consultation with infectious disease specialists is recommended and is likely to improve appropriate empiric therapy (Baddour, 2015).

Of growing concern is the rise in incidence of multidrug-resistant organisms (Peterson, 2009). Of most concern are the "ESCAPE" pathogens: *Enterococcus faecium, Staphylococcus aureus, Clostridium difficile, Acinetobacter baumannii, Pseudomonas aeruginosa*, and Enterobacteriaceae. *Staphylococcus aureus* and enterococci comprise a significant portion of infective endocarditis cases (see Table 1). In addition, *Staphylococcus aureus* and *Pseudomonas aeruginosa* are common pathogens in injection drug users with infective endocarditis (see Table 2). Many organizations have identified multidrug-resistant pathogens to be a global health concern including the Infectious Diseases Society of America, Centers for Disease Control, the Whole Health Organization, and the United States White House. Methods proposed to attenuate the rise in resistance include limiting antibiotic consumption to only those needing therapy (e.g. antimicrobial stewardship), developing new drugs, and limiting antibiotic use in livestock (United States, 2015). Unfortunately, few new antibiotics are being developed in order to combat this rise in resistance. Attempts to increase antimicrobial stewardship are ongoing but have been mainly focused in the hospital setting and efforts to curtail antibiotic consumption in livestock are only slowly being adopted. Patients with infective endocarditis infected with multidrug-resistant pathogens have limited treatment options and are at a higher risk of mortality and morbidity.

TREATMENT

General Principles

This section will focus on advances that have occurred in recent years for treatment of two of the most common bacteria responsible for infective endocarditis: *Staphylococcus aureus* and enterococci. The goal of treatment is sterilization of the infected heart tissue, particularly the infected vegetation. Drug penetration into the vegetation can be limited and therapeutic activity may be altered as some microorganis are metabolically inactive. Altered antimicrobial activity in this instance is called the inoculum effect; in particular, drugs that act on the cell wall (i.e. beta-lactams) may have reduced activity in large inoculums when bacteria near the center of the vegetation are metabolically inactive. Cell wall agents have activity on growing and rapidly dividing cells; however, in this instance, some cell wall agents may have reduced activity. In addition, host immune defenses may be altered due to constant activation and the inability to penetration into the vegetation. Due to some of these concerns, long durations of intravenous (iv) antimicrobial therapy is preferred. In addition, bactericidal antibiotics are recommended (Baddour, 2015). In order to achieve bactericidal activity, combination therapy is required or helpful in certain situations.

Optimizing Pharmacodynamic Parameters

When designing antimicrobial therapy, special attention should be given to optimizing the pharmacodynamic parameters of certain antimicrobials. For example, prolonged or continuous infusion of beta-lactam antibiotics has been shown to decrease mortality in certain populations (Lodise, 2007), although this has not been evaluated in infective endocarditis. Other antibiotics of interest include vancomycin with efficacy maximized when the 24-hour area under the curve to minimum inhibitory concentration (AUC_{24}:MIC) ratio exceeds 400. Several retrospective reports have identified this target to result in improved mortality and greater clinical success in *Staphylococcus aureus* bacteremia (Kullar, 2011; Holmes, 2013). These results have yet to be confirmed in infective endocarditis or by prospective trials. The current standard for vancomycin dosing is to target a serum trough level of 15-20 mg/L in serious infections (Rybak, 2009). Unfortunately, AUC and trough are poorly correlated with trough not being recommended as a reliable surrogate by some groups (Patel, 2011; Neely, 2014). Several different methods are available to determine optimal vancomycin dose to target a specific AUC; unfortunately, none of these methods have been robustly tested in prospective trials (Pai, 2014; Fuchs, 2013). Further research is desperately needed in this field; currently, it appears prudent to attempt to calculate the AUC for a vancomycin dosage regimen instead of relying on the vancomycin target trough concentration. This holds true in cases where vancomycin is needed for treatment of infective endocarditis.

Daptomycin is frequently used in infective endocarditis caused by certain bacteria. While the Food and Drug Administration (FDA) approved dosing is 6 mg/kg for serious infections including right-sided infective endocarditis, higher doses are increasingly being used across the United States. Daptomycin is a lipopeptide with concentration dependent activity (optimizing the maximum concentration to minimum inhibitory concentration [MIC] ratio improves microbiological efficacy). As such, higher doses may result in better clinical efficacy. Daptomycin is often used in cases where vancomycin and other agents cannot and is considered one of the last feasible options for some microorganisms. Confirming daptomycin susceptibility prior to treatment is important due to a correlation between reduced daptomycin susceptibility and vancomycin-intermediate *Staphylococcus aureus* (Cui, 2006). As such, treatment failure with daptomycin may have serious consequences. Efforts to improve daptomycin efficacy have focused on utilizing higher than FDA approved doses to limit treatment failure and to limit the development of resistance. Several analyses have concluded that doses up to 12 mg/kg of daptomycin are safe with limited adverse reactions (Lai, 2013; Benvenuto, 2006). While some data suggest high-dose daptomycin to be safe, data are not available suggesting enhanced efficacy. While daptomycin has been studied in infective endocarditis, large prospective trials evaluating its safety and efficacy are not available. Unfortunately, in many instances, daptomycin is one of the only remaining options for some patients and must be used despite the paucity of data.

Treatment of Staphylococcal Infective Endocarditis

As mentioned in previous sections, *Staphylococcus aureus* is the microorganism responsible for the largest percentage of cases of infective endocarditis. It is common in all subtypes of infective endocarditis, including injection drug users. During its widespread introduction in World War II, penicillin had high activity against *Staphylococcus aureus*. Unfortunately, in 1942, penicillin-resistant *Staphylococcus aureus* (with resistance mediated by production of a penicillinase) was identified in hospitals and, later, in the general community (Rammelkamp, 1942). By the 1960s, over 80% of all clinically isolated *Staphylococcus aureus* was resistant to penicillin (Chambers, 2001). In 1961, a new class of antibiotics was introduced with the approval of methicillin. This class of antibiotics resists hydrolysis by the penicillinase produced by *Staphylococcus aureus*; unfortunately, resistance to methicillin was rapidly identified and was later called methicillin-resistant *Staphylococcus aureus* (MRSA). Once uncommon in the 1960s, some geographical areas report methicillin-resistance in excess of 50% of all *Staphylococcus aureus* isolates currently. New therapeutic options have been developed over the last several decades.

Therapeutic options for treatment of infective endocarditis caused by *Staphylococcus aureus* are listed in Table 3 (see Appendix). For methicillin-susceptible *Staphylococcus aureus* (MSSA), nafcillin or oxacillin are the preferred options with cefazolin being recommended for those patients unable to tolerate primary therapy (Baddour, 2015). In other infections caused by MSSA, cefazolin is a primary therapy as well as nafcillin and oxacillin. While susceptible in *in vitro* testing, the presence of a large inoculum of MSSA, may lead to higher rates of cefazolin failure as compared to that of nafcillin or oxacillin. In an *in vitro* study in 2009, it was shown that high production of a penicillinase (type A beta-lactamase) could be responsible for cefazolin failure (Nannini, 2009). This report suggested that 19% of MSSA displayed this inoculum effect and potential for inducing cefazolin failure. As a high number of organisms are present in vegetations, the chance of cefazolin failure because of the inoculum effect could be substantial. For this reason, cefazolin should be used only as an alternative to nafcillin or oxacillin. The increased rate of potential cefazolin failure, in comparison to that of nafcillin or oxacillin, has not been readily shown in other severe diseases such as in MSSA bacteremia. In a retrospective cohort study, treatment with cefazolin was not associated with higher rates of treatment failure in comparison to nafcillin; however, cefazolin was much better tolerated with nafcillin discontinuation rates of almost 20% (Lee, 2011). In a separate study, 34% of patients requiring long-term therapy discontinued nafcillin as compared to only 7% of patients treated with cefazolin (Youngster, 2014). Common adverse effects for nafcillin included rash, renal dysfunction, and liver abnormalities. All patients experiencing an adverse reaction with nafcillin that were switched to cefazolin completed their treatment (Youngster, 2014). In summary, while there may be a higher potential failure in patients treated with cefazolin due to the inoculum effect, it is much more likely that patients will tolerate and be able to finish therapy when treated with cefazolin as compared to nafcillin or oxacillin.

The US guidelines recommend vancomycin to be used for MSSA only when a patient is unable to receive nafcillin, oxacillin, or cefazolin. Multiple retrospective studies have examined the efficacy of vancomycin versus nafcillin, oxacillin, or cefazolin, and these data are generally considered to be overall poor in quality (Holland, 2014). In general, studies have found that treatment of MSSA bacteremia with nafcillin, oxacillin, or cefazolin results in better overall clinical efficacy as compared to treatment with vancomycin. One study of patients with MSSA bacteremia found 79% lower mortality in those treated with cefazolin or nafcillin; in patients treated initially with vancomycin and then switched to cefazolin or nafcillin, they identified a 69% lower mortality in comparison to those receiving therapy with vancomycin alone (Schweizer, 2011).

For patients with MRSA infective endocarditis, the US guideline recommends vancomycin or daptomycin. For those patients infected with vancomycin intermediate *Staphylococcus aureus* (VISA), daptomycin or ceftaroline may be options. While vancomycin has been the standard therapy for MRSA for over 5 decades, daptomycin has only recently been approved in 2003. The FDA approved indications include treatment of *Staphylococcus aureus* bacteremia and also right-sided infective endocarditis. While the study that led to his FDA approval was small, the results suggested that daptomycin had similar efficacy to comparative drugs (vancomycin for MRSA and nafcillin, oxacillin, cloxacillin, or flucloxacillin for MSSA) including those with right-sided infective endocarditis (Cubicin, 2006). Not enough patients with left-sided infective endocarditis were enrolled in the study in order to perform a formal analysis. In a separate analysis published in 2013, patients treated with daptomycin with either left or right-sided endocarditis had good clinical outcomes with success of 89% (Kullar, 2013). Patients generally received high doses of daptomycin in this study with a median dose of 9.8 mg/kg/day (in comparison to the FDA approved dosage of 6 mg/kg/day). No patients required discontinuation of daptomycin therapy because of adverse events. In 2013, a retrospective analysis (n=170) evaluated the difference in clinical outcomes between patients treated with vancomycin or daptomycin for MRSA bacteremia with a vancomycin MIC > 1 mg/L. They identified a higher mortality and also a longer time to bacteremia clearance in those treated with vancomycin. The authors suggest that in scenarios when the vancomycin MIC is > 1 mg/L, daptomycin may be preferred (Murray, 2013). In contrast to this report, a multicenter study found a similar composite failure rate between vancomycin and daptomycin of 39% and 31% ($P = 0.259$). While they did note a few outcomes that favored daptomycin, overall, no difference was found (Moise, 2016). A meta-analysis that included a total of 38 studies of *Staphylococcus aureus* bacteremia found that mortality did not differ between patients with high vancomycin MICs (≥ 1.5 mg/L) and those with low vancomycin MICs (< 1.5 mg/L) (Kalil, 2014). In addition, some have suggested that regardless of the vancomycin MIC, switching therapy should be considered in those patients that fail to have an adequate response with vancomycin after 3-4 days (Kullar, 2014).

Currently, there is still debate on which therapy is the treatment of choice in MRSA infective endocarditis, particularly in those with vancomycin MICs > 1.0 mg/L. In cases of VISA or failure of vancomycin or daptomycin therapy, a paucity of evidence exists. However, anecdotal evidence suggests that combination therapy, often involving the newly approved ceftaroline, should be considered (Kullar, 2016; Sakoulas & Moise, 2014). Ceftaroline is a fifth generation cephalosporin with activity similar to ceftriaxone with one major difference; ceftaroline is the only beta-lactam with activity against MRSA. It is currently only approved for treatment of MRSA in the setting of skin and soft tissue infections; however, it has been used off-label in a number of cases with good success (Ho, 2012). Despite lack of high quality clinical evidence, its use continues to grow in refractory cases and could be considered as a viable alternative.

Treatment of Enterococcal Infective Endocarditis

Enterococci are the third most common pathogens in patients with infective endocarditis (see Table 1) with *Enterococcus faecalis as* the most frequently isolated. These organisms have low virulence in comparison to *Staphylococcus aureus* but can carry significant resistance genes making successful treatment of invasive disease, such as infective endocarditis, difficult (Mundy, 2000). Enterococci have reduced susceptibility to penicillins relative to streptococci but are still considered to have intrinsic susceptibility to penicillin, ampicillin, and piperacillin. Resistant to the penicillins is mediated by alteration of the penicillin binding protein (PBP) or production of a penicillinase. They express low levels of PBP4 and PBP5 to which cephalosporins bind, rendering this class ineffective when used as monotherapy. Additionally, some enterococci produce an aminoglycoside modifying enzyme causing these microorganisms to be highly resistant to this class.

Historically, a vast majority of treatment failures with enterococcal endocarditis occurred with patients receiving penicillin monotherapy. In order to achieve bactericidal activity and decrease treatment failure, the US guidelines recommend combination therapy for penicillin-susceptible enterococci (see Table 3). In the past few years, several major studies have been published which have led to treatment advances. In 1999 and 2001, studies demonstrated the efficacy of ampicillin plus ceftriaxone in *in vitro* and animal models with *Enterococcus faecalis* that expressed high-level gentamicin resistance (Gavalda, 1999; Desbiolles, 2001). The rationale for using ceftriaxone for synergy stems from data suggesting that enterococci upregulate PBP2 and PBP3, to which ceftriaxone binds, in the presence of ampicillin; the combination of agents provides enhanced saturation of PBP leading to bactericidal activity (Gavalda, 1999). In 2003, a study suggested that ampicillin plus ceftriaxone led to similar efficacy when compared to ampicillin plus gentamicin in enterococci that were susceptible to gentamicin (Gavalda, 2003). Finally, in 2007 and 2013, clinical studies confirmed that ampicillin plus ceftriaxone was just as effective, but with less renal toxicity, as ampicillin plus gentamicin in enterococcal endocarditis caused by gentamicin susceptible and resistant strains (Gavalda, 2007; Fernandez-Hidalgo, 2013). The US guidelines currently recommend ampicillin plus ceftriaxone to be used in those with impaired renal function or in cases of high-level gentamicin resistance (Baddour, 2015). While some experts recommend this combination in all scenarios of enterococcal infective endocarditis (Fernandez-Hidalgo, 2013), data are lacking to substantiate this recommendation.

As gentamicin can cause up to 25% of patients to discontinue therapy due to new renal failure when treating enterococcal endocarditis, there has been interest in limiting the duration of gentamicin combination therapy. In 2002, a retrospective report of 93 cases of enterococcal endocarditis from Sweden concluded that utilizing ampicillin plus gentamicin for 2 weeks followed by ampicillin alone for 2-4 weeks led to excellent treatment success (Olaison, 2002). Based partly on this study, Sweden changed their national guidelines to recommend only 2 weeks of gentamicin therapy. In 2013, a quasi-experimental report from Sweden described the treatment outcomes of 84 patients with enterococcal endocarditis with approximately half being treated with longer duration and half being treated with only 2 weeks of gentamicin therapy (Dahl, 2013). They identified no difference in clinical outcomes with the exception that those receiving longer duration of gentamicin therapy had more significant decreases in renal function. While this option was not recommended in the US guidelines, it appears to be an acceptable alternative.

For vancomycin-resistant enterococci (VRE), daptomycin and linezolid are viable treatment options. Linezolid is an oxazolidinone that binds to the bacterial ribosome leading to bacteriostatic activity. While susceptibility to linezolid remains high (>97%), resistance has been detected, particularly during treatment (Baddour, 2015). Linezolid has been used in multiple cases of infective endocarditis including treatment of VRE. In a review of case reports including 6 cases of VRE endocarditis, treatment with linezolid led to clinical cure in 5 patients but only improvement, and eventual death, in the 6th (Falagas, 2006). Several other cases have reported the outcomes of linezolid with one reporting treatment failure (Tsigrelis, 2007).

Daptomycin is a cyclic lipopeptide that has bactericidal activity against enterococci via bacterial membrane disruption. It is FDA approved for treatment of right-sided infective endocarditis caused by *Staphylococcus aureus*, but not enterococci. Despite this lack of indication, daptomycin has been used for treatment of VRE infective endocarditis. In a case series of 49 patients with infective endocarditis treated with daptomycin, 9 were infected with VRE with 6 achieving clinical success (Levine, 2007). One analysis of high-dose daptomycin (median 8.2 mg/kg) for treatment of enterococcal infections found clinical success of 89% and limited adverse events suggesting this dosage to be safe (Casapao, 2013). In the largest study to date, investigators retrospectively compared treatment with linezolid to that of daptomycin for VRE bacteremia (n=644) (Britt, 2015). Included in the study were 39 cases of endocarditis, although a formal analysis was not conducted on this subgroup. The study concluded that daptomycin resulted in superior clinical outcomes including treatment success and mortality, but not recurrence of bacteremia. As substantial differences existed in the baseline characteristics of the study groups, the investigators performed a propensity score-matched analysis. The results of this analysis were similar to the other analyses showing daptomycin to be superior.

While clinical efficacy has been shown for VRE infections, development of daptomycin resistance has been documented, particularly during treatment (Kanafani, 2007). Due to the isolation of VRE with high daptomycin MICs, several have suggested combination therapy to be preferred in this scenario. The use of non-susceptible antibiotics in combination with daptomycin has been shown to be synergistic and enhance daptomycin binding and activity. This phenomenon, known as the seesaw effect, is also described for treatment of daptomycin non-susceptible *Staphylococcus aureus* (Dhand, 2011). In the case of enterococci, the development of daptomycin non-susceptibility has been accompanied by a paradoxical enhanced susceptibility to typically resistant ampicillin or ceftaroline (hence "seesaw") (Sakoulas, 2012; Sakoulas, 2013; Sakoulas & Rose, 2014). Use of combination therapy with daptomycin plus ampicillin or ceftaroline leads to bactericidal activity. While shown *in vitro*, limited cases have been published to demonstrate the clinical utility of these combinations. While there is a substantial lack of clinical data, US guidelines suggest that prescribers consider use of combination therapy in cases with high daptomycin MICs in which no reliable agents exist (Baddour, 2015). Based on these data, daptomycin has become the preferred agent for treatment of VRE infections, including infective endocarditis. While not well established, high-dose daptomycin (>6 mg/kg) is recommended (Baddour, 2015) and is generally considered safe.

FUTURE RESEARCH

While advances have been made in recent years, emerging technology to identify microorganisms directly from blood samples will greatly enhance pathogen identification. Some of these tools have yet to be developed but will likely be built on platforms of genomic, proteomic, or antigen based systems. The ability to detect a pathogen immediately upon drawing a blood sample would reduce unnecessary antibiotic use, improve time to optimal therapy, and further aid in definitive diagnosis of infective endocarditis. New treatments have been recently explored for infective endocarditis caused by *Staphylococcus aureus* and enterococci. Despite this, there is a paucity of national or international trials evaluating different treatment options. While certain medical fields, such as oncology, enroll patients into national studies funded by either governmental or organizational grants, research on infectious diseases, including infective endocarditis, are often performed by single centers or geographically limited multicenter studies. Future work needs to be done, particularly in diseases with relatively low incidence such as VRE infective endocarditis.

CONCLUSION

Infective endocarditis continues to carry substantial risk of mortality and morbidity despite recent advances in pathogen identification and treatment. While some investigational advances have been made, these have to be confirmed by well-designed clinical trials. Due to this, clinicians are often left with the necessity of following recommendations based on overall poor quality evidence.

REFERENCES

Baddour, L. M., Wilson, W. R., Bayer, A. S., Fowler, V. G. Jr, Tleyjeh, I. M., Rybak, M. J., & Taubert, K. A. et al. (2015). Infective Endocarditis in Adults: Diagnosis, Antimicrobial Therapy, and Management of Complications: A Scientific Statement for Healthcare Professionals From the American Heart Association. *Circulation*, *132*(15), 1435–1486. doi:10.1161/CIR.0000000000000296 PMID:26373316

Baron, E. J., Scott, J. D., & Tompkins, L. S. (2005). Prolonged Incubation and Extensive Subculturing Do Not Increase Recovery of Clinically Significant Microorganisms from Standard Automated Blood Cultures. *Clinical Infectious Diseases*, *41*(11), 1677–1680. doi:10.1086/497595 PMID:16267743

Benvenuto, M., Benziger, D. P., Yankelev, S., & Vigliani, G. (2006). Pharmacokinetics and tolerability of daptomycin at doses up to 12 milligrams per kilogram of body weight once daily in healthy volunteers. *Antimicrobial Agents and Chemotherapy*, *50*(10), 3245–3249. doi:10.1128/AAC.00247-06 PMID:17005801

Britt, N. S., Potter, E. M., Patel, N., & Steed, M. E. (2015). Comparison of the Effectiveness and Safety of Linezolid and Daptomycin in Vancomycin-Resistant Enterococcal Bloodstream Infection: A National Cohort Study of Veterans Affairs Patients. *Clinical Infectious Diseases*, *61*(6), 871–878. doi:10.1093/cid/civ444 PMID:26063715

Casapao, A. M., Kullar, R., Davis, S. L., Levine, D. P., Zhao, J. J., Potoski, B. A., & Rybak, M. J. et al. (2013). Multicenter study of high-dose daptomycin for treatment of enterococcal infections. *Antimicrobial Agents and Chemotherapy*, *57*(9), 4190–4196. doi:10.1128/AAC.00526-13 PMID:23774437

Chambers, H. F. (2001). The changing epidemiology of Staphylococcus aureus? *Emerging Infectious Diseases*, *7*(2), 178–182. doi:10.3201/eid0702.010204 PMID:11294701

Cubicin®: FDA Briefing Document for Anti-Infective Drugs Advisory Committee Meeting. (2006). Retrieved on 2/23/2016 from http://www.fda.gov/ohrms/dockets/ac/06/briefing/2006-4209B1_02_01-FDA-Background.pdf

Cui, L., Tominaga, E., Neoh, H., & Hiramatsu, K. (2006). Correlation Between Reduced Daptomycin Susceptibilities and Vancomycin Resistance in Vancomycin-Intermediated *Staphylococcus aureus*. *Antimicrobial Agents and Chemotherapy*, *50*(3), 1079–1082. doi:10.1128/AAC.50.3.1079-1082.2006 PMID:16495273

Dahl, A., Rasmussen, R. V., Bundgaard, H., Hassager, C., Bruun, L. E., Lauridsen, T. K., & Bruun, N. E. et al. (2013). Enterococcus faecalis infective endocarditis: A pilot study of the relationship between duration of gentamicin treatment and outcome. *Circulation*, *127*(17), 1810–1817. doi:10.1161/CIRCULATIONAHA.112.001170 PMID:23543002

Desbiolles, N., Piroth, L., Lequeu, C., Neuwirth, C., Portier, H., & Chavanet, P. (2001). Fractional maximal effect method for in vitro synergy between amoxicillin and ceftriaxone and between vancomycin and ceftriaxone against Enterococcus faecalis and penicillin-resistant Streptococcus pneumoniae. *Antimicrobial Agents and Chemotherapy*, *45*(12), 3328–3333. doi:10.1128/AAC.45.12.3328-3333.2001 PMID:11709304

Dhand, A., Bayer, A. S., Pogliano, J., Yang, S. J., Bolaris, M., Nizet, V., & Sakoulas, G. et al. (2011). Use of antistaphylococcal beta-lactams to increase daptomycin activity in eradicating persistent bacteremia due to methicillin-resistant Staphylococcus aureus: Role of enhanced daptomycin binding. *Clinical Infectious Diseases*, *53*(2), 158–163. doi:10.1093/cid/cir340 PMID:21690622

Durack, D. T., & Beeson, P. B. (1972). Experimental bacterial endocarditis. I. Colonization of a sterile vegetation. *British Journal of Experimental Pathology*, *53*, 44–49. PMID:5014243

Durack, D. T., Beeson, P. B., & Petersdorf, R. G. (1972). Experimental endocarditis. 3. Production and progress of the disease in rabbits. *British Journal of Experimental Pathology*, *54*, 142–151. PMID:4700697

Erbel, R., Rohmann, S., Drexler, M., Mohr-Kahaly, S., Gerharz, C. D., Iversen, S., & Meyer, J. et al. (1988). Improved diagnostic value of echocardiography in patients with infective endocarditis by transesophageal approach: A prospective study. *European Heart Journal*, *9*, 43–53. PMID:3345769

Falagas, M. E., Manta, K. G., Ntziora, F., & Vardakas, K. Z. (2006). Linezolid for the treatment of patients with endocarditis: A systematic review of the published evidence. *The Journal of Antimicrobial Chemotherapy*, *58*(2), 273–280. doi:10.1093/jac/dkl219 PMID:16735427

Fernández-Hidalgo, N., Almirante, B., Gavaldà, J., Gurgui, M., Peña, C., de Alarcón, A., & Pahissa, A. et al. (2013). Ampicillin plus ceftriaxone is as effective as ampicillin plus gentamicin for treating enterococcus faecalis infective endocarditis. *Clinical Infectious Diseases*, *56*(9), 1261–1268. doi:10.1093/cid/cit052 PMID:23392394

Fowler, V. G. Jr, Scheld, W. M., & Bayer, A. S. (2015). Endocarditis and Intravascular Infections. In J. E. Bennett, R. Dolin, & M. J. Blaser (Eds.), *Mandell, Douglas, and Bennett's Principles and Practices of Infectious Diseases* (pp. 990–1028). Philadelphia, PA: Elsevier Saunders.

Frontera, J. A., & Gradon, J. D. (2000). Right-sided endocarditis in injection drug users: Review of proposed mechanisms of pathogenesis. *Clinical Infectious Diseases*, *30*(2), 374–379. doi:10.1086/313664 PMID:10671344

Fuchs, A., Csajka, C., Thoma, Y., Buclin, T., & Widmer, N. (2013). Benchmarking therapeutic drug monitoring software: A review of available computer tools. *Clinical Pharmacokinetics*, *52*(1), 9–22. doi:10.1007/s40262-012-0020-y PMID:23196713

Gavaldà, J., Len, O., Miró, J. M., Muñoz, P., Montejo, M., Alarcón, A., & Pahissa, A. et al. (2007). Brief communication: Treatment of Enterococcus faecalis endocarditis with ampicillin plus ceftriaxone. *Annals of Internal Medicine*, *146*(8), 574–579. doi:10.7326/0003-4819-146-8-200704170-00008 PMID:17438316

Gavaldá, J., Onrubia, P. L., Gómez, M. T., Gomis, X., Ramírez, J. L., Len, O., & Pahissa, A. et al. (2003). Efficacy of ampicillin combined with ceftriaxone and gentamicin in the treatment of experimental endocarditis due to Enterococcus faecalis with no high-level resistance to aminoglycosides. *The Journal of Antimicrobial Chemotherapy*, *52*(3), 514–517. doi:10.1093/jac/dkg360 PMID:12917251

Gavaldà, J., Torres, C., Tenorio, C., López, P., Zaragoza, M., Capdevila, J. A., & Pahissa, A. et al. (1999). Efficacy of ampicillin plus ceftriaxone in treatment of experimental endocarditis due to Enterococcus faecalis strains highly resistant to aminoglycosides. *Antimicrobial Agents and Chemotherapy*, *43*, 639–646. PMID:10049280

Habib, G., Lancellotti, P., Antunes, M. J., Bongiorni, M. G., Casalta, J. P., Del Zotti, F., & Zamorano, J. L. et al. (2015). 2015 ESC Guidelines for the management of infective endocarditis: The Task Force for the Management of Infective Endocarditis of the European Society of Cardiology (ESC). Endorsed by: European Association for Cardio-Thoracic Surgery (EACTS), the European Association of Nuclear Medicine (EANM). *European Heart Journal*, *36*(44), 3075–3128. doi:10.1093/eurheartj/ehv319 PMID:26320109

Ho, T. T., Cadena, J., Childs, L. M., Gonzalez-Velez, M., & Lewis, J. S. II. (2012). Methicillin-resistant Staphylococcus aureus bacteraemia and endocarditis treated with ceftaroline salvage therapy. *The Journal of Antimicrobial Chemotherapy*, *67*(5), 1267–1270. doi:10.1093/jac/dks006 PMID:22311935

Holland, T. L., Arnold, C., & Fowler, V. G. Jr. (2014). Clinical management of Staphylococcus aureus bacteremia: A review. *Journal of the American Medical Association*, *312*(13), 1330–1341. doi:10.1001/jama.2014.9743 PMID:25268440

Holmes, N. E., Turnidge, J. D., Munckhof, W. J., Robinson, J. O., Korman, T. M., OSullivan, M. V., & Johnson, P. D. et al. (2013). Vancomycin AUC/MIC ratio and 30-day mortality in patients with Staphylococcus aureus bacteremia. *Antimicrobial Agents and Chemotherapy*, *57*(4), 1654–1663. doi:10.1128/AAC.01485-12 PMID:23335735

Huang, A. M., Newton, D., Kunapuli, A., Gandhi, T. N., Washer, L. L., Isip, J., & Nagel, J. L. et al. (2013). Impact of rapid organism identification via matrix-assisted laser desorption/ionization time-of-flight combined with antimicrobial stewardship team intervention in adult patients with bacteremia and candidemia. *Clinical Infectious Diseases*, *57*(9), 1237–1245. doi:10.1093/cid/cit498 PMID:23899684

Kalil, A. C., Van Schooneveld, T. C., Fey, P. D., & Rupp, M. E. (2014). Association between vancomycin minimum inhibitory concentration and mortality among patients with Staphylococcus aureus bloodstream infections: A systematic review and meta-analysis. *Journal of the American Medical Association*, *312*(15), 1552–1564. doi:10.1001/jama.2014.6364 PMID:25321910

Kanafani, Z. A., Federspiel, J. J., & Fowler, V. G. Jr. (2007). Infective endocarditis caused by daptomycin-resistant Enterococcus faecalis: A case report. *Scandinavian Journal of Infectious Diseases*, *39*(1), 75–77. doi:10.1080/00365540600786465 PMID:17366018

Kullar, R., Casapao, A. M., Davis, S. L., Levine, D. P., Zhao, J. J., Crank, C. W., & Rybak, M. J. et al. (2013). A multicentre evaluation of the effectiveness and safety of high-dose daptomycin for the treatment of infective endocarditis. *The Journal of Antimicrobial Chemotherapy*, *68*(12), 2921–2926. doi:10.1093/jac/dkt294 PMID:23928022

Kullar, R., Davis, S. L., Levine, D. P., & Rybak, M. J. (2011). Impact of vancomycin exposure on outcomes in patients with methicillin-resistant Staphylococcus aureus bacteremia: Support for consensus guidelines suggested targets. *Clinical Infectious Diseases*, *52*(8), 975–981. doi:10.1093/cid/cir124 PMID:21460309

Kullar, R., McKinnell, J. A., & Sakoulas, G. (2014). Avoiding the perfect storm: The biologic and clinical case for reevaluating the 7-day expectation for methicillin-resistant Staphylococcus aureus bacteremia before switching therapy. *Clinical Infectious Diseases*, *59*(10), 1455–1461. doi:10.1093/cid/ciu583 PMID:25048852

Kullar, R., Sakoulas, G., Deresinski, S., & van Hal, S. J. (2016). When sepsis persists: A review of MRSA bacteraemia salvage therapy. *The Journal of Antimicrobial Chemotherapy*, *71*(3), 576–586. doi:10.1093/jac/dkv368 PMID:26565015

Kwong, J. C., McCallum, N., Sintchenko, V., & Howden, B. P. (2015). Whole genome sequencing in clinical and public health microbiology. *Pathology*, *47*(3), 199–210. doi:10.1097/PAT.0000000000000235 PMID:25730631

Lai, C. C., Sheng, W. H., Wang, J. T., Cheng, A., Chuang, Y. C., Chen, Y. C., & Chang, S. C. (2013). Safety and efficacy of high-dose daptomycin as salvage therapy for severe gram-positive bacterial sepsis in hospitalized adult patients. *BMC Infectious Diseases*, *13*(1), 66. doi:10.1186/1471-2334-13-66 PMID:23379510

Lamas, C. C., & Eykyn, S. J. (2000). Bicuspid aortic valveA silent danger: Analysis of 50 cases of infective endocarditis. *Clinical Infectious Diseases*, *30*(2), 336–341. doi:10.1086/313646 PMID:10671338

Lee, S., Choe, P. G., Song, K. H., Park, S. W., Kim, H. B., Kim, N. J., & Oh, M. D. et al. (2011). Is cefazolin inferior to nafcillin for treatment of methicillin-susceptible Staphylococcus aureus bacteremia? *Antimicrobial Agents and Chemotherapy*, *55*(11), 5122–5126. doi:10.1128/AAC.00485-11 PMID:21825299

Levine, D. P., & Lamp, K. C. (2007). Daptomycin in the treatment of patients with infective endocarditis: Experience from a registry. *The American Journal of Medicine*, *120*(10), S28–S33. doi:10.1016/j.amjmed.2007.07.011 PMID:17904948

Lodise, T. P. Jr, Lomaestro, B., & Drusano, G. L. (2007). Piperacillin-tazobactam for Pseudomonas aeruginosa infection: Clinical implications of an extended-infusion dosing strategy. *Clinical Infectious Diseases*, *44*(3), 357–363. doi:10.1086/510590 PMID:17205441

Moise, P. A., Culshaw, D. L., Wong-Beringer, A., Bensman, J., Lamp, K. C., Smith, W. J., & Zervos, M. J. et al. (2016). Comparative Effectiveness of Vancomycin Versus Daptomycin for MRSA Bacteremia With Vancomycin MIC >1 mg/L: A Multicenter Evaluation. *Clinical Therapeutics*, *38*(1), 16–30. doi:10.1016/j.clinthera.2015.09.017 PMID:26585355

Moss, R., & Munt, B. (2003). Infection drug use and right sided endocarditis. *Heart (British Cardiac Society)*, *89*(5), 577–581. doi:10.1136/heart.89.5.577 PMID:12695478

Mundy, L. M., Sahm, D. F., & Gilmore, M. (2000). Relationships between Enterococcal Virulence and Antimicrobial Resistance. *Clinical Microbiology Reviews*, *13*(4), 513–522. doi:10.1128/CMR.13.4.513-522.2000 PMID:11023953

Murdoch, D. R., Corey, G. R., Hoen, B., Miró, J. M., Fowler, V. G. Jr, Bayer, A. S., & Cabell, C. H. et al. (2009). Clinical presentation, etiology, and outcome of infective endocarditis in the 21st century: The International Collaboration on Endocarditis-Prospective Cohort Study. *Archives of Internal Medicine*, *169*(5), 463–473. doi:10.1001/archinternmed.2008.603 PMID:19273776

Murray, K. P., Zhao, J. J., Davis, S. L., Kullar, R., Kaye, K. S., Lephart, P., & Rybak, M. J. (2013). Early use of daptomycin versus vancomycin for methicillin-resistant Staphylococcus aureus bacteremia with vancomycin minimum inhibitory concentration >1 mg/L: A matched cohort study. *Clinical Infectious Diseases*, *56*(11), 1562–1569. doi:10.1093/cid/cit112 PMID:23449272

Mylonakis, E., & Calderwood, S. B. (2001). Infective endocarditis in adults. *The New England Journal of Medicine*, *345*(18), 1318–1330. doi:10.1056/NEJMra010082 PMID:11794152

Nannini, E. C., Stryjewski, M. E., Singh, K. V., Bourgogne, A., Rude, T. H., Corey, G. R., & Murray, B. E. et al. (2009). Inoculum effect with cefazolin among clinical isolates of methicillin-susceptible Staphylococcus aureus: Frequency and possible cause of cefazolin treatment failure. *Antimicrobial Agents and Chemotherapy*, *53*(8), 3437–3441. doi:10.1128/AAC.00317-09 PMID:19487449

Neely, M. N., Youn, G., Jones, B., Jelliffe, R. W., Drusano, G. L., Rodvold, K. A., & Lodise, T. P. (2014). Are vancomycin trough concentrations adequate for optimal dosing? *Antimicrobial Agents and Chemotherapy*, *58*(1), 309–316. doi:10.1128/AAC.01653-13 PMID:24165176

Olaison, L., & Schadewitz, K. (2002). Enterococcal endocarditis in Sweden, 19951999: Can shorter therapy with aminoglycosides be used? *Clinical Infectious Diseases*, *34*(2), 159–166. doi:10.1086/338233 PMID:11740702

Pai, M. P., Neely, M., Rodvold, K. A., & Lodise, T. P. (2014). Innovative approaches to optimizing the delivery of vancomycin in individual patients. *Advanced Drug Delivery Reviews*, *77*, 50–57. doi:10.1016/j.addr.2014.05.016 PMID:24910345

Patel, N., Pai, M. P., Rodvold, K. A., Lomaestro, B., Drusano, G. L., & Lodise, T. P. (2011). Vancomycin: We cant get there from here. *Clinical Infectious Diseases*, *52*(8), 969–974. doi:10.1093/cid/cir078 PMID:21460308

Perez, K. K., Olsen, R. J., Musick, W. L., Cernoch, P. L., Davis, J. R., Peterson, L. E., & Musser, J. M. (2014). Integrating rapid diagnostics and antimicrobial stewardship improves outcomes in patients with antibiotic-resistant Gram-negative bacteremia. *The Journal of Infection*, *69*(3), 216–225. doi:10.1016/j.jinf.2014.05.005 PMID:24841135

Peterson, L. R. (2009). Bad bugs, no drugs: No ESCAPE revisisted. *Clinical Infectious Diseases*, *49*(6), 992–993. doi:10.1086/605539 PMID:19694542

Petti, C. A., Bhally, H. S., Weinstein, M. P., Joho, K., Wakefield, T., Reller, L. B., & Carrol, K. C. (2006). Utility of Extended Blood Culture Incubation for Isolation of Haemophilus, Actinobacillus, Cardiobacterium, Eikenella, and Kingella Organisms: A Retrospective Multicenter Evaluation. *Journal of Clinical Microbiology*, *44*(1), 257–259. doi:10.1128/JCM.44.1.257-259.2006 PMID:16390985

Pibarot, P., & Dumesnil, J. G. (2009). Prosthetic heart valves: Selection of the optimal prosthesis and long-term management. *Circulation*, *119*(7), 1034–1048. doi:10.1161/CIRCULATIONAHA.108.778886 PMID:19237674

Rammelkamp, C. H., & Maxon, T. (1942). Resistance of Staphylococcus aureus to the action of penicillin. *Proc Royal Soc Exper Biol Med*, *51*(3), 386–389. doi:10.3181/00379727-51-13986

Rybak, M. J., Lomaestro, B. M., Rotschafer, J. C., Moellering, R. C. Jr, Craig, W. A., Billeter, M., & Levine, D. P. et al. (2009). Therapeutic monitoring of vancomycin in adults summary of consensus recommendations from the American Society of Health-System Pharmacists, the Infectious Diseases Society of America, and the Society of Infectious Diseases Pharmacists. *Pharmacotherapy*, *29*(11), 1275–1279. doi:10.1592/phco.29.11.1275 PMID:19873687

Sakoulas, G., Bayer, A. S., Pogliano, J., Tsuji, B. T., Yang, S. J., Mishra, N. N., & Moise, P. A. et al. (2012). Ampicillin enhances daptomycin- and cationic host defense peptide-mediated killing of ampicillin- and vancomycin-resistant Enterococcus faecium. *Antimicrobial Agents and Chemotherapy*, *56*(2), 838–844. doi:10.1128/AAC.05551-11 PMID:22123698

Sakoulas, G., Moise, P. A., Casapao, A. M., Nonejuie, P., Olson, J., Okumura, C. Y., & Nizet, V. et al. (2014). Antimicrobial salvage therapy for persistent staphylococcal bacteremia using daptomycin plus ceftaroline. *Clinical Therapeutics*, *36*(10), 1317–1333. doi:10.1016/j.clinthera.2014.05.061 PMID:25017183

Sakoulas, G., Nonejuie, P., Nizet, V., Pogliano, J., Crum-Cianflone, N., & Haddad, F. (2013). Treatment of high-level gentamicin-resistant Enterococcus faecalis endocarditis with daptomycin plus ceftaroline. *Antimicrobial Agents and Chemotherapy*, *57*(8), 4042–4045. doi:10.1128/AAC.02481-12 PMID:23689728

Sakoulas, G., Rose, W., Nonejuie, P., Olson, J., Pogliano, J., Humphries, R., & Nizet, V. (2014). Ceftaroline restores daptomycin activity against daptomycin-nonsusceptible vancomycin-resistant Enterococcus faecium. *Antimicrobial Agents and Chemotherapy*, *58*(3), 1494–1500. doi:10.1128/AAC.02274-13 PMID:24366742

Schweizer, M. L., Furuno, J. P., Harris, A. D., Johnson, J. K., Shardell, M. D., McGregor, J. C., & Perencevich, E. N. et al. (2011). Comparative effectiveness of nafcillin or cefazolin versus vancomycin in methicillin-susceptible Staphylococcus aureus bacteremia. *BMC Infectious Diseases*, *11*(1), 279. doi:10.1186/1471-2334-11-279 PMID:22011388

Selton-Suty, C., Célard, M., Le Moing, V., Doco-Lecompte, T., Chirouze, C., Iung, B., & Hoen, B. et al. (2012). Preeminence of Staphylococcus aureus in infective endocarditis: A 1-year population-based survey. *Clinical Infectious Diseases*, *54*(9), 1230–1239. doi:10.1093/cid/cis199 PMID:22492317

Spellberg, B., Bartlett, J. G., & Gilbert, D. N. (2013). The Future of Antibiotics and Resistance. *The New England Journal of Medicine*, *368*(4), 299–302. doi:10.1056/NEJMp1215093 PMID:23343059

Spellberg, B., Guidos, R., Gilbert, D., Bradley, J., Boucher, H. W., Scheld, W. M., & Edwards, J. Jr et al.. (2008). The epidemic of antibiotic resistant infections: A call to action for the medical community from the Infectious Diseases Society of America. *Clinical Infectious Diseases*, *46*(2), 155–164. doi:10.1086/524891 PMID:18171244

Szabo, S., Lieberman, J. P., & Lue, Y. A. (1990). Unusual pathogens in narcotic-associated endocarditis. *Reviews of Infectious Diseases*, *12*(3), 412–415. doi:10.1093/clinids/12.3.412 PMID:2359905

Tribouilloy, C., Rusinaru, D., Sorel, C., Thuny, F., Casalta, J. P., Riberi, A., & Habib, G. et al. (2010). Clinical characteristics and outcome of infective endocarditis in adults with bicuspid aortic valves: A multicentre observational study. *Heart (British Cardiac Society)*, *96*(21), 1723–1729. doi:10.1136/hrt.2009.189050 PMID:20478858

Tsigrelis, C., Singh, K. V., Coutinho, T. D., Murray, B. E., & Baddour, L. M. (2007). Vancomycin-resistant Enterococcus faecalis endocarditis: Linezolid failure and strain characterization of virulence factors. *Journal of Clinical Microbiology*, *45*(2), 631–635. doi:10.1128/JCM.02188-06 PMID:17182759

Unites States White House. (2015). *National action plan for combating antibiotic-resistant bacteria.* Retrieved on 2/23/2016 from https://www.whitehouse.gov/sites/default/files/docs/national_action_plan_for_combating_antibotic-resistant_bacteria.pdf

Von Reyn, C. F., Levy, B. S., Arbeit, R. D., Friedland, G., & Crumpacker, C. S. (1981). Infective endocarditis: An analysis based on strict case definitions. *Annals of Internal Medicine*, *94*(4_Part_1), 505–518. doi:10.7326/0003-4819-94-4-505 PMID:7011141

Youngster, I., Shenoy, E. S., Hooper, D. C., & Nelson, S. B. (2014). Comparative evaluation of the tolerability of cefazolin and nafcillin for treatment of methicillin-susceptible Staphylococcus aureus infections in the outpatient setting. *Clinical Infectious Diseases*, *59*(3), 369–375. doi:10.1093/cid/ciu301 PMID:24785233

ADDITIONAL READING

Baddour, L. M., Wilson, W. R., Bayer, A. S., Fowler, V. G. Jr, Tleyjeh, I. M., Rybak, M. J., & Taubert, K. A. et al. (2015). Infective Endocarditis in Adults: Diagnosis, Antimicrobial Therapy, and Management of Complications: A Scientific Statement for Healthcare Professionals From the American Heart Association. *Circulation*, *132*(15), 1435–1486. doi:10.1161/CIR.0000000000000296 PMID:26373316

Fernández-Hidalgo, N., Almirante, B., Gavaldà, J., Gurgui, M., Peña, C., de Alarcón, A., & Pahissa, A. et al. (2013). Ampicillin plus ceftriaxone is as effective as ampicillin plus gentamicin for treating enterococcus faecalis infective endocarditis. *Clinical Infectious Diseases*, *56*(9), 1261–1268. doi:10.1093/cid/cit052 PMID:23392394

Fowler, V. G. Jr, Scheld, W. M., & Bayer, A. S. (2015). Endocarditis and Intravascular Infections. In J. E. Bennett, R. Dolin, & M. J. Blaser (Eds.), *Mandell, Douglas, and Bennett's Principles and Practices of Infectious Diseases* (pp. 990–1028). Philadelphia, PA: Elsevier Saunders.

Habib, G., Lancellotti, P., Antunes, M. J., Bongiorni, M. G., Casalta, J. P., Del Zotti, F., & Zamorano, J. L. et al. (2015). 2015 ESC Guidelines for the management of infective endocarditis: The Task Force for the Management of Infective Endocarditis of the European Society of Cardiology (ESC). Endorsed by: European Association for Cardio-Thoracic Surgery (EACTS), the European Association of Nuclear Medicine (EANM). *European Heart Journal*, *36*(44), 3075–3128. doi:10.1093/eurheartj/ehv319 PMID:26320109

Holland, T. L., Arnold, C., & Fowler, V. G. Jr. (2014). Clinical management of Staphylococcus aureus bacteremia: A review. *Journal of the American Medical Association*, *312*(13), 1330–1341. doi:10.1001/jama.2014.9743 PMID:25268440

Kalil, A. C., Van Schooneveld, T. C., Fey, P. D., & Rupp, M. E. (2014). Association between vancomycin minimum inhibitory concentration and mortality among patients with Staphylococcus aureus bloodstream infections: A systematic review and meta-analysis. *Journal of the American Medical Association*, *312*(15), 1552–1564. doi:10.1001/jama.2014.6364 PMID:25321910

Lee, S., Choe, P. G., Song, K. H., Park, S. W., Kim, H. B., Kim, N. J., & Oh, M. D. et al. (2011). Is cefazolin inferior to nafcillin for treatment of methicillin-susceptible Staphylococcus aureus bacteremia? *Antimicrobial Agents and Chemotherapy*, *55*(11), 5122–5126. doi:10.1128/AAC.00485-11 PMID:21825299

Murdoch, D. R., Corey, G. R., Hoen, B., Miró, J. M., Fowler, V. G. Jr, Bayer, A. S., & Cabell, C. H. et al. (2009). Clinical presentation, etiology, and outcome of infective endocarditis in the 21st century: The International Collaboration on Endocarditis-Prospective Cohort Study. *Archives of Internal Medicine*, *169*(5), 463–473. doi:10.1001/archinternmed.2008.603 PMID:19273776

Rybak, M. J., Lomaestro, B. M., Rotschafer, J. C., Moellering, R. C. Jr, Craig, W. A., Billeter, M., & Levine, D. P. et al. (2009). Therapeutic monitoring of vancomycin in adults summary of consensus recommendations from the American Society of Health-System Pharmacists, the Infectious Diseases Society of America, and the Society of Infectious Diseases Pharmacists. *Pharmacotherapy*, *29*(11), 1275–1279. doi:10.1592/phco.29.11.1275 PMID:19873687

Unites States White House. (2015). National action plan for combating antibiotic-resistant bacteria, 1-62. Retrieved on 2/23/2016 from https://www.whitehouse.gov/sites/default/files/docs/national_action_plan_for_combating_antibotic-resistant_bacteria.pdf

APPENDIX

Table 1. Etiology of infective endocarditis

Microorganism	Percent Isolated
Staphylococci *Staphylococcus aureus* Coagulase-negative staphylococci	41.3% 30.5% 10.7%
Streptococci	30.4%
Enterococci	10.2%
Culture-negative	9.2%
Fungi	1.6%
HACEK	1.5%
Polymicrobial	1.1%
Other pathogens	4.6%

HACEK = *Haemophilus* sp, *Actinobacillus actinomycetemcomitans*, *Cardiobacterium hominis*, *Eikenella corrodens*, *Kingella kingae*
Data adapted from 2 previous studies (Selton-Suty, 2012; Murdoch, 2009)

Table 2. Etiology of infective endocarditis in intravenous drug users

Microorganism	Percent Isolated
Staphylococcus aureus	38-60%
Pseudomonas aeruginosa	14%
Fungi (*Candida* spp.)	14%
Streptococci	6-16%
Other aerobic Gram-negative bacilli	2-15%
Culture-negative	12.9%
Enterococci	8%
Polymicrobial	1-8%
Coagulase-negative staphylococci	2%

Data adapted from 2 sources (Fowler, 2015; Szabo, 1990)

Table 3. Treatment for common causes of native infective endocarditis

Microorganism	Antimicrobial Options	Duration of Therapy
Staphylococcus aureus MSSA MRSA hVISA or VISA	nafcillin, oxacillin, or cefazolin vancomycin or daptomycin daptomycin or ceftaroline	≥ 6 weeks
Enterococcus Susceptible to penicillin Resistant to penicillin/ampicillin and susceptible to vancomycin Resistant to vancomycin	Ampicillin plus gentamicin OR Penicillin plus gentamicin OR Ampicillin plus ceftriaxone Vancomycin plus gentamicin Linezolid or daptomycin	4-6 weeks 4-6 weeks 6 weeks 6 weeks > 6 weeks

Adapted from Baddour, 2015

Chapter 11
Advancements in Cardiovascular Diagnostics

Yan Li
Cleveland Clinic, USA

Karen L. Fang
Cleveland Clinic, USA

Zhi Huang
Cleveland Clinic, USA

Yun Lu
No. 1 Hospital of Lanzhou University, China

Bin Zhang
Mayo Clinic, USA

Yali Yao
No. 1 Hospital of Lanzhou University, China

ABSTRACT

The cardiology diagnostic are the methods of identifying current or past heart conditions, which can advise caregivers on patient diagnosis and provide a proper therapy plan, nowadays couple new diagnostic methods have been developed and some of them like radionuclide myocardial perfusion imaging, coronary computed tomography angiogram, cardiac magnetic resonance imaging, intravascular ultrasonography, optical coherence tomography, intravascular thermography, intravascular elastography, and near-infrared spectroscopy have been approved for clinical use. Not only the advanced technologies, the new biomarkers, and genetic markers may provide new potential targets for the diagnosis, therapy, and prevention of heart diseases.

INTRODUCTION

Since the x-ray was first applied to the chest in 1895 and the original galvanometer electrocardiogram was created by Dr. Willem Einthoven in 1902, cardiologists have been working to augment their history and physical exam with new objective information gleaned by the various technological advancements of each historical era. The first three-lead electrocardiographic machine was bought for everyday clinical use in 1908 by Sir Edward Schafer of the University of Edinburgh, and was used primarily to study arrhythmias. The idea of the myocardial infarction developed in 1910, and it was found by 1930 that the readout from an electrocardiogram could often produce patterns pathognomonic enough to diagnose cardiac-related chest pain. By 1954, the electrocardiogram had gradually developed into the 12-lead

DOI: 10.4018/978-1-5225-2092-4.ch011

system used ubiquitously today by family practitioners and cardiologists alike (AlGhatrif & Lindsay, 2012). From these beginnings, the field of cardiovascular diagnosis has burst forth in leaps and bounds: within the last 25 years, ever-improving imaging techniques and laboratory assays for increasingly sensitive and specific biomarkers for cardiac muscle disruption have taken their places next to the electrocardiogram as pillars of cardiovascular diagnosis and care (Dolci & Panteghini, 2006). This chapter works to provide an updated snapshot of the current field, with a focus on areas in which great improvements have been made in the last few decades and a nod to the great discoveries now visible just beyond the next bend in the road.

Advancements in Disease Diagnosis

Real-Time Cardiac Monitors

The electrocardiogram (EKG) excels as a first-line diagnostic tool in cardiology because it is a noninvasive, inexpensive, and well-established test capable of providing a wealth of diagnostic information. The 12-lead system may not have changed in the last 60 years, but improvements and new applications are always of interest. One new direction in which the use of EKGs has been rapidly expanding is in monitoring at-risk patients in the community as they go about their daily lives. There is only so much any stress test in the hospital can show – many arrhythmias have previously gone undetected until they cause severe cardiac events, because it has been impossible to analyze a patient's intermittent arrhythmia unless the EKG is performed while the pathologic heart rhythm is actively happening.

The Holter monitor, a small battery-operated recorder that is capable of recording 2 or 3 channels of the standard 12-lead EKG, has been the mainstay of ambulatory monitoring since its inception in the 1980's(Barry, Campbell, Nabel, Mead, & Selwyn, 1987). The Holter can record patient-activated event markers, and it is cheap and records continuously, thereby allowing for the detection of asymptomatic arrhythmias. Unfortunately, monitoring in this way is limited, usually to 24-48 hours at a time. Wearing the device, with its external electrodes, may do more than inconvenience the patients for a day or two; it may also deter patients from going about all of their normal daily activities, thus causing the Holter to miss any arrhythmias generated by motions or situations which the patient avoids out of discomfort(Giada, Bertaglia, Reimers, Noventa, & Raviele, 2012).

Since then, new devices have been developed which are capable of transmitting information via telephone lines to the hospital, of storing and sending information recorded in the minutes before activation (loop recording), and of recognizing when an arrhythmia is occurring and activating automatically, then sending the information to a real-time station monitored by medical personnel.

Most recently developed and approved by the Food and Drug Administration of the United States (FDA) is the implantable cardiac monitor (ICM) (Rome, Kramer, & Kesselheim, 2014). These monitors combine the loop recording abilities of previous monitors with automatic detection of arrhythmias and wireless transmission of data. They are no different from their un-implantable cousins in storing a one-lead ECG tracing but have the added capability for long-term monitoring up to 36 months (Giada & Bartoletti, 2015; Giada et al., 2012). The other monitors mentioned above have had a maximum of 3-4 weeks' monitoring life, so this is a more than 36-fold improvement.

The ICM implantation procedure is minimally invasive and simple enough to be done in the outpatient setting. A subcutaneous pocket is created by a small skin incision, the monitor is inserted and anchored to the muscular plane, and then the pocket is closed and an external programmer used to make sure the

ECG trace is satisfactory. Implantation is usually in the left parasternal area of the chest, but can also be done at the fourth intercostal space along the left anterior axillary line, and in young girls can be done at the inferior and medial border of either breast. External ECG mapping done before the implantation will determine the optimal area and alignment for the device to rest on each individual patient.

The ICM is not without limitations: it is more invasive than external monitoring and does present a risk of insertion-site complications such as infection and bleeding. The research thus far suggests that, rather than being wholly better than other monitor types, it adds to the field by broadening the diagnostic toolbox. It provides an option for patients with symptoms of possible arrhythmic origin that are so infrequent or transient that other monitoring methods have failed. Like external loop recording monitors, its automatic activation allows for its use with possibly debilitating symptoms, but the ICM is unique in that it can be used even in situations of poor patient compliance (Giada et al., 2012).

Currently, the implantable cardiac monitor is indicated for patients with syncope or palpitations whose symptoms have failed to be elucidated with a standard history, physical, and EKG (Giada et al., 2012). There is also beginning to be a consideration for its use in difficult epilepsy cases and unexplained falls, as it may well be an excellent tool for distinguishing between true epilepsy and syncope occurring with myoclonic movements.

There are now two major ICM models on the market: the Reveal XT, made by Medtronic, and the Confirm, made by St. Jude Medical ("St. Jude's Confirm Implantable Cardiac Monitor Wins FDA Approval.,"). The Reveal has a validated algorithm to both detect atrial fibrillation (AF) and monitor the amount of time spent in AF (Hindricks et al., 2010). Follow-up with patients implanted with the Reveal can be done remotely by an automatic transmitter with Web-based software. The Confirm also has an algorithm for the detection of AF, but this algorithm has yet to be validated, and follow-up can be done remotely through a telephone line (Giada et al., 2012).

Advancements of Cardiovascular Diagnostic Imaging

In severe cases, the EKG is often not conclusive enough to effectively guide physicians through the entire diagnostic decision tree. Fortunately, like the musculoskeletal system, the cardiovascular system performs its function on a scale visible to the human eye. Thus, it has been possible to develop imaging techniques which improve diagnostic accuracy to an ever-increasing degree.

Today, well-studied, ubiquitous methods for cardiac imaging and diagnosis include the echocardiogram, radionuclide myocardial perfusion imaging (rMPI), and coronary angiography. The echocardiogram uses ultrasound waves to image the heart, and Doppler technology now allows for the careful inspection of blood flow. Furthermore, 3-D echocardiography has been steadily advancing since the development of the first matrix array transducer in 2003, and it is now used in clinics to assess the dimensions and volumes of cardiac chambers with a considerable improvement in accuracy over its 2-D counterpart (Aggeli et al., 2015). The rMPI involves injecting a radioactive tracer into the bloodstream, then recording the signal via SPECT or PET imaging and mapping out perfusion deficits within the heart. The echocardiogram and rMPI can both be done at rest or with stress testing, and if they fail to safely rule out significant cardiovascular disease, the next step is to visualize the coronary artery lumen via angiogram. Angiography in the traditional sense involves catheterizing the coronary arteries, usually via the femoral vein, and injecting a radioopaque dye to visualize the patency of the lumen along each vessel. The percentage of luminal stenosis seen on angiography has been a longstanding essential determining factor in the decision to proceed with further intervention, and should intervention be needed, its success can be immediately measured without removing the catheter. The use of nanotechnology to create new contrast dyes is where today's angiography improves on tradition. Gadofosvaset trisodium, the first blood-pool agent, binds to albumin and stays in the circulation with a half-life of 16 hours, long enough to reach steady-state. It and other blood-pool agents such as gold nanoparticles and gold nanoshells are capable of improving angiogram image quality significantly, and are particularly useful in patients with anomalous or post-surgical cardiovascular anatomy. Most exciting of all, these nanoparticles may just be the contrast agent that is finally capable of visualizing plaques. Because nanoparticle movement is determined mostly by convective forces rather than being patterned after simple diffusion, and because these particles' half-lives are so long, these particles tend to 1) extravasate at areas of inflammation or leakage, and to 2) stay there until taken up by macrophages (Annapragada, 2015).

Unfortunately, until the full potential of these particles is realized and FDA-approved, invasive coronary angiography still reveals insufficient information about the presence and composition of plaques for which vessels can compensate via dilation. Physicians are left with very little information about the condition of the artery walls themselves, a thing of crucial interest in assessing patients for coronary artery dissection. One early study of 23 patients who developed a second infarction after a previous cardiac catheterization showed a median percent stenosis of only 48%(Fenning & Wilensky, 2014) – 70% of acute coronary occlusions happen in areas that were previously angiographically insignificant (Schaar et al., 2007). A myriad of studies since have come together to reveal several criteria which appear to characterize these "vulnerable plaques," called such because they are at high risk for rupture whether or not they cause significant artery stenosis. In tandem, a myriad of diagnostic measures have appeared as well to gauge levels of these new characteristics in vivo.

Among these recently developed diagnostic procedures are several new tools of the "uninvasive" category. The coronary computed tomography angiogram (CTA) and vascular MRI aim to perform the function of the invasive angiogram without the associated fuss and risk, and ultrasound has been repurposed for gauging patient status as a point-of-care transthoracic procedure in the emergency department as well as for the measurement of the carotid intima-media thickness (Andrew Taylor et al., 2012; O'Leary et al., 1999). Advancements in the signal analysis have picked up on ways to record backscattering of the US signal to later differentiate offline between the various components of plaques. Compared to histology, integrated backscatter ultrasound has a sensitivity of 80-85% and a specificity of 78-91% for detecting thrombi, lipid pools, and fibrous tissue (Soloperto, 2012).

Computed tomography based angiography has been extensively compared to invasive angiography in the literature and is now beginning to see clinical use. Although it does not possess the ability of invasive angiography to immediately visualize the effects of revascularization efforts, studies have shown that only 40% of such procedures actually proceed to intervention (Gorenoi, Schonermark, & Hagen, 2012). It has been proposed, therefore, to make CTA a "gatekeeper" for catheterization in future; this would protect the remaining 60% of patients from unnecessary invasive therapy (Marwick, Cho, ó Hartaigh, & Min, 2015). The spatial resolution of CTA is about 400 um, and with the standard 64-slice multidetector scanner and iodinated contrast, CTA can distinguish plaques as calcified, non-calcified, or partially calcified, thereby directing treatment considerably more appropriately than its invasive cousin (Fenning & Wilensky, 2014). Its greatest strength, however, is its 97-99% negative predictive value (Marwick et al., 2015). Overall, CTA has shown a 94-99% sensitivity and 64-83% specificity for coronary stenoses, and meta-analysis has recommended pretest probability of disease as the most important determining factor in its use over invasive angiography (Gorenoi et al., 2012; Marwick et al., 2015). At a pretest probability of coronary heart disease of 50% or below, CTA came out on top with a lower cost per true positive patient, likely due to its impressive negative predictive power. Above a pretest probability of 70%, invasive coronary angiography is the test of choice (Gorenoi et al., 2012).

Cardiac magnetic resonance imaging (CMR) is becoming solidly established in the field of cardiovascular diagnostics for the identification of structural abnormalities and the assessment of ventricular function, myocardial perfusion, and myocardial viability (Dastidar, Rodrigues, Ahmed, Baritussio, & Bucciarelli-Ducci, 2015; Pilz et al., 2009). MRI's high reproducibility and precision, excellent image quality, lack of radiation risk, and high native contrast between myocardium and blood are often enough to justify its relatively high cost, especially in difficult and previously inconclusive cases. MR coronary angiography, however, is still a work in progress. It is markedly inferior to CTA and not yet available for clinical use(Pilz et al., 2009).

As mentioned above, the vulnerability of a plaque has been correlated to a multitude of variables. These include the thickness of its fibrous cap, the size of its lipid core, the presence of inflammatory cells, the extent of vessel wall remodeling involved, the amount of plaque-free vessel wall, and its 3D morphology (Fenning & Wilensky, 2014; O'Leary et al., 1999; Schaar et al., 2007; Suh et al., 2011; Soloperto 2012). The remainder of new developments in cardiovascular diagnostics involve improvements on the quality of information about these variables acquired during coronary catheterization. These include angioscopy, intravascular ultrasonography (IVUS), optical coherence tomography (OCT), intravascular thermography, intravascular elastography, and near-infrared spectroscopy.

Angioscopy has a spatial resolution of 50-200 μm and involves using a fiber-optic bundle attached to a guidewire to directly visualize the vessel luminal surface (Fenning & Wilensky, 2014). This shows atherosclerotic plaques as white, yellow, or orange protrusions, with a higher intensity of yellow associated with thinner fibrous caps. Deep yellow most commonly signifies a lipid-rich atheroma with a necrotic core, yellow-red coloring denotes a plaque with a vulnerable, thin fibrous cap, and white or gray colored lesions represent fibrous plaques (Fenning & Wilensky, 2014).

IVUS and OCT use ultrasound and visible light, respectively, to analyze vessel wall and plaque composition from within the artery. Intravascular ultrasonography is done by inserting a catheter with a miniature ultrasound transducer into the vessel in question and capturing an image as the catheter is pulled backward at a steady pace along the luminal wall. IVUS uses ultrasound frequencies between 30 and 50MHz and is capable of an axial resolution of about 150-250 um and a lateral resolution of 250 um (Fenning & Wilensky, 2014). Because the media is sonolucent and the delineation between the media and intima difficult to distinguish, the "plaque burden" as seen on IVUS consists of the thickness of the intima and the media combined. Unsatisfied with just this "gray-scale" image, the field has since come up with various techniques for further sorting and analyzing IVUS data in order to differentiate between the various components of plaques. For example, radiofrequency tissue characterization uses the detection of radiofrequency waves with an autoregression model to sort the signal and characterize tissue as fibrous, fibrofatty, part of the necrotic core, or calcified (Iwamoto; Suh, Seto, Margey, Cruz-Gonzalez, & Jang, 2011). Virtual Histology IVUS (VH-IVUS) uses backscatter detection and analysis as mentioned above with the transthoracic ultrasound, but with the added benefit of being able to accomplish its analysis in real-time rather than offline (Soloperto, 2012). Clinically, VH-IVUS has the potential to improve patient outcomes by inspecting and measuring vessel size, evaluating side-branch anatomy, and assessing plaque length and calcification before percutaneous intervention is attempted. Recent studies of retrospective data have reported that IVUS done in conjunction with carotid artery stenting resulted in precise disease assessment and efficient surgery planning, with no adverse events (n=110) and higher accuracy in confirming adequate stent expansion than offered by angiography (Bandyk & Armstrong, 2009).

Optical coherence tomography was first developed by Huang et al. at the Massachusetts Institute of Technology in 1991(Huang et al., 1991), and Tearney, Brezinski et al. first suggested its use as a methodology for intravascular imaging in 1997(Tearney, 1997). The fundamental principle of OCT is very similar to that of IVUS, the difference being that OCT uses near-infrared light in the wavelength range of 1250-1350 nm. As a result, OCT provides a roughly tenfold improvement over IVUS in resolution, with images resolved to 10-20 μm, but the light it utilizes can penetrate only 1-3 mm into the vessel wall, versus an 8 mm penetration by the sound waves of IVUS. In addition, the light used by OCT is subject to scattering and attenuation by blood cells, thus requiring a balloon catheter and saline flush to operate at peak performance and subjecting the patient to an increased risk of further ischemic damage (Roleder et al., 2015). OCT has, thus far, been most successful in the assessment of coronary stents, as its high resolution allows for careful study of stent expansion, peri-procedural vessel trauma, and stent-vessel interaction down to the level of minor amounts of tissue coverage of individual stent struts (Regar, Ligthart, Bruining, & van Soest, 2011).

Further techniques include intravascular thermography and intravascular ultrasound elastography/palpography, which use changes in temperature and wall strain, respectively, to infer the presence of inflammation and plaque formation along the artery walls (C. L. de Korte, Pasterkamp, van der Steen, Woutman, & Bom, 2000; Chris L. De Korte, Schaar, Mastik, Serruys, & Van Der Der Steen, 2003; Chris L. de Korte & van der Steen, 2002; Schaar et al., 2007). Intravascular MRI (IVMRI) is currently still in the preliminary stages of development, but has shown a spatial resolution as low as 100 um and may someday be superior to IVUS in the identification of lipid, fibrous, and calcified areas of plaque (Soloperto, 2012).

Finally, near-infrared spectroscopy measures molecular vibrational transitions in response to emitted infrared light in the 750-2500 nm region. It has been used, for the most part, to quantify the amount of lipid in plaques: it has shown a sensitivity of 90% and specificity of 93% for lipid pools (Schaar et al., 2007). It has also demonstrated a sensitivity of 77% and specificity of 93% for thin fibrous caps and a sensitivity of 84% and specificity of 89% for inflammatory cells, but it still has room to grow in terms of acquisition time, resisting the influence of changes in pH and temperature, and handling the same scattering experienced by OCT by blood cells (Schaar et al., 2007).

Cholesterol, Cardiac Biomarkers, and Genetic Biomarkers

Cholesterol

Cholesterol is a steroltype substance that is found in animal cells and circulatory system. It plays a significant role in many functions, including supporting cell membranes, as substance in vitamin D synthesis, and playing critical role in the biogenesis of steroid hormones. The homeostasis of cholesterol is an indicator to evaluate the subsequent consequences of its aleration, such as in disease like diabetes, obesity, and heart disease. If the level of cholesterol increases, the risk of dangerous consequences such as atherosclerosis also rises. Blood cholesterol level is also important to heart health. High-level cholesterol in the blood also increases the risk of heart disease. When cholesterol level increases too high in blood, the walls of the arteries in the heart become thicker. In the same time, it causes narrow of the arteries and slows down even blocks the blood flow in the heart. Once blockage of heart blood supply appears, subsequent heart attack followed. So the cholesterol level in the blood is a critical indicator of heart health. Keeping lower cholesterol level can reduce the risk of heart disease for everyone.

During the cholesterol transportation to the whole body, cholesterol must bind to lipoproteins because most cholesterol could not be transported directly in blood. There are two types of lipoproteins in the circulatory system, including low-density lipoprotein (LDL) and high-density lipoprotein (HDL) (Nicholls, 2009). The roughly total cholesterol amount is composed of LDL cholesterol (LDL-C), HDL-cholesterol (HDL-C) and triglyceride (TG). LDL-C is easier to form a thick, hard deposit to narrow the arteries. So LDL-C is assigned to "bad" cholesterol. In contrast, HDL-C belongs to "good" cholesterol due to its function as a scavenger to clean LDL-C back to the liver. Besides these two kinds of cholesterol, one other class of lipids found in blood is triglycerides. High levels of TG may be related to complex diseases, such as atherosclerosis and obesity.

LDL-C, HDL-C, TG, and their relative ratios can be used as predictors of cardiovascular disease. The ratio of plasma TG/HDL-C can be used to evaluate the risk of cardiovascular disease in the hypertensive patients. Analysis of data from a study in a community between 2003 and 2012 shows that the people with the small ratio of TG/HDL-C have the low risk of cardiovascular disease (Salazar et al., 2013). The health cut-point of the ratio of TG/HDL-C is 2.5 in women or 3.5 in men. However, hypertensive people have the high risk of cardiovascular disease. They need to keep the ratio of TG/HDL-C in the lower level than that in normotensive people. The recent study also evaluates the relation between TG/HDL-C ratio and cardiovascular disease risk in obese patients with type 2 diabetes. In most normal weight population, the ratio of TG/HDL-C keeps in the lower level (<1.9). However, in people with obese this ratio increases, subsequently increasing the risk of coronary heart disease and cardiovascular disease. Other studies show that HDL-C itself also can be an independent predictor for evaluation of the risk of cardiovascular disease. The risk of cardiovascular disease will reduce 2-3 percent if the level of HDL-C in the blood increases 10 mg/L.

People with the mutation in HDL-C regulating gene have a low level of HDL-C, resulting in early atherosclerosis and increasing the risk of cardiovascular disease. Development of therapy that directly targets and increases the HDL-C level may be a new strategy to reduce the risk of cardiovascular disease. However, recent studies show that increase of HDL-C only in blood causes side effects related to inflammation, hemostasis and cell apoptosis. The LDL-C/HDL-C ratio is another reliable indicator for predicting the risk of cardiovascular disease since LDL-C and HDL-C play the opposite role functions in cardiovascular disease. In the patients with hypertriglyceridemia, high LDL-C/HDL-C ratio leads to higher risk of coronary heart disease. Beside LDL-C, some cholesterol exists in the blood of people like a very LDL-C fraction. Both of them are "bad" cholesterol. Thus, only calculating LDL-C/HDL-C ratio does not offer an accurate evaluation of the risk of cardiovascular disease. New algorithms have been created to elevate the total cholesterol (TC), and the new TC/HDL-C ratio can be used to estimate the risk of cardiovascular disease. In a similar way, the total non-HDL-C level has been used as a predictor to estimate the risk of cardiovascular disease (Zuo et al., 2015). A recent study shows that non-HDL-C is a better predictor than LDL-C in evaluating the cardiovascular disease mortality.

Cardiac Biomarkers

Cardiac biomarkers are measurable and quantifiable biological parameters that can evaluate heart damage and heart function with a degree of specificity. Over half a century ago, biomarkers for ischemic cardiac damage had been applied to diagnose acute myocardial infarction (AMI). After that, more and more cardiac biomarkers of necrosis, inflammation, hemodynamics stress and platelet function are found to estimate heart damage and function. Understanding the biological mechanism, measuring technology and clinical evidence of those biomarkers are important to apply those biomarkers into clinical care.

Traditional Cardiac Biomarkers

Creatinine is one kind of non-protein nitrogenous waste product, which comes from the breakdown of creatine and phosphocreatine. The muscle cells produce the majority of the creatinine. The serum creatinine level is relative to cardiovascular disease mortality. Elevated serum creatinine level in the elderly or hypertensive persons increases the risk of mortality. The serum enzymes creatine kinase (CK), and the myocardial specific isoform (CK-MB) have been used to be indicators for the clinical decision over several decades (Masugata et al., 2011). However, these enzymes also exist in other tissues, such as skeletal muscle, smooth muscle, and brain. Thus, increased serum level of these enzymes could arguably be caused by a non-heart condition.

Troponin is a protein complex, consisting of troponin I, troponin T, and troponin C, which regulates contraction in cardiac muscle cells. Once muscle cell damage occurs, for instance, due to myocardial infarction, the subunit of troponin will be released into circulation. Early detectable Troponin could lead to a more accurate earlier diagnosis. The early recognition that a cardiac arrest has occurred is key to survival, for every minute a patient stays in cardiac arrest, their chances of survival drop by roughly 10% (Mellor & Woollard, 2010). If the myocardium is damaged, only certain subunits of troponin (troponin I and troponin T) will be released. These two troponin subunits in circulation can serve as biomarkers for myocardial infarction diagnosis. Recent studies demonstrate that the level of cardiac troponin in blood is indeed strongly associated with cardiovascular mortality (Pohlhammer et al., 2014). Improving the sensitivity of troponin assays is important for early diagnosis of AMI. High sensitive troponin test has been developed to measure the extremely low level of troponin. However, more accurate parameters should be established based on new high-sensitivity troponin assay.

Myoglobin is another biomarker for myocardial infarction. It is a red protein in muscle cells which can bind to specific iron and oxygen. Once muscle cells are damaged, myoglobin will release into the blood from damaged cells (Sun et al., 2014). However, myoglobin is not a specific indicator for myocardial damage; it is also found in acute renal failure. So myoglobin is used to combine with other indicators troponin or CK and CK-MB for diagnosis of AMI.

Lipoprotein A, an oxidation-specific biomarker, is a subunit resembling the LDL complex. High concentration of lipoprotein A in blood can leads to the increased thickness of the arterial wall. So lipoprotein A can be used as an independent indicator of a risk of atherosclerotic diseases (Schmitz & Orso, 2015), including coronary heart disease and stroke. As a biomarker, lipoprotein A is more sensitive in the cardiovascular disease than that in stroke. Recent studies focus on the potential therapeutic target of lipoprotein A in the treatment of cardiovascular disease and illustrate the benefit of lowering lipoprotein A to cardiovascular disease.

Myocardiocytes secrete brain natriuretic peptide and N-Terminal Brain Natriuretic peptide (BNP/NT-proBNP) from heart ventricles, triggered by excessive stretching of myocardiocytes. They are another important prognostic predictor for all stages of heart failure, including postoperative recovery (Kara et al., 2015). Because elevated BNP/NT-proBNP level has remained for more than three months in the acute catecholamine-induced myocardial inflammatory condition of Tako-Tsubo cardiomyopathy (TTC).

Osteopontin, as known as bone sialoprotein I, is highly expressed in myocardiocytes in patients with hypertensive heart disease or heart failure comparing to that in normal people (Lopez et al., 2013). Osteopontin expression increases under a variety of conditions of the heart, and is close associated with increased myocyte apoptosis and myocardial dysfunction (Singh, Dalal, & Singh, 2014). Patients in NYHA class above than II revealed a significant induction, which suggests that osteopontin is a marker for advanced heart failure. Moreover, osteopontin emerged as an independent predictor of 4-year death and added significant information for the risk assessment of patients with heart failure. The risk of death within 48 months was almost 6-fold greater in patients assigned to a low-risk group according to whose osteopontin levels were above the average (Rosenberg et al., 2008). Which make osteopontin as a potential biomarker for heart failure and predicts death in patients with heart failure (Rosenberg et al., 2008; Singh, Foster, Dalal, & Singh, 2010).

Inflammation plays central roles in cardiovascular disease. The pathogenesis of atherosclerosis is accompanied by vascular inflammation in all stages. Since inflammatory markers can reflect the changing of inflammatory process of atherosclerosis, specific inflammatory biomarkers may be useful predictors for evaluating the risk of atherosclerosis. Examples of sthese imprtant biomarkers include Tumor necrosis factors-α (TNF-α), IL-6, Intercellular Adhesion Molecule 1 (ICAM-1, also known as CD54), vascular cell adhesion molecule 1 (VCAM-1, also known as CD106), C-reactive protein (CRP) and Fibrinogen. Among those inflammatory biomarkers, CRP is a most important one to estimate the risk of coronary artery disease (Ogita et al., 2015). Overpass several decades, many studies have demonstrated that CRP is an efficient indicator of the risk of cardiovascular disease. Unstable angina often accompanies the patients with increasing plasma level of CRP (≥3 mg/L). For the patients with acute coronary syndromes, high-sensitivity CRP is an efficient indicator to evaluate the damage of myocardiocytes. We can more accurately evaluate myocardial infarction with combining the use of two high sensitivity markers CRP and troponin T biomarkers.

New Cardiac Biomarkers

Asymmetric dimethylarginine (ADMA) is an endogenous small molecular found in circulation. Since its molecular structure is similar to L-arginine, ADMA is a natural inhibitor of nitric oxide synthesis by competitive substitution with L-arginine in the context of the production of nitric oxide. ADMA has been reported to be a predictor of atherosclerosis risk [6]. Recent studies also demonstrate that ADMA increases in the patients with ischemic chronic heart failure. ADMA also can be used as an excellent indicator of short-term or long-term mortality in patients with chronic heart failure. Beside ADMA in blood, the urinary ADMA level can also be used as a potential predictor for diagnosis of cardiac dysfunction. F2-isoprostanes (prostaglandin F2-like compounds) is another oxidative stress maker which also associated with cardiovascular disease. However, the detailed mechanism will need to be demonstrated.

Another novel cardiac biomarker is myeloperoxidase (MPO) which has been found to be associated with heart failure (Andreou et al., 2010). MPO produces hypochlorous acid which is used by the neutrophil to kill bacteria and other pathogens. As a peroxidase enzyme, MPO oxidizes the lipoprotein, including LDL and HDL. HDL may be converted into a dysfunctional form by oxidation modification. Recently studies also verify the relationship between MPO activity and cardiovascular disorder. MPO and CRP measurement provided more accuracy for the risk prediction than CRP itself (Heslop, Frohlich, & Hill, 2010).

Matrix metalloproteinases (MMPs) are zinc-dependent proteases that regulate digestion of collagen and extracellular matrix (ECM) homeostasis. The MMPS play different roles in various physiological and pathological processes such as tissue repair, metastasis, morphogenesis and arthritis. Different members of MMPs are diverse biomarkers in heart damage. For example, compared to BNP, MMP-2 is a better predictor for identification of Heart Failure with a preserved Ejection Fraction (HFpEF). MMP-1, as known as interstitial collagenase, is another useful biomarker to evaluate the mortality risk of chronic HF. However, the lack of significant clinical studies limit the clinical application of MMPs as biomarkers, because of the slow elevation of MMP levels after ACS. (Soejima et al., 2003; Zakynthinos & Pappa, 2009). Although, MMPs family are non-cardiac specific biomarkers by using them individually, but combining different MMPs family members with other biomarkers, as tissue inhibitors of metalloproteinases (TIMP-1 or TIMP-4), placental growth factor (PlGF) (Autiero, Luttun, Tjwa, & Carmeliet, 2003; Heeschen et al., 2004) or A2 phospholipases(Caslake et al., 2000), can increase the accurate of evaluation or identification of cardiac disease (Zakynthinos & Pappa, 2009).

So far, there are so many biomarkers have been identified as predict risk factor of heart disease. However, none of them can accurately predict the condition of heart health. There are two strategies to develop a new accurate prediction of heart disease, including screening new, efficient cardiac biomarkers and analysis of the efficiency of the combination of two or three exit cardiac biomarkers.

Genetic Biomarkers

CVD has the higher rate of mortality than cancer in the world. Some environmental factors can cause CVD, including smoking, lack of exercise, and obesity. It is well known that genetic mutations play a central role in the development of CVD (Anthony, George, & Eaton, 2014). A genome-wide screen for the mutations of cardiovascular disease associated genes has found many important gene mutations in CVD (Ito et al., 2014; Kathiresan & Srivastava, 2012; Newton-Cheh & Smith, 2010), for example, parental cardiovascular disease independently predicted future offspring events, CVD risk have 2-3 fold increase to offspring (Lloyd-Jones et al., 2004). New therapeutic or prevention strategies will probably be developed in accordance with these CVD associated genes.

Cardiomyopathy, a commonly inherited disorder affecting myocardiocytes, may cause some serious consequences such as sudden cardiac death, arrhythmias, and heart failure. Recent studies demonstrate that more than 50% patients with cardiomyopathy have multiple genetic mutations. Genetic cardiomyopathies lead to high pediatric mortality if the CVD affects younger individuals. Thus, investigating the genetic background of the patient's family and identification of genetic mutations relative to cardiomyopathies can promote prevention and therapy of cardiovascular disease. Over several decades, some genetic mutations have been identified in common in cardiomyopathies. Mutation of the heart muscle relative protein troponin I (TNNI3) has been found and causes the occurrence of cardiomyopathies. Up to now, over 50 gene mutations have been reported to be relative to cardiomyopathies, including titin (TNN), lamin A/C (LMNA), β-myosin heavy chain (MYH7) and troponin t (TNNT2).

Coronary heart disease (CHD) is a cardiovascular disease with high mortality rate. Studies show the association between CHD and specific genetic mutations. For example, a mutation in ALOX5AP (This gene encodes a protein, 5-lipoxygenase, is required for leukotriene synthesis) has been reported contributes to CHD in patients with familial hypercholesterolemia (van der Net et al., 2009). Mutation of ALOX5AP gene was reported contributes to CHD risk in patients with familial hypercholesterolemia (van der Net et al., 2009; Zhang et al., 2012). Mutations in some hypercholesterolemia related genes, such as the LDL receptor gene (LDLR), proprotein convertase subtilisin/Kexin type 9 gene (PCSK9), and the ligand-binding domain of apolipoprotein B100 (APOB) genes have also been reported to be associated with CHD. Another study demonstrates that HDL-C metabolism associated genes, including ATP-binding cassette A1 (ABCA1), apolipoprotein A1 (APOA1), and lecithin-cholesterol acyltransferase (LCAT) are potential biomarker candidates of CHD. Lipid related genetic mutations are one of the most important predictors for coronary heart disease (Global Lipids Genetics et al., 2013; Isaacs et al., 2013). In the past 5 years, several research confirmed that 9p21 is a common risk factor for CHD in different races, which include Asian, Caucasian, and African (Assimes et al., 2008; Broadbent et al., 2008; Helgadottir et al., 2008; Helgadottir et al., 2007; Hinohara et al., 2008; Kotani et al., 2009; McPherson et al., 2007; Roberts & Stewart, 2012; Samani et al., 2007; Wellcome Trust Case Control, 2007). Those abnormal result even can be caught at birth. Nowadays, the inherited disease center had been set in some hospitals, genetic screening and counseling service are provided. Although the earlier clinic treatment program can be made earlier and more individually, identify the familial diseases and slow their progression through preventative care.

MicroRNAs are small, noncoding RNA sequences in cells that can regulate the expression of target genes, and play diverse roles in development and disease (Chang & Mendell, 2007; Mendell & Olson, 2012; Obad et al., 2011; Small & Olson, 2011). It is well known that specific classes of microRNAs play a critical role in angiogenesis, cholesterol metabolism, and myocardiocytes biogenesis, which could be the novel potential genetic biomarker for diagnosis of CVD(Kingwell, 2011). miRNA has been shown its expression is necessary for the development and maintenance of vascular smooth muscle cells (VSMC), miR-143 and miR-145 promote a contractile VSMC phenotype and are required for maintenance of normal vascular function. Human genome-wide association studies have identified single nucleotide polymorphisms in the miRNA binding sites of several renin angiotensin aldosterone system (RAAS) -associated genes that correlate with a dysregulation of blood pressure (Albinsson et al., 2011; Albinsson et al., 2010; Quiat & Olson, 2013). A recent study shows that the level of some microRNAs in serum/plasma, such as miR-122 and 126 decreases after the patients suffer the heart attack, suggesting that these microRNAs can be the novel potential biomarkers for the diagnosis, therapy and prevention of CVD (Quiat & Olson, 2013). miR-21, miR-130a, miR-27b, and miR-210, whereas miR-221 and miR-222 have been published that close associated with peripheral arterial disease (Bronze-da-Rocha, 2014; Bronze-da-Rocha et al., 2012). And Li C et al. reported that serum microRNAs might be a good target biomarker for diagnosis of acute myocardial infarction and angina pectoris (Li et al., 2013).

Altogether, recent studies have identified many genetic mutations that are significantly associated with the changing of biomarkers in CVD, and further studies need to focus on figuring out the function and mechanism of these genetic mutations and the risk of CVD. These studies may provide new potential targets for the diagnosis, therapy, and prevention of CVD.

Recently research results show more and more critical risk factors for cardiac-related disease. Hypercholesterolemia, as one of the independent risk factor, has been demonstrated accelerate cardiovascular diseases, and widely used in current clinical diagnosis and therapies selection. So very well-controlled cholesterol level bring significant benefit, such as satins family compounds been used. However, some diseases are non-cholesterol related, such as aging-related aortic valve stenosis. For those diseases, cardiac risk biomarkers and genetic cardiac biomarkers may become alternative options. Unfortunately, many of those biomarkers wildly exist in whole circulation system and tightly related to multiple organs and tissue. Those will limited transfer laboratory research achievements to clinic use. Since cross-talking between different pathways are very common, biomarker targeting treatment still needs more and more evidence supporting in the future.

REFERENCES

Aggeli, C., Felekos, I., Kastellanos, S., Panagopoulou, V., Oikonomou, E., Tsiamis, E., & Tousoulis, D. (2015). Real-time three-dimensional echocardiography: Never before clinical efficacy looked so picturesque. *International Journal of Cardiology*, *198*, 15–21. doi:10.1016/j.ijcard.2015.06.052 PMID:26149331

Albinsson, S., Skoura, A., Yu, J., DiLorenzo, A., Fernandez-Hernando, C., Offermanns, S., & Sessa, W. C. et al. (2011). Smooth muscle miRNAs are critical for post-natal regulation of blood pressure and vascular function. *PLoS ONE*, *6*(4), e18869. doi:10.1371/journal.pone.0018869 PMID:21526127

Albinsson, S., Suarez, Y., Skoura, A., Offermanns, S., Miano, J. M., & Sessa, W. C. (2010). MicroRNAs are necessary for vascular smooth muscle growth, differentiation, and function. *Arteriosclerosis, Thrombosis, and Vascular Biology*, *30*(6), 1118–1126. doi:10.1161/ATVBAHA.109.200873 PMID:20378849

AlGhatrif, M., & Lindsay, J. (2012). A brief review: History to understand fundamentals of electrocardiography. *J Community Hosp Intern Med Perspect*, *2*(1). doi:10.3402/jchimp.v2i1.14383 PMID:23882360

Andreou, I., Tousoulis, D., Miliou, A., Tentolouris, C., Zisimos, K., Gounari, P., & Stefanadis, C. et al. (2010). Effects of rosuvastatin on myeloperoxidase levels in patients with chronic heart failure: A randomized placebo-controlled study. *Atherosclerosis*, *210*(1), 194–198. doi:10.1016/j.atherosclerosis.2009.10.046 PMID:19962701

Andrew Taylor, R., Oliva, I., Van Tonder, R., Elefteriades, J., Dziura, J., & Moore, C. L. (2012). Point-of-care Focused Cardiac Ultrasound for the Assessment of Thoracic Aortic Dimensions, Dilation, and Aneurysmal Disease. *Academic Emergency Medicine*, *19*(2), 244–247. doi:10.1111/j.1553-2712.2011.01279.x PMID:22288871

Annapragada, A. (2015). Advances in nanoparticle imaging technology for vascular pathologies. *Annual Review of Medicine*, *66*(1), 177–193. doi:10.1146/annurev-med-042513-125551 PMID:25587649

Anthony, D., George, P., & Eaton, C. B. (2014). Cardiac risk factors: biomarkers and genetic tests to determine cardiovascular risk. *FP Essent, 421*, 11-15. Retrieved from http://www.ncbi.nlm.nih.gov/pubmed/24936714

Assimes, T. L., Knowles, J. W., Basu, A., Iribarren, C., Southwick, A., Tang, H., & Quertermous, T. et al. (2008). Susceptibility locus for clinical and subclinical coronary artery disease at chromosome 9p21 in the multi-ethnic ADVANCE study. *Human Molecular Genetics*, *17*(15), 2320–2328. doi:10.1093/hmg/ddn132 PMID:18443000

Autiero, M., Luttun, A., Tjwa, M., & Carmeliet, P. (2003). Placental growth factor and its receptor, vascular endothelial growth factor receptor-1: Novel targets for stimulation of ischemic tissue revascularization and inhibition of angiogenic and inflammatory disorders. *Journal of Thrombosis and Haemostasis*, *1*(7), 1356–1370. doi:10.1046/j.1538-7836.2003.00263.x PMID:12871269

Bandyk, D. F., & Armstrong, P. A. (2009). Use of intravascular ultrasound as a "Quality Control" technique during carotid stent-angioplasty: Are there risks to its use? *The Journal of Cardiovascular Surgery*, *50*(6), 727–733. PMID:19935603

Barry, J., Campbell, S., Nabel, E. G., Mead, K., & Selwyn, A. P. (1987). Ambulatory monitoring of the digitized electrocardiogram for detection and early warning of transient myocardial ischemia in angina pectoris. *The American Journal of Cardiology*, *60*(7), 483–488. doi:10.1016/0002-9149(87)90290-6 PMID:3115078

Broadbent, H. M., Peden, J. F., Lorkowski, S., Goel, A., Ongen, H., Green, F., & Watkins, H. et al. (2008). Susceptibility to coronary artery disease and diabetes is encoded by distinct, tightly linked SNPs in the ANRIL locus on chromosome 9p. *Human Molecular Genetics*, *17*(6), 806–814. doi:10.1093/hmg/ddm352 PMID:18048406

Bronze-da-Rocha, E. (2014). MicroRNAs expression profiles in cardiovascular diseases. *Biomed Res Int*, *985408*. doi:10.1155/2014/985408 PMID:25013816

Bronze-da-Rocha, E., Novoa, A., Teixeira, N., Vasconcelos, C. S., Cerveira, C., Castro e Melo, J., & Carvalho, M. C. (2012). Evaluation of the reactivity of sera from patients with systemic lupus erythematosus against the human MCP1. *Journal of Clinical Immunology*, *32*(4), 721–728. doi:10.1007/s10875-012-9665-4 PMID:22371290

Caslake, M. J., Packard, C. J., Suckling, K. E., Holmes, S. D., Chamberlain, P., & Macphee, C. H. (2000). Lipoprotein-associated phospholipase A(2), platelet-activating factor acetylhydrolase: A potential new risk factor for coronary artery disease. *Atherosclerosis*, *150*(2), 413–419. Retrieved from http://www.ncbi.nlm.nih.gov/pubmed/10856534 doi:10.1016/S0021-9150(99)00406-2 PMID:10856534

Chang, T. C., & Mendell, J. T. (2007). microRNAs in vertebrate physiology and human disease. *Annual Review of Genomics and Human Genetics*, *8*(1), 215–239. doi:10.1146/annurev.genom.8.080706.092351 PMID:17506656

Dastidar, A. G., Rodrigues, J. C. L., Ahmed, N., Baritussio, A., & Bucciarelli-Ducci, C. (2015). The Role of Cardiac MRI in Patients with Troponin-Positive Chest Pain and Unobstructed Coronary Arteries. *Current Cardiovascular Imaging Reports*, *8*(8), 28. doi:10.1007/s12410-015-9345-x PMID:26146527

de Korte, C. L., Pasterkamp, G., van der Steen, A. F. W., Woutman, H. A., & Bom, N. (2000). Characterization of Plaque Components With Intravascular Ultrasound Elastography in Human Femoral and Coronary Arteries In Vitro. *Circulation*, *102*(6), 617–623. doi:10.1161/01.CIR.102.6.617 PMID:10931800

De Korte, C. L., Schaar, J. A., Mastik, F., Serruys, P. W., & Van Der Der Steen, A. F. W. (2003). Intravascular Elastography. From Bench to Bedside. *Journal of Interventional Cardiology*, *16*(3), 253–259. doi:10.1034/j.1600-0854.2003.8049.x PMID:12800404

de Korte, C. L., & van der Steen, A. F. W. (2002). Intravascular ultrasound elastography: an overview. *Ultrasonics, 40*(1-8), 859-865. doi:10.1016/s0041-624x(02)00227-5

Dolci, A., & Panteghini, M. (2006). The exciting story of cardiac biomarkers: From retrospective detection to gold diagnostic standard for acute myocardial infarction and more. *Clinica Chimica Acta*, *369*(2), 179–187. doi:10.1016/j.cca.2006.02.042 PMID:16698005

Fenning, R. S., & Wilensky, R. L. (2014). New Insights into the Vulnerable Plaque from Imaging Studies. *Current Atherosclerosis Reports*, *16*(3), 397. doi:10.1007/s11883-014-0397-1 PMID:24477795

Giada, F., & Bartoletti, A. (2015). Value of Ambulatory Electrocardiographic Monitoring in Syncope. *Cardiology Clinics*, *33*(3), 361–366. doi:10.1016/j.ccl.2015.04.004 PMID:26115822

Giada, F., Bertaglia, E., Reimers, B., Noventa, D., & Raviele, A. (2012). Current and Emerging Indications for Implantable Cardiac Monitors. *Pacing and Clinical Electrophysiology*, *35*(9), 1169–1178. doi:10.1111/j.1540-8159.2012.03411.x PMID:22530875

Global Lipids Genetics, C., Willer, C. J., Schmidt, E. M., Sengupta, S., Peloso, G. M., Gustafsson, S., & Abecasis, G. R. et al. (2013). Discovery and refinement of loci associated with lipid levels. *Nature Genetics*, *45*(11), 1274–1283. doi:10.1038/ng.2797 PMID:24097068

Gorenoi, V., Schonermark, M. P., & Hagen, A. (2012). CT coronary angiography vs. invasive coronary angiography in CHD. *GMS Health Technol Assess*, *8*, Doc02. doi:10.3205/hta000100 PMID:22536300

Heeschen, C., Dimmeler, S., Fichtlscherer, S., Hamm, C. W., Berger, J., Simoons, M. L., & Investigators, C. et al. (2004). Prognostic value of placental growth factor in patients with acute chest pain. *Journal of the American Medical Association*, *291*(4), 435–441. doi:10.1001/jama.291.4.435 PMID:14747500

Helgadottir, A., Thorleifsson, G., Magnusson, K. P., Gretarsdottir, S., Steinthorsdottir, V., Manolescu, A., & Stefansson, K. et al. (2008). The same sequence variant on 9p21 associates with myocardial infarction, abdominal aortic aneurysm and intracranial aneurysm. *Nature Genetics*, *40*(2), 217–224. doi:10.1038/ng.72 PMID:18176561

Helgadottir, A., Thorleifsson, G., Manolescu, A., Gretarsdottir, S., Blondal, T., Jonasdottir, A., & Stefansson, K. et al. (2007). A common variant on chromosome 9p21 affects the risk of myocardial infarction. *Science*, *316*(5830), 1491–1493. doi:10.1126/science.1142842 PMID:17478679

Heslop, C. L., Frohlich, J. J., & Hill, J. S. (2010). Myeloperoxidase and C-reactive protein have combined utility for long-term prediction of cardiovascular mortality after coronary angiography. *Journal of the American College of Cardiology*, *55*(11), 1102–1109. doi:10.1016/j.jacc.2009.11.050 PMID:20223364

Hindricks, G., Pokushalov, E., Urban, L., Taborsky, M., Kuck, K. H., Lebedev, D., & Purerfellner, H. et al. (2010). Performance of a New Leadless Implantable Cardiac Monitor in Detecting and Quantifying Atrial Fibrillation Results of the XPECT Trial. *Circulation: Arrhythmia and Electrophysiology*, *3*(2), 141–147. doi:10.1161/CIRCEP.109.877852 PMID:20160169

Hinohara, K., Nakajima, T., Takahashi, M., Hohda, S., Sasaoka, T., Nakahara, K., & Kimura, A. et al. (2008). Replication of the association between a chromosome 9p21 polymorphism and coronary artery disease in Japanese and Korean populations. *Journal of Human Genetics*, *53*(4), 357–359. doi:10.1007/s10038-008-0248-4 PMID:18264662

Huang, D., Swanson, E., Lin, C., Schuman, J., Stinson, W., Chang, W., & et, et al.. (1991). Optical coherence tomography. *Science*, *254*(5035), 1178–1181. doi:10.1126/science.1957169 PMID:1957169

Isaacs, A., Willems, S. M., Bos, D., Dehghan, A., Hofman, A., Ikram, M. A., & van Duijn, C. M. et al. (2013). Risk scores of common genetic variants for lipid levels influence atherosclerosis and incident coronary heart disease. *Arteriosclerosis, Thrombosis, and Vascular Biology*, *33*(9), 2233–2239. doi:10.1161/ATVBAHA.113.301236 PMID:23766260

Ito, K., Bick, A. G., Flannick, J., Friedman, D. J., Genovese, G., Parfenov, M. G., & Seidman, C. et al. (2014). Increased burden of cardiovascular disease in carriers of APOL1 genetic variants. *Circulation Research*, *114*(5), 845–850. doi:10.1161/CIRCRESAHA.114.302347 PMID:24379297

Iwamoto, T. a. Acoustical Imaging. http://link.springer.com/chapter/10.1007/978-1-4020-8823-0_21, 5.

Kara, K., Lehmann, N., Neumann, T., Kalsch, H., Mohlenkamp, S., Dykun, I., & Mahabadi, A. A. et al. (2015). NT-proBNP is superior to BNP for predicting first cardiovascular events in the general population: The Heinz Nixdorf Recall Study. *International Journal of Cardiology*, *183*, 155–161. doi:10.1016/j.ijcard.2015.01.082 PMID:25666125

Kathiresan, S., & Srivastava, D. (2012). Genetics of human cardiovascular disease. *Cell*, *148*(6), 1242–1257. doi:10.1016/j.cell.2012.03.001 PMID:22424232

Kingwell, K. (2011). Cardiovascular disease: microRNA protects the heart. *Nature Reviews. Drug Discovery*, *10*(2), 98. doi:10.1038/nrd3380 PMID:21283101

Kotani, K., Fujiwara, S., Tsuzaki, K., Sano, Y., Matsuoka, Y., Hamada, T., & Sakane, N. (2009). An association between angiotensin II type 2 receptor gene A/C3123 polymorphism and glycemic control marker in a general Japanese population. *Molecular Biology Reports*, *36*(5), 917–920. doi:10.1007/s11033-008-9263-y PMID:18437528

Li, C., Fang, Z., Jiang, T., Zhang, Q., Liu, C., Zhang, C., & Xiang, Y. (2013). Serum microRNAs profile from genome-wide serves as a fingerprint for diagnosis of acute myocardial infarction and angina pectoris. *BMC Medical Genomics*, *6*(1), 16. doi:10.1186/1755-8794-6-16 PMID:23641832

Lloyd-Jones, D. M., Nam, B. H., DAgostino, R. B. Sr, Levy, D., Murabito, J. M., Wang, T. J., & ODonnell, C. J. et al. (2004). Parental cardiovascular disease as a risk factor for cardiovascular disease in middle-aged adults: A prospective study of parents and offspring. *Journal of the American Medical Association*, *291*(18), 2204–2211. doi:10.1001/jama.291.18.2204 PMID:15138242

Lopez, B., Gonzalez, A., Lindner, D., Westermann, D., Ravassa, S., Beaumont, J., & Diez, J. et al. (2013). Osteopontin-mediated myocardial fibrosis in heart failure: A role for lysyl oxidase? *Cardiovascular Research*, *99*(1), 111–120. doi:10.1093/cvr/cvt100 PMID:23619422

Marwick, T. H., Cho, I., ó Hartaigh, B., & Min, J. K. (2015). Finding the Gatekeeper to the Cardiac Catheterization Laboratory. *Journal of the American College of Cardiology*, *65*(25), 2747–2756. doi:10.1016/j.jacc.2015.04.060 PMID:26112200

Masugata, H., Senda, S., Inukai, M., Himoto, T., Murao, K., Hosomi, N., & Goda, F. et al. (2011). Seasonal variation in estimated glomerular filtration rate based on serum creatinine levels in hypertensive patients. *The Tohoku Journal of Experimental Medicine*, *224*(2), 137–142. Retrieved from http://www.ncbi.nlm.nih.gov/pubmed/21617334 doi:10.1620/tjem.224.137 PMID:21617334

McPherson, R., Pertsemlidis, A., Kavaslar, N., Stewart, A., Roberts, R., Cox, D. R., & Cohen, J. C. et al. (2007). A common allele on chromosome 9 associated with coronary heart disease. *Science*, *316*(5830), 1488–1491. doi:10.1126/science.1142447 PMID:17478681

Mellor, R., & Woollard, M. (2010). Skill acquisition by health care workers in the Resuscitation Council (UK) 2005 Guidelines for Adult Basic Life Support. *International Emergency Nursing*, *18*(2), 61–66. doi:10.1016/j.ienj.2009.08.003 PMID:20382366

Mendell, J. T., & Olson, E. N. (2012). MicroRNAs in stress signaling and human disease. *Cell*, *148*(6), 1172–1187. doi:10.1016/j.cell.2012.02.005 PMID:22424228

Newton-Cheh, C., & Smith, J. G. (2010). What can human genetics teach us about the causes of cardiovascular disease? *Journal of the American College of Cardiology*, *55*(25), 2843–2845. doi:10.1016/j.jacc.2009.11.097 PMID:20579541

Nicholls, S. J. (2009). Relationship between LDL, HDL, blood pressure and atheroma progression in the coronaries. *Current Opinion in Lipidology*, *20*(6), 491–496. doi:10.1097/MOL.0b013e32832ec396 PMID:19593124

Obad, S., dos Santos, C. O., Petri, A., Heidenblad, M., Broom, O., Ruse, C., & Kauppinen, S. et al. (2011). Silencing of microRNA families by seed-targeting tiny LNAs. *Nature Genetics*, *43*(4), 371–378. doi:10.1038/ng.786 PMID:21423181

Ogita, M., Miyauchi, K., Kasai, T., Doi, S., Wada, H., Naito, R., & Daida, H. et al. (2015). Impact of preprocedural high-sensitive C-reactive protein levels on long-term clinical outcomes of patients with stable coronary artery disease and chronic kidney disease who were treated with drug-eluting stents. *Journal of Cardiology*, *66*(1), 15–21. doi:10.1016/j.jjcc.2014.10.010 PMID:25572020

OLeary, D. H., Polak, J. F., Kronmal, R. A., Manolio, T. A., Burke, G. L., & Wolfson, S. K. Jr. (1999). Carotid-Artery Intima and Media Thickness as a Risk Factor for Myocardial Infarction and Stroke in Older Adults. *The New England Journal of Medicine*, *340*(1), 14–22. doi:10.1056/NEJM199901073400103 PMID:9878640

Pilz, G., Graw, M., Heer, T., Klos, M., Ali, E., & Hoefling, B. (2009). Myocardial hypoperfusion due to hypoplastic coronary arteries: A cause for false-positive results during adenosine stress Cardiac Magnetic Resonance Imaging. *Journal of Cardiovascular Magnetic Resonance*, *11*(Suppl 1), 155. doi:10.1186/1532-429X-11-S1-P155

Pohlhammer, J., Kronenberg, F., Rantner, B., Stadler, M., Peric, S., Hammerer-Lercher, A., & Kollerits, B. et al. (2014). High-sensitivity cardiac troponin T in patients with intermittent claudication and its relation with cardiovascular events and all-cause mortalitythe CAVASIC Study. *Atherosclerosis*, *237*(2), 711–717. doi:10.1016/j.atherosclerosis.2014.10.097 PMID:25463110

Quiat, D., & Olson, E. N. (2013). MicroRNAs in cardiovascular disease: From pathogenesis to prevention and treatment. *The Journal of Clinical Investigation*, *123*(1), 11–18. doi:10.1172/JCI62876 PMID:23281405

Regar, E., Ligthart, J., Bruining, N., & van Soest, G. (2011). The diagnostic value of intracoronary optical coherence tomography. *Herz*, *36*(5), 417–429. doi:10.1007/s00059-011-3487-7 PMID:21744151

Roberts, R., & Stewart, A. F. (2012). 9p21 and the genetic revolution for coronary artery disease. *Clinical Chemistry*, *58*(1), 104–112. doi:10.1373/clinchem.2011.172759 PMID:22015375

Roleder, T., Jąkała, J., Kałuża, G., Partyka, Ł., Proniewska, K., Pociask, E.,... Dudek, D. (2015). The basics of intravascular optical coherence tomography. *PWKI, 2*, 74-83. doi:10.5114/pwki.2015.52278

Rome, B. N., Kramer, D. B., & Kesselheim, A. S. (2014). FDA Approval of Cardiac Implantable Electronic Devices via Original and Supplement Premarket Approval Pathways, 19792012. *Journal of the American Medical Association, 311*(4), 385. doi:10.1001/jama.2013.284986 PMID:24449317

Rosenberg, M., Zugck, C., Nelles, M., Juenger, C., Frank, D., Remppis, A., & Frey, N. et al. (2008). Osteopontin, a new prognostic biomarker in patients with chronic heart failure. *Circulation: Heart Failure, 1*(1), 43–49. doi:10.1161/CIRCHEARTFAILURE.107.746172 PMID:19808269

Salazar, M. R., Carbajal, H. A., Espeche, W. G., Aizpurua, M., Leiva Sisnieguez, C. E., March, C. E., & Reaven, G. M. et al. (2013). Identifying cardiovascular disease risk and outcome: Use of the plasma triglyceride/high-density lipoprotein cholesterol concentration ratio versus metabolic syndrome criteria. *Journal of Internal Medicine, 273*(6), 595–601. doi:10.1111/joim.12036 PMID:23331522

Samani, N. J., Erdmann, J., Hall, A. S., Hengstenberg, C., Mangino, M., Mayer, B., & Schunkert, H. et al. (2007). Genomewide association analysis of coronary artery disease. *The New England Journal of Medicine, 357*(5), 443–453. doi:10.1056/NEJMoa072366 PMID:17634449

Schaar, J., Mastik, F., Regar, E., den Uil, C., Gijsen, F., Wentzel, J.,... van der Stehen, A. (2007). Current Diagnostic Modalities for Vulnerable Plaque Detection. *CPD, 13*(10), 995-1001. doi:10.2174/138161207780487511

Schmitz, G., & Orso, E. (2015). Lipoprotein(a) hyperlipidemia as cardiovascular risk factor: Pathophysiological aspects. *Clinical Research in Cardiology; Official Journal of the German Cardiac Society, 10*(Suppl), 21–25. doi:10.1007/s11789-015-0074-0 PMID:25708587

Singh, M., Dalal, S., & Singh, K. (2014). Osteopontin: At the cross-roads of myocyte survival and myocardial function. *Life Sciences, 118*(1), 1–6. doi:10.1016/j.lfs.2014.09.014 PMID:25265596

Singh, M., Foster, C. R., Dalal, S., & Singh, K. (2010). Role of osteopontin in heart failure associated with aging. *Heart Failure Reviews, 15*(5), 487–494. doi:10.1007/s10741-010-9158-6 PMID:20127409

Small, E. M., & Olson, E. N. (2011). Pervasive roles of microRNAs in cardiovascular biology. *Nature, 469*(7330), 336–342. doi:10.1038/nature09783 PMID:21248840

Soejima, H., Ogawa, H., Sakamoto, T., Miyamoto, S., Kajiwara, I., Kojima, S., & Kishikawa, H. et al. (2003). Increased serum matrix metalloproteinase-1 concentration predicts advanced left ventricular remodeling in patients with acute myocardial infarction. *Circulation Journal, 67*(4), 301–304. Retrieved from http://www.ncbi.nlm.nih.gov/pubmed/12655159 doi:10.1253/circj.67.301 PMID:12655159

Soloperto, G. (2012). Progress in atherosclerotic plaque imaging. *World Journal of Radiology, 4*(8), 353. doi:10.4329/wjr.v4.i8.353 PMID:22937215

St. Jude's Confirm Implantable Cardiac Monitor Wins FDA Approval. (n.d.). Retrieved from http://www.medgadget.com/2008/09/saint_judes_confirm_implantable_cardiac_monitor_wins_fda_approval.html

Suh, W. M., Seto, A. H., Margey, R. J. P., Cruz-Gonzalez, I., & Jang, I. K. (2011). Intravascular Detection of the Vulnerable Plaque. *Circulation: Cardiovascular Imaging*, *4*(2), 169–178. doi:10.1161/CIRCIMAGING.110.958777 PMID:21406663

Sun, Z., Wu, W., Liu, J., Ma, N., Zheng, Z., Li, Q., & Miao, J. et al. (2014). Influence of glucose-lowering rate on CKMB and myoglobin serum levels in type-2 diabetes patients with coronary heart disease. *Human Immunology*, *75*(12), 1182–1187. doi:10.1016/j.humimm.2014.10.006 PMID:25454625

Tearney, G. J. (1997). In Vivo Endoscopic Optical Biopsy with Optical Coherence Tomography. *Science*, *276*(5321), 2037–2039. doi:10.1126/science.276.5321.2037 PMID:9197265

van der Net, J. B., Versmissen, J., Oosterveer, D. M., Defesche, J. C., Yazdanpanah, M., Aouizerat, B. E., & Sijbrands, E. J. et al. (2009). Arachidonate 5-lipoxygenase-activating protein (ALOX5AP) gene and coronary heart disease risk in familial hypercholesterolemia. *Atherosclerosis*, *203*(2), 472–478. doi:10.1016/j.atherosclerosis.2008.07.025 PMID:18775537

Wellcome Trust Case Control, C. (2007). Genome-wide association study of 14,000 cases of seven common diseases and 3,000 shared controls. *Nature*, *447*(7145), 661–678. doi:10.1038/nature05911 PMID:17554300

Zakynthinos, E., & Pappa, N. (2009). Inflammatory biomarkers in coronary artery disease. *Journal of Cardiology*, *53*(3), 317–333. doi:10.1016/j.jjcc.2008.12.007 PMID:19477372

Zhang, S. Y., Xu, M. L., Zhang, C. E., Qu, Z. Y., Zhang, B. B., Zheng, Z. Y., & Zhang, L. M. (2012). Association of ALOX5AP gene single nucleotide polymorphisms and cerebral infarction in the Han population of northern China. *BMC Medical Genetics*, *13*(1), 61. doi:10.1186/1471-2350-13-61 PMID:22849376

Zuo, P. Y., Chen, X. L., Liu, Y. W., Zhang, R., He, X. X., & Liu, C. Y. (2015). Non-HDL-cholesterol to HDL-cholesterol ratio as an independent risk factor for the development of chronic kidney disease. *Nutrition, Metabolism, and Cardiovascular Diseases*, *25*(6), 582–587. doi:10.1016/j.numecd.2015.03.003 PMID:25921842

Chapter 12
Immunosuppressive Therapy in Heart Transplantation

Yan Li
Cleveland Clinic, USA

Zhi Huang
Cleveland Clinic, USA

April Yingfang Li
Northeast Ohio Medical University, USA

Bin Zhang
Mayo Clinic, USA

Ifeyinwa S. Nwankwo
Case Western Reserve University School of Medicine, USA

Yun Lu
No. 1 Hospital of Lanzhou University, China

Yali Yao
No. 1 Hospital of Lanzhou University, China

ABSTRACT

Heart transplantation is a surgical procedure performed on patients with end-stage heart failure or other irreversible heart disease, Heart transplant prolongs the life of severe heart disease patients. Most of the receipts could survive more than 2-3 years, five-year survival rate could reach 70-80% with immunosuppressive therapy, rejection still an important problem after transplantation. Currently, traditional calcineurin inhibitors, antimetabolite agents, and steroids, wildly used after transplantation, the new generation of immunosuppressive medicines have been developed, and cell-based immunotherapy, as mesenchymal stem cell, myeloid-derived suppressor cells, dendritic cells, pluripotent cells and Treg cells are promising to be used in cellular immunotherapy in organ transplantation.

INTRODUCTION

The chapter focused on heart transplantation indication, prognosis, traditional and new generation immunosuppressive medicine, cell immunotherapy in adult and pediatric heart transplantation.

DOI: 10.4018/978-1-5225-2092-4.ch012

Transplantation Opportunity and Clinical Prognosis

Indications

Congestive heart failure (CHF) affects 7.5 million people in North America and 23 million people worldwide(Alraies & Eckman, 2014). 550,000 patients develop heart failure (HF) each year, and the incidence is increasing, doubling with each decade after 45 years of age (Mozaffarian et al., 2015).

It has been reported that about 20% lifetime risk after midage for heart failure and while more patients are surviving the early stages of cardiac disease 10% of patients with HF are in the advanced stage (Deng, 2002). Based on 2011 mortality data from the American Heart Association, CHF contributes more than 30% of any-mention deaths attributable to cardiovascular disease(Mozaffarian et al., 2015). Cardiac transplantation has become the primary course of treatment for those in the last phases of this disease (Jung et al., 2011).

Heart failure is a complex syndrome defined by elevated cardiac filling pressure at rest or when under stress, also characterized by inadequate peripheral oxygen delivery, caused by cardiac dysfunction (Tse, 2011). HF is normally characterized by cardiac muscle dilation (dilated cardiomyopathy) or hypertrophy (Leclercq, 2007). There are two types of heart failure, reduced ejection fraction (systolic dysfunction), and preserved ejection fraction (diastolic dysfunction) (Lilly, 2012). Ejection fraction (EF) is a measurement of how well the heart is pumping each time it contracts. If this is low, it is an indication that the heart is not contracting during systole as well as it should be and, therefore, cannot pump blood to the periphery effectively. When EF is "preserved", it means that while the fraction of blood being pumped is the same, there is an overall decrease in the amount of blood being pumped, even though the percentage of blood being ejected from the ventricles is the same(Lilly, 2012).

Some conditions that can lead to a reduced EF include coronary artery disease, chronic volume overload as is seen in aortic or mitral valve regurgitation, dilated cardiomyopathies, advanced aortic stenosis, and uncontrolled severe hypertension. Conditions that can lead to preserved EF are all as a result of impaired filling of the ventricles during diastole. These can include left ventricular hypertrophy, restrictive cardiomyopathy, myocardial fibrosis, transient myocardial ischemia, and pericardial constriction or tamponade(Lilly, 2012). According to research studies, the most common diagnoses associated with heart transplantation were dilated cardiomyopathy, ischemic cardiomyopathy, and hypertrophic cardiomyopathy (Jung et al., 2011).

Systolic dysfunction heart failure comprises 50% of all heart failure patients (Alraies & Eckman, 2014). Congestive heart failure (CHF) is a form of systolic dysfunction, and its prevalence has increased over the years as a result of improved longevity of the population and better-quality management of acute coronary syndromes (Deng, 2002).

The first heart transplant was successfully done in 1967 in Groote-Schuur-Hospital, Kapstadt, South Africa. The U.S. accomplished its first successful heart transplant at Stanford University in 1968 (Deng, 2002). Currently, tens of thousands of heart transplants are being performed worldwide and due to major advancements in immunosuppression, rejection control, and infection control, the results of the procedures have improved dramatically since its inception (Deng, 2002; Jung et al., 2011) (Table 1).

The indications for heart transplantation are many and varied. Common indications such as having advanced heart disease unaltered by optimal medical therapy or failure of cardiac resynchronization therapy to improve symptoms of the underlying pathology are often considered in the stratification of patients on extensive waiting lists. There are criteria, however, in the determination of eligible patients

Table 1. Advancement in heart transplants

Year	Advancement in Heart Transplants
1966	Temporary Assist Device, the booster pump was successfully implanted by Dr. DeBakey (**April 21st, 1966**).
1967	First successful heart transplant completed by Dr. Christian Banard in Cape Town, South Africa (**Dec 3rd, 1967**).
1969	First successful temporary artificial heart transplant in a human by Dr. Denton Cooley, the patient lived for 65 hours.
1970s	Discovery of cyclosporine, an immunosuppressant drug derived from soil fungus by Jean Borel.
1982	First successful permanent artificial heart: "**Jarvik-7**", designed by Dr. Robert Jarvik.
1984	First successful pediatric heart transplant.
1994	Discovery of tacrolimus, another instrumental immunosuppressant drug derived from a fungus.

based on the classifications of severity of HF by the New York Association Class (NYHA) and another system generated by the American College of Cardiology and American Heart Association (ACC/AHA). The NYHA has classes I-IV, each based on the functional capabilities of the patients. Class I indicates there is no limitation to activities, class II is regular activity limited due to mild shortness of breath, class III specifies those with symptoms under minimal exertion, and class IV patients have symptoms at rest (Alraies & Eckman, 2014).

The ACC/AHA has four stages of classification as well, A-D. Stage A includes patients with a high of developing the cardiac disease based on significant family history but without structural heart disease or symptoms of heart failure and stage D includes those in advanced stages of heart failure optimal therapy notwithstanding. The refractory patients in need of specialized interventions, stage D patients, have the options of end-of-life-care or extraordinary measures like heart transplantation, mechanical circulatory machinery, or pharmaceutical therapy (Alraies & Eckman, 2014; Jessup et al., 2009).

There are several indications for heart transplantation dictated by the ACC/AHA guidelines including:

1. In refractory cases of cardiogenic shock that require left ventricular assist device (LVAD) or intra-aortic balloon pump counterpulsation cardiac transplantation can be indicated (Alraies & Eckman, 2014). Refractory Cardiogenic shock is when the heart fails to pump enough blood to the organs to function, leading to multiorgan system failure if not remedied immediately. The LVAD is a device that uses electromagnetic energy to pump oxygenated blood to the body in patients with advanced heart failure(Milla, Pinney, & Anyanwu, 2012). While it is not a replacement for the heart, its assistance can be critical for those waiting for a heart transplant.
2. Instances of cardiogenic shock that necessitate continuous intravenous inotropic therapy such as digoxin, dobutamine, or milrinone (Alraies & Eckman, 2014). Inotropic drugs act to increase the contractility of the heart through stimulation of the sympathetic and adrenergic receptors on the heart, leading to an increase in the amount of blood that can be pumped out. Prolonged use of this is dangerous, however, and indicative of heart transplant necessity.
3. When a patient has a peak VO2 less than ten mL/kg per min after reaching the anaerobic threshold, they are highly indicated for the procedure. This is the gold standard of cardiac transplant indications. Peak VO2 is defined as the maximum rate of oxygen consumption measured during a monitored exercise activity (typically on a treadmill). When below a certain level, this means the

cardiac reserve and adaptation of peripheral tissues are inadequate; this serves as one of the best predictors of when an individual can become a candidate for cardiac transplantation (Jessup et al., 2009; Milla et al., 2012). Compensated CHF patients with a peak oxygen consumption of less than 14 mL/kg/min or <50% predicted, in particular, are considered sick enough for transplantation (Alraies & Eckman, 2014). Research studies show that the cut-off point of <10 mL/kg/min is a more accurate threshold when identifying most eligible candidates for heart transplantation. In one study including 715 patients referred for cardiac transplantation due to advanced HF, one year event-free survival was 87% in patients with Vo2 >14 mL/kg/min, 77% in those with Vo2 between 10.1 and 14 mL/kg/min, and 65% of patients with less than 10 mL/kg/min (Milla et al., 2012).

4. Those patients with an NYHA class III or IV in spite of maximized resynchronization treatment or other medical therapies are considered sick enough for cardiac transplants (Alraies & Eckman, 2014). Arrhythmias, or irregular heart rhythms, can be found in patients with severe heart failure. Resynchronization therapy is when this rhythm is "reset" by a pacemaker, a small machine implanted in the heart. According to the AHA, cardiac resynchronization therapy such as the Implantable Cardioverter Defibrillator (ICD), can improve the blood flow in the heart, as well as its efficiency("Cardiac Resynchronization Therapy (CRT)., " 2015; Lund et al., 2014). This can reduce the symptoms in such patients, for example, shortness of breath, as well as decrease morbidity. However, recent studies have shown that Cardiac Resynchronization Therapy (CRT) does not decrease the rate of mortality or hospitalization, and actually possibly increases mortality in individuals with systolic heart failure and a narrow QRS duration.
5. Those experiencing recurrent life-threatening left ventricular arrhythmias despite an implantable cardiac defibrillator, antiarrhythmic therapy, or catheter-based ablation are also indicated for cardiac transplantation(Alraies & Eckman, 2014). As stated above, implantable cardiac defibrillators or other methods of cardiac resynchronization therapy has been proven to reduce total mortality by a reduction in sudden cardiac death in patients with NHA functional class III or IV despite optimal medical treatment("Cardiac Resynchronization Therapy (CRT)., " 2015). However, should these methods fail to suppress life-threatening left ventricular arrhythmias, these patients should be referred for cardiac transplantation.
6. Patients with end-stage congenital HF and no evidence of pulmonary hypertension can be indicated for transplantation(Alraies & Eckman, 2014). Certain congenital anomalies can predispose an individual to heart failure if not remedied. An example would be a congenital bicuspid aortic valve, where the aortic valve is comprised of only two leaflets, instead of the normal three. In its advanced stages, it can lead to chronic pressure overload on the heart, disabling its ability to pump effectively during systole(Lilly, 2012). Valve replacement is the only treatment for this condition.
7. Patients with refractory angina lacking effective medical or surgical therapeutic options can be indicated for surgery(Alraies & Eckman, 2014; Deng, 2002). Angina pectoris is a very common manifestation of ischemic heart disease, presenting with symptoms of chest discomfort and pressure. Stable angina is this feeling of discomfort during physical exertion. It is considered unstable angina if the symptoms present at rest and last for a longer amount of time. If unstable angina persists, risks of myocardial infarction, heart attack, increases substantially after 15-20 seconds (Lilly, 2012). When ischemic heart disease is not controlled, and there is neither potential medical or surgical options a patient can go into refractory angina and be a likely candidate for cardiac transplantation.

8. Another important factor is the hemodynamic management of pulmonary vascular resistance (PVR), which when below 4 Wood units (320 dynes-sec/cm^5) (normal is $\leq$ 1.5 Wood units) are considered for transplantation (Gallino, Eugster, Schneider, Furrer, & Turina, 1988). During the postoperative period, the healthy donor right ventricle is acutely subjected to substantially increased workload; thusly, it is critical to be pharmacologically able to reduce the PVR acutely. A non-reversible PVR greater than 6 Wood units is a major excluding factor. One report has shown that mortality rate over three months was higher in patients with PVR greater than 2.5 Wood units compared to those with lower values, but if the initially high PVR could be reduced pharmacologically, the mortality rate decreased dramatically (Gallino et al., 1988).

Due to the very complex nature of heart failure, including its varying neurohormonal, hemodynamic, and electrophysiologic properties that contribute to the morbidity and mortality of the disease, it is critical to recognize that basing of the selection process on one sole indication can be highly erroneous.

There are probable cardiac transplantation criteria as well as inadequate indication criteria, and it is important that this risk stratification be in place so that these transplants are going to the most appropriate candidate (Alraies & Eckman, 2014; Deng, 2002). The United Network of Organ Sharing (UNOS) is the organization that assigns transplant candidates a status according to their medical conditions. IA is the highest status, assigned to the sickest, longest waiting patients. With respect to UNOS status, the national median waiting time for status 1A is 49 days (Alraies & Eckman, 2014).

Donor criteria have changed significantly in recent decades, expanding from a very narrow, specific criteria to a very broad, inclusive one. This has occurred because of the increasing demand and stagnant availability of donor's hearts (Gallino et al., 1988). The extended criteria include advanced donor heart dysfunction, donor heart structural changes, donor malignancies, donor-recipient size match, donor age, and donor infection. In spite of the size of the donor recipient, a normal sized adult male has become suitable for most candidates (Alraies & Eckman, 2014).

Prognosis

According to the International Society for Heart and Lung Transplantation (ISHLT) registry, the 1-year survival rate post cardiac transplantation is approximately 90%, with those in a favorable functional status within 1-3 years also approaching 90% (Alraies & Eckman, 2014; Lund et al., 2014). These patients generally can do normal activities and can return to work during that 1-3 year period (Lund et al., 2014). It has even been reported that despite cardiac denervation, many of these patients can perform very well athletically (Kemp W.L., 2008). Survival has improved for the first year after cardiac transplantation compared to the 1980s and 1990s, due to vast improvements in immunosuppression, relaxed donor requirements and the stringent, risk-based stratification of recipients (Hillebrands et al., 2001; MX). Even still, this improvement is mostly applicable to the initial 6-12 months post-transplant, after which mortality rate remains equal to that prior to these advancements in healthcare (Hillebrands et al., 2001). The 5-year survival rate is 69%, and the median survival of all cardiac transplantation patients is 11 years. Median survival increases to 14 years if the patient survives the first year post-transplant (MX).

There are many causes of morbidity in post heart transplant recipients. Some leading causes for all transplant recipients and retransplant beneficiaries who occur particularly during the early period after transplantation include graft failure, infection, and multiple organ failures (Alraies & Eckman, 2014; MX). During the following 3-5 years, some common post-transplant morbidities include coronary artery vasculopathy (CAV), malignancy, renal dysfunction, hypertension, hyperlipidemia, and diabetes. Malignancy is the most common cause of death in post-transplant recipients.

Coronary artery vasculopathy is a panarterial disease that is of both immunologic and nonimmunologic origin (Hillebrands et al., 2001; MX). This multifactorial disease occurred in the epicardial coronary arteries and characterized by diffuse intimal hyperplasia. The nature of the hyperplasia is concentric and longitudinal and confined to the areas of the allograft (Grauhan et al., 1998; Montgomery, Cozzi, West, & Warren, 2011; MX). The immunologic factors play a major role in this disease, especially considering that the antibody-mediated rejection takes place solely in the donor's arteries and not the recipients. After these initial years, the incidence of death related to this decreases. Recent studies indicate that the greater the HLA mismatch between donors and recipients, the greater incidence there is of CAV in patients (Eisen Howard J; Grauhan et al., 1998; Hillebrands et al., 2001; MX). Approximately 30-40% of patients will develop this disease within five years post-transplantation(Alraies & Eckman, 2014). Although only 11% of deaths post-transplantation are as a result of acute rejection within the initial three years, ISHLT recognizes that both acute and chronic immune reactions are important factors involved in allograft rejection and a leading cause of death for retransplant patients.

Rejection of allograft transplantation is considered an adaptive immunologic reaction to a foreign tissue, or the donor tissue. It is necessary to understand the different classifications of rejection of cardiac allograft transplants that can occur post transplantation. Rejection can be either a cellular or humoral immune response as a result of the alloantigen, with cellular rejection being facilitated by T cells and humoral via antibodies (Kemp W.L., 2008; Montgomery et al., 2011). The other classification for rejection is based on timing after the transplantation procedure is completed: hyperacute, acute, and chronic(Kemp W.L., 2008). Cellular rejection can be a result of the recipient's $CD4^{+}$ T cells being hypersensitive, leading to graft tissue damage via the release perforin by cytotoxic T cells. These T cells have matured from CD8 T cells and can be stimulated through a direct or indirect pathway. The direct pathway involves major histocompatibility complex (MHC) molecules, which play the primary role in rapid rejection reactions (Kemp W.L., 2008; Lilly, 2012; Montgomery et al., 2011). Every person has polymorphic genes encoding for histocompatibility proteins like MHC molecules that are responsible for the immunologic response to the allografts (Montgomery et al., 2011). In this direct pathway, the molecules are on the surface of the alloantigen cells and are recognized by the body. Indirectly, the recipient's antigen presenting cells presents these antigens, leading to the activation of the adaptive immune system and subsequent attack on the graft tissue, resulting in rejection.

The humoral, or vascular rejection is due to preformed antibodies against the vasculature of the graft. Specifically, human leukocyte antigens (HLA) are the human form of histocompatibility complex (MHC) molecules involved in these rapid, potent reactions (Montgomery et al., 2011). It is only when these HLA antigens between the donor and recipient are mismatched on all cells of the graft that this rejection occurs. Associated with the worst prognosis, this form of rejection can increase the risk of CAV almost tenfold.

Acute allograft rejection can be cellularly or humoral mediated. Experiments have demonstrated changes in specificity and memory as mediated by lymphocytes, occurring approximately ten days after transplantation in an acute allograft rejection (Jung et al., 2011; Kemp W.L., 2008; Lilly, 2012; Montgomery et al., 2011). Clinically, there are typically lesions found, infiltrated with large numbers of lymphocytes and macrophages, which cause damage to the tissue. The microscopic morphology varies between the cellular and the humoral graft rejection. The acute, cellularly mediated rejection morphology presents with interstitial mononuclear infiltrate, hemorrhaging, edema, and swollen endothelial cells, or endothelialitis. The acute humoral morphology includes parenchymal infarcts, necrotizing vasculitis, and neutrophilic infiltrate. This humoral rejection can happen more rapidly if there is a second transplant with the same organ, and the recipient has developed a memory of the grafted tissue (Lilly, 2012; Montgomery et al., 2011). The diagnosis of acute cellular rejection can be made by endomyocardial biopsy, which can be accomplished via routine inspection or if suggestive symptoms are present (Abbas, 2003). An acute allograft rejection does respond excellently to cyclosporine, an immunosuppressant, however.

If this pathology presents during the first 24 hours after transplantation, it is considered hyperacute rejection (HAR). Induced in most cases by preformed donor-specific HLA antibodies (DSA), this humoral mediated immunologic response occurs so rapidly that vascularization of the tissue cannot occur. Some sources of these preformed DSA include the stimulation via allo-presensitization during pregnancy, transfusions, and previous transplants (20). These antibodies bind to the antigens present in the allograft tissue, leading to characteristic thrombotic occlusion and interstitial hemorrhage. Histologically, HAR is also defined by edema and intermittent loss of vascular integrity(Deng, 2002). There can also be neutrophils found within the arterioles and infarcts of parenchyma. Irreparable damage and cessation of function secondary to ischemia can occur within minutes to hours of the transplantation. Grossly, this can manifest as cyanosis of the organ with discolored parenchyma.

Chronic rejection is the last type of chronologically classified allograft rejection and can occur between 4-6 months and initial years post-transplantation. The exact mechanism for this form of rejection is unclear, however, indirect, cellularly-mediated reactions are implicated in the process. Changes in microscopic morphology include changes in the vasculature, interstitial mononuclear infiltrate, interstitial fibrosis, and eventual loss of tissue (Abbas, 2003; Deng, 2002; Kemp W.L., 2008; Montgomery et al., 2011; MX).

Immunosuppressive Medicines

Immunosuppressant drugs are essential in the prevention of allograft rejection and ensuring long-term success postoperatively (Table 2). This can be achieved through a variety of mechanisms of action, and often several are implemented per patient.(Darst JR, 2012; Lindenfeld et al., 2004) Each category of drug offers fundamentally unique benefits, though complications, such as medication-specific adverse effects or therapy failure in the form of rejection, are possible even in combination. However, several novel therapies are in development or clinical trial phases and may provide new avenues for post-transplantation care and continued success. Such options will be addressed toward the end of this section.

Most Widely Used Immunosuppressant

The primary goal of immunosuppressive therapy is to prevent rejection of a cardiac allograft. In addition, an ideal regimen will not hinder the ability of the immune system to respond to infectious agents. Thus, most immunosuppressants are aimed at T-cell-mediated mechanisms rather than those of B-cells. Drugs to reduce B-cell function via the lowering of antibody load are available, but only feasible in individuals whose existing antibody levels are high or who have developed antibodies to donor tissue. (Gruessner A.C., 2014). Currently, the most commonly used immunosuppressants can be divided into three categories: calcineurin inhibitors, antimetabolite/antiproliferative agents, and steroids. Drugs from each class are commonly used in combination though the exact regimen varies depending on preferences

Table 2. Immunosuppressive agents used in heart transplant recipients

Commonly used Immunosuppressive Agents in Heart Transplant Recipients		
	Class	**Common Side Effects**
Prednisone	corticosteroid	Aggression, agitation, Anxiety, blurred vision, dizziness, irregular, etc.
Methylprednisolone	corticosteroid	Aggression, agitation, Anxiety, blurred vision, dizziness, irregular, etc.
Azathioprine	immunosuppressant	Black, tarry stools, bleeding gums, blood in the urine or stools, chest pain, cough or hoarseness, etc.
Mycophenolate Mofetil	immunosuppressant	respiratory tract infection, urinary tract infection, herpes simplex infection, viremia, etc.
Cyclosporine	immunosuppressant	hypertension, hirsutism, tremor, nephrotoxicity, increased blood urea nitrogen, etc.
Tacrolimus	immunosuppressant	Infection, diabetes mellitus, headache, tremor, hyperglycemia, etc.
Sirolimus	immunosuppressant	urinary tract infection and upper respiratory tract infection, etc.
Everolimus	immunosuppressant	Stomatitis, increased serum glucose, decreased hemoglobin, and lymphocytopenia, etc.
Basiliximab	chimeric (murine/human) monoclonal antibody	Abdominal pain, coughing, dizziness, fever or chills, weakness, painful urination, etc.

of the operative location and needs of the patient. The objective of this chapter is the focus on which therapies are most commonly utilized in current practice.

Calcineurin Inhibitors

The gold standard for primary immunosuppression in cardiac transplant recipients has long been calcineurin inhibitors (CNIs), namely cyclosporine and tacrolimus. Both inhibit interleukin-2 (IL-2) production in T cells by forming complexes with endogenous proteins and binding calcineurin, which prevents its phosphatase activity.(Schonder K.S., 2014) Since the development of cyclosporine in the 1980s, post-transplantation outcomes significantly improved. Most notably, three-year survival rates increased to 70%, which is an impressive 30% increase prior to the use of cyclosporine.(Lindenfeld J, 2004)

Despite the undeniable benefits, long-term use of CNIs contributes to several comorbidities, which may ultimately lead to mortality or irreversible harms. The effects of CNIs on the renal system have been well studied. Nephrotoxicity caused by these medications is usually permanent, even after a decrease in therapy or complete withdrawal.(Mudge, 2007) These damages are not only associated with the impaired renal function but also with the development of diabetes and hypertension. Tacrolimus is associated with lower risk of renal toxicity compared to cyclosporine, but also with a higher risk for neural symptoms and hyperglycemia. CNIs may also promote tumor formation by enhancing production of growth factors that cause tumor growth and angiogenesis. However, this is currently only a postulation and has not yet been established.(Lindenfeld J, 2004)

Antimetabolite and Antiproliferative Agents

The two most commonly used drugs in this category, azathioprine (AZA) and mycophenolate mofetil (MMF), work by inhibiting DNA synthesis in T- and B-cells. AZA is first converted to its active metabolic form, thio-inosine-monophosphate, which acts as a purine analog in DNA. MMF inhibits de novo purine synthesis, which is an essential process in lymphocytes specifically. While AZA is typically used post-operatively for maintenance therapy in combination with a CNI and steroid, MMF is mainly given as rejection prophylaxis. Both have similar efficacies though MMF shows slightly better one-year and three-year survival rates. Since the action of AZA is less specific to lymphocytes than MMF, it is associated with a broad range of myelosuppressive effects, such as thrombocytopenia and anemia. (Lindenfeld J, 2004)

Steroids

Some of the earliest immunosuppressants used for transplantation are steroids, such as prednisone, and methylprednisolone. These drugs have a wide-spread effect, suppressing not only lymphocytes, but also granulocytes, monocytes, and macrophages.(Lindenfeld J, 2004; Schonder K.S., 2014). This is achieved through their ability to regulate the transcription of genes responsible for immune responses. They first diffuse freely into the cell and bind to intracellular glucocorticoid receptors. These complexes translocate to the nucleus and bind to regulatory sequences of DNA. In lymphocytes, the genes affected are those for growth factors, cytokines, CD40 ligand, and adhesion molecules, among others. In non-lymphocytes, genes for adhesion to endothelial cells and differentiation are down-regulated. Because of these potent generalized effects, steroids are often used in induction and maintenance therapy, or to combat moderate rejection. (Lindenfeld et al., 2004) However, continued use of steroids is associated with "Cushingoid" symptoms, such as weight gain, hirsutism, and accumulation of fat in the face and posterior neck (which are known as moon face and buffalo hump, respectively). Thus, there is an attempt to limit the duration of steroid therapies and dosages are carefully tapered off.(Gruessner A.C., 2014)

Advancement of Drugs in Allograft Rejection

Therapies to enhance immunosuppression, limit adverse effects and improve overall outcomes are constantly being developed and tested. Among the forefront are sirolimus and its derivative everolimus, the former receiving FDA approval in 1999 and the latter awaiting approval after showing success in clinical trials. Sirolimus is a macrolide antibiotic with a structure similar to that of tacrolimus. However, rather than targeting calcineurin, sirolimus inhibits the activation of TOR. This not only prevents the proliferation of T- and B-cells, but also that of arterial smooth muscle cells and endothelial cells.5 The significance of this mechanism is that allograft atherosclerosis and tumor growth become negated, giving sirolimus an advantage over CNIs in this instance.(Mudge, 2007) Noted adverse effects include hypercholesterolemia, hyperlipidemia, and hypertriglyceridemia. Moderate thrombocytopenia is also possible though all of these effects are reversible. In trials, the same anti-proliferative effects of sirolimus have been demonstrated with everolimus, though the occurrence of bacterial infections is higher in comparison to AZA.(Lindenfeld J, 2004)

Monoclonal antibodies are being thoroughly investigated due to their potential to be safer and more efficient than other options, especially CNIs Alefacept, in particular, may improve long-term resistance to rejection by decreasing numbers of T-memory cells. Both are indicated for the treatment of psoriasis, and trials for transplant cases have thus far been limited to kidney allografts.4 Anti-CD25 antibodies, such as daclizumab and basiliximab, lower T-cell production of IL-2 and are approved by the FDA for immunosuppression in renal transplantations when combined with cyclosporine and steroids. Trials with cardiac allograft recipients have shown a promising reduction in the number of acute rejection episodes in comparison to traditional therapies through studies with basiliximab have been more ambiguous. Antibodies to target CD28, which is involved in T-cell activation, are also being developed. The chimeric molecule CTLA4Ig seems promising, as it has a greater affinity for CD28 than its endogenous ligands, B7-1 and -2.1 another antibody therapy, Campath-1H, is awaiting approval by the FDA for transplant immunosuppression. It targets CD25, which has an unknown function but is found in high concentrations in lymphocytes, suggesting it has a pivotal role in immune response. Trials have shown that when paired with sirolimus, Campath-1H produces nearly 100% three-year survival rates, despite having a relatively high early rejection rate (28%) (Mehra, Uber, & Kaplan, 2006).

Another immunosuppressive agent used in the prevention of rejection episodes is anti-thymocyte globulin (ATG). Its various mechanisms include inhibiting the process of leukocyte adhesion to microvascular endothelium and subsequent extravasation of effector cells, as well as induction of apoptosis of leukocytes infiltrating grafts. Additionally, ATG works to modulate the activity of dendritic cells in vivo. A prospective randomized study was done by Faggian et. al in 2010 determined that high-dose ATG lead to a lower rate of early and late complications, specifically with graft vasculopathy (Faggian et al., 2010). Muromonab-CD3 (OKT3) is a murine antibody that recognizes the epsilon chain of CD3 molecule on T cells and was used primarily in the treatment of refractory acute allograft rejection (Circulation, 2004). However, due to serious side effects, this drug was removed from the market in 2009. Some of the side effects included but are not limited to hemodynamic compromise, cytokine releasing syndrome, aseptic meningitis, and encephalopathy.

Cell Therapy

During the solid organ transplantation, short-term and long-term acceptance of allografts can be achieved by inducing recipients' immunosuppression via continuous treatment with traditional immunosuppressive drugs. However, long-term treatment with traditional drugs not only causes the heavy economic burden to patients but also lead to serious side effects on patient's metabolism, resulting in diabetes and hyperlipidemia. So it is urgent to develop the novel immunosuppressive therapy for solid organ transplantation. Cellular immunotherapy base on all kinds of cells with immunosuppressive function is a potential one (Fandrich, 2010). More and more studies have demonstrated that mesenchymal stem cell (MSCs), myeloid-derived suppressor cells (MDSC), dendritic cells, pluripotent cells and Treg cells have an immunosuppressive function, and they are promising to be used in cellular immunotherapy in organ transplantation.

Mesenchymal Stem Cells (MSCs)

More than 40 years ago, MSCs were first identified and isolated from bone marrow. After that, more and more studies show that MSCs have emerged as one of the most promising candidates for cell therapy in tissue injury because of their self-renewal ability and potential differentiation into three principal lineages, such as osteoblastic, adipocytic and chondrocyte lineages. For their property of treating cardiac repair, numerous studies demonstrate that human MSCs transdifferentiate into cardiomyocytes by coculturing of ventricular myocytes in vitro or being injected into mouse heart in vivo.

In addition to their treatment in tissue injury, MSCs can be applied to treat some immune disorders because MSCs also play a critical role in regulating the immune response (Aggarwal & Pittenger, 2005). MSCs themselves can escape host immune response after being infused into an allogeneic host because they do not express some molecules human leukocyte antigen (HLA) major histocompatibility complex (MHC) class I, B7-1, B7-2, CD40 and CD40 ligand in the cell surface. Now more and more studies show that MSCs have a powerful immunomodulatory in vivo. For examples, the infusion of BM-derived MSCs can alleviate graft-versus-host disease (GVHD) both in mice and in humans. In systemic lupus erythematosus (SLE) patients, umbilical cord (UC)-derived MSCs were able to inhibit inflammation and reduce damage to the bowel. Similarly in Crohn's disease patient, autologous BM-derived MSCs could reduce inflammation and protect the kidneys. For skin allograft, infusion of allogeneic MSCs could extend the survival of skin allograft in immunocompetent baboons. In the allogeneic small bowel transplantation, treatment of bone marrow mesenchymal stem cells (BMMSCs) treatment can prolong the survival of allograft by reducing acute cellular rejection and apoptosis.

Heart transplantation, one kind of solid organ transplantation has more severe immunologic rejection. MSCs have been used as an immunosuppressive therapy in animal models and clinical trials of some organ transplantation, including heart transplantation models (Wu et al., 2013). The evidence for recent studies demonstrated that transfusion of MSCs into recipients could be a new immunosuppressive therapy in heart transplantation since they can reduce immunologic rejection and prolong the survival of allografts. The scientists demonstrate that transfusion of donor-derived MSCs into recipients indeed can prolong the survival of cardiac allografts by promoting the expansion of Treg cells and reducing the production of pro-inflammatory cytokines. In control group without transfusion of donor MSCs, all the cardiac allografts are rejected within 13 days. However, in the treatment group, transfusion of donor MSCs dramatically prolong the survival time of cardiac allografts. Another study confirms this result. Transfusion of MSCs before heart transplantation or one day after transplantation can promote an accumulation of CD4+ CD25+ Foxp3+ Treg cells which induce immune tolerance. However, coinjection donor MSCs and hematopoietic stem cells (HSCs) can block the MSCs-induced immune tolerance, indicating HSCs can block the immune tolerance induced by MSCs. So researchers may further investigate how HSCs negative regulate MSCs-induced immunosuppression in heart transplantation. In the chronic rejection of heart transplantation, alloreactive CD4+ T cells cause the vascular stenosis in the cardiac graft, finally resulting in cardiac allograft rejection. After cardiac transplantation, transfusion of MSCs can promote the T cell population change from Th1/Th2 to anti-inflammatory Th2, resulting in the inhibition of chronic rejection. Recent studies focus on the conjoint effect of combining MSCs with traditional anti-immune drugs in heart transplantation. MSCs transfusion combined with low-dose rapamycin treatment significantly induce immunosuppression and prolong the long-term survival of cardiac allografts (H. Wang et al., 2014). This function relies on the expression of B7-H1 on the surface of MSCs. The effect of MSC treatment combining with other clinical immunosuppressive drugs, including sirolimus (Srl), ciclosporin A (CiA) and mycophenolate mofetil (MMF) have been investigated.

Although MSCs treatment in heart transplantation has a promising therapeutic effect, the extending survival time still is too short. We know that MSCs can escape the immune response. Once MSCs differentiated in vivo, the immune attack will come back. So cellular immunotherapy based on MSCs should be developed. Combination MSCs immunotherapy with traditional immunosuppressive drugs is a feasible way to improve the therapeutic efficiency. A Recent study demonstrates the conjoint effect on combination MSCs with MMF or rapamycin in immune tolerance during heart transplantation. Combined treatment with MSCs and other type immunosuppressive cells may be another potential therapy in future.

Myeloid-Derived Suppressor Cells (MDSC)

More than 20 years ago MDSC were first described in tumor-bearing mice or cancer patients. The increasing MDSC population was detected in the peripheral blood of patients with different types of cancer, promoting tumor escape from host immune response. In addition to cancers, MDSC accumulation also found in some inflammation relative diseases, including various acute and chronic inflammation, bacterial infection, sepsis, traumatic stress and autoimmunity. Collectively, all above evidence suggests that MDSC accumulation is a common phenotype in all kinds of inflammation.

MDSC are a heterogeneous cell population which including progenitor cells of macrophages, granulocytes, dendritic cells and immature myeloid cells, defined by a function of immune suppressive activity and phenotype with expression of characteristics relate to hematopoietic cell precursors. MDSC can be identified by the high level of myeloid cell surface marker CD11b and the low level of MHC class II molecules. Phenotypically, MDSCs include two different subsets monocytic and granulocytic.

The primary function of MDSC is to mediate immune suppression via suppressing proliferation and cytokine production in both T and NK cells. MDSC also can induce the apoptosis of some subpopulation of T cells. Further studies show that multiple signal pathways were involved in MDSC mediated immune suppression(Nagaraj, Schrum, Cho, Celis, & Gabrilovich, 2010), such as inducible nitric oxide synthetase (iNOS), hemeoxygenase 1 (HO-1), Arginase-1 (Arg-1), NADPH oxidase (NOX2) and TGFβ. Because of the negative regulation of immune response, MDSC may be a useful resource to regulate transplantation tolerance in organ transplantation.

The relation between MDSC and transplantation tolerance was first described in kidney allografting model in rat(Boros, Ochando, Chen, & Bromberg, 2010). In this model, treatment with anti-CD28 antibodies can induce the immune tolerance to rat kidney allograft. In the same time, an accumulation of $CD3^-$ class II^- $CD11b^+$ $CD80/86^+$ cells were found in the blood of tolerant recipients. Further studies identified those cells as MDSC by function to inhibit the proliferation of effector T cells and to induce apoptosis in effector T cells. Inhibition of the activity of iNOS by iNOS inhibitor amino guanidine promoted the allografts rejection. Another study shows the similar result, both granulocytic and monocytic MDSC suddenly increase in recipients after renal transplantation. These observations demonstrate that the expansion of MDSC during kidney transplantation indeed participate in the induction of transplantation tolerance. However, an only adoptive transfer of MDSC to transplanted recipients cannot induce kidney allograft tolerance in the rat model, suggesting MDSC themselves are not enough to induce this allograft tolerance. The similar results were reported in renal transplant patients. After transplantation $CD11b^+$ $CD33^+$ and HLA^-DR^- MDSC population increased in patients and suppressed the proliferation of $CD4^+$ T cells. In graft-versus-host disease (GVHD), expansion of donor-derived T cells can induce anti-recipient immune attack and lead to the death of the recipient. Pre-injection of MDSC can reduce the lethality of GVHD by inducing the differentiation of donor-derived T cells into Th2 T cells in the mouse model.

In heart transplantation mouse model, mammalian target of rapamycin (mTOR) inhibitors can be used to induce immunosuppression, contributing to the survival of cardiac allograft. The results show that the number of MDSC in recipients with rapamycin treatment rapidly increases compared to that in control mice (Zhang et al., 2014). At the same time, the iNOS level also increases in those MDSC. Further study reveals that mTOR and its downstream Raf/MEK/ERK signal pathway play a critical role in the recruitment and expansion of MDSC. In another study, use of anti-CD200 antibody also can promote the survival of cardiac allograft. In this cardiac transplantation model, treatment with anti-CD200 antibody also can promote the production of Treg cells and MDSC. In another chronic cardiac rejection mouse model, donor hearts from B6.C-H2bm12/KhEg mice are transplanted into recipients, MHC class II-mismatched C57BI/6J mice. Treatment with interleukin-33 (IL-33) can inhibit chronic cardiac rejection and significantly prolong the survival of cardiac allografts(Gajardo, Morales, Campos-Mora, Campos-Acuna, & Pino-Lagos, 2015). Results show that pretreatment with IL-33 decreases the level of IL-17A but increases the production of IL5, IL-10, and IL-13. At the same time, evidence from flow cytometry assay shows that IL-33 treatment induces the CD4+ Foxp3+ Treg cells and CD11b (high) Grl (intermediate) MDSC. Collectively, the expansion of MDSC plays a central role in extending the long-term survival of cardiac allografts by treatment with some drugs or other factors. That means MDSC could also play a significant role in cardiac transplantation. Investigation of the detailed mechanism of the expansion of MDSC in cardiac transplantation can better understand the function of MDSC in cardiac transplantation and finally promote the application of MDSC in human cardiac transplantation.

Other Immunosuppressive Cells

Beside MSC and MDSC, there are other types of cells involved in immunosuppression, including Dendritic cells (DCs)(van Kooten et al., 2011), Treg cells(Chai et al., 2015) and pluripotent cells(Imberti, Monti, & Casiraghi, 2015). In the mammalian immune system, DCs are one kind of antigen-presenting cells which process antigens and present them to T cells or B cells. In the beginning, it is well-known that DCs can promote the immune response. Activation of DCs enhances anti-tumor immune response. DCs can be activated by Toll-like receptor (TLR) and then inhibit Treg cells function, finally resulting in activation of the immune response. However, among the DCs, some subpopulation of regulatory DCs play a priority role in the control of autoimmune disease by suppressing the immune response. A recent study shows that the subpopulation of CD11b(high) la(low) regulatory DCs that come from hematopoietic stem cells or mature DCs can inhibit the immune response in a feedback way. Activated Fas signal in the regulatory DCs promotes them to secrete IL-10 and IP-10, and then significantly inhibits the proliferation of CD4+ T cells (Y. Wang, Bi, Wu, & Wang, 2011). At the same time, CD4+ T cells themselves can Secret Fas ligand to promote regulatory DCs-induced inhibition of CD4+ T cells in a negative feedback mechanism. Immunological rejection is one of the significant problems in Allogeneic tooth transplantation. One recent study focuses on the application of immature DCs in immune tolerance of mice allogenic tooth transplantation. Donor bone marrow-derived immature DCs are injected into recipients with allogenic or autogenic tooth transplantation. No blatant rejection is found in both autogenic transplantation groups without or with the treatment of immature DCs. However, in allogeneic transplantation groups, treatment with immature DCs significantly reduces rejection compared to control treatment. Indoleamine 2, 3-dioxygenase (IDO) can inhibit allograft rejection by suppressing T cell response (Yu et al., 2008). The subpopulation of IDO+ DCs has been confirmed to inhibit the expansion of CD4+ CD25- T cells in vitro. Treatment with 3-HAA can enhance this inhibition induced by IDO+ DCs. Further study in mouse small bowel transplantation model confirms this fact that treatment with IDO+ DCs and 3-HAA dramatically prolong the survival time of allograft. A recent survey shows the migration of host-derived and donor-derived DCs in heart transplantation model. The results demonstrate that host-derived DCs are induced to migrate into the cardiac allograft quickly after transplantation. However, later both host-derived and donor-derived DCs can be found in host spleen and hepatic lymph nodes. This evidence indicates that DCs could be associated with the survival of cardiac allografts. Different subpopulations of DCs present the opposite functions in heart transplantation. In heart transplantation, the organs from older donor have shorter survival time than the one from the young donor because there are CD11c+ DCs in the older heart can trigger the production of IL-17A in recipients which induce expansion of CD4+ CD8+ T cells and alloimmune response. The survival time of older allografts will be extended by depletion of CD11c+ DCs before transplantation or blockade of IL-17A. Another study demonstrates that mir-155 can accelerate cardiac allograft rejection by induced differentiation of DCs. This evidence verifies the existence of the anti-transplantation DCs. In contrast, some subsets of DCs that inhibit immune response during heart transplantation have also been found. One subpopulation of DCs, named Tolerogenic DCs (Tol-DCs) is a group of immature DCs. Transfusion of Tol-DCs into recipients can induce immune tolerance and prolong the survival of cardiac allografts in heart transplantation model. Tol-DCs can induce the proliferation of Treg cells, inhibit the effect of cytotoxic lymphocytes and promote Th2 cells differentiation. Combined treatment fms-like tyrosine kinase three ligands (Flt3L) with low-dose rapamycin can dramatically prolong the survival of cardiac allografts compared to untreated group. The mechanism is that this combined treatment can induce the expansion of Tol-DCs and Treg cells. Now we know that Tol-DCs can be obtained from four methods, such as gene modification, drug induction, cytokine induction and isolation of liver or spleen. Treatment with drug NK026680, a novel triazolopyridine derivative, induces the production of Tol-DCs that prolong the survival of cardiac allografts by inhibiting the immune response. Soluble CD83 also can induce the production of Tol-DCs, resulting in heart transplant tolerance and longtime survival of heart allografts. Other studies show that Tol-DCs also can be induced by the blockade of CD40-CD40L costimulation, NBD-peptide and LF15-0195. Altogether, Tol-DCs play the key roles in transplantation immune tolerance. Further studies of the mechanism of Tol-DCs can contribute to the survival of cardiac transplantation.

The functions of Treg cells in immune tolerance have been well-described. Numerous studies based on animal transplantation model demonstrate that Treg cells play an effective role in transplantation immune tolerance and promote the survival of allograft. Adoptive transfusion of TCRαβ (+) CD3 (+) $CD4^{-}CD8^{-}NK1.1^{-}$ (double negative, DN) T cells can induce expansion of CD4+ Foxp3+ Treg cells that contribute to long-term cardiac allograft survival. Combined treatment simvastatin with aspirin dramatically promotes the survival time of cardiac allograft by the accumulation of CD4+ CD25+ Treg cells in recipients. Depletion of CD4+ CD25+ Treg cells in recipients promotes the cardiac allograft rejection. Another study shows that IL10 inhibit allograft rejection and prolong the long-term survival of allograft by regulation of CD4+ CD25+ Treg cells (Lu et al., 2014). ECP (extracorporeal photopheresis) has been applied for the treatment of cardiac allograft rejection for several decades. Now scientists demonstrate that ECP-induced immunosuppression depends on promoting the accumulation of Treg cells and the lymphocyte apoptosis. Since the promising function of Treg cells in immunosuppression, the mechanisms of immunosuppression by Treg cells have been verified. Treg cells constitutive express cytotoxic T-lymphocyte antigen-4 (CTLA-4) which inhibits the interaction between CD28 and B7 ligands and block the activation of APC. High-affinity IL-2 receptor CD25 on the surface of Treg cells can consume IL-2 and promote IL-2 depletion-induced the apoptosis of effector T cell. Treg cells also directly secret some immunosuppressive cytokines, such as IL-10, IL-35 and transforming growth factor β (TGF β) to induce immune tolerance. So the transfusion of Treg cells into recipients or induced expansion of Treg cells in recipients by drugs or cytokines may be a potential immunosuppressive therapy in heart transplantation. However, the application of Treg cells in transplantation tolerance is a double-edged sword. They also increase the incidence rate of cancer in recipients.

Although all above kinds of immunosuppressive cells have been verified to play promising functions in solid organ transplantation, the big problem with them is how to obtain enough amount cells for therapy or further studies. The induced pluripotent stem (iPS) cells that are created from patient's somatic cells will be a useful resource for cell therapy. iPS cells can be used for some tissue damage repair like myocardial repair. It is possible to induce directly iPS cells to differentiate into those kinds of immunosuppressive cells. It will overcome the problem of the limitation of those immunosuppressive cells.

Future Role of Nanotechnology in Cardiomyopathies and Transplants

Nanotechnology is defined by the National Nanotechnology Initiative as the understanding and control of matter at dimensions between approximately 1 and 100 nm, where unique phenomena enable novel applications (Buxton, 2011). There have been many recent advances in this field with respect to drug delivery, molecular imaging, and cell labeling (Kim, Ahn, Dvir, & Kim, 2014). For example, it has been discovered that small molecule drugs can be loaded or encapsulated into nanoparticles, and when target ligands are conjugated to the surface of these nanoparticles, they are taken up by target cells, inside which the nanoparticles unload their drug cargo. (Kim et al., 2014) Another study investigated engraftment of a nanoridged polyethylene glycol-based hydrogel scaffold in a myocardial infarction model. In the rat model employed, this scaffold was found to promote retention and growth of transplanted heart cells and their integration into host tissue (Kim, E. 2014). The future of nanotechnology is expanding rapidly, with high hopes of broader amplification in its application to assess valvular disease, predict the expansion of aortic aneurysm, and to assess transplant rejection (Buxton, 2011).

Immunosuppressive Therapy and Immune Globin in Pediatric Heart Transplant

Heart transplantation is a potentially life-saving procedure for children with end-stage heart disease and no other options for survival. Though transplant is not a guaranteed cure and may be followed by multiple complications, expected a lifespan of the patient can be drastically prolonged. This is in part due to immunosuppressive regimens specifically tailored to pediatric needs, which improves patient and allograft survival and overall outcomes. More recently, an increasing number of therapies have been developed to minimize toxicity while boosting efficacy. Such improvements combat the inherent limitations of immunosuppressants, such as susceptibility to infection and failure to prevent allograft rejection.

Indications, Prognosis, and Complications

Due to the number of risks associated with cardiac transplantation in children, this option is only considered when all other forms of treatment have been exhausted. Indications include progressive heart failure that remains unresponsive to medical treatment, congenital heart disease that cannot be feasibly repaired with surgery, and unresponsive malignant arrhythmias. (Darst JR, 2012) All conditions result in end-stage heart disease and lower the life expectancy of the patient to less than two years.(Fish R.M., 2011) The current estimated life expectancy for all pediatric patients following a cardiac transplant is over fourteen years though exact numbers cannot be determined since the procedure was only recently introduced in the mid-1980s.(Benden et al., 2012)

Immediately following surgery, the quality of life and prognosis are typically good. Immunosuppressive therapies do leave the recipient susceptible to infections, most commonly with cytomegalovirus or reactivation of latent viruses. Such infections are life threatening and are the second leading cause of death within the first year following a pediatric heart transplant. Live and attenuated vaccinations are thus avoided immediately following surgery. (Fish R.M., 2011)

Cardiac allograft vasculopathy, also called graft coronary artery disease, is one of the most concerning long-term complications following pediatric heart transplantation. The proliferation of the intima in coronary arteries causes narrowing or complete occlusion of the lumen and can diffuse to distal vessels, making treatments such as stents, bypass grafting, or angioplasty obsolete. The direct relationship to immunosuppressive therapy remains unknown. Thus, adjustments to avoid the development of cardiac allograft vasculopathy are difficult to make. (Darst JR, 2012)

Chronic immunosuppressive therapy with CNIs such as cyclosporine and tacrolimus may also cause renal impairment. Treatment with alternatives, namely sirolimus and everolimus, may lessen nephrotoxic effects and the development of long-term complications. (Fish R.M., 2011)

In adolescent patients, non-compliance with immunosuppressant regimens may be the leading cause of cause of death post-operatively. New medications and administration strategies are being implemented to raise adherence in these individuals. (Darst JR, 2012)

Current Immunosuppressive Therapy Protocol

Various combinations of immunosuppressants exist as possible therapy options in pediatric recipients. Regimens include monotherapies, dual therapies, and triple therapies, and a CNI (cyclosporine or tacrolimus) is always included. (Khimji, Kazmerski, & Webber, 2008) Avoidance of steroids, especially in cardiac transplants, is becoming increasingly common due to side effects such as growth retardation, impaired wound healing, and Cushingoid symptoms.(Darst JR, 2012) Therefore, dual therapies may instead contain AZA, MMF, or sirolimus/everolimus in accompaniment to a CNI. Triple therapies typically consist of a CNI, steroid, and either AZA/MMF or sirolimus/everolimus.(Khimji et al., 2008)

New Immunosuppressive Therapies in Pediatric Heart Transplantation

While several new medications are in development, most have not been extensively tested in pediatric patients. Promising data has been gathered in adult trials that can be extrapolated to pediatric situations, and hopefully, will lead to successful applications in the near future.

Alemtuzumab, a monoclonal antibody targeting CD52 found on T- and B-cells, natural killer cells, and monocytes, is becoming a preferred induction agent in transplantation surgeries though it has not yet been FDA approved for this purpose. Studies in children are few in number, but existing evidence in kidney transplants shows alemtuzumab is equally as effective as other inducing agents, based on one-year survival rates and kidney function. (Nguyen & Shapiro, 2014)

A fusion protein of CTLA4 and IgG1, belatacept acts as an inhibitor of T-cell activation and may be an option for pediatric heart transplant recipients. Currently, use has been limited to adult patients, and data has shown that while acute graft rejection rates were higher in comparison to cyclosporine, patient and allograft survival rates were comparable while renal function was significantly better. Furthermore, intravenously administered drugs such as belatacept may remedy non-compliance issues with adolescent patients. (Nguyen & Shapiro, 2014)

Though most immunosuppressants used currently attempt to target T-cell mechanisms, an increasing number of therapies aimed at B-cell alloantibody production has appeared. In particular, bortezomib, which is approved by the FDA for the treatment of multiple myelomas, seems promising. It functions as a proteasome inhibitor and ultimately lowers the number of plasma cells, preventing the production of alloantibodies. (Nguyen & Shapiro, 2014) A study conducted in 2011 by the University of Cincinnati analyzed allograft survival with the use of bortezomib in both adults and pediatric heart transplant recipients. Results showed a substantial decrease in humoral activity, solidifying the potential of bortezomib in immunosuppressive therapies. (Woodle, Walsh, Alloway, Girnita, & Brailey, 2011)

REFERENCES

Abbas, A. (2003). Transplantation Immunology. *Cellular & Molecular Immunology*, 359–381.

Aggarwal, S., & Pittenger, M. F. (2005). Human mesenchymal stem cells modulate allogeneic immune cell responses. *Blood, 105*(4), 1815–1822. doi:10.1182/blood-2004-04-1559 PMID:15494428

Alraies, M. C., & Eckman, P. (2014). Adult heart transplant: Indications and outcomes. *Journal of Thoracic Disease*, *6*(8), 1120. PMID:25132979

Benden, C., Edwards, L. B., Kucheryavaya, A. Y., Christie, J. D., Dipchand, A. I., Dobbels, F., & Hertz, M. I. et al. (2012). The Registry of the International Society for Heart and Lung Transplantation: Fifteenth pediatric lung and heart-lung transplantation report2012. *The Journal of Heart and Lung Transplantation, 31*(10), 1087–1095. doi:10.1016/j.healun.2012.08.005 PMID:22975098

Boros, P., Ochando, J. C., Chen, S. H., & Bromberg, J. S. (2010). Myeloid-derived suppressor cells: Natural regulators for transplant tolerance. *Human Immunology, 71*(11), 1061–1066. doi:10.1016/j.humimm.2010.08.001 PMID:20705113

Chai, J. G., Ratnasothy, K., Bucy, R. P., Noelle, R. J., Lechler, R., & Lombardi, G. (2015). Allospecific CD4(+) T cells retain effector function and are actively regulated by Treg cells in the context of transplantation tolerance. *European Journal of Immunology*, *45*(7), 2017–2027. doi:10.1002/eji.201545455 PMID:25944401

Darst, C. K. Jr, & Miyamoto, S. D. (2012). Cardiovascular Diseases. *CURRENT Diagnosis & Treatment. Pediatrics*, *21e*, 20.

Deng, M. C. (2002). Cardiac transplantation. *Heart (British Cardiac Society)*, *87*(2), 177–184. doi:10.1136/heart.87.2.177 PMID:11796563

Faggian, G., Forni, A., Milano, A. D., Chiominto, B., Walpoth, B. H., Scarabelli, T., & Mazzucco, A. (2010). Antithymocyte globulin induction therapy in heart transplantation: Prospective randomized study of high vs standard dosage. *Transplantation Proceedings*, *42*(9), 3679–3687. doi:10.1016/j.transproceed.2010.06.036 PMID:21094838

Fandrich, F. (2010). Cell therapy approaches aiming at minimization of immunosuppression in solid organ transplantation. *Current Opinion in Organ Transplantation*, *15*(6), 703–708. doi:10.1097/MOT.0b013e328340669a PMID:20930635

Fish, R. M. M. M. G. (2011). The Transplant Patient. Tintinalli's Emergency Medicine: A Comprehensive Study Guide. Academic Press.

Gajardo, T., Morales, R. A., Campos-Mora, M., Campos-Acuna, J., & Pino-Lagos, K. (2015). Exogenous interleukin-33 targets myeloid-derived suppressor cells and generates periphery-induced Foxp3(+) regulatory T cells in skin-transplanted mice. *Immunology*, *146*(1), 81–88. doi:10.1111/imm.12483 PMID:25988395

Gallino, A., Eugster, W., Schneider, K., Furrer, M., & Turina, M. (1988). Indications and contra-indications for heart transplantation. *Schweizerische Medizinische Wochenschrift*, *118*(14), 522–524. PMID:3287606

Grauhan, O., Müller, J., Volk, H., Fietze, E., Cohnert, T., Meyer, R.,... Warnecke, H. (1998). Treatment of humoral rejection after heart transplantation. *The Journal of Heart and Lung Transplantation: The Official Publication of the International Society for Heart Transplantation, 17*(12), 1184-1194.

Hillebrands, J.-L., Klatter, F. A., van den Hurk, B. M., Popa, E. R., Nieuwenhuis, P., & Rozing, J. (2001). Origin of neointimal endothelium and α-actin–positive smooth muscle cells in transplant arteriosclerosis. *The Journal of Clinical Investigation*, *107*(11), 1411–1422. doi:10.1172/JCI10233 PMID:11390423

Imberti, B., Monti, M., & Casiraghi, F. (2015). Pluripotent stem cells and tolerance induction in organ transplantation. *Current Opinion in Organ Transplantation*, *20*(1), 86–93. doi:10.1097/MOT.0000000000000144 PMID:25522138

Jessup, M., Abraham, W. T., Casey, D. E., Feldman, A. M., Francis, G. S., Ganiats, T. G., & Silver, M. A. et al. (2009). 2009 focused update: ACCF/AHA guidelines for the diagnosis and management of heart failure in adults: a report of the American College of Cardiology Foundation/American Heart Association Task Force on Practice Guidelines developed in collaboration with the International Society for Heart and Lung Transplantation. *Journal of the American College of Cardiology*, *53*(15), 1343–1382. doi:10.1016/j.jacc.2008.11.009 PMID:19324967

Jung, S.-H., Kim, J. J., Choo, S. J., Yun, T.-J., Chung, C. H., & Lee, J. W. (2011). Long-term mortality in adult orthotopic heart transplant recipients. *Journal of Korean Medical Science*, *26*(5), 599–603. doi:10.3346/jkms.2011.26.5.599 PMID:21532848

Khimji, I. A., Kazmerski, T. M., & Webber, S. A. (2008). Immunosuppressive Agents in Pediatric Heart Transplantation. In Handbook of Pediatric Cardiovascular Drugs (pp. 190-214). Springer Science + Business Media.

Kim, E. S., Ahn, E. H., Dvir, T., & Kim, D. H. (2014). Emerging nanotechnology approaches in tissue engineering and regenerative medicine. *International Journal of Nanomedicine*, *9*(Suppl 1), 1–5. doi:10.2147/IJN.S61212 PMID:24872698

Leclercq, C. (2007). New guidelines for cardiac resynchronisation therapy: Simplicity or complexity for the doctor? *Heart (British Cardiac Society)*, *93*(9), 1017–1019. doi:10.1136/hrt.2007.122267 PMID:17699167

Lilly, L. S. (2012). *Pathophysiology of heart disease: a collaborative project of medical students and faculty*. Lippincott Williams & Wilkins.

Lindenfeld, J., Miller, G. G., Shakar, S. F., Zolty, R., Lowes, B. D., Wolfel, E. E., & Kobashigawa, J. et al. (2004). Drug therapy in the heart transplant recipient: part I: cardiac rejection and immunosuppressive drugs. *Circulation*, *110*(24), 3734–3740. doi:10.1161/01.CIR.0000149745.83186.89 PMID:15596559

Lindenfeld, J. M. G., Shakar, S. F., Zolty, R., Lowes, B. D., Wolfel, E. E., Mestroni, L., & Kobashigawa, J. et al. (2004). Drug therapy in the heart transplant recipient–Part II: Immunosuppressive drugs. *Circulation, 110*, 7. PMID:15611389

Lu, X., Yang, X., Zhou, Q., Wang, Y., Feng, S., Jin, J., & Chen, J. et al. (2014). Cardiac allograft tolerance induced by isogeneic CD4+CD25+ regulatory T cells. *Experimental and Clinical Transplantation, 12*(2), 133–138. Retrieved from http://www.ncbi.nlm.nih.gov/pubmed/24702146 PMID:24702146

Lund, L. H., Edwards, L. B., Kucheryavaya, A. Y., Benden, C., Christie, J. D., Dipchand, A. I., & Meiser, B. et al. (2014). The registry of the International Society for Heart and Lung Transplantation: thirty-first official adult heart transplant report—2014; focus theme: retransplantation. *The Journal of Heart and Lung Transplantation, 33*(10), 996–1008. doi:10.1016/j.healun.2014.08.003 PMID:25242124

Mehra, M. R., Uber, P. A., & Kaplan, B. (2006). Immunosuppression in cardiac transplantation: Science, common sense and the heart of the matter. *American Journal of Transplantation, 6*(6), 1243–1245. doi:10.1111/j.1600-6143.2006.01326.x PMID:16686745

Milla, F., Pinney, S. P., & Anyanwu, A. C. (2012). Indications for heart transplantation in current era of left ventricular assist devices. *Mount Sinai Journal of Medicine: A Journal of Translational and Personalized Medicine, 79*(3), 305-316.

Montgomery, R. A., Cozzi, E., West, L. J., & Warren, D. S. (2011). Humoral immunity and antibody-mediated rejection in solid organ transplantation. *Seminars in Immunology, 23*(4), 224–234. doi:10.1016/j.smim.2011.08.021 PMID:21958960

Mozaffarian, D., Benjamin, E. J., Go, A. S., Arnett, D. K., Blaha, M. J., Cushman, M., & Stroke Statistics, S. et al. (2015). Heart disease and stroke statistics2015 update: A report from the American Heart Association. *Circulation, 131*(4), e29–e322. doi:10.1161/CIR.0000000000000152 PMID:25520374

Mudge, G. H. (2007). Sirolimus and Cardiac Transplantation: Is It the Magic Bullet? *Circulation, 116*(23), 2666–2668. doi:10.1161/CIRCULATIONAHA.107.737965 PMID:18056538

Nagaraj, S., Schrum, A. G., Cho, H. I., Celis, E., & Gabrilovich, D. I. (2010). Mechanism of T cell tolerance induced by myeloid-derived suppressor cells. *Journal of Immunology (Baltimore, MD.: 1950), 184*(6), 3106–3116. doi:10.4049/jimmunol.0902661 PMID:20142361

Nguyen, C., & Shapiro, R. (2014). New immunosuppressive agents in pediatric transplantation. *Clinics (Sao Paulo), 69*(Suppl 1), 8–16. doi:10.6061/clinics/2014(Sup01)03 PMID:24860853

Tse, H. (2011). *Oxford desk reference*. Oxford, UK: Oxford University Press. doi:10.1093/med/9780199568093.001.0001

van Kooten, C., Lombardi, G., Gelderman, K. A., Sagoo, P., Buckland, M., Lechler, R., & Cuturi, M. C. (2011). Dendritic cells as a tool to induce transplantation tolerance: Obstacles and opportunities. *Transplantation, 91*(1), 2–7. doi:10.1097/TP.0b013e31820263b3 PMID:21452405

Wang, H., Qi, F., Dai, X., Tian, W., Liu, T., Han, H., & Du, C. et al. (2014). Requirement of B7-H1 in mesenchymal stem cells for immune tolerance to cardiac allografts in combination therapy with rapamycin. *Transplant Immunology, 31*(2), 65–74. doi:10.1016/j.trim.2014.06.005 PMID:24978830

Wang, Y., Bi, Y., Wu, K., & Wang, C. (2011). Dendritic cell co-transfected with FasL and allergen genes induces T cell tolerance and decreases airway inflammation in allergen induced murine model. *Molecular Biology Reports*, *38*(2), 809–817. doi:10.1007/s11033-010-0170-7 PMID:20373028

Woodle, E. S., Walsh, R. C., Alloway, R. R., Girnita, A., & Brailey, P. (2011). Proteasome inhibitor therapy for antibody-mediated rejection. *Pediatric Transplantation*, *15*(6), 548–556. doi:10.1111/j.1399-3046.2011.01543.x PMID:21884344

Wu, S. M., Zhang, W. X., Wang, M. H., Zhang, H. Z., Wu, D. G., Zhou, Z. J., & Xiong, L. H. (2013). Proteomic analysis of the immunosuppressive effects of mesenchymal stem cells in a rat heart transplantation model. *Adv Clin Exp Med, 22*(6), 785-794. Retrieved from http://www.ncbi.nlm.nih.gov/pubmed/24431306

Yu, G., Fang, M., Gong, M., Liu, L., Zhong, J., Feng, W., & Gong, F. et al. (2008). Steady state dendritic cells with forced IDO expression induce skin allograft tolerance by upregulation of regulatory T cells. *Transplant Immunology*, *18*(3), 208–219. doi:10.1016/j.trim.2007.08.006 PMID:18047928

Zhang, Y., Bi, Y., Yang, H., Chen, X., Liu, H., Lu, Y., & Liu, G. et al. (2014). mTOR limits the recruitment of CD11b+Gr1+Ly6Chigh myeloid-derived suppressor cells in protecting against murine immunological hepatic injury. *Journal of Leukocyte Biology*, *95*(6), 961–970. doi:10.1189/jlb.0913473 PMID:24569105

Section 3

The Recent Technological Advancements in Cardiovascular Sciences

Chapter 13
Recent Innovations in Coronary Stents

Poulomi Sengupta
CSIR-National Chemical Laboratory, India

ABSTRACT

In heart diseases, there are frequent incidents of narrowing or blocking coronary arteries by fatty plaque deposition. As a result, blood pressure rises and the arteries weaken. This can lead to rapid rupture of the blood vessels, also known as heart attack or brain stroke. In some cases the arteries lose elasticity over old age. Heart stent or coronary stent inserts in the blocked/fragile region of coronary artery. It helps to expand the artery to allow free flow of blood and consequently, reduces blood pressure. Over past 20 years there are many modifications and innovations in the field of cardiac stents, in this chapter we will discuss few of those.

INTRODUCTION

Heart: the most important organ for mammals and birds. Heart muscles pump oxygenated blood from its left cavities (Figure 1) to different vital organs (like brain, liver, kidney) and tissues to support various cellular activities. After regional utilities, when the carbondioxide-rich blood reaches the heart (right side), it is transported to lungs to get re-oxygenated. Blood enters left ventricles of heart on its way back and again delivers oxygen to remote tissues.

In this way heart constantly works as a pumping machine that is responsible for our healthy life. With the advancement of technology, less exercise, consumption of ready-to-eat fatty food, smoking, alcoholism and stress, blood gradually develops lower ability to carry oxygen. Or, due to elevated body weight and less physical movements, oxygen carried by the blood is not sufficient to meet the cumulative demand. To combat this, heart tries to pump more blood which creates a lateral pressure on the arteries. Years after year's relatively high pressure pushes the artery walls towards sacrificing its elasticity, they become more rigid progressively. In certain cases, there is plaque like growth (mostly from fatty food) along the inner wall of the arteries. These plaques contain varying amounts of cholesterol, calcium, muscle cells, and connective tissues, a process called 'arteriosclerosis' (also atherosclerosis). Due to this

DOI: 10.4018/978-1-5225-2092-4.ch013

Figure 1. Circulation of blood through heart
Image adapted from http://www.bodylanguageholistic.com/

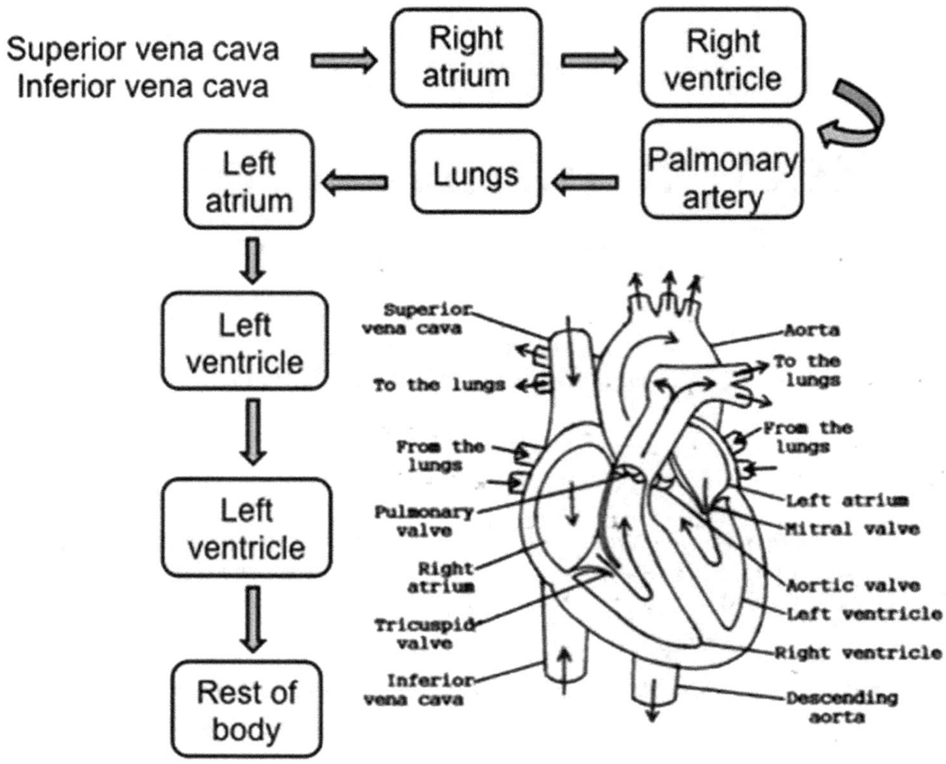

unwanted deposition when coronary arteries narrow more than 50% to 70%, the blood supply beyond the plaque becomes inadequate to meet the increased oxygen demand of the heart muscle during heavy work. Constant flow-in and flow-out push the arteries and veins towards huge pressure on the inner wall. This results in chest pain in 75% cases including shortness of breath (which comes from half functional lungs). These patients are said to have silent angina and are equally prone to a heart attack.

This even results in high-pressure build-up, which can lead to i) rupture of the arteries ii) deoxygenated heart and remote organs/tissues. Either of which, in absence of proper on-time medical intervention can bring up death in few hours. There could also be blood clot in the vessels, which can move around and while in brain can cause partial or total blockage in the arteries leading to a 'brain stroke' (also knows as, ischemic stroke). A brain stroke can be as simple as a mere dementia (partial shut off of few functions as the brain cells are dead due to lack of oxygen). In some cases a hemorrhagic stroke can also take place when a blood vessel within the brain bursts. The reason is mostly uncontrolled hypertension. This can lead up to a whole body paralysis or brain death. In addition to these major problems there are equally life-threatening complications in heart disease like arrhythmia, dysfunctional heart valve etc.

These unfortunate prognoses of cardiovascular diseases are very prevalent in any region, gender making it the most common reason for death in the world. In United States alone almost 610,000 people die from heart disease every year (Xu *et al.*, 2016), that is almost 1 in 4 deaths. Every year at least 735, 000 Americans have a heart attack, of these 525,000 is a first attack. Consequently, cardiovascular procedures performed in the United States have increased to more than three times in last decade. This increased

Figure 2. Timeline of cardiovascular disease treatments

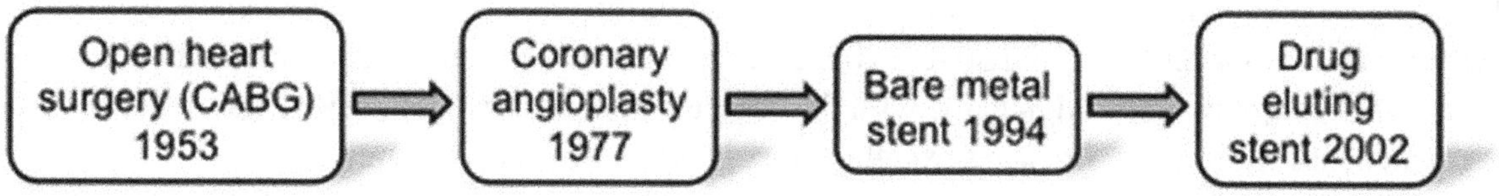

trend is expected to continue with the aging of the population, coupled with epidemics of obesity and diabetes mellitus (Rao *et al.*, 2008). Luckily, with on time proper medical intervention many unfortunate incidents can be avoided. With the tremendous advancement of medical science in past few decades, especially in tackling cardiovascular diseases there are both invasive and non-invasive procedures. Interventions to restore blood flow include: (a) atherectomy (catheter based device to remove the plaque), (b) angiogenesis (use of laser catheter or through gene therapy), (c) brachytherapy (optimum delivery system of gamma or beta radiations), (d) angioplasty (removal or compression of the plaque by use of catheter, balloon or stent) and (e) bypass grafting (detouring around the blockage). In this chapter, we plan to focus on procedure mentioned in (d).

Percutaneous Coronary Intervention (PCI), also recognized as 'angioplasty' is a non-surgical procedure that opens blocked or narrowed coronary arteries. Looking at the severity of a blockage cardiologists take the right decision for a proper intervention. In this method a partial or full body anesthesia is required but dehospitalization is a fast procedure. After the intervention the patient can have a low risk better quality of life through long years. So it is necessary to have an in-depth knowledge about the types of stents, their merits and demerits. We plan to discuss the progress of stent designs, materials and properties. Still, PCI is a recent technique; physicians are challenging cardiovascular disease since long by the following ways.

HISTORY OF CARDIOVASCULAR DISEASES

How was the Treatment Earlier

For long time (first successful open heart surgery being performed in 1953) open heart bypass surgery (coronary artery bypass grafting or CABG) was the only solution for a blocked artery. In this method an active vein from leg or hand is surgically removed and replaced the blocked artery. One of the major interventions performed today is called PCI or percutaneous coronary intervention. It reduced the prevalence of bypass surgery in 90-95% cases. The oldest form of PCI is balloon angioplasty.

Balloon Angioplasty

Balloon angioplasty was first tried in 1977. In this method a long catheter is inserted into the artery through groin or wrist. The tip of the catheter has a balloon, which is inflated as soon as it reaches the area of blocked artery. The inflated balloon can compress the plaque and restore the necessary blood flow with the result of more oxygen delivery to the heart muscles. This was good up until few years when the physicians realized that as soon as the catheter was removed the artery came back to its original shape – also known as elastic recoil. This may lead to the need of emergency bypass graft surgery (CABG). Most importantly, around 30% to 40% cases the plaque also came back with time (or it is called restenosis). A major breakthrough came with the advancement of stents. However, before going to stent like permanent fixture let us browse through some plaque removal techniques.

Plaque Removal Techniques

Various plaque removal devices were devolved in order to remove plaques from the arteries. These are performed using PCI. These include the use of excimer laser for photoablation of plaque, rotational atheroctomy (use of high speed diamond-encrusted drill) for mechanical ablation of plaque, and directional atherectomy for cutting and removal of plaques. These methods were thought to be very effective initially but now a days only used in selective cases as an adjunct to standard percutaneous coronary intervention.

Balloon angioplasty as well as plaque removal techniques are temporary solutions. For a longer relief cardiologists recommend employment of stents.

WHAT ARE 'STENTS'

Stents are thin mesh like tubular metallic structures (Figure 3) which can be inserted in place of a ruptured artery. Coronary stenting is a more permanent form of PCI. With the intercoronary stents, atherectomy, as well as newer pharmacologic agents it reduced complications related to atherosclerosis and reduced recurrence after percutaneous coronary interventions. Currently the recurrence after stenting is lower than 10%.

Figure 3. How coronary stents expand in artery
Image adapted from http://www.telegraph.co.uk/news/uknews/theroyalfamily/8977422/Coronary-stenting-how-does-it-work.html

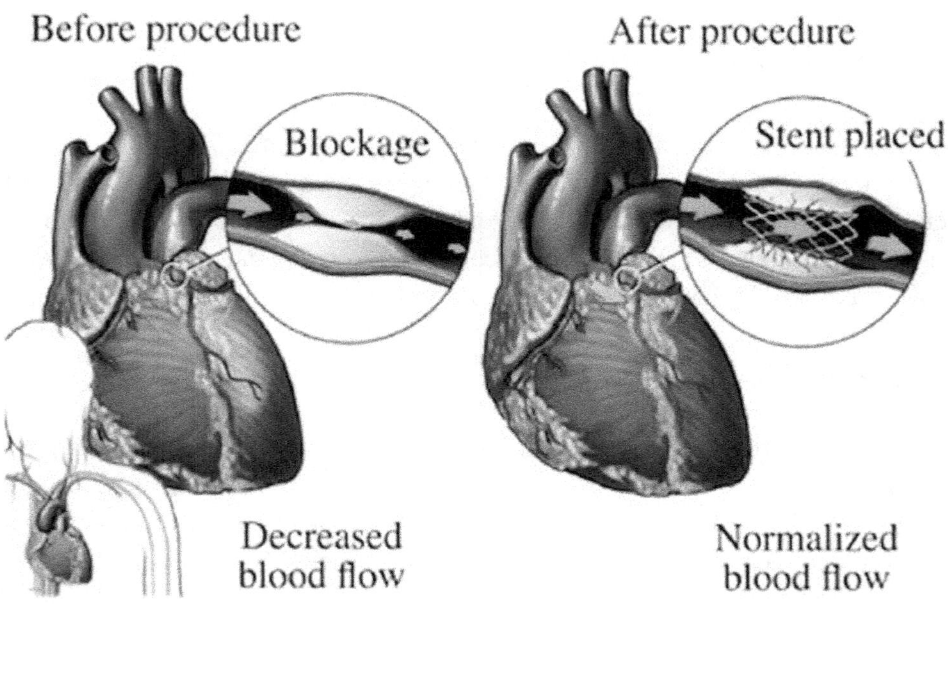

Figure 4. REBEL: Platinum-chromium coronary stent system from Boston Scientific

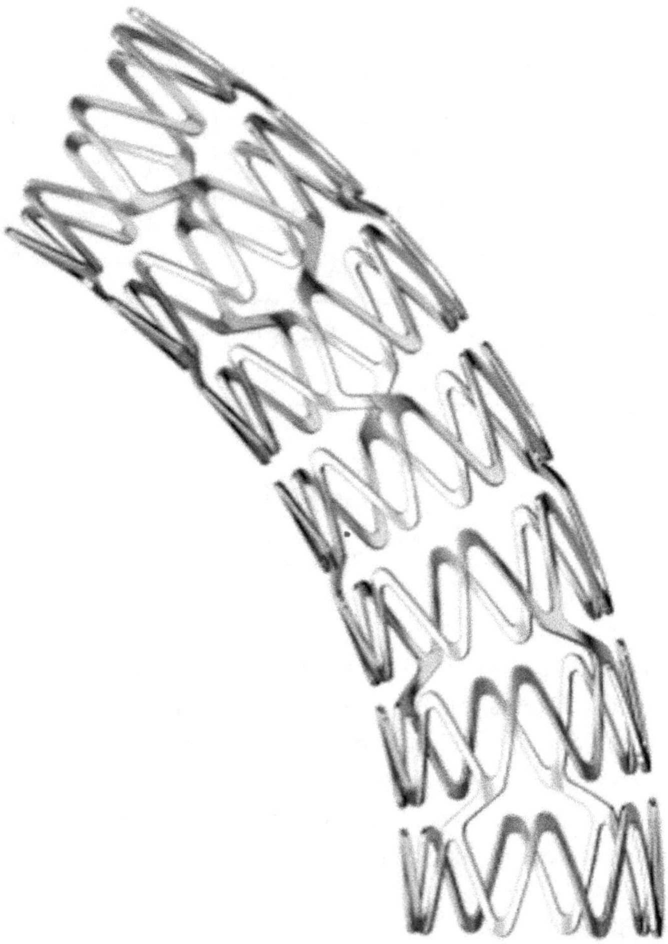

During 1980s it was around 30 years that research on stent was going on. Scientists and cardiologists were waiting for the clinical trial results on the very first stents. In 1986 a French cardiologist first installed a stent. But in the decade of eighties, stents were installed only in the case of abrupt vessel closure and dissections. It could also be employed following angioplasty to avoid restenosis. Now-a-days coronary stents have nearly eliminated the problem of abrupt occlusion, which occurs in 5% of patients where balloon angioplasty is employed. Coronary stenting has reduced the chance of restenosis by more than 50% (Kulick *et al.*, 2010). Most satisfactory from a patient's point of view, no open-heart surgery is at all required during PCI. When successful, it can relieve severe chest pain or angina, improve the prognosis of individuals with unstable angina, and minimize or stop a heart attack without having the patient undergo a open heart coronary artery bypass graft surgery.

In 1994 FDA accepted stents and subsequently more and more patients were treated with stents that are employed by PCI balloon but remain in the artery as 'scaffolds'. This has markedly reduced the chances of emergency CABG to below 1%. At present, the only patients that require just balloon angioplasty are the ones with vessel size lower than 2 mm (minimum diameter stents available). In some cases balloon

Figure 5. Classification of stents

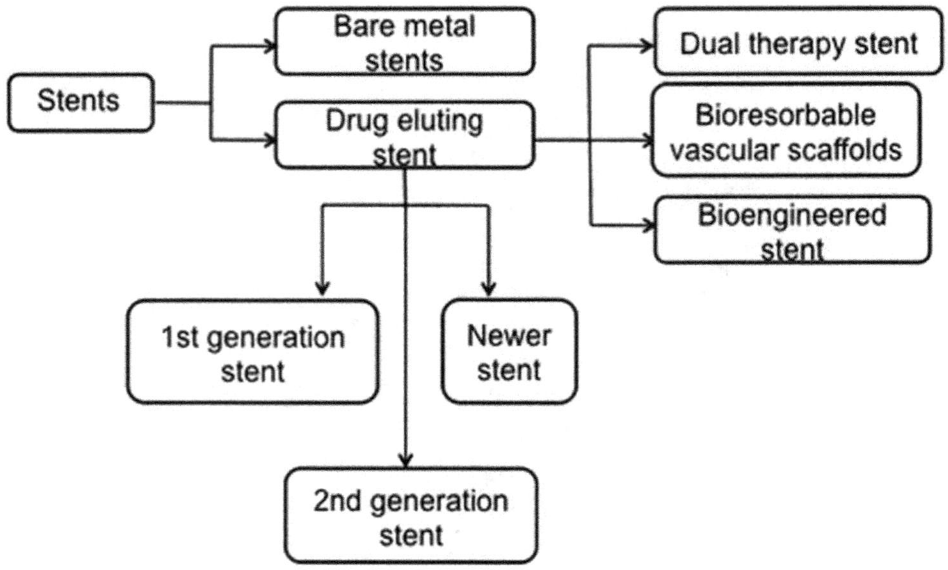

mediated interventions are still necessary. For example, in narrower branches of coronary artery, having scar tissue in already employed stents, for cases where patients are unable to take blood thinners.

Generally after stent employment, patients are prescribed oral blood thinners (like clopidogrel, aspirin) for around a year. To overcome the cumbersome process of pills taking and for better delivery of medications, researchers have come up with drug eluting stents where drug is automatically eluted with time for a long time period. Based on this, stents can be classified in two categories.

Bare Metal Stents (BMS)

Bare metal stents are usually stainless steel stents and have no special coating. They are preloaded in a collapsed form onto a catheter balloon. They act as scaffolding to prop open blood vessels after they are widened with angioplasty. As the artery heals, tissue grows around the stent, holding it in place *(Dangas et al.*, 2002). BMS generally results extremely favourable during the initial clinical results. However, long-term results have been shattered by the dual problems of in-stent restenosis (ISR) or scar tissue formation and stent thrombosis (along with excessive neointimal proliferation) in the arterial lining increasing the risk of re-blockage. Grossly 20-30% patients show eventual re-narrowing of the artery while using BMS.

Drug Eluting Stent (DES)

As discussed in the previous paragraph, incidents of restenosis can take place even after performing a stent. Although patients are prescribed to take anticoagulants, with a considerable time period there is accumulation of plaque or scar tissue inside the employed stent. In some cases the fibrosis or ingression of scar tissue is up to such an extent the tissue slowly covers that metallic mesh of the stent. In these cases deployment of a stent also becomes a challenge. To combat this, the upgraded version of stents has come up with many modifications. The modern stent is a combination of metallic structure along with a thin polymer film. The polymeric film may contain embedded blood thinning drugs, which on slow sustained release removes the clots from arteries. The polymeric film is designed to disappear by slow degradation leaving metallic stent structure alive. With drug eluting stent, the chances of restenosis have been brought under 10%.

Drug Eluting Stents (DES) are coated with medication that is released to help prevent the growth of scar tissue in the artery lining. This helps the artery remain smooth and open, ensuring good blood flow and reduces the chances of the artery re-narrowing or restenosis. The commonly used drugs must be anti-inflammatory, antithrombogenic, antiproliferative and immunosuppressive. However, it also leads to a higher chance of blood clots (stent thrombosis). Commonly used drugs are everolimus, paclitaxel, sirolimus/rapamycin, zotarolimus, biolimus, actinomycin etc (Luscher *et al.*, 2007). Their release profile has been widely investigated in order to establish a slow and sustained release mechanism in presence of proper chemical triggers. Release kinetics and applied dose plays a major role in the duration and magnitude of arterial drug uptake, equally important is the mechanism by which the drug is released.

There have been modifications and up gradation of drug eluting stents. Grossly they are of 3 types:

Dual Therapy Stent (DTS)

Dual Therapy Stent (DTS) is the latest type of coronary stent. The inner wall and outer wall of the stent are differently treated. It is the first stent designed to (i) reduce the likelihood of the re-narrowing of the artery, (ii) help the healing process of the artery by endothelial coverage. It combines the benefit of DES and bio-engineered stents and is the only stent to contain a drug with active healing technology. The stent surface facing the artery wall contains endothelial progenitor cells (EPCs). This plays a pivotal role in stent endothelialization of the artery. EPCs are unique in their ability to promote endothelial regeneration and proper healing of vascular lesions by migrating to lesion sites and differentiating into mature endothelial cells. EPCs are captured by probing with anti-CD34 antibodies. This ultimately promotes natural healing and helps the healthy artery function properly. Simultaneously, it also releases drug that stops the artery blockage without any worry of swelling or an inflammatory response. The drug (generally sirolimus) is delivered from a bioresorbable polymer that will degrade over time. Genous Bio-engineered stent, OrbusNeich Medical Technologies are the pioneers in this technology (Baber *et al.*, 2012).

Bioresorbable Vascular Scaffold (BVS)

The Bio-Vascular Scaffold (BVS) is a drug eluting stent on a dissolvable type of scaffold platform that can be absorbed by the body over time. Before the emergence of drug eluting stents, patients after PCI were subjected to dual antiplatelet therapy (coumadin, clopidogrel). Staying under timely medication is cumbersome. In addition to that, a 'traceless stent' gives some psychological benefits. Like some of the currently available Drug Eluting Stents (DES), BVS is coated with a drug released from a polymer that disappears over time to reduce the likelihood of the artery re-narrowing (restenosis). The scaffold itself is absorbed overtime. Unlike DTS, there is no active element to promote artery healing.

Abbott's bioresorbable stent Absorb™ is made of poly-L-lactide and coated with everolimus. It shows slow degradation over 6 months to 2 years. It has shown very good results in clinical trial as well. Table 1 shows the comparison of different absorbable stents.

Table 1. Comparison of different commercial stents

Absorption Time	2 Years	<4 Months	<4 Months	2 Years	6 Months
Strut Thickness μm	170	165	156	200	200
Deployment	Self expanding and heated balloon	Balloon	Balloon	Balloon	Balloon
Radio opacity	Gold markers	Nil	Pt markers	Iodine impregnated	Nil
Drug elution	Nil	Nil	Everolimus	Nil	Sirolimus salicylate
Absorption products	Lactic acid, CO_2, and H_2O	NA	Lactic acid, CO_2, and H_2O	Amino acids, ethanol,CO_2	Salicylate, CO_2, and H_2O
Design	Zig-zag helical coils with straight bridges	Sinusoidal in phase hoops linked by straight bridges	Cohort A: out-of-phase sinusoidal hoops, straight and direct links; Cohort B: in-phase hoops with straight links	Side and lock	Tube with lasercut voids
Coating material	Nil	Nil	Poly-D,L-lactide	Nil	Salicylate_ different linker
Strut material	Polymer-poly-l-lactic acid	Metal magnesium alloy	Polymer-poly-l-lactide	Polymer tyrosine-Derived Polycarbonate polymer	Polymer salicylate_linker
Stent	Igaki-Tamai	Bioabsorbable Mg alloy	BVS Bioabsorbable vascular solutions	REVA	BTI bioabsorbable Therapeutics inc

Bio-Engineered Stent

Bio-engineered Stent is also known as antibody-coated stent. This type of stent differs from DES because it does not contain a polymer and does not use a drug. As a result, it helps to speed up the cell lining of the artery (endothelialization), promoting natural healing. The antibody on the stent's surface attracts circulating Endothelial Progenitor Cells (EPCs) which come from human bone marrow and help speed up the formation of healthy endothelium. This provides rapid coverage over the stent's surface helping to reduce the risk of early and late thrombosis (blood clots). GenousCoCr from OrbusNeich is marketed using this technology (Lim *et al.*, 2011).

The drug eluting stents again can also be classified into three broad categories (Figure 5). 1. 1st generation stents 2. 2nd generation stents and 3. Newer stents. All DES currently approved in the United States have the same general components, although they differ with respect to the stent platform, polymer, and antirestenotic drug type. Differences may be observed with respect to deliverability (ease of placement), efficacy (prevention of restenosis), and safety (rates of stent thrombosis and myocardial infarction).

The first two DES to be approved in the United States were the sirolimus-eluting stent (SES) in 2003 and paclitaxel-eluting stent (PES) in 2004. They are now often referred to as "first generation" DES. SES are no longer available in the United States and Europe and PES are infrequently used due to superiority of second generation stents (Cutlip *et al.*). In 2008, the zotarolimus-eluting stent (ZES) and the everolimus-eluting stent (EES) were approved for use and now they are referred to as "second generation" DES. The ZES has undergone further modification with a change in polymer to achieve improved pharmacokinetics and has largely replaced the earlier version of ZES. The newer DES has a stent platform of a cobalt-chromium or platinum-chromium alloy, thinner and more deliverable than the first generation DES. In addition, second generation DES are more biocompatible than the first generation DES: They may generate less inflammatory response and have more rapid vessel endothelialization. This biocompatibility and associated reduced inflammatory response is likely due to improvements in polymer technology and may translate into lower rates of myocardial infarction and stent thrombosis. However, despite this potential improvement in biocompatibility, the recommended duration of dual antiplatelet therapy with aspirin and a $P2Y_{12}$ receptor blocker is 12 months, similar to the first generation DES.

PROBLEMS AND RISKS WITH STENTS

Installation of a stent comes with few 'professional hazards'. There are cases of bleeding, fracture of stents, dislodgement, hypersensitivity, stent thrombosis, infection etc. But their occurrence in most cases is lower than 2%. In case of DES implanted patients, due to a relatively slower healing process, they must strictly follow their doctor's recommendation on drug therapy (DAPT) to help reduce risk of stent thrombosis. Current American Heart Association recommendations are for a minimum DAPT therapy of at least 12 months after DES implantation (Levine *et al.*, 2011).

Table 2. Comparison of different drug eluting stents

Special features	Superior to BMS in reducing the magnitude of neointimal proliferation and clinical restenosis • Late stent thrombosis is more likely to occur with these stents		Stent exhibiting clearly lower thrombosis rates as compared to first generation DES			Polymer free DES and biodegradable stents
Polymers	Nonerodable polymer-polyethylene-co-vinyl acetate and poly-n-butyl methacrylate	Soft elastomeric polymer-poly(styrene-bisobutylene-b-styrene)	Persistent, nonerodible, two polymers (a) Polyvinylidene fluoride cohexafluoropropylene and (b) poly-n-butyl methacrylate	Persistent, Biolinx polymer, blend of 3 polymers: hydrophobic C10, hydrophilic C19 and polyvinyl pyrrolidone	Persistent-phosphorylcholine	Biodegradable/ polymer free Poly(styrene-b-isobutylene-b-styrene)
Platform	Stainless steel	Stainless steel	Platinum chromium	Cobalt–chromium	Cobalt–chromium	Cobalt chromium, nickel-titanium, Platinum chromium etc.
Drugs	Sirolimus,	Paclitaxel	Everolimus	Zotarolimus	Zotarolimus	Biolimus, Sirolimus, Everolimus
Examples	Cypher (Cordis Corporation)	Taxus (Boston Scientific)	Xience/Promus (Boston Scientific)	Endeavor Resolute (Medtronic)	Endevour ZES (Medtronic)	Axxess stent NEVO stent Translute™
Types of stents	First generation DES		Seconds generation DES			Other stents

CONCLUSION AND FUTURE DIRECTION

The use of stents has definitely lowered down the occurrence of MACE (major cardiac adverse events). Especially upon the usage of DES there has been a significant reduction in MACE. Although there are huge amount of controversy regarding the efficacy of drug eluting stents, a clinical trial conducted in 2010 indicates reduction in (i) probability of death or myocardial infarction, (ii) probability of stent thrombosis, and also (iii) probability of target vessel revascularization (Kaiser *et al.* 2010). Gershlick *et al.* (2007) pooled outcomes from the first several ZES clinical studies including 1,317 patients and reported that, despite varied baseline clinical and angiographic characteristics, treatment with the ZES was associated with consistently low rates of TVR, stent thrombosis, and overall MACE at 2-year follow-up. In past few years several clinical trials have been conducted worldwide (like SPIRIT and ENDEAVOR trial series) which compare the efficacy of EES over ZES or PES. Still, cardiac disease is not fully manageable. The new age clinicians and scientists should work together and focus on the following points: (i) assessment whether stent thrombosis rates plateau or continue to increase over time; (ii) assessment of the incidence rate of cardiac death and myocardial infarction (MI); (iii) gather information on antiplatelet therapy use; and (iv) study routine clinical use of DES. The extent of thrombosis should also be uniformly measured. Given the huge diversity of patients and clinicians, it is hard to maintain uniformity. The focus of next generation stents should be on further development towards long-term safety and efficacy along with excellent extent of endothelialization and rapid arterial healing.

Stents in past few years have rapidly changed the picture of cardiovascular patients. They are more tension free and can lead a normal lifestyle. Morbidity, mortality due to cardiac arrest has also gone down too. Patients no longer have to come back for cardiac catheterizations due to ISR. We hope for an even better future with the advancement of cardiac stents.

ABBREVIATIONS

DES: Drug eluting stent.
MI: Myocardial infarctions.
BMS: Bare metallic stent.
DTS: Dual therapy stent.
BVS: Bioresorbable vascular scaffold.
EES: Everolimus eluting stent.
ZES: Zotarolimus eluting stent.
PES: Paclitaxel eluting stent.
PTCA: Percutaneous transluminal coronary angioplasty.
PCI: Percutaneous coronary intervention.
CABG: coronary artery bypass grafting.
TVR: Target vessel revascularization.
TLR: Target lesion revascularization.
MACE: Major adverse cardiac events.
ISR: In-stent restenosis.
DAPT: Dual antiplatelet therapy.

REFERENCES

Baber, U., Brener, S., Sergie, Z., Yu, J., Xu, K., Dangas, G., & Stone, G. et al. (2012). Impact of bivalirudin on access and non-access related bleeding in patients undergoing balloon aortic valvuloplasty: Results from A 2 center registry. *Journal of the American College of Cardiology*, *59*, E42.

Cutlip, D. (n.d.). *Comparison of drug-eluting intracoronary stents*. Retrieved from http://www.uptodate.com/contents/drug-eluting-compared-to-bare-metal-intracoronary-stents?source=see_link

Dangas, G., & Kuepper, F. (2002). Restenosis: Repeat Narrowing of a Coronary Artery. *Circulation*, *220*(105), 2586–2587. doi:10.1161/01.CIR.0000019122.00032.DF PMID:12045160

Gershlick, A., Kandzari, D. E., Leon, M. B., Wijns, W., Meredith, I. T., Fajadet, J., & Kuntz, R. E. et al. (2007). InvestigatorsZotarolimus-eluting stents in patients with native coronary artery disease: Clinical and angiographic outcomes in 1,317 patients. *The American Journal of Cardiology*, *100*(8), 45M–55M. doi:10.1016/j.amjcard.2007.08.021 PMID:17950832

Kaiser, C., Galatius, S., Erne, P., Eberli, F., Alber, H., Rickli, H., & Pfisterer, M. et al. (2010). Drug-Eluting versus Bare-Metal Stents in Large Coronary Arteries. *The New England Journal of Medicine*, *363*(24), 2310–2319. doi:10.1056/NEJMoa1009406 PMID:21080780

Levine, G. N. (2011). *ACCF/AHA/SCAI Guideline for Percutaneous Coronary Intervention (*2011). *Circulation*, *12*, e574–e651. PMID:22064601

Lim, W. H., Seo, W. W., Choe, W., Kang, C.-K., Park, J., Cho, H.-J., & Kim, H.-S. et al. (2011). Stent Coated With Antibody Against Vascular Endothelial-Cadherin Captures Endothelial Progenitor Cells, Accelerates Re-Endothelialization, and Reduces Neointimal Formation. *Arteriosclerosis, Thrombosis, and Vascular Biology*, *31*(12), 2798–2805. doi:10.1161/ATVBAHA.111.226134 PMID:22015656

Luscher, T. F., Steffel, J., Eberli, F. R., Joner, M., Nakazawa, G., Tanner, F. C., & Virmani, R. (2007). Drug-Eluting Stent and Coronary Thrombosis Biological Mechanisms and Clinical Implications. *Circulation*, *115*(8), 1051–1058. doi:10.1161/CIRCULATIONAHA.106.675934 PMID:17325255

Rao, S. V., Califf, R. M., Kramer, J. M., Peterson, E. D., Gross, T. P., Pepine, C. J.,... Kulick, D. (2010). *Coronary Balloon Angioplasty and Stents (Percutaneous Coronary Inverention, PCI)*. Retrieved from http://www.medicinenet.com/coronary_angioplasty/article.htm

Waksman, R., Mehran, R., & Krucoff, M. W. (2008). Postmarket evaluation of breakthrough technologies. *American Heart Journal*, *156*(2), 201–208. doi:10.1016/j.ahj.2008.01.036 PMID:18657647

Xu, J., Murphy, S. L., Kochanek, K. D., & Bastian, B. A. (2016). *Deaths: Final Data for 2013*. Retrieved from http://www.cdc.gov/nchs/data/nvsr/nvsr64/nvsr64_02.pdf

KEY TERMS AND DEFINITIONS

Angioplasty: A non-invasive procedure to widen the narrowed or blocked artery.

Arrhythmia: Irregular heartbeat, either too fast or too slow.

Atherosclerosis: Closing of vessels by plaque formation.

Infarctions: Tissue death caused by local lack of oxygen.

Ischemic Stroke: Stroke arising of blood vessel blockage.

Plaque: Insoluble solid deposits.

Restenosis: (Inside stent) blocking because of solid deposits.

Scar Tissue: An area with new tissue after a wound. In context of heart stent, it is newly formed tissue inside stent.

Stent: Metallic cage like object, which goes inside a blood vessel to aid in improved blood flow.

Thrombosis: Generation of a blood clot inside blood vessel.

Chapter 14
Nanoparticle-Based Drug Delivery Systems for Cardiovascular Applications

Arti Patel
University of South Florida, USA

Yashwant V. Pathak
University of South Florida, USA

ABSTRACT

Nanomedicine has vastly improved the treatment and diagnosis of many cardiovascular conditions such as atherosclerosis, myocardial ischemia, myocardial infarction, restenosis, and thrombosis. A few nanoparticle drug delivery systems that are currently being tested and used in clinical trials include lipid-based drug delivery, controlled drug release, and specific targeting. The chapter describes the various drug delivery methods, the various nanoparticles, and their application on specific cardiovascular conditions. This chapter compiles examples of specific clinical trials that are being conducted, using nanoparticles for therapy of cardiovascular conditions.

INTRODUCTION

The application of nanotechnology in medicine has greatly increased over the past couple decades. Nanotechnology uses and manipulates materials of nano-scale to assist with drug delivery in the body, as well as detecting and diagnosing diseases. Nanoparticles possess unique physical properties such as large surface area to mass ratio, high reactivity, and nano-size, which allow them to overcome many limitations presented by traditional drug delivery methods (Zhang et al., n.d.). Nanoparticles are a practical method of drug delivery because they can be modified to target specific areas, therefore increasing affectivity.

Current drug delivery methods that are used for cardiovascular applications include lipid-based oral delivery, drug delivery via the coronary venous system, microbubbles, and nanoparticles for controlled-release delivery. Nanoparticles are currently being used for diagnosis and therapy of various cardiovas-

DOI: 10.4018/978-1-5225-2092-4.ch014

cular conditions such as atherosclerosis, thrombosis, myocardial infarction, myocardial ischemia, and restenosis. Clinical studies show that polyglycolic acid-polymer (PLGA) and liposome nanoparticles are an effective drug delivery system to help treat these cardiovascular conditions. Surface-level modification of nanoparticles is being tested to help with drug targeting to specific regions of inflammation and injury. These advancements with nanotechnology allow for more specific and controlled drug treatment options, therefore improving therapeutics in cardiovascular applications.

TYPES OF CARDIOVASCULAR DRUG DELIVERY SYSTEMS

Cardiovascular drug delivery is unique because the vascular system provides drugs for systemic effects, as well as to specific organs. Local administration of drugs include methods such as drug delivery into the myocardium, drug delivery via the coronary venous system, injection into coronary arteries using a cardiac catheter, intrapericardial drug delivery, and the release of drugs into arterial lumen using stents (Jain, 2008). Drug delivery to the cardiovascular system is administered and mediated through various means. The main types of cardiovascular drug delivery include the use of microbubbles, ultrasound, lipid-based oral delivery, controlled-release drug delivery, and nanoparticle delivery.

Microbubble Drug Delivery Systems

Microbubbles are 1μm-1mm in size and are used as contrast agents for ultrasound imaging and targeted drug delivery. An example of a therapeutic application of microbubbles includes microbubble-enhanced sonothrombolysis. Clinical trials of microbubble-enhanced sonothrombolysis treatment are being conducted in acute ischemic stroke and acute myocardial infarction. Microbubbles can be used to target antigenic determinants expressed on endothelial cells by incorporating targeting ligands onto the surface of the microbubbles (Unger, Porter, Lindner, & Grayburn, 2014). Microbubbles can be loaded with therapeutic agents and can be delivered to specific areas of the cardiovascular system. Delivery of therapeutics can be achieved by; microbubbles being manufactured to incorporate bioactive substances in the microbubble shell, microbubbles being incubated with bioactive substances so the substance attaches to the microbubble shell, and microbubbles and bioactive substances being co-administered (Mayer & Bekeredjian, 2008).

Lipid-Based Drug Delivery Systems

Lipid-based drug delivery systems are used for improving oral bioavailability, sustaining and controlling drug release, improving drug stability, reducing food intake effect, targeting injured sites, and for combination therapy. Lipid based drug delivery systems optimize oral delivery of cardiovascular drugs (Rao, Tan, Thomas, & Prestidge, 2014). A specific type of lipid-based drug delivery system is self-emulsifying drug delivery systems (SEDDS), which are commonly used for cardiovascular drugs. Self-emulsifying drug delivery systems incorporate more hydrophilic surfactants and co-solvents in order to reduce oil and water tension of emulsion droplets. SEDDSs can reduce the re-dispersed emulsion droplet size and therefore create a small, localized, dispersion (Rao, Tan, Thomas, & Prestidge, 2014).

Controlled Drug Delivery

Controlled drug release provides a means for reducing the risk of cardiovascular disease at certain specific times. The continuous and controlled drug release is accomplished through the incorporation of cellulose-based substances (Rao, Tan, Thomas, & Prestidge, 2014). Controlled drug release can be accomplished through physical mechanisms such as diffusion of drugs through a polymer layer, deterioration of the polymer that is controlling drug release, regulation of osmotic pressure for drug release, and the use of ion exchange. Chemical mechanisms that break bonds between drug molecules and their delivery mechanism include polymer chains that undergo chemical degradation (Acharya & Park, 2006). The two types of controlled-release drug delivery systems include orally active and transcutaneous, which are regulated by diffusion, bioerosion, and generation of osmotic pressure. These allow for short-acting therapeutic drugs to be administered daily with greater efficiency and fewer side effects (Katz, Rosenberg, & Frishman, 1995). Studies are being conducted using hollow microspheres for controlled release of cardiovascular drugs. The drug-loaded microspheres have low densities and allow for buoyancy, which helps them sustain continuous drug release for over 12 hours (Soppimath, Kulkarni, & Aminabhavi, 2001).

Nanoparticle Drug Delivery

A more recent cardiovascular drug delivery system that is being researched and clinically applied is the nanoparticle drug delivery. Nanoparticle drug delivery uses materials that are 1-100nm in diameter. Some of the various types of nanoparticles that are being used are micelles, liposomes, and nanocrystals. These nanoparticles adjust drug kinetics of vascular permeability (Matoba & Egashira, 2014).

TYPES OF NANOPARTICLE DRUG DELIVERY SYSTEMS

As previously discussed, nanoparticles are used as a drug delivery system for drugs that have poor solubility in water (Zhang et al., n.d.). Specific types of nanoparticles include micelles, liposomes, and nanocrystals that are 1-100nm in size. These nanoparticles can be used as a drug delivery system to increase bioavailability. The large surface area to mass ratio of nanoparticles improves drug dissolution, which increases absorption because a high drug concentration gradient is created (Lee, Yun, & Park, 2015).

Micelles

Various nanoparticles can be used for drug delivery systems, such as micelles, which assemble in aqueous solutions because of their hydrophilic heads and hydrophobic tails. Micelles are used to overcome solubility issues because they incorporate hydrophobic drugs in their centers. Liposomes are composed of a lipid bilayer that encapsulate hydrophilic drugs inside. Similarly, Macromolecule polymers can create polymeric nanospheres and dendrimers that encapsulate drugs. Silk Fibroin is an example of a naturally occurring protein polymer that is used for the delivery of drugs and small biomolecules (Mottaghitalab, Farokhi, Shokrgozar, Atyabi, & Hosseinkhani, 2015). Carbon nanotubes are cylindrical shaped and hold therapeutic drugs inside them. Nano-sized crystalline structures can be used for drug delivery as well as for imaging purposes (Matoba & Egashira, 2014).

Nanoparticle Specialized Targeting

Nanoparticles are created to assist with specialized targeting, using ligands and antibodies on the surface of the nanoparticle. Modifications on the lipid head of polymer nanoparticles can create "stealth" nanoparticles. These nanoparticles, such as polyethylene glycol can circumvent mononuclear phagocyte systems, and inhibit blood proteins from binding to the lipid head surface (Schiener et al., 2014). Nanoparticles can circulate for different time periods depending on size, length, surface density, and surface charge. Nanoparticles that have modifications made to help increase circulation time increases the ability of the nanoparticle to reach its target (Schiener et al., 2014). The two types of targeting include passive and active. Passive targeting does not allow for the nanoparticle removal through body mechanisms such as metabolism and excretion. This allows for the drug to stay in circulation in the blood stream, and find its targets through properties such as pH, temperature, molecular size and shape (Khanna, 2012). Passive targeting is when the drug-enclosed nanoparticle is passively contained in an area of increased microvascular permeability. Active targeting is when the surface of the nanoparticle is modified with a ligand to help target specific cells. The active targeting method is usually used when there is a greater gradient of drug concentration between the damaged area and the unharmed area (Galagudza et al., 2012).

Nanofluids

A nanoparticle suspension in a fluid such as water creates nanofluids that can be used for various applications. The advantages of using nanofluid include an minimal clogging, microchannel cooling, a decrease in the system size, while still increasing the heat transfer of the system (Tripathi, & Bég, 2014). Biomedical engineering has facilitated the use of magnetic nanoparticles to assist in drug delivery to specific region of the body. Magnetic nanoparticles that make up a nanofluid can assist drugs to be guided through the bloodstream with the use of an external magnet (Abbasi, Hayat, & Alsaedi, 2015). Copper-water nanofluid that has a magnetic force applied to it is an example of a peristaltic transport method.

APPLICATION OF NANOTECHNOLOGY IN CARDIOVASCULAR DRUG DELIVERY SYSTEMS

Nanotechnology allows for earlier detection and improved therapeutic drug delivery systems for cardiovascular conditions. Current research is focusing on using nanoparticle drug delivery systems for the diagnosis and treatment of atherosclerosis, thrombosis, myocardial infarction, myocardial ischemia, and restenosis.

Atherosclerosis

Arteriosclerosis is a cardiovascular condition where the blood vessels inside the body become thick and stiff leading to atherosclerosis, myocardial infarction, and stroke. The inflammation of the vascular lumen in atherosclerosis can lead to the formation of atheromatous plaque (Psarros, Lee, Margaritis, & Antoniades, 2012). Atherosclerosis is the thickening of the vascular lumen and the accumulation of white blood cells. This narrowing of the blood vessel leads to a decrease in blood flow, which can cause a myocardial infarction and thrombosis. The plaque deposit in the blood vessel can dislodge and move through the blood stream, leading to a stroke. Computed tomography (CT) is currently being used to image coronary arteries to detect the narrowing of vascular lumen. One study being conducted uses a nanoparticle drug delivery system to deliver polyglycolic acid (PLGA) polymer, and crystalline metal nanoparticles to atherosclerotic plaques. These nanoparticle drug delivery systems have been found to successfully aid with CT detection as well as plaque destabilization (Matoba & Egashira, 2014). Nanoparticles that are being used for atherosclerosis therapy include, liposomes, peroflourocarbons, anionic micelles, nanoparticle–protein conjugates, RNA delivery, fullerenes, and theranostic. Liposome nanoparticles target macrophages and help reduce inflammation and suppress neointimal growth. Perflourocarbons are used with imaging of plaques with MRI. Anionic micelles, nanoparticle–protein conjugates, and specific fullerenes, target low-density lipoproteins which play a major role in atherogenesis when they are oxidized. Preclinical research conducted using a rat model, showed that RNA-delivery nanoparticles reduced neointimal formation after a balloon angioplasty. Theranostic nanoparticles composed of dextran and iron target macrophages, furthermore aiding with MRI imaging, as well as elimination of macrophages that construct plaque (Psarros, Lee, Margaritis, & Antoniades, 2012). Specific glucocorticoids can help decrease inflammation and prevent atheroprogression. In a study using a mouse model, liposome-encapsulated dexamethasone was able to deliver the drug to an atherosclerotic plaque by reducing the side effects and increasing the drug affectivity (Sureddi, & Mehta, 2011).

As mentioned previously, nanoparticles that have surface modifications made to them can be directed towards their target cells. To aid with nanoparticle targeting in the treatment of atherosclerosis, nanoparticles have surface modifications made by adding antibodies, peptides, or aptamers. Specialized nanoparticles can target the extracellular matrix and clotted plasmid proteins on plaques. Other specific target sites that have been identified for nanoparticle delivery include the junction adhesion molecule-A, monocytes, and neutrophils (Schiener et al., 2014). Magnetoflourescent nanoparticles are also currently being studied for their diagnostic and therapeutic characteristics. Magnetoflourescent properties harness properties that eradicate macrophage atheroma's and further stabilize lesions. Through intravenous administration, the nanoparticles can target macrophage rich areas (Sureddi, & Mehta, 2011). These various nanoparticles and targeting techniques will be able to aid in the decrease of atherosclerosis progression.

Thrombosis

Thrombosis is the formation of blood clots that form in blood vessels, eventually leading to the obstruction of blood flow. Blood clots can form under specific conditions or if the blood vessel is injured. Thrombosis is a serious cardiovascular condition that can lead to anoxia, hypoxia, and infarction. Currently, nanoparticle drug delivery systems are being studied to effectively reduce to the effect of thrombosis.

Antithrombotic agents have many clinical uses but they have disadvantages such as low targeting ability and short life-span in plasma. *In vitro* and *in vivo* studies are being conducted to show how drug encapsulated nanoparticles create a good affinity to thrombi and have strong thrombolytic enhancing effects (Zapotoczny, Szczubiałka, & Nowakowska, 2015). These nanoparticles are can detect changes and inflammation in the endothelium, as well as target drugs to lesions furthermore reducing atherosclerotic plaque or thrombosis formation. *In vitro* studies show that chitosan coated liposome nanoparticles that encapsulate tissue plasminogen activators (tPA) dissolve clots more efficiently than tPA in solution. Modifying the surface of the liposome nanoparticles with RGD increases thrombolysis (Zapotoczny, Szczubiałka, & Nowakowska, 2015). Fibrin is a non-globular protein found in blood clotting. Nanoparticles that target fibrin can help increase the efficiency of drugs compared to free drug administered for clot lysis. Thrombolytic agents such as tissue plasminogen activator have been found to more effectively destroy clots using fibrin-targeted, streptokinase-loaded nanoparticles (Fibrin-targeted perfluorocarbon nanoparticles for targeted thrombolysis, n.d.). Specific nanoparticle targeting of tissue shows promise in treating thrombosis.

Myocardial Infarction and Myocardial Ischemia-Reperfusion Injury

With acute myocardial infarctions, a percutaneous coronary intervention is the leading preventative method, which is done by placing multiple stents in a stenotic coronary artery. In an *in vivo* study, Chan et al. (2011) developed a paclitaxel-encapsulated nanoparticle to target damaged vasculature that had formed from smooth muscle proliferation and intravascular thrombosis, following a Percutaneous Coronary Intervention (PCI). These nanoparticles are specialized with collagen-IV targeting peptides in an effect to suppress stenosis. The study was conducted using a rat model and showed a 50% reduction of arterial stenosis using the nanoparticle drug treatment (Rakesh & Soonjo, 2007).

Nanoparticle drug delivery systems are also being used for acute myocardial infarction and myocardial ischemia-reperfusion injury. Myocardial ischemia can cause inflammation, tissue damage, and decay. Myocardial ischemia-reperfusion produces reactive oxygen species, calcium abundance, and changes in pH, which lead to mitochondrial injury and eventually necrosis (Matoba & Egashira, 2014). Clinical studies show that nanoparticle drug delivery systems can aid with myocardial ischemia by administering a drug during reperfusion. This nanoparticle drug delivery system can target inflammatory monocytes and ischemic myocardium.

In a study being conducted by Takahama *et al.* (2009), liposome nanoparticle delivery of adenosine during myocardial reperfusion has increased the concentration of adenosine in the myocardium compared to free adenosine. PLGA nanoparticles are being tested as a drug delivery system for myocardial ischemia-reperfusion injury with mice models to see if they enhance therapeutic performance (Matoba & Egashira, 2014). A study by Galagudza *et al.*(2014), investigated silica nanoparticles as drug delivery system to carry adenosine to ischemic-reperfused heart. As mentioned previously, nanoparticles can be used to target specific areas passively or actively. A passive targeting approach with adenosine on the surface of the silica nanoparticle was found to be more effective compared to free adenosine.

In myocardial ischemia, a portion of the heart is deprived of oxygen and the ATP level decreases. One study done in isolated ischemic rat hearts as well as *in-vivo* rabbits showed that ATP-loaded liposomes and immunoliposomes protected the myocardium from ischemic-reperfusion damage. Targeting exogenous ATP to damaged myocytes using nanoparticle liposomes that have antimyosin antibodies on the surface of liposomes, is an effective passive drug delivery system (Hartner, Verma, Levchenko, Bernstein, & Torchilin, n.d.).

Restenosis

Restenosis is the reoccurrence of stenoses that occur from procedures that are done to treat damaged arteries and blood vessels. The reobstruction of a blood vessel follows procedures that are done to remove original blockages and narrowing. Some strategies that are being used for decreasing the manifestation of restenosis include, local drug delivery, adventitial drug implants, stents, and catheter based drug delivery. There are various types of nanoparticle drug delivery systems that could be used for restonisis, such as biopolymers and synthetic polymers. These nanoparticles can be created to be diffusion based, biodegradable, as well as set to release the drug at specific time incraments or continuously. Biodegradable polymer nanoparticles that contain theraputic drugs are being used for intra-arterial localization. These specific nanoparticles are a co-polymer named polylactic polyglycolic acid(PLGA). PLGA biodegrades through the hydrolysis of the ester linkage, producing lactic acid and glycolic acid. In this process, the nanoparticles will undergo hydrolysis in the arterial wall and continuously release the drug. This will repair the arterial wall and reduce the occurance of restenosis. Nanoparticle in vivo studies have been conducted using rat, dog, and pig models along with ex vivo studies being conducted with a dog carotid artery (Labhasetwar, Song, & Levy, 1997). A specific drug that is being tested and studied by Westedt et al. (2007) is Paclitaxel. The drug concentrations delievered to prevent restenosis must be very high,localized, and have a long duration. The nanoparticle encapsulated Paclitaxel was tested on white rabits that had balloon cathetar mechanical induced damage to the illiac artery. The higher concentration of Paclitaxel-loaded nanoparticle in this study showed a decrease in neointimal formation, therefore decreasing the chances of restenosis (Westedt et al., 2007).

FUTURE PERSPECTIVES

Nanoparticles have helped overcome many limitations and have increased bioavailability of therapeutic drugs, however there are disadvantages of using nanomedicine. Some of these disadvantages include, limited infusibility, increased toxicity, and immunosuppression (Schiener et al., 2014). Specifically with nanoparticle treatment of atherosclerosis, there have been studies showing an increase of immunogenicity with PEG polymer nanoparticles after repetitive treatment (Schiener et al., 2014). Nanoparticle use in atherosclerosis shows potential for personalized medicine, but improvements must be made with tissue-specific targeting to help decrease toxicity for individual patients (Schiener et al., 2014). Clinical trials would like to conduct further experimentation in order to enhance dosage and physiochemical characteristics to create better infusibility (Galagudza et al., 2012).

Early diagnosis with nanoparticles drug delivery systems is key to improving treatment of thrombosis and atherosclerosis, therefore enhancing clinical outcomes (Zapotoczny, Szczubiałka, & Nowakowska, 2015). Nanoparticle drug delivery methods that are used for cardiovascular conditions also show promise for inflammatory diseases such as obstructive pulmonary disease and asthma (Buxton, 2009). Even though there are disadvantages to nanoparticle based drug delivery systems, most are advantages that improve bioavailability, and specifically target drugs to the effected area.

CONCLUSION

Current applications of nanoparticle drug delivery systems successfully allow for the detection, diagnosis, and treatment of many cardiovascular conditions. Treatment of conditions such as atherosclerosis, restenosis, thrombosis, myocardial infarction, and myocardial ischemia have largely benefitted through the use of nanoparticle drug delivery systems. The various different types of nanoparticles such as micelles, nanofluids, and liposomes have helped target and increase bioavailability of therapeutic drugs. Nanoparticles help with the diagnosis of cardiovascular conditions, as well as help us better understand drug delivery pathways. This allows researchers to create new advancements with nanoparticle structure and targeting capabilities.

REFERENCES

Abbasi, F., Hayat, T., & Alsaedi, A. (2015). Peristaltic transport of magneto-nanoparticles submerged in water: Model for drug delivery system. *Physica E, Low-Dimensional Systems and Nanostructures, 123*. doi:10.1016/j.physe.2014.12.026

Acharya, G., & Park, K. (2006). Mechanisms of controlled drug release from drug-eluting stents. *Advanced Drug Delivery Reviews, 58*, 387-401. doi:10.1016/j.addr.2006.01.016

Buxton, D. B. (2009). Nanomedicine for the management of lung and blood diseases. *Nanomedicine (London), 4*(3), 331–339. doi:10.2217/nnm.09.8 PMID:19331540

Chan, J., Rhee, J., & Farokhzad, O. (2011). In vivo prevention of arterial restenosis with paclitaxel-encapsulated targeted lipid—polymeric nanoparticles. *Proceedings of the National Academy of Sciences of the United States of America*.

Fibrin-targeted perfluorocarbon nanoparticles for targeted thrombolysis. (n.d.). Retrieved May 20, 2013, from http://www.ncbi.nlm.nih.gov/pubmed/17716136

Galagudza, M., Korolev, D., Postnov, V., Naumisheva, E., Grigorova, Y., Uskov, I., & Shlyakhto, E. (2012). Passive targeting of ischemic-reperfused myocardium with adenosine-loaded silica nanoparticles. *International Journal of Nanomedicine, 71671*. doi:10.2147/IJN.S29511 PMID:22619519

Hartner, W., Verma, D., Levchenko, T., Bernstein, E., & Torchilin, V. (n.d). ATP-loaded liposomes for treatment of myocardial ischemia. *Wiley Interdisciplinary Reviews-Nanomedicine And Nanobiotechnology, 1*(5), 530-539.

Jain, K. (2008). Drug Delivery Systems. In *Drug Delivery Systems* (p. 16). Totowa, NJ: Humana. doi:10.1007/978-1-59745-210-6_1

Katz, B., Rosenberg, A., & Frishman, W. H. (1995). Controlled-release drug delivery systems in cardiovascular medicine. *American Heart Journal, 129*(2), 359–368. doi:10.1016/0002-8703(95)90019-5 PMID:7832110

Khanna, V. K. (2012). Targeted Delivery of Nanomedicines. *ISRN Pharmacology, 2012*, 1–9. doi:10.5402/2012/571394

Labhasetwar, V., Song, C., & Levy, R. J. (1997, February 15). *Nanoparticle drug delivery system for restenosis*. Retrieved from http://ac.els-cdn.com/S0169409X96004838/1-s2.0-S0169409X96004838-main.pdf?_tid=6f3e82c6-0f13-11e5-a92a-00000aab0f6c&acdnat=1433901365_efc2bb3176ba31c69419d-1000d79c27f

Lee, B. K., Yun, Y. H., & Park, K. (2015). Smart nanoparticles for drug delivery: Boundaries and opportunities. *Chemical Engineering Science, 125*, 158-164. doi:10.1016/j.ces.2014.06.042

Matoba, T., & Egashira, K. (2014). Nanoparticle-Mediated Drug Delivery System for Cardiovascular Disease. *International Heart Journal, 55*(4), 281–286. doi:10.1536/ihj.14-150 PMID:24942639

Mayer, C. R., & Bekeredjian, R. (2008). Ultrasonic gene and drug delivery to the cardiovascular system. *Advanced Drug Delivery Reviews, 60*, 1177-1192. doi:10.1016/j.addr.2008.03.004

Mottaghitalab, F., Farokhi, M., Shokrgozar, M. A., Atyabi, F., & Hosseinkhani, H. (2015). Review: Silk fibroin nanoparticle as a novel drug delivery system. *Journal of Controlled Release*, 206161–206176. doi:10.1016/j.jconrel.2015.03.020

Psarros, C., Lee, R., Margaritis, M., & Antoniades, C. (2012). Review: Nanomedicine for the prevention, treatment and imaging of atherosclerosis. *Maturitas, 73*, 52-60. doi:10.1016/j.maturitas.2011.12.014

Rao, S., Tan, A., Thomas, N., & Prestidge, C. A. (2014). Review: Perspective and potential of oral lipid-based delivery to optimize pharmacological therapies against cardiovascular diseases. *Journal of Controlled Release, 193*, 174–187. doi:10.1016/j.jconrel.2014.05.013

Schiener, M., Hossann, M., Viola, J. R., Ortega-Gomez, A., Weber, C., Lauber, K., & Soehnlein, O. et al. (2014). Review: Nanomedicine-based strategies for treatment of atherosclerosis. *Trends in Molecular Medicine*, 20271–20281. doi:10.1016/j.molmed.2013.12.001 PMID:24594264

Sharma & Kwon. (2007). New applications of nanoparticles in cardiovascular imaging. *Journal of Experimental Nanoscience, 2*(1-2), 115-126. DOI: 10.1080/17458080601101176

Soppimath, K., Kulkarni, A., & Aminabhavi, T. (2001). Development of Hollow Microspheres as Floating Controlled-Release Systems for Cardiovascular Drugs: Preparation and Release Characteristics. *Drug Development and Industrial Pharmacy, 27*(6), 507–515. doi:10.1081/DDC-100105175 PMID:11548857

Sureddi, R., & Mehta, J. L. (2011). Nanomedicine in Cardiovascular Diseases: Emerging Diagnostic and Therapeutic Potential. *Journal Of Nanotechnology In Engineering And Medicine, 2*(3), 031012. doi:10.1115/1.4005490

Takahama, H., Minamino, T., Asanuma, H., Fujita, M., Asai, T., Wakeno, M., & Kitakaze, M. et al. (2009). Prolonged targeting of ischemic/reperfused myocardium by liposomal adenosine augments cardioprotection in rats. *Journal of the American College of Cardiology, 53*(8), 709–717. doi:10.1016/j.jacc.2008.11.014 PMID:19232905

Tripathi, D., & Bég, O. A. (2014). A study on peristaltic flow of nanofluids: Application in drug delivery systems. *International Journal of Heat and Mass Transfer*, 7061–7070. doi:10.1016/j.ijheatmasstransfer.2013.10.044

Unger, E., Porter, T., Lindner, J., & Grayburn, P. (2014). Cardiovascular drug delivery with ultrasound and microbubbles. *Advanced Drug Delivery Reviews*, 72110–72126. doi:10.1016/j.addr.2014.01.012 PMID:24524934

Westedt, U., Kalinowski, M., Wittmar, M., Merdan, T., Unger, F., Fuchs, J., & Kissel, T. et al. (2007). Poly(vinyl alcohol)-graft-poly(lactide-co-glycolide) nanoparticles for local delivery of paclitaxel for restenosis treatment. *Journal of Controlled Release*, 11941–11951. doi:10.1016/j.jconrel.2007.01.009 PMID:17346845

Zapotoczny, S., Szczubiałka, K., & Nowakowska, M. (2015). Review article: Nanoparticles in endothelial theranostics. *Pharmacological Reports, 67*(4), 751–755. doi:10.1016/j.pharep.2015.05.018

Zhang, L., Gu, F., Chan, J., Wang, A., Langer, R., & Farokhzad, O. (2008, May). Nanoparticles in medicine: Therapeutic applications and developments. *Clinical Pharmacology and Therapeutics, 83*(5), 761–769. doi:10.1038/sj.clpt.6100400 PMID:17957183

Section 4
Alternative Medicine and Cardiovascular Therapy

Chapter 15
Complementary and Alternative Medicine Use in Hypertension:
The Good, the Bad, and the Ugly: Hypertension Treatment From Nature - Myth or Fact?

Aymen Shatnawi
University of Charleston School of Pharmacy, USA

Alison Shafer
Pacific University, USA

Hytham Ahmed
Damanhour University, Egypt

Fawzy Elbarbry
Pacific University, USA

ABSTRACT

Thirty six percent of people in USA and Canada regularly use complementary and alternative medicine (CAM) for the prevention and treatment of different diseases, including hypertension. Generally, majority of the hypertensive patients do not disclose the use of such remedies, and also health care providers do not usually ask their hypertensive patients if they use CAM. The widespread consumption of CAM in hypertension requires clear understanding of their underlying mechanism of action, efficacy and safety. This chapter will provide a comprehensive list of CAM commonly used by Americans for the prevention and treatment of hypertension as well as their postulated mechanism of action. Modulation of drug metabolizing enzymes and their safety will also be covered along with the clinical consequences, i.e. drug-herb or herb-disease interactions. patients and healthcare providers should also be careful with using CAM therapies, because not only is there minimal evidence that several CAM products work to treat hypertension, but their safety hasn't been well-established.

DOI: 10.4018/978-1-5225-2092-4.ch015

INTRODUCTION

Definition

Blood pressure (BP) is a measurement of the pressure in the blood vessels, both when the heart contracts (systolic blood pressure, SBP) and when it is filling with blood between beats (diastolic blood pressure, DBP). Hypertension (HTN), or high blood pressure, is defined as SBP of 140 mmHg or above and/or DBP of 90 mmHg or above, or currently taking medication to lower blood pressure (NHLBI, 2015).HTN is a major predictor for coronary heart disease, stroke, and renal failure. Starting at an ideal BP of 115/75, every 20/10 mmHg (systolic/diastolic) increase in BP doubles the risk of cardiovascular diseases. As HTN can be directly linked with more than 360,000 American deaths annually and 17.3 million annual deaths globally, the disease and its associated complications are the most common cause of death in the world (Mozaffarian et al., 2015).

Elevated BP can be classified into three different categories, with ever increasing risks of complications: pre-HTN is systolic blood pressure from 120-139 mmHg or diastolic blood pressure from 80-89 mmHg, Stage I HTN is SBP from 140-159 mmHg or DBP from 90-99 mmHg, and Stage II HTN is SBP ≥ 160 mmHg or DBP ≥ 100 mmHg (NHLBI, 2015). High BP is the most common reason for American adults to both visit their healthcare providers and to take medications, but only 51.4% of Americans who are being treated for HTN are considered to be controlled, usually to a goal BP of <140/90 mmHg for most patients, including those with diabetes and chronic kidney disease. Current recommended goal BP for patients older than 60 years is <150/90 mmHg, though this is a matter of some debate. Blood pressure goals for the general public and those with comorbid conditions may be revised with future updates to HTN guidelines, as recent evidence has shown that tighter control of BP leads to lower rates of MI, heart failure, stroke, and death. Resistant HTN can be diagnosed when a patient is on optimal doses of 3 classes of anti-HTN medications but their BP remains ≥140/90, or if they are using medications from ≥4 classes of anti-HTN medications regardless of resulting BP (Group, 2015; James et al., 2014; Mozaffarian et al., 2015).

Uncontrolled BP can lead to various complications that usually include end-organ damage, like left-ventricular hypertrophy (LVH), heart failure, stroke (ischemic and/or hemorrhagic), chronic kidney disease (CKD), and end-stage renal disease (ESRD). When DBP is greater than 120 mmHg, it can lead to many complications, including hypertensive urgency (DBP > 120 with no end-organ damage) or hypertensive emergency (DBP > 120 with acute, ongoing organ damage, usually to the brain, eyes, kidneys, or heart). At the opposite end of the spectrum, when treatment is too effective and brings BP too low (DBP < 55-60 mmHg), a patient may be at increased risk of myocardial infarction or stroke. Therefore, when a patient is being treated for HTN, it is important to monitor their BP closely while initiating treatment, changing doses of medications, or changing treatments (Jan Basile & Michael J Bloch, 2015).

When a patient is diagnosed with pre-HTN or greater, it is usually recommended that lifestyle modifications are either started before or in concert with any pharmacological therapy, as these can have a marked impact on lowering BP. These lifestyle changes include sodium restriction, weight loss, a diet similar to that outlined by DASH (Dietary Approaches to Stop HTN), 30 minutes of exercise most days, moderate alcohol intake, and patient education (Jan Basile & Michael J Bloch, 2015).

Pathophysiology and Causes

HTN is usually classified as *essential* (primary), or *secondary*. More than 90% of people with HTN fall into the first category, where the exact underlying pathological cause of the elevated BP is not known. However, genetic factors are thought to play an important role in the development of primary HTN. For example, the risk of becoming hypertensive when a person has a family history of one or two hypertensive parents is twice as high as the general population. Additional risk factors for primary HTN include age, obesity, race, excessive dietary salt intake, excess alcohol consumption, physical inactivity, diabetes, dyslipidemia, and low Vitamin D levels (Tabassum & Ahmad, 2011).

Less than 10% of hypertensive patients are diagnosed with secondary HTN, where the underlying cause of elevated BP is identifiable. Secondary HTN is usually drug-induced, disease-related (e.g., diabetes), or physiologically induced (e.g., reduced number of nephrons due to fetal malformation, kidney damage, or other causes). Normally the first step in treating this type of HTN is to remove the offending agent(s) or treat the underlying disease(s) or physiological condition(s). Chronic kidney disease (CKD), Cushing syndrome, hyper- or hypo-thyroid, hyperparathyroidism, obstructive sleep apnea, pheochromocytoma, and primary hyper-aldosteronism are the most common and well-recognized comorbid diseases related to secondary HTN. Several agents have been also correlated with elevated BP, including prescription drugs (e.g., amphetamines, corticosteroids, oral contraceptives, anti-depressant medications, calcineurin inhibitors, decongestants, and non-steroidal anti-inflammatory drugs), street drugs (e.g., cocaine, methamphetamine, and ephedra alkaloids), and food substances (e.g., sodium, ethanol, and licorice) (Jan Basile & Michael J Bloch, 2015; Tabassum & Ahmad, 2011).

Although there is still uncertainty about the pathophysiology of primary HTN, many interrelated factors have been found to contribute to persistent blood pressure elevation. Among the proposed factors are vascular resistance, oxidative stress, endothelial dysfunction, and salt sensitivity. Abnormalities in any of the homeostatic neuro-hormonal mechanisms such as the sympathetic nervous system (SNS), renin-angiotensin-aldosterone system (RAAS), peripheral autoregulation, electrolyte balance, and natriuretic hormones have also been associated with HTN pathophysiology.

Nitric oxide (NO), endothelium-derived relaxing factor, is a paracrine vasodilator that has been implicated in vascular tone regulation. Many *in vitro* and *in vivo* studies suggest that chronic HTN reduces endothelium dependent responses of peripheral vasculature, probably due to decreased availability of NO (Doggrell & Brown, 1998). On the other hand, NO derived from inducible isoform of the enzyme nitric oxide synthase (iNOS) has been considered to enhance the tissue damage, due to accelerated reactive nitrogen species formation (Tsai, Tsai, Yu, & Ho, 2007).

Mathematically, blood pressure is the product of systemic vascular resistance (SVR) and cardiac output (CO). Therefore, increased SVR and/or CO will likely result in HTN. For example, a rise in intracellular calcium concentration is believed to cause contraction of the smooth muscle cells and increase SVR, which may explain the vasodilatory effect of calcium channel blockers. On the other hand, CO rises in response to factors such as increased sympathetic nervous system activity, stimulation of the renin-angiotensin-aldosterone system (RAAS), and elevated intravascular volume resulting from excessive sodium intake and/or renal sodium retention. Therefore, these systems are the targets of most current conventional pharmacological therapies. (Ernst, 2012)

Prevalence and Epidemiology

Hypertension affects about one billion people globally, with approximately 80 million people in the United States alone. Blood pressure has been shown to increase in a linear fashion with age. While only 7.3% of US adults ages 18-39 are hypertensive, approximately 65% of adults over age 60 are hypertensive. This large number is expected to grow as more of the US population begins to live more than 60 years, due to improvements in treatment of chronic disease and diseases of the elderly. Additionally, as obesity rates both in the US and globally continue to rise, HTN rates are expected to rise, as well (Jan Basile & Michael J Bloch, 2015). In 2008, 17.3 million deaths were attributed to HTN and its complications, and it is anticipated that this number will increase to greater than 23.6 million by 2030 (Tabassum & Ahmad, 2011).

Strong evidence from several studies indicates that African Americans, who develop HTN earlier in life and have a higher average BP than white Americans, are also more susceptible to salt-sensitive HTN. Thus, HTN in African Americans is more responsive to dietary salt restriction. Conversely, African Americans tend to have a less successful response to the recommended first-line pharmacotherapy of angiotensin-converting enzyme inhibitors (ACE-I) and angiotensin receptor blockers (ARB), indicating differences in the (RAAS) signaling cascade which seem to be correlated with higher numbers of African Americans with HTN than white Americans (43% & 45.7% African American men and women vs. 33.9% & 32.7% white American men and women). It is interesting to note that there is a greater proportion of African American women than men with HTN, while the opposite is true in white Americans (Papademetriou, Narayan, & Kokkinos, 2004; Tabassum & Ahmad, 2011).

Cost to the Healthcare System

According to data from the National Center for Health Statistics (NCHS) in 2011-2012, 82.7% of adults with HTN were aware of their condition and 75.6% reported taking prescribed medication(s) to lower their blood pressure. The total cost of treatment and medical services for American adults with HTN exceeded $42.9 billion, with an expected increase to $274 billion by 2030 when it has been estimated that 41.4% of Americans will have HTN. Almost half of the money paid for HTN treatment and complications is spent on prescription medications, but the cost of cardiovascular disease (CVD) and stroke far exceeds this cost, at greater than $320 billion annually. Globally, the cost of HTN, both controlled and uncontrolled, exceeded $863 billion in 2011, but by 2030 is expected to rise to over a trillion dollars annually, while the cost of CVD and stroke will be an additional estimated $980 billion (Mozaffarian et al., 2015). HTN has become both a health crisis and an economic strain, not just in the US, but all over the world.

TREATMENT

Conventional Therapy

There are many classes of conventional medications that can be used to treat HTN, including angiotensin-converting enzyme inhibitors (ACE-I), angiotensin receptor blockers (ARBs), calcium channel blockers (CCBs), and diuretics which reduce total blood volume by increasing urinary water and sodium excretion. These medications are commonly used in varying combinations to achieve optimal dosing and BP control. Additionally, beta blockers, which are usually used in heart conditions, can be used as add-on therapy in resistant HTN, as well as several other classes of medications (James et al., 2014).

The benefits of using these medications are well-studied, so their effects and possible drug-drug or drug-food interactions are well-described. There have been many large randomized, controlled trials to investigate their effectiveness in lowering BP, and in preventing HTN complications such as heart failure, myocardial infarction, stroke, and death.

However, many people in both developing and developed countries do not have easy access to these medications. They may also prefer to use natural medicines or traditional therapies, and this choice may be attributed to the high cost of conventional medicines, lack of prescription drug insurance, fear of side effects of the medicines, cultural beliefs, or a belief that herbal remedies are "safer".

Complementary and Alternative Medicine (CAM)

According to the World Health Organization (WHO), traditional herbal medicines are getting significant attention in global health discussions, and it can be safely presumed that traditional herbal medicines and other alternative therapies will play a significant role in future strategies to alleviate and treat chronic illnesses, such as HTN. The WHO is working to ensure that these treatments are affordable, accessible, trustworthy, and culturally accepted. In 1999, for example, only 19 countries had research institutes for the study of CAM treatments, but by 2012, there were 73 countries having such research organizations. There are several risks associated with the use of CAM treatments, including adulterated/poor-quality/counterfeit products, misleading or unreliable information about the effects, delaying conventional treatment and risking a worsening of the condition, and possible adverse effects of the treatments. The WHO is committed to reduce these risks by improving the global knowledge base about CAM therapy. This may also have a large economic impact because the worldwide annual market for these products and services approaches $ 60 billion, as 75-80% of the world population uses them, primarily in developing countries, and with improved information the market will only be increasing in coming years (Tabassum & Ahmad, 2011; WHO, 2013).

In 2007, in the United States, a survey by the NCCAM (National Center for Complementary and Alternative Medicines) estimated that approximately 83 million people (approximately 34% of the US population) used CAM therapies, which included herbal medications and oral supplements, with spending exceeding $33.9 billion in out-of-pocket costs (not reimbursed by health insurance) (Nahan, Barnes, Stussman, & Bloom, 2011). This amount reflects visits to practitioners ($11.9 billion), non-vitamin/non-mineral supplements and treatments ($14.8 billion), and other CAM therapies ($7.2 billion on practices such as yoga and acupuncture), Figure 1. It is worth noting that most Americans use CAM therapies as a complementary to their conventional care, but only 5% of people using CAM treatments, alone (Clarke, Black, Stussman, Barnes, & Nahin, 2015).

Also noteworthy is that CAM usage in the U.S. is most prevalent among college-educated people. Almost 43% of respondents to a survey in 2012 who reported having a college education were purchasing these treatments, while only 15.6% of people with a high school education or lower were using them. More of the college educated users of CAM are women than men, and more have private insurance (38%) than public insurance (24.8%) or a lack of insurance (22.9%) (Clarke et al., 2015). In the US, the use of CAM varies by region, as seen in Figure 2. In developing countries, CAM therapies are a much more common form of treatment, such as in China where 90% of hospitals have a Traditional

Figure 1. Out-of-pocket spending on conventional and alternative (CAM) therapies as a portion of total healthcare spending, 2007
(Ernst, 2012)

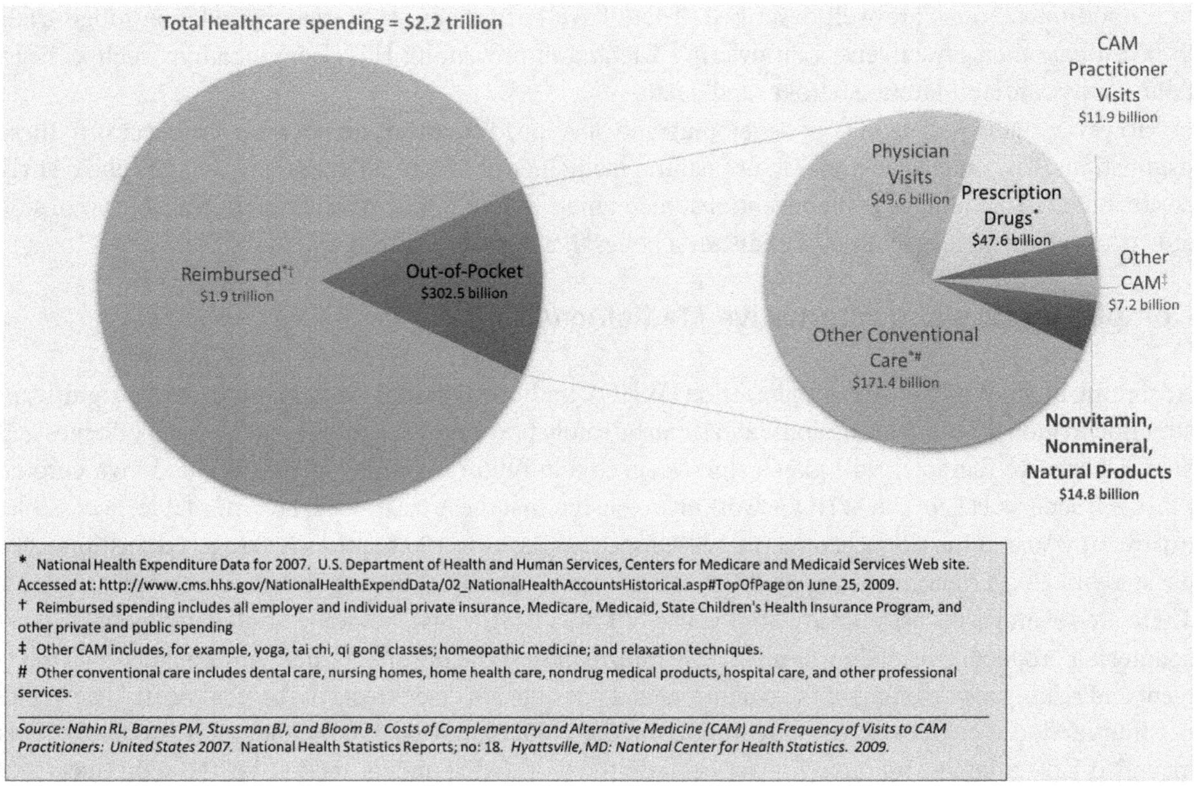

and Complimentary Medicine (T&CM) department. In fact, HTN was the 5th most common reason for admission to T&CM hospitals in 2008 (WHO, 2013).

The American Heart Association (AHA) performed a literature review in 2013 of several studies involving alternative modalities of HTN treatment, and concluded that "it is reasonable for all individuals with blood pressure levels >120/80 to consider trials of alternative approaches as adjunct methods to help lower BP when clinically appropriate." Additionally, they developed a treatment algorithm for when or if it may be appropriate to add these CAM options. These recommendations can be found in the American Heart Association June 2013 report (Brook et al., 2013).

This chapter will present the evidence for or precautions against the use of several dietary supplements and herbal options for treating HTN, but it is worth noting that there are additional, non-dietary therapies being used and tested for effectiveness against HTN, as well, such as acupuncture, meditation, regulated breathing practices, and others. Currently, the best evidence for these non-supplement therapies is in support of breathing and meditation, but research is ongoing. The AHA recently concluded that transcendental meditation and biofeedback techniques "may be considered" as adjunct therapy to conventional HTN treatment because of some supporting evidence and a lack of health risks (Brook et al., 2013).

Figure 2. Regional use of CAM therapy, 2012
(Ernst, 2012)

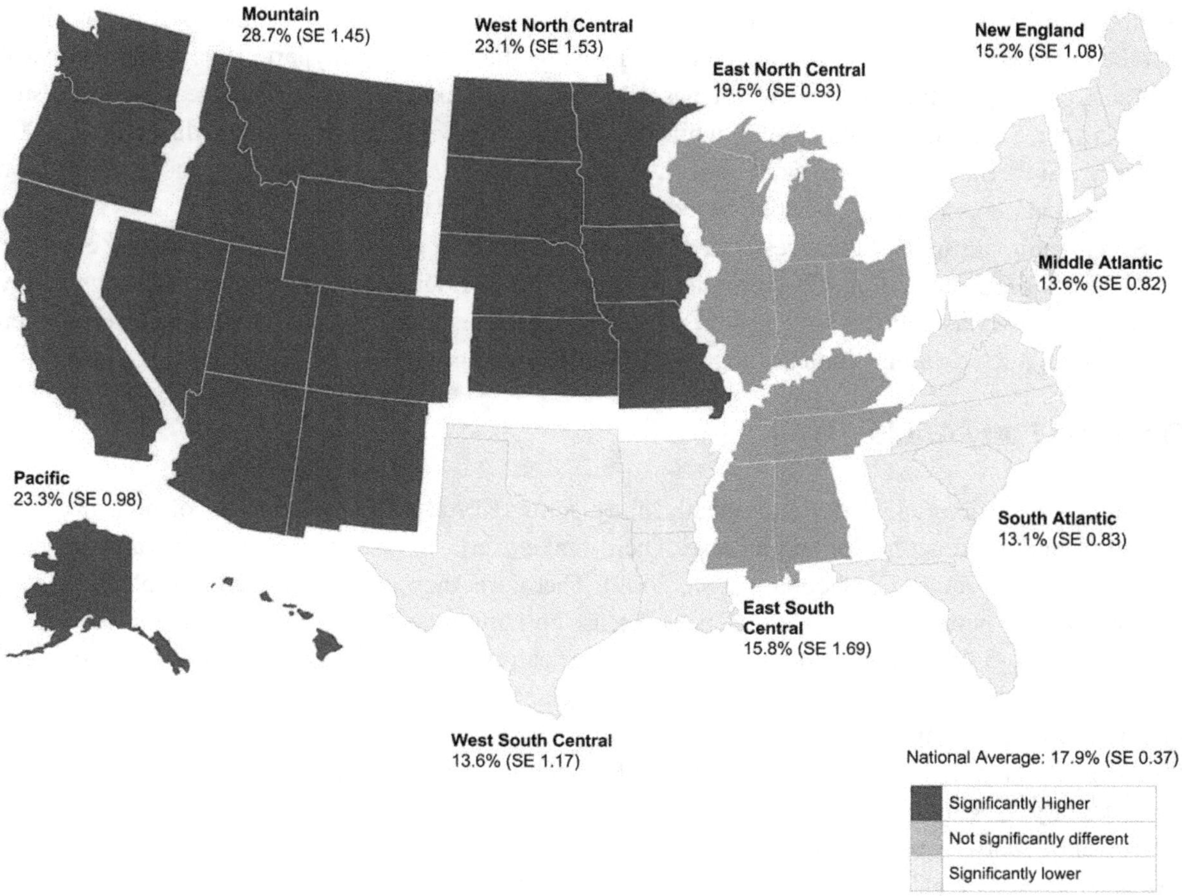

Garlic

Garlic, *Allium sativum L. (Liliaceae)*, is a member of the family *Alliaceae*. Several human and animal studies have shown favorable cardiovascular effects after using garlic in its raw or processed forms. These effects include antihypertensive, anti-atherosclerotic, lipid-lowering and antioxidant properties (Dhawan & Jain, 2005; Durak et al., 2004). Garlic has been used as a safe and alternative antihypertensive remedy for many years by almost 50% of the hypertensive patients (Kwak et al., 2014; Stabler, Tejani, Huynh, & Fowkes, 2012a; Xiong et al., 2015). Several mechanisms have been postulated to explain the antihypertensive activity of garlic including angiotensin-converting enzyme inhibition (Asdaq & Inamdar, 2010), reduction of vasoconstrictor prostanoids compounds synthesis (Al-Qattan, Khan, Alnaqeeb, & Ali, 2001), increasing nitric oxide activity and concentration, enhancing hydrogen sulfide generation (Al-Qattan et al., 2006), and upregulation of the growth suppressor p27 and the reduction of ERK 1/2 phosphorylation that leads to reverse arterial remodeling (Castro, Gil Lorenzo, Gonzalez, & Cruzado, 2010).

Allicin, which gives garlic its unique odor, is the most active component of garlic and responsible for several garlic medicinal properties. Meta-analysis of several clinical trials have shown that garlic indeed has antihypertensive effect, but, with varied biological response (Duda, Suliburska, & Pupek-Musialik,

2008; L. A. Simons et al., 1995). The suggested reasons behind this variability are preparation methods, deficiencies in methodology, dosage variations of *garlic* and differences in treatment durations (S. Simons, Wollersheim, & Thien, 2009; Stabler, Tejani, Huynh, & Fowkes, 2012b). Furthermore, it was shown that the initial BP level is an important factor influencing the garlic's antihypertensive effect (Qidwai & Ashfaq, 2013). Therefore, patients with a baseline SBP ≥ 140 mmHg usually displayed positive results (Holzgartner, Schmidt, & Kuhn, 1992), while others with SBP < 140 mmHg didn't (Macan et al., 2006; Williams, Sutherland, McCormick, Yeoman, & de Jong, 2005). This may indicate that garlic is more effective in patients with high systolic blood pressure than other types of HTN.

Several animal studies have investigated the potential effect of garlic on drug metabolizing enzymes. In rats it has been shown that the expression level of CYP2E1, an isoform with a procarcinogen activity, was significantly reduced and several phase 2 proteins, especially glutathione S-transferase were upregulated. Such data may indicate a chemo-preventive potential of garlic (Le Bon et al., 2003).

Omega-3 Fatty Acids

Omega-3 fatty acids (ω-3 FAs) are essential fatty acids (EFAs) with wide variety of pharmacological behaviors in human health and disease. Their intake exerts a clear improvement in cardiovascular morbidity and mortality (Yashodhara et al., 2009). Therefore, they are widely used as food and dietary supplements for patients with wide variety of disease conditions such as cardiovascular, endocrine, and neurological. ω-3 FAs can be found in high content in seafood, fish particularly fatty fish (albacore tuna, mackerel, salmon, sardines), fish oils and in many vegetable oils such as canola, flaxseed and wheat germ oils. Interestingly, people in Greenland and Japan, where fish is an essential part in their diet, showed low rates of coronary heart disease (CHD). Other dietary sources of ω-3 FAs include walnuts, human milk and organ meats.

The antihypertensive effect of ω-3 FAs is showed in both hypertensive (Geleijnse, Giltay, Grobbee, Donders, & Kok, 2002; Ueshima et al., 2007) and normotensive (Ueshima et al., 2007) subjects. In contrast to garlic, it was proven that ω-3 FAs normalizes blood pressure in both systolic and diastolic HTN (Geleijnse et al., 2002). Furthermore, it has been shown that regular intake of ω-3 FAs prevent the development of HTN (Dallongeville et al., 2003).

The mechanism of action of ω-3 FAs in HTN is not fully understood. However, oxidative stress and inflammation have been shown as contributing factor in HTN development. Recent studies showed that ω-3 FAs have antioxidative activity and improved cardiac function. In addition ω-3 FAs also control the synthesis of immune modulators such as prostaglandins and leukotrienes, which ultimately regulate the arachidonic acid pathway and other pro-inflammatory molecules (Yueqin Liu et al., 2014).

ω-3 FAs when used appropriately are considered safe. However, it is also reported that ω-3 FAs have anticoagulant activity and excessive intake might increase the risk of bleeding. Therefore, extra caution should be taken during concomitant administration with anticoagulant drugs such as warfarin(Sanders, Vickers, & Haines, 1981).

Green Tea (GT)

Green tea extract or its purified flavonoids and polyphenols have shown evidence of protection against HTN and reduce the risk for stroke and inflammation (Nantz, Rowe, Bukowski, & Percival, 2009;

Dirk Taubert, Roesen, & Schoemig, 2007). Several animal studies and experimental interventions in humans have indicated a favorable effect of GT consumption on reducing the risk of development of atherosclerosis and reducing the incidence of cardiovascular events such as ischemic heart disease and stroke (Clement, 2009; Kuriyama, 2008). A longitudinal study utilizing data from 1109 Chinese reported an inverse association between GT consumption and 5-year BP change among Chinese adults (Tong, Taylor, Giles, Wittert, & Shi, 2014; C. S. Yang & Pan, 2012). The data also revealed that the effect of GT was nullified by smoking and obesity. GT mechanism of action is believed to be through improvement of endothelial function and blood flow enhancement (Nagaya et al., 2004). Furthermore, GT enhances metabolism and energy expenditure and reduces weight in obese patients. Moreover, GT lowers LDL cholesterol and total cholesterol, and reduces LDL oxidation. It should be also noted that GT polyphenols, especially catechins, may significantly impact the activity of important drug metabolizing enzymes, and hence, influence pharmacokinetics of a wide array of drugs used by patients with HTN (C. S. Yang & Pan, 2012).

Ginger

Ginger (GR) or rhizome of the perennial herb *Zingiber officinale Roscoe* is a famous spice plant, commonly used as a food additive to enhance its taste and smell. Indo-Pak subcontinent is the biggest exporter of ginger in the world (Shoji, Iwasa, Takemoto, Ishida, & Ohizumi, 1982). Ginger contains gingerol, shogaol, zingerone, zingiberol and paradol which exert its sharply strong taste or smell (Connell & McLachlan, 1972; Varma, Jain, & Bhattacharyya, 1962). Ginger has been used historically in the treatment of many diseases including gastrointestinal disorders (such as diarrhea, constipation, colic, anorexia, dyspepsia, nausea, vomiting, motion sickness) and HTN (Ghayur & Gilani, 2005). For example, in the traditional medicine practice of Pakistan, herbalists prescribe ginger to hypertensive patients to be taken after dinner, mostly because of its diuretic effect.

Rat studies with crude extract of ginger have indicated dose-dependent reduction in blood pressure (Fugh-Berman, 2000). The exact mechanism by which ginger reduces BP is not clear yet. One proposed mechanisms is blockade of voltage-dependent Ca^{2+} channels. Because of the anti-thrombotic potential of ginger, it may interact with blood-thinning drugs such as warfarin and must be used carefully in patients with blood clotting disorders.

Quercetin

Quercetin is a polyphenolic flavonoid that can be found in many plant-based foods, such as berries, apples, onions and red wine. Similar to other polyphenolic compounds, an inverse association was reported between Quercetin consumption and the risk of cardiovascular diseases. Recently, it was demonstrated that quercetin intake by hypertensive patients (>140 mmHg systolic and >90 mmHg diastolic) led to a decrease in blood pressure (Larson, Symons, & Jalili, 2012). The blood pressure lowering effect of quercetin was also evident in spontaneously hypertensive and Dahl salt-sensitive rats(Mackraj, Govender, & Ramesar, 2008) as well as rats that consume a high-fat, high-sucrose diet (Yamamoto & Oue, 2006), rats deficient in NO (Duarte et al., 2002), rats infused with angiotensin I (Häckl, Cuttle, Dovichi, Lima-Landman, & Nicolau, 2002), or have experimentally induced pressure overload using aortic constriction (Jalili et al., 2006). Many mechanisms have been proposed to explain the observed blood pressure lowering effect of quercetin including antioxidant effects, angiotensin-converting enzyme inhibition, and endothelium-dependent and -independent function improvement. Due to its vasorelaxant effect, co-administration of quercetin with other vasodilating agents may precipitate significant pharmacodynamics interactions (Vrolijk et al., 2015)

Wilde Thyme

Thymus serpyllum L. (wild thyme, TE) is an aromatic herb from the Lamiaceae family (genus Thymus) traditionally used as a culinary herb. Certain species of this genus are used in traditional medicine for the prevention or treatment of some diseases (*Herba thymi. In: Zhang X (ed) WHO monographs on selected medicinal plants*, 1999a; Mihailovic-Stanojevic et al., 2013). The family Lamiaceae exhibits significant polymorphism in morphological characteristics and composition of ethereal oils. Phenolic monoterpenes, thymol and carvacrol are the main constituents of essential oil of thyme (Cosentino et al., 1999; *Herba thymi. In: Zhang X (ed) WHO monographs on selected medicinal plants*, 1999b), while phenolic acid (rosmarinic acid) and flavonoids (quercetin, eriocitrin, luteolin, and apigenin) are proposed to be the polyphenolic compounds responsible for the antioxidant effects of aqueous tea infusions (Kulisic, Krisko, Dragovic-Uzelac, Milos, & Pifat, 2007; Yao et al., 2004). Rosmarinic and caffeic acids as predominant phenols presented in the TE.

In animal study, it was shown that the intake of TE significantly elevated the plasma NO as well as the total plasma nitrate/nitrite concentrations in spontaneously hypertensive rats (SHR) compared to normotensive control (WKY) (AlaghbandZadeh et al., 1996). In addition, *in vitro* studies have also shown that TE has antioxidant property and free radical scavenging activity, which might contribute to TE anti-hypertensive effect (Doggrell & Brown, 1998). Although *in vitro* and *in vivo* animal studies may indicate a promising use of TE as a dietary supplement to reduce BP in human, further investigation needed to elucidate the effectiveness of each TE components in HTN as well as their exact mechanisms of action.

TE is considered one of the safest CAM products and has Generally Recognized as Safe (GRAS) status in US if taken as recommended. So far no significant risks have been reported due to its regular consumption (Regulations, 2015).

Cinnamon

Cinnamon is a spice with pleasant aromatic flavor obtained from the peeled, dried, and brown bark of a southeast Asian tree genus *Cinnamomum*. Available clinical studies, although limited, have shown a blood pressure lowering effect of cinnamon in diabetic patients (Preuss, Echard, Polansky, & Anderson, 2006). Consumption of 2g of cinnamon for 12 weeks significantly reduces both systolic and diastolic blood pressures in Type 2 diabetic patients compared to control groups (Akilen, Tsiami, Devendra, & Robinson, 2010). Despite the fact that the underlying mechanism behind this effect is not fully elucidated, it seems that cinnamon lessens the levels of circulating insulin, which may clarify why it's compelling for those with diabetes (Akilen et al., 2010). As the tested dose was safe and well tolerated over the 12 weeks of treatment, cinnamon intake could be considered as an additional dietary supplement option for regulation of blood pressure, especially when no evidence in the literature indicates a potential effect of cinnamon on drug metabolizing enzymes (Akilen et al., 2010).

Persimmon

Persimmon (Diospyros kaki L) is a plant native to China and generally distributed in tropics and subtropics of East Asia, such as, Japan and Korea (Xie, Xie, Xu, & Yang, 2015) that is famous for its sweet fruits. "Shiye" is the fresh or dry leaves of persimmon. The leaves of the persimmon have been traditionally used to treat HTN in Japan. Many flavonoids, such as astragallin, which are isolated from persimmon Leaves have shown moderate inhibition of angiotensin-converting enzyme activity. For example, 300 µg/mL of astragalin showed an enzyme inhibition by 67%. Furthermore The IC_{50} of astragalin is 180 µg/mL (Kenji Kameda et al., 1987).

Origanum Majorana (OM) Leaves

Origanum majorana Linn (sweet marjoram), Family-Lamiaceae, is an essential aromatic plant native to the Mediterranean and southern Europe (Novak et al., 2000). OM is usually utilized as a part of cookery as condiment and a spice which is used to flavor meats, sausages, soups and salads. OM is also used in cosmetics and in the creation of vermouths and sharp flavoring. As a restorative plant, sweet marjoram has generally been utilized as stimulant and tonic. Marjoram volatile oil has already appeared to show antifungal activity (Pimple, Kadam, & Patil, 2012).

Traditionally, OM is used for the treatment of diabetes, catarrh, asthma, insomnia and anxiety. Exploratory examination has demonstrated many useful effects of leaves such as, antioxidant (Jun et al., 2001; Suhaj, 2006), hepatoprotecitve (El-Ashmawy, El-Nahas, & Salama, 2005), antibacterial (Darwish & Aburjai, 2010), antifungal (Manohar et al., 2001), antihypertensive (Tahraoui, El-Hilaly, Israili, & Lyoussi, 2007) and antiplatelet aggregation properties (Yazdanparast & Shahriyary, 2008). Moreover, other species of the same genus Origanum, i.e. Origanum vulgare has antihyperglycemic effect (Lemhadri, Zeggwagh, Maghrani, Jouad, & Eddouks, 2004) and antioxidant activities (Chun, Vattem, Lin, & Shetty, 2005).

OM is available in different extract forms such as hydrodistilled volatile oil extract (OMO), methanolic extract (OMM), petroleum ether extract (OMPE) and aqueous extract (OMW) and each of them has different biological effect. For example, the volatile oil (OMO, 100 mg/kg p.o.) is less significant ($p<0.05$) in bringing down the raised triglyceride and cholesterol levels. On the other hand, methanolic (OMM, 200 and 400 mg/kg p.o.) and aqueous (OMW, 200 and 400 mg/kg p.o.) extracts considerably demonstrated antihyperlipidemic effect, which may have indirectly contributed to its use as antihypertensive plant.

OM has Generally Recognized as Safe (GRAS) status in US if used in amount commonly found in foods.

Therefore, its consumption as recommended is free of side effects (Regulations, 2015).

Coenzyme Q10

Coenzyme Q10 or CoQ10 (2,3 dimethoxy-5 meth-6-decaprenyl benzoquinone) is a fat-soluble vitamin-like compound that is mainly derived from mevalonic acid and phenylalanine and almost found in every single human cells. The compound was first isolated in 1957 from beef mitochondria. Compared to the rest of human body, organs with high-energy turnover such as kidney, heart, liver and pancreas contain the highest amount. Normally, the human body produces sufficient amounts of CoQ10 that is needed for many physiological processes. However, CoQ10 can also be supplemented by oral intake or by the consumption of animal derived foods such as beef, poultry and seafood. It has been shown that regular daily intake of such foods provides approximately 3-5 mg. Following oral ingestion, CoQ10 is mainly absorbed in the small intestine and its bioavailability enhanced by the presence of oily rich meal. Following absorption, CoQ10 molecule forms a complex with low-density lipoprotein (LDL) in the liver and then transported and stored in various tissues. Interestingly, It has been shown that CoQ10 reaches its highest level during childhood, and it continues to decline with age progression, reaching its lowest level at age 80 and older. Although it has been shown that CoQ10 could prolong the lifespan of *Caenorhabditis elegans* soil worm, yet, there is no clear evidence to support this effect in humans (Ishii et al., 2004).

CoQ10 gains its powerful antioxidant activity due to presence of benzooquinone group within its chemical structure. The compound is capable of quenching free radicals generated from various biological pathways, works as a membrane stabilizer and a cofactor in several vital metabolic pathways such as ATP production in oxidative respiration.

The advantage of oral intake of CoQ10 supplements has been well studied in various diseases such as angina, congestive heart failure, aged macular degeneration and Parkinson's disease. Importantly, The effect of CoQ10 on blood pressure in hypertensive patients has been also demonstrated by several preliminary clinical studies. Indeed, patients who received either CoQ10 alone or along with their conventional antihypertensive agents have shown a statistically significant reduction in their overall blood pressure compared to control groups. In a 12-week, double blind, placebo controlled clinical study done by Burke and associates on patient with isolated systolic HTN, they have demonstrated that daily intake of 120 mg of CoQ10 significantly reduced the systolic blood pressure (SBP) by 17.8 mmHg compare to 1.7 mmHg reduction in the placebo group (Burke, Neuenschwander, & Olson, 2001). Singh and his team have also conducted an 8-week randomized, double blind clinical trial on hypertensive patients with coronary artery disease and who were taking their conventional antihypertensive agents for at least one year. The participants were given either 120 mg per day of CoQ10 or a placebo. In fact, oral supplementation of CoQ10 showed a reduction in SBP by 16 mmHg and diastolic blood pressure (DBP) by 9 mmHg compared to placebo group (Singh, Niaz, Rastogi, Shukla, & Thakur, 1999). In addition, they have reported that insulin resistance, serum glucose levels, triglycerides, lipid peroxides were also reduced in CoQ10 treated patients. Digiesi and associates conducted a 10-week crossover study on patient with essential HTN. In his study, patients were given 100 mg per day of CoQ10 with 2-week washout period prior to CoQ10 initiation. Both, SBP and DBP significantly reduced by 17 and 12 mmHg respectively (Digiesi et al., 1994). Finally, Langsjoen and colleagues conducted a study on individuals with established essential HTN. Instead of giving patients a fixed dose of CoQ10, each individual received an adjusted dose of CoQ10 that is required to maintain CoQ10 serum concentration of ≥ 2.0 µg / ml. Consistent with previous studies, they have found that CoQ10 reduced the SBP by 11.4 mmHg and DBP by 9 mmHg (Langsjoen, Langsjoen, Willis, & Folkers, 1994). Interestingly, they also have found that in some patient's, oral supplementation of CoQ10 led to either dose reduction or discontinuation of their conventional antihypertensive therapy. Conversely, in a small, double blind, placebo controlled clinical trial; the lowering blood pressure effect of 100 mg CoQ10 daily intake in patients with HTN and metabolic syndrome was not significant suggesting that the complexity level of the disease in those patients overrides the CoQ10 benefits (Young et al., 2012).

As mentioned earlier, the increase in the oxidative stress is well documented as a key factor in the development of HTN. Those changes cause significant alterations in the endothelium contraction and vascular resistance. The imbalance between reactive oxygen species (ROS) production and nitric oxide (NO) bioavailability both contribute to HTN development (Y. K. Yang et al., 2015). Notably, CoQ10 levels have been shown to be low in patients who are identified to have a greater prevalence of HTN. However, the exact mechanism of CoQ10 action in HTN is not fully understood. Yet, its powerful antioxidant activity has been attributed as a key factor in reducing the peripheral resistance and improving the endothelial-independent arterial relaxation by decreasing the levels of peroxidation, attenuation of endothelial nitric oxide synthase down-regulation and eventually maintaining nitric oxide bioavailability (Folkers et al., 1981; Pepe et al., 2007). In addition, it has been suggested that CoQ10 might also boost the synthesis of prostacyclin PGI2, a potent vasodilator, or increase the arterial smooth muscle sensitivity to PGI2 leading to peripheral vascular resistance reduction and ultimately to blood pressure (BP) reduction (Lonnrot et al., 1998). It is also though that CoQ10 might interfere with aldosterone-angiotensin pathway by decreasing the secretion of aldosterone and compromises the effect of angiotensin in sodium and water retention(Fabre, Banks, McIsaac, & Farrell, 1965).

CoQ10 is generally well tolerated and has no significant adverse effects if taken as recommended. However, administration of statins have been shown to reduce CoQ10 levels in dose dependent manner (Rundek, Naini, Sacco, Coates, & DiMauro, 2004). The mechanism of CoQ10 levels reduction is partially understood and could be due to the cholesterol lowering effect by statins; yet, the clinical significance of such reduction is not fully understood. Some researchers believe that CoQ10 reduction might have a role in the development of statin related myopathy. Despite CoQ10 has a similar chemical structure as vitamin K derivative menaquinon, the effect of CoQ10 and warfarin co-administration on blood clotting is still controversial. However, close monitoring of INR is highly recommended.

Vitamin C

Vitamin C or Ascorbic acid is a water-soluble antioxidant found in high concentration in citrus fruits and rosehip. Although it can be produced by many mammals, human must obtain vitamin C by other sources like food or as an oral supplement. The vitamin is labile and decomposed upon air or heat exposure or cooking, and food storage causes a significant vitamin amount reduction. Vitamin C has a key role in many biological pathways such as cellular respiration, carbohydrate metabolism and lipid and protein synthesis. It is also involved in the synthesis of various endogenous factors like dopamine, norepinephrine and thyroxin. Following oral intake, vitamin C is readily absorbed from the intestine by an active process. The percentage of absorbed amount is dose dependent, for example, approximately 50% of a 1250 mg dose is absorbed, compare to 87% of a 30 mg oral dose. Vitamin C is distributed very well in human body including the central nervous system and metabolized to an active compound dehydroascorbic acid. Both vitamin C and its active metabolite are eliminated by renal excretion. Daily intake of 400 mg of vitamin C or higher attain a steady state of 80 µmol/L serum concentration, However, doses higher than 2g/day may increase the risk of developing renal oxalate calculi(Urivetzky, Kessaris, & Smith, 1992).

Vitamin C is traditionally used to boost the immune system against viral infection such as flue. However, the role of vitamin C in HTN management has been studied by several small and short-term clinical studies. Interestingly, it has been shown that vitamin C deficiency is associated with increases of both SBP and DBP(Block et al., 2001; Kim et al., 2002). Yet, daily oral intake of 500 mg of vitamin C alone has no significant effect on both SBP and DBP in hypertensive patients(Block et al., 2001; Kim et al., 2002). Instead, It appears that vitamin C has a beneficial effect only in patients, who take vitamin C along with their conventional antihypertensive medications. In those patients, vitamin C appears to reduce their SBP modestly, while the effects on DBP have been inconsistent. In randomized, one-month double blind clinical trial conducted by Duffy and associates, hypertensive patients were given either

500 mg of vitamin C daily or placebo along with their antihypertensive medications. Interestingly, SBP was significantly reduced by 13 mmHg in treated groups compared to placebo, but no significant effect on DBP(Duffy et al., 1999). Sato and colleagues also conducted another randomized clinical study in elderly patients. They have noticed that patients who received 600 mg /daily of vitamin C for six months showed a significant reduction in their SBP by 20 mmHg compared to placebo, however, they also did not observe any significant effect on DBP(Sato et al., 2006). Fotherby and his team also conducted a 6-month double blind crossover study in which elderly patients were given either 500 mg of vitamin C or placebo with a one-week washout period, and reported that daily intake of vitamin C has modest lowering effects on high SBP(Fotherby, Williams, Forster, Craner, & Ferns, 2000).

The exact mechanism of vitamin C in HTN is not fully understood. However, It has been suggested that, the inhibition of endothelium-derived nitric oxide (NO), a potent vasodilator, by superoxide anions is a major contributing cause of HTN development. Possibly, the antioxidant activity of vitamin C and its free radical scavenging roles, reverse the superoxide inhibition activity; allow vasodilatation and eventually leading to BP reduction. Furthermore, it has been shown that vitamin C works also as an enzyme modulator on the vascular wall by increasing the bioavailability of endothelial nitric oxide synthase (eNOS) and decreasing NADPH oxidase (Ulker, McKeown, & Bayraktutan, 2003).

Vitamin C appears to be safe and its effect is dose related. Generally, It has been found that oral intake of more than 2 g per day might be associated with several adverse effects such as osmotic diarrhea and gastrointestinal upset. In addition, vitamin C may also enhance the precipitation of oxalate and urate in urine and increases the possibility of forming kidney stones. The incidence of hyperoxaluria risk is significantly higher in people with oxalate kidney stones history and who tend to take 1 g and more of vitamin C per day. Other reports have shown that vitamin C might also increase the risk of cardiovascular mortality in postmenopausal diabetic women, carotid inner wall thickening in men, and DNA damage by increasing the production of reactive oxygen molecules and hemolysis in people with glucose-6-phosphate dehydrogenase deficiency.

Dark Chocolate and Cocoa Products

Traditionally, cocoa products are widely used in food industry and in manufacturing of various cosmetic and pharmaceutical preparations. The plant extract is highly enriched with flavonoids such as epicatechin and catechin, which have shown various benefits in reducing cardiovascular diseases incidences and in the managements of hypercholesterolemia. The Cocoa also contains many other ingredients such as caffeine, theobromine, tyramine, fat and carbohydrates. Interestingly, the benefits of cocoa consumption in HTN got greater attention following the observational studies conducted on Kuna Indians people who live in San Blas Island of Panama, a place that is traditionally well known for cocoa trees and unprocessed cocoa drinks. Researcher have noticed that Kuna Indians people who drank at least three cups daily of cocoa drinks have lower blood pressure compared to the ones who migrated to the mainland and stopped consuming cocoa drinks. These observations encouraged scientist to conduct various clinical trials to identify the possible roles of cocoa in HTN management. However, the Cocoa effect appears to be significant in both pre-hypertensive and hypertensive patients rather than normotensive individuals. Indeed, the BP reduction with dark chocolate, a product which is highly rich in polyphenols, is not as robust as other supplementary products such CoQ10 or DASH diets.

The effect of Cocoa on blood pressure reduction was conducted by various clinical trials. Taubert and his associate conducted an 18-week, randomized single blind, parallel study on a small group of patients whom their ages ranging from 56 through 73 years and with either untreated pre-hypertensive state or stage 1 HTN and had no other concomitant risk factors (D. Taubert, Roesen, Lehmann, Jung, & Schomig, 2007). Patients were randomly assigned to get either 6.3 g daily of rich polyphenol containing dark chocolate or polyphenol-free white chocolate. Indeed, the patients who were given dark chocolate showed a significant reduction in their both SBP and DBP by 2.9 and 1.9 mmHg respectively. The investigators related the reduction in the BP to the activation of endothelial nitric oxide synthesis. In addition, and to support his findings, Taubert also conducted another study on small group of elderly patients with mild untreated stage 1 isolated systolic HTN (D. Taubert, Berkels, Roesen, & Klaus, 2003). Patients were randomly assigned to get 100 g of dark chocolate that contain at least 500 mg of polyphenols and 90 g of polyphenol free white chocolate for 14 days. SBP was significantly declined by 5.1 mmHg and DBP by 1.8 mmHg in patients given dark chocolate compared to white chocolate group. Furthermore, Grassi and his colleagues, conducted a 15-day randomized single blind, crossover study in patients with essential HTN. The patients were given either a 100 g of dark chocolate and 90 g of polyphenol free white chocolate. Ambulatory 24 hours BP decreased by 11.9 mmHg and DBP by 8.5 mmHg respectively in patient who received dark chocolate, while no effect on BP was noticed in patients who received white chocolate (Grassi et al., 2005). Grasssi has also showed that dark chocolate polyphenols decrease insulin resistance, LDL and cholesterol levels in hypertensive patients. Interestingly, the effect of dark chocolate on BP in healthy subjects seems to be not significant. In this context, Engler conducted a 2-week study on healthy volunteers to evaluate the effect of daily intake of high flavonoid rich dark chocolate on the endothelial function and its effect on blood pressure reduction (Engler et al., 2004). Although there was an improvement in individual's endothelial function; their BP was not significantly affected. Rostami and his associate conducted an 8-week, randomized, placebo-controlled double blind study on individuals with type 2 diabetes and HTN. Patients were given either 25 g of dark chocolate or equivalent amount of white chocolate. Dark chocolate induced significant reduction in both SBP and DBP by 5.93 and 6.4 mmHg respectively compared to the white chocolate group. Interestingly, the triglycerides levels in patients who received dark chocolate were also effectively reduced. Yet, no effect on insulin resistance or glycemic control was observed in both groups(Rostami et al., 2015).

Conversely, Muniyappa and his team conducted a 2-week randomized, double blind, placebo controlled, crossover study in individuals with essential HTN and who were taking their conventional antihypertensive drugs (Muniyappa et al., 2008). Patients were asked to stop their conventional medications prior to the study initiation. Then, the patients were given flavanol-rich cocoa drink (900 mg of flavonols per day) for 2 weeks followed by 7 days washout period prior placebo treatment initiation. In fact, the result generated from study was conflicting and despite the fact that consumption of falvonol-rich cocoa enhanced insulin mediated vasodilation yet it has no significant effect on BP reduction or insulin resistance.

Many studies suggested that Cocoa improve the endothelial function and increase production of nitric oxide, a potent vasodilator, possibly through up-regulation of endothelial nitric oxide synthase (eNOS), an effect which was reversed by a competitive inhibitor of eNOS such as L-G monomethyl arginine(Heiss et al., 2005; D. Taubert et al., 2003; D. Taubert et al., 2007). The role of oxidative stress in HTN is also well documented as mentioned before. It has been also suggested that flavonols can work as an antioxidant during the oxidative stress through reducing the nitric oxide (NO) breakdown by reactive oxygen species. Furthermore, the ability of chocolate- flavanols to inhibit angiotensin-converting enzymes (ACE) was also supported by several *in vivo* and *in vitro* studies (Persson, Persson, Hagg, & Andersson, 2011).

Modest consumption of cocoa is considered safe. However, cocoa also contain other ingredient such caffeine, theobromine and calories and excessive consumption might cause undesirable side effects such as increase in heart rate, GI upset and weight gain. Cocoa might also inhibit platelets aggregation and adhesion and decreases iron absorption. In addition, caffeine has been found to inhibit CYP450 1A2 enzyme, and such effect might decrease the metabolism of many drugs such as clozapine and might increase their possible side effects. Caffeine might affect the serum lithium levels and abrupt consumption of cocoa might lead to increase serum levels and thereby potentiate lithium side effects such as tremors(Mester et al., 1995). However, the clinical significance of cocoa on lithium needs further investigation.

L-Arginine

L-arginine (2-amino-5-guanidinopentanoic acid) is a non-essential amino acid that is required for protein synthesis. The amino acid is naturally found in high amount in many foods such as fish, beef, eggs and dairy products. Following oral intake, the arginine is well absorbed in the jejunum by special carries, then subjected to extensive metabolism by enterocytes. Arginine homeostasis is mainly regulated by hepatic metabolism and urinary excretion. Human pharmacokinetic studies showed that excessive intake activate both hepatic arginase and renal clearance. L- arginine is able to stimulate the release of growth hormone (GH), prolactin, glucagon, insulin, and gastrin in stomach and inhibit the tubular reabsorption of protein. Arginine is also a natural substrate for nitric oxide synthase that converts the amino acid into a potent vasodilator nitric oxide, which involved in many regularity function of the cardiovascular system. Also it has been shown that arginine conversion to nitric oxide improves endothelial function, reduces monocyte endothelial adhesion and increases coronary blood flow in patient with coronary artery diseases (Lerman, Burnett, Higano, McKinley, & Holmes, 1998). L-arginine may also act as an antioxidant by decreasing the production of vascular super-oxidase, improving nitric acid availability and decreases the incidence of nitrate tolerance (Parker, Parker, Caldwell, Farrell, & Kaesemeyer, 2002). The roles of arginine in several cardiovascular diseases, erectile dysfunction and many others were investigated. However, The benefits of oral intake of arginine on blood pressure reductions were also conducted in both healthy individuals and diseased patients. Interestingly, it has been shown that people with normal diet who have adequate concentration of L-arginine that ensures optimum NO production by NOS enzyme do not respond to supplementation compared to people with L-arginine deficient diet. Therefore, L-arginine supplementation appears to be more effective in patients who do not consume enough L-arginine in their diet (Wu & Meininger, 2000).

To investigate the role of L-arginine in HTN, Ast and his team, conducted a 4-week, randomized, parallel, double blind, clinical trial to study the effect of arginine consumption on BP in healthy volunteers and in patients with mild HTN (Ast et al., 2010). Individuals in each group were randomized to receive either 6 or 12 g daily of arginine or placebo. The result showed a significant reduction in both SBP and DBP in patients with mild HTN and who received 12 g of arginine daily compared to placebo control. Neri and his colleagues also conducted another 12-week, randomized double blind study in female with gestational HTN (Neri et al., 2010). In his study, women were randomized to receive 4 g daily of oral arginine versus placebo and then submitted to 24 h ambulatory BP monitoring. Although supplementation with L-arginine does not significantly affect the overall blood pressure; it has been shown that L-arginine daily consumption is associated with improved health outcomes, less need for antihypertensive medications and fewer neonatal and maternal complications. Martina and associate conducted a 6-month clinical trial to study the effect of oral intake of L-arginine along with N-acetyl cysteine, a precursor of glutathione, in type two diabetic patients with HTN (Martina et al., 2008). The combination treatment caused statistically significant reduction in both SBP and DBP mean arterial pressure by improving the endothelial function, reducing the oxidative stress and increasing NO availability. Morris and his team also studied the role of arginine in pulmonary HTN secondary to sickle cell anemia (Morris et al., 2003). It has been shown that NO, a potent vasodilator is deficient during the sickle cell crises. Oral intake of L-arginine produced 15.2% mean reduction in pulmonary artery systolic pressureby donating nitrogen for NO synthesis and decreeing the serum levels of the potent vasoconstrictor endotheilin-1. Palloshi and his team conducted a 4-week clinical trial in hypertensive patients with angina. Patients were given 6 g of L-arginine along with their conventional antihypertensive and anti-angina drugs. L-arginine significantly reduced SBP by 20 mmHg(Palloshi et al., 2004).

Appropriate L-arginine consumption appears to be safe, however side effects such as bloating, diarrhea and abdominal pain have been reported. Importantly, in patients with renal insufficiency or failure, arginine causes hyperkalemia, which might lead to cardiac arrhythmia, and possibly death. As a result, L-arginine Supplementation in those patients is not recommended.

Ginkgo Biloba

Ginkgo biloba, commonly known as ginkgo, has been widely used in Asia for more than 2000 years in traditional medicine. In addition, its seeds served as an important food source during the 1930-1960 food shortage in Japan. Both, gingko seeds and leaf extracts are of the top selling medicinal plant products worldwide. Gingko biloba leaf extract (GBE) contain many compounds such as flavonoids, terpenoids, organic acids, carbohydrate, lipid and many others. Also, both seeds and leaf extracts contain ginkotoxin, a toxic product that might cause seizures if ingested in excessive amount. Interestingly, The plant extracts has been shown to improve brain energy supply, enhance nerve growth and communication function that have beneficial effects in several medical conditions like dementia, sexual dysfunction, depression and attention deficit hyperactivity disorder.

The role of GBE in HTN was also investigated *in vitro* and *in vivo*. However, the results in human were conflicting. In one large-scale and long-term clinical trial, Brinkley and his team found that the ingestion of 240 mg of GBE in elderly patients with either HTN or pre-HTN stage has no significant effect on BP compared to the ones who received placebo(Brinkley et al., 2010). Kudolo conducted a small clinical trial to study the effect of GBE on pancreatic beta cell function. In addition to GBE ability to increase the rate of insulin clearance, it has been shown that GBE also significantly decrease both SBP and DPB by 9 and 18 mmHg respectively (Kudolo, 2000).Furthermore, Wang et al, published a systematic review on Chinese clinical trials and the benefits of Chinese herbal products including GBE in HTN management(Wang et al., 2013). Wang concluded that many Chinese clinical trials have shown that flavonol glycosides of GBE significantly lower blood pressure and improve the quality of life in hypertensive patient.

The mechanism by which GBE reduces BP in hypertensive patients is not fully understood. However, it was proposed that GBE has a vasodilation activity that inhibits the rise in BP by its ability to counteract the endothelium dysfunction and restore the vascular sensitivity to endothelium-dependent relaxants. In addition, GBE is highly rich with flavonoids the most available active ingredients, which have been reported to modulate ACE system (Actis-Goretta, Ottaviani, & Fraga, 2006; K. Kameda et al., 1987). Furthermore, experiments in hypertensive rat models supported those finding and showed that GBE inhibits the angiotensin-converting enzyme and preserve vascular reactivity, which attenuates the increase in BP (Mansour, Bahgat, El-Khatib, & Khayyal, 2011). The anti-oxidant activity of GBE in oxidative stress is another possible mechanism by which GBE exert its antihypertensive effect.

In tissue culture experiment, flavonoids were found to decreases the intracellular production of ROS while increasing the levels of ROS in the culture media, a phenomena that might explain the increase of Malondialdehyde (MDA), a marker for oxidative stress, in rats treated with GBE extract (Choi, Chee, & Lee, 2003; Robaszkiewicz, Balcerczyk, & Bartosz, 2007). It is also worth noting that the differences in quality and composition of the GBE may also affect the bioavailability of the active ingredients and therefore affect the GBE biological effects (Kressmann, Muller, & Blume, 2002).

GBE if used appropriately and as recommended is considered safe and well tolerated. However, it can cause mild gastrointestinal upset, headache, dizziness, constipation, and sometimes-allergic skin reactions. Moreover, excessive consumption of leaf extract or seeds can be life threatening. Although the number of roasted seeds that can be eaten safely is not defined, yet it has been suggested that ingesting more than ten to fifteen roasted seeds per day can cause several side effects including difficulty of breathing, seizures, loss of consciousness, and even shock. In addition, fresh ginkgo seed is highly toxic and oral consumption should be avoided since it might cause serious side effects including death. Furthermore, numerous analytical and phytochemical studies *in vitro* and *in vivo* using animal models were performed on gingko leaf extract and have shown that CYP 1A2, 2C9, 2C19, 2D6, 2E1 and 3A4 are all inhibited by GBE to variable degrees. However, the clinical significant effect of GBE on most human CYP enzymes appears to be minimal. GBE also seems to inhibit p-glycoprotein in vivo and organic anion transporting polypeptide (OATP) in vitro (Naccarato, Yoong, & Gough, 2012). Yet, it has been shown that in healthy volunteers, ginkgo does not appear to significantly alter the pharmacokinetics of the OATP substrates such as ticlopidine.

Psyllium

Psyllium is a dietary fiber supplement that is commonly used as stool softener, treatment for diarrhea, blood cholesterol lowering agent and in many other clinical conditions. The product is also used in food industry as food thickener and stabilizer. The seeds and the seed husk are the most applicable part of psyllium and both are rich in water-soluble fibers that form a viscous gel when mixed with water. Despite the fact that soluble fibers might undergo partial fermentation by intestinal bacteria in the colon, yet the bulking effect of psyllium is mainly due to the intact material.

The role of dietary fiber consumption in HTN has been studied in both animal and human. In fact, It has been shown that daily intake of fibers in a form of food or as an oral supplements may decrease the risk of HTN development. In addition, it has been reported that with the risk of higher blood pressure may be related to low dietary fiber intake (Stamler, Caggiula, & Grandits, 1997). As a result, the world health organization (WHO) recommend an increase in dietary fiber intake as a safe and effective approach to reduce CVD in hypertensive population ("Diet, nutrition and the prevention of chronic diseases," 2003).

In many clinical trials psyllium appears to reduce blood pressure significantly. Burke and his associates conducted an 8-week, parallel randomized, controlled clinical study on hypertensive patients and who were taking their conventional antihypertensive medication for at least six months. Patients were given either low fiber diet or asked to consume an additional 15 g of psyllium, fiber rich diet, per day along with soy protein diet (V. Burke et al., 2001). Interestingly, systolic blood pressure was significantly reduced by 5.9 mmHg in patients treated with fiber and protein diet compared to control diet subjects. Cicero and his team conducted a 6-month randomized clinical trial in overweight patients with HTN. Daily intake of 3.5 g three times a day was associated with a significant decrease in both SBP and DBP by 5.2 and 2.2 mmHg respectively (Cicero et al., 2007). Pal and associates conducted another 12-week, randomized, single blind, parallel clinical study in overweight and obese individuals (Pal, Khossousi, Binns, Dhaliwal, & Radavelli-Bagatini, 2012). Subjects were randomized into three groups, a) the control group who were supplemented with placebo in addition to their regular diet; b) fiber supplemented group; and c) the healthy eating and placebo supplemented group. Fiber supplement group were given 12 gm of Metamucil® containing 7 g of psyllium three times a day. Both SBP and DBP were lower in fiber diet group by approximately 7% compared to control group at week six. Yet, there was no significant difference in either SBP or DBP between the groups at 12 week. The lack of differences at the end of the experiment was attributed to psychological stress or day-to-day variability in BP.

The mechanism by which psyllium is reducing the BP is not fully understood. It has been shown that hypercholesterolemia impairs the endothelial dependent dilatation and associated with NO-induced vasodilation loss, which ultimately leads to an increase in BP and HTN. Therefore, it was proposed that the indirect effect of psyllium on BP could be due to its ability to improve the patient lipid profile through increasing intestinal viscosity and decreasing lipid absorption (Jenkins, Kendall, Axelsen, Augustin, & Vuksan, 2000). Furthermore, it has been shown that the increase in insulin resistance might be also involved in the development of HTN (Ferrannini et al., 1987). Interestingly, the ability of water-soluble fiber has been shown to decrease insulin resistance in both healthy and diabetic patient and might be a contributing factor in psyllium BP reduction (Anderson et al., 1991; Fukagawa, Anderson, Hageman, Young, & Minaker, 1990)

Appropriate use of psyllium is considered safe. However transient flatulence, constipation and GI upset have been reported. In addition some patients are allergic to psyllium, a reaction that might be sever and could lead to anaphylactic shock. In addition, psyllium can reduce the digestion of fat, decrease its absorption and increase fat fecal content (Ganji & Kies, 1994).

CONCLUSION

It is very clear that CAM therapies are used by a lot of people worldwide including Americans with large out-of pocket expenses for prevention or treatment of various health conditions. While, most Americans use CAM as a complementary to their conventional therapy, a small percentage of people are also using CAM treatments, alone. However, despite their clinical effectiveness and lower cost, the lack of scientific information regarding the safety for some, and the false impression by the general public that "natural" products are generally safe, yet many of them required further investigation. Importantly, CAM products can be easily introduced to the US market and sold without FDA restriction or any safety testing requirements. Indeed, the widespread consumption, the lack of quality control, adulterated/counterfeit products and unethical marketing could add further risks to CAM users. Consequently, it is crucial that the health care providers should familiarize themselves with CAM and CAM products efficacy and safety, question their patients if they are using these remedies and evaluate the current clinical studies so they can deliver evidence-based advice to their patients accordingly. Generally, the use of CAM products in this chapter can be considered for all hypertensive patients and for many their use is supported by clinical studies but not as robust as that for conventional pharmacotherapy. CAM products such as CoQ10, psyllium, dark chocolate, cinnamon, garlic and thyme are considered safe and can be taken alone or together with conventional therapies. However, Ginkgo biloba, can cause serious adverse effects through drug-herb interaction or by itself. As a result, both patients and health care providers should be aware of recommended doses, treatment duration, CAM possible side effects and if any drug-herbal or herbal-disease interactions exist. A summary of our findings is presented in Table 2.

Table 1. List of abbreviations

Abbreviation	Term
ACEi	angiotensin-converting enzyme inhibitors
ARBs	angiotensin receptor blockers
BP	Blood pressure
CAM	Complementary & Alternative Medicine
CCBs	calcium channel blockers
CKD	Chronic kidney disease
CO	cardiac output
CoQ10	Coenzyme Q10
CVD	cardiovascular disease
DBP	Diastolic blood pressure
ESRD	end-stage renal disease
GBE	Gingko biloba leaf extract
GRAS	Generally Recognized as Safe
HTN	Hypertension
NO	nitric oxide
RAAS	renin-angiotensin-aldosterone system
SBP	Systolic blood pressure
SNS	sympathetic nervous system
SVR	systemic vascular resistance
TE	wild thyme

Table 2. Summary of findings

Product	Clinical Effect on BP	Common Adverse Effects	Comments	Reference
Cinnamon	↓ SBP and DBP	No significant adverse effects reported, well tolerated	Significant BP reduction effect mainly in HT patients with Type 2 diabetes.	Akilen and Robinson, 2010
Coenzyme Q10	↓ SBP and DBP	Possible GI upset	• Statin reduce CoQ10 levels (possible mechanism of statin myopathy adverse effect). • Interfere with warfarin (monitor INR)	Singh 1999 Burke 2001 Degesie 1994 Langsjoen 1994 Rundek 2004
Dark Chocolate	↓ SBP and DBP	• Excessive ingestion: o GI upset. o Weight gain. o Caffeine cause CNS stimulation and increase heart rate.	• Decrease iron absorption. • Inhibit platelet aggregation. • Inhibits CYP450 1A2 enzyme and increase many drugs adverse effects (e.g clozapine). • Abrupt consumption might increase serum level of lithium in patients taking the drug.	D.taubert, berkels 2003 Grassi 2005 Person, 2011 Mester 1995
Garlic	Effective in SBP ≥ 140 mmHg	• Breath and body odor. • GI irritation and heart burn.	• Interfere with anticoagulant function • Inhibit CYP2E1 and increase levels of its substrates (e.g acetaminophen, ethanol, theophylline).	Holzgartner, 1992 Macan 2006 Williams,2005

continued on following page

Table 2. Continued

Product	Clinical Effect on BP	Common Adverse Effects	Comments	Reference
Ginger	Dose dependent in BP reduction	Abdominal discomfort	May interact with anticoagulant/antiplatelet (e.g warfarin) and increase the risk of bleeding.	Fugh-berman 2000
Ginko Biloba	↓ SBP and DBP	• Excessive ingestion: o GI upset. o Headache. o Seizures. o Shock.	• Inhibit and induce many CYP 450 enzymes (1A2, 2C9, 2C19, 2D6, 2E1, 3A4) and interact with many drug metabolism (e.g. TCA, Bupropion, statins) • Inhibit drug transporters P-glycproteins and OATP, lead to multiple drug interactions (e.g. ticlopidine)	Wang, 2013 Actis, 2006 Kameda 1987 Naccarato, 2012 Choi, Chee (2003)
Green Tea	Consumption has inverse association with HT risk	• High dosses: o GI upset o CNS stimulation, sleep disturbance due to caffeine.	• Benefit in HT is nullified by smoking and obesity. • Affect many CYP enzymes (1A2, 3A4) and influence the clearance of wide array of drugs (e.g Clozapine, warfarin)	Tong, tyalor 2014 Yan and pan 2012
L-arginine	↓SBP and DBP, ↓Pulmonary HT	• Bloating • Diarrhea • Abdominal pain	• If used in gestational HT: Fewer neonatal and maternal complications. • C/I: renal insufficiency (leads to hyperkalemia)	Ast 2010 Neri, 2010 Morris 2003 Martina, 2008 Palloshi, 2004
Omega 3-fatty acids	↓ SBP and DBP	• Very well tolerated. • Increase risk of bleeding • Might increase triglycerides	• Interfere with anticoagulant agents and increase risk of bleeding (e.g. warfarin)	Geleijnse, 2002 Ueshima 2007 Sanders and Vickers 1981
Origanum Majorana	↓ SBP and DBP	• GRAS	• Different extract forms available with different pharmacodynamic properties	Tahraoui, 2007 Regulation, 2015
Persimmon	↓ SBP and DBP	• N/A	• N/A	Kenji kameda 1987
Psyllium	↓ SBP and DBP	• GI upset • Constipation • Reduce fat digestion and absorption	• Might delay or decrease the absorption of several drugs (lithium).	Burke 2001 Cicero 2007 Ganji 1994
Quercetin	↓SBP and DBP	• Headache • Possible tingling	• Interact with vasodilators and enhance their effects	Larson, Symons 2012 Mackraj, 2008 Vrolijk 2015
Vitamin C	↓ SBP	• High doses: o GI upset o Osmotic diarrhea. o Hyperoxaluria. o Kidney stones.	• Decompose upon heat or air exposure. • GI absorption is dose dependent. • Avoid in G6PD deficiency.	Urivetzky, 1992 Duffy 1999 Sato 2006 Fotherby 2000

REFERENCES

Actis-Goretta, L., Ottaviani, J. I., & Fraga, C. G. (2006). Inhibition of angiotensin converting enzyme activity by flavanol-rich foods. *Journal of Agricultural and Food Chemistry*, *54*(1), 229–234. doi:10.1021/jf052263o PMID:16390204

Akilen, R., Tsiami, A., Devendra, D., & Robinson, N. (2010). Glycated haemoglobin and blood pressure-lowering effect of cinnamon in multi-ethnic Type 2 diabetic patients in the UK: A randomized, placebo-controlled, double-blind clinical trial. *Diabetic Medicine*, *27*(10), 1159–1167. doi:10.1111/j.1464-5491.2010.03079.x PMID:20854384

Al-Qattan, K. K., Khan, I., Alnaqeeb, M. A., & Ali, M. (2001). Thromboxane-B2, prostaglandin-E2 and hypertension in the rat 2-kidney 1-clip model: A possible mechanism of the garlic induced hypotension. *Prostaglandins, Leukotrienes, and Essential Fatty Acids*, *64*(1), 5–10. doi:10.1054/plef.2000.0232 PMID:11161580

Al-Qattan, K. K., Thomson, M., Al-Mutawa'a, S., Al-Hajeri, D., Drobiova, H., & Ali, M. (2006). Nitric oxide mediates the blood-pressure lowering effect of garlic in the rat two-kidney, one-clip model of hypertension. *The Journal of Nutrition*, *136*(3), 774S–776S. PMID:16484561

Alaghband-Zadeh, J., Das, I., Hanson, M. R., MacGregor, C. A., de Wardener, H. E., & Laycock, J. F.AlaghbandZadeh. (1996). Hypothalamic and plasma total nitrate/nitrite concentrations in spontaneously hypertensive rats. *Experimental Physiology*, *81*(5), 881–883. doi:10.1113/expphysiol.1996.sp003984 PMID:8889485

Anderson, J. W., Zeigler, J. A., Deakins, D. A., Floore, T. L., Dillon, D. W., & Wood, C. L. (1991). Metabolic effects of high-carbohydrate, high-fiber diets for insulin-dependent diabetic individuals. *The American Journal of Clinical Nutrition*, *54*(5), 936–943. PMID:1659172

Asdaq, S. M., & Inamdar, M. N. (2010). Potential of garlic and its active constituent, S-allyl cysteine, as antihypertensive and cardioprotective in presence of captopril. *Phytomedicine*, *17*(13), 1016–1026. doi:10.1016/j.phymed.2010.07.012 PMID:20739164

Ast, J., Jablecka, A., Bogdanski, P., Smolarek, I., Krauss, H., & Chmara, E. (2010). Evaluation of the antihypertensive effect of L-arginine supplementation in patients with mild hypertension assessed with ambulatory blood pressure monitoring. *Medical Science Monitor*, *16*(5), CR266–CR271. PMID:20424555

Basile & Bloch. (2015). *Overview of hypertension in adults*. Retrieved from http://www.uptodate.com/contents/overview-of-hypertension-in-adults?source=search_result&search=hypertension+overview&selectedTitle=1~150

Block, G., Mangels, A. R., Norkus, E. P., Patterson, B. H., Levander, O. A., & Taylor, P. R. (2001). Ascorbic acid status and subsequent diastolic and systolic blood pressure. *Hypertension*, *37*(2), 261–267. doi:10.1161/01.HYP.37.2.261 PMID:11230282

Brinkley, T. E., Lovato, J. F., Arnold, A. M., Furberg, C. D., Kuller, L. H., Burke, G. L., & Williamson, J. D. et al. (2010). Effect of Ginkgo biloba on blood pressure and incidence of hypertension in elderly men and women. *American Journal of Hypertension*, *23*(5), 528–533. doi:10.1038/ajh.2010.14 PMID:20168306

Brook, R. D., Appel, L. J., Rubenfire, M., Ogedegbe, G., Bisognano, J. D., Elliott, W. J., & Rajagopalan, S. et al. (2013). Beyond medications and diet: Alternative approaches to lowering blood pressure a scientific statement from the American heart association. *Hypertension*, *61*(6), 1360–1383. doi:10.1161/HYP.0b013e318293645f PMID:23608661

Burke, B. E., Neuenschwander, R., & Olson, R. D. (2001). Randomized, double-blind, placebo-controlled trial of coenzyme Q10 in isolated systolic hypertension. *Southern Medical Journal*, *94*(11), 1112–1117. doi:10.1097/00007611-200111000-00015 PMID:11780680

Burke, V., Hodgson, J. M., Beilin, L. J., Giangiulioi, N., Rogers, P., & Puddey, I. B. (2001). Dietary protein and soluble fiber reduce ambulatory blood pressure in treated hypertensives. *Hypertension*, *38*(4), 821–826. doi:10.1161/hy1001.092614 PMID:11641293

Castro, C., Gil Lorenzo, A., Gonzalez, A., & Cruzado, M. (2010). Garlic components inhibit angiotensin II-induced cell-cycle progression and migration: Involvement of cell-cycle inhibitor p27(Kip1) and mitogen-activated protein kinase. *Molecular Nutrition & Food Research*, *54*(6), 781–787. doi:10.1002/mnfr.200900108 PMID:19904760

Choi, E. J., Chee, K. M., & Lee, B. H. (2003). Anti- and prooxidant effects of chronic quercetin administration in rats. *European Journal of Pharmacology*, *482*(1-3), 281–285. doi:10.1016/j.ejphar.2003.09.067 PMID:14660033

Chun, S.-S., Vattem, D. A., Lin, Y.-T., & Shetty, K. (2005). Phenolic antioxidants from clonal oregano (Origanum vulgare) with antimicrobial activity against Helicobacter pylori. *Process Biochemistry*, *40*(2), 809–816. doi:10.1016/j.procbio.2004.02.018

Cicero, A. F., Derosa, G., Manca, M., Bove, M., Borghi, C., & Gaddi, A. V. (2007). Different effect of psyllium and guar dietary supplementation on blood pressure control in hypertensive overweight patients: A six-month, randomized clinical trial. *Clinical and Experimental Hypertension (New York, N.Y.)*, *29*(6), 383–394. doi:10.1080/10641960701578378 PMID:17729055

Clarke, T. C., Black, L. I., Stussman, B. J., Barnes, P. M., & Nahin, R. L. (2015). Trends in the use of complementary health approaches among adults: United States, 2002–2012. *National Health Statistics Reports*, (79): 1–16. PMID:25671660

Clement, Y. (2009). Can green tea do that? A literature review of the clinical evidence. *Preventive Medicine*, *49*(2-3), 83–87. doi:10.1016/j.ypmed.2009.05.005 PMID:19465043

Connell, D. W., & McLachlan, R. (1972). Natural pungent compounds: IV. Examination of the gingerols, shogaols, paradols and related compounds by thin-layer and gas chromatography. *Journal of Chromatography. A*, *67*(1), 29–35. doi:10.1016/S0021-9673(01)97144-4

Cosentino, S., Tuberoso, C. I. G., Pisano, B., Satta, M., Mascia, V., Arzedi, E., & Palmas, F. (1999). In-vitro antimicrobial activity and chemical composition of Sardinian Thymus essential oils. *Letters in Applied Microbiology*, *29*(2), 130–135. doi:10.1046/j.1472-765X.1999.00605.x PMID:10499301

Dallongeville, J., Yarnell, J., Ducimetiere, P., Arveiler, D., Ferrieres, J., & Montaye, M. (2003). Fish consumption is associated with lower heart rates. *Circulation*, *108*(7), 820–825. doi:10.1161/01.CIR.0000084542.64687.97 PMID:12912821

Darwish, R. M., & Aburjai, T. A. (2010). Effect of ethnomedicinal plants used in folklore medicine in Jordan as antibiotic resistant inhibitors on Escherichia coli. *BMC Complementary and Alternative Medicine*, *10*(1), 9. doi:10.1186/1472-6882-10-9 PMID:20187978

Dhawan, V., & Jain, S. (2005). Garlic supplementation prevents oxidative DNA damage in essential hypertension. *Molecular and Cellular Biochemistry*, *275*(1-2), 85–94. doi:10.1007/s11010-005-0824-2 PMID:16335787

Diet, nutrition and the prevention of chronic diseases. (2003). *World Health Organ Tech Rep Ser, 916*, i-viii, 1-149.

Digiesi, V., Cantini, F., Oradei, A., Bisi, G., Guarino, G. C., Brocchi, A., & Littarru, G. P. et al. (1994). Coenzyme Q10 in essential hypertension. *Molecular Aspects of Medicine*, *15*(Suppl), s257–s263. doi:10.1016/0098-2997(94)90036-1 PMID:7752838

Doggrell, S. A., & Brown, L. (1998). Rat models of hypertension, cardiac hypertrophy and failure. *Cardiovascular Research*, *39*(1), 89–105. doi:10.1016/S0008-6363(98)00076-5 PMID:9764192

Duarte, J., Jimenez, R., OValle, F., Galisteo, M., Perez-Palencia, R., Vargas, F., & Tamargo, J. et al. (2002). Protective effects of the flavonoid quercetin in chronic nitric oxide deficient rats. *Journal of Hypertension*, *20*(9), 1843–1854. doi:10.1097/00004872-200209000-00031 PMID:12195128

Duda, G., Suliburska, J., & Pupek-Musialik, D. (2008). Effects of short-term garlic supplementation on lipid metabolism and antioxidant status in hypertensive adults. *Pharmacological Reports*, *60*(2), 163–170. PMID:18443377

Duffy, S. J., Gokce, N., Holbrook, M., Huang, A., Frei, B., Keaney, J. F. Jr, & Vita, J. A. (1999). Treatment of hypertension with ascorbic acid. *Lancet*, *354*(9195), 2048–2049. doi:10.1016/S0140-6736(99)04410-4 PMID:10636373

Durak, I., Kavutcu, M., Aytac, B., Avci, A., Devrim, E., Ozbek, H., & Öztürk, H. S. (2004). Effects of garlic extract consumption on blood lipid and oxidant/antioxidant parameters in humans with high blood cholesterol. *The Journal of Nutritional Biochemistry*, *15*(6), 373–377. doi:10.1016/j.jnutbio.2004.01.005 PMID:15157944

El-Ashmawy, I. M., El-Nahas, A. F., & Salama, O. M. (2005). Protective effect of volatile oil, alcoholic and aqueous extracts of Origanum majorana on lead acetate toxicity in mice. *Basic & Clinical Pharmacology & Toxicology*, *97*(4), 238–243. doi:10.1111/j.1742-7843.2005.pto_136.x PMID:16176560

Engler, M. B., Engler, M. M., Chen, C. Y., Malloy, M. J., Browne, A., Chiu, E. Y., & Mietus-Snyder, M. L. et al. (2004). Flavonoid-rich dark chocolate improves endothelial function and increases plasma epicatechin concentrations in healthy adults. *Journal of the American College of Nutrition*, *23*(3), 197–204. doi:10.1080/07315724.2004.10719361 PMID:15190043

Ernst, E. (2012). Complementary and alternative medicine (CAM) for disease prevention. *Preventive Medicine*, *55*(6), 558–559. doi:10.1016/j.ypmed.2012.06.027 PMID:22809872

Fabre, L. F. Jr, Banks, R. C., McIsaac, W. M., & Farrell, G. (1965). Effects of Ubiquinone and Related Substances on Secretion of Aldosterone and Cortisol. *The American Journal of Physiology*, *208*, 1275–1280. PMID:14301392

Ferrannini, E., Buzzigoli, G., Bonadonna, R., Giorico, M. A., Oleggini, M., Graziadei, L., & Bevilacqua, S. et al. (1987). Insulin resistance in essential hypertension. *The New England Journal of Medicine*, *317*(6), 350–357. doi:10.1056/NEJM198708063170605 PMID:3299096

Folkers, K., Drzewoski, J., Richardson, P. C., Ellis, J., Shizukuishi, S., & Baker, L. (1981). Bioenergetics in clinical medicine. XVI. Reduction of hypertension in patients by therapy with coenzyme Q10. *Research Communications in Chemical Pathology and Pharmacology*, *31*(1), 129–140. PMID:7255868

Fotherby, M. D., Williams, J. C., Forster, L. A., Craner, P., & Ferns, G. A. (2000). Effect of vitamin C on ambulatory blood pressure and plasma lipids in older persons. *Journal of Hypertension*, *18*(4), 411–415. doi:10.1097/00004872-200018040-00009 PMID:10779091

Fugh-Berman, A. (2000). Herbs and dietary supplements in the prevention and treatment of cardiovascular disease. *Preventive Cardiology*, *3*(1), 24–32. doi:10.1111/j.1520-037X.2000.80355.x PMID:11834913

Fukagawa, N. K., Anderson, J. W., Hageman, G., Young, V. R., & Minaker, K. L. (1990). High-carbohydrate, high-fiber diets increase peripheral insulin sensitivity in healthy young and old adults. *The American Journal of Clinical Nutrition*, *52*(3), 524–528. PMID:2168124

Ganji, V., & Kies, C. V. (1994). Psyllium husk fibre supplementation to soybean and coconut oil diets of humans: Effect on fat digestibility and faecal fatty acid excretion. *European Journal of Clinical Nutrition*, *48*(8), 595–597. PMID:7957006

Geleijnse, J. M., Giltay, E. J., Grobbee, D. E., Donders, A. R. T., & Kok, F. J. (2002). Blood pressure response to fish oil supplementation: Metaregression analysis of randomized trials. *Journal of Hypertension*, *20*(8), 1493–1499. doi:10.1097/00004872-200208000-00010 PMID:12172309

Ghayur, M. N., & Gilani, A. H. (2005). Ginger lowers blood pressure through blockade of voltage-dependent calcium channels. *Journal of Cardiovascular Pharmacology*, *45*(1), 74–80. doi:10.1097/00005344-200501000-00013 PMID:15613983

Grassi, D., Necozione, S., Lippi, C., Croce, G., Valeri, L., Pasqualetti, P., & Ferri, C. et al. (2005). Cocoa reduces blood pressure and insulin resistance and improves endothelium-dependent vasodilation in hypertensives. *Hypertension*, *46*(2), 398–405. doi:10.1161/01.HYP.0000174990.46027.70 PMID:16027246

Group, S. R. (2015). A randomized trial of intensive versus standard blood-pressure control. *The New England Journal of Medicine*, *373*(22), 2103–2116. doi:10.1056/NEJMoa1511939 PMID:26551272

Häckl, L. P. N., Cuttle, G., Dovichi, S. S., Lima-Landman, M. T., & Nicolau, M. (2002). Inhibition of angiotensin-converting enzyme by quercetin alters the vascular response to bradykinin and angiotensin I. *Pharmacology*, *65*(4), 182–186. doi:10.1159/000064341 PMID:12174832

Heiss, C., Kleinbongard, P., Dejam, A., Perre, S., Schroeter, H., Sies, H., & Kelm, M. (2005). Acute consumption of flavanol-rich cocoa and the reversal of endothelial dysfunction in smokers. *Journal of the American College of Cardiology*, *46*(7), 1276–1283. doi:10.1016/j.jacc.2005.06.055 PMID:16198843

Herba thymi. (1999). In *WHO monographs on selected medicinal plants* (Vol. 1). Geneva: WHO.

Holzgartner, H., Schmidt, U., & Kuhn, U. (1992). Comparison of the efficacy and tolerance of a garlic preparation vs bezafibrate. *Arzneimittel-Forschung/Drug Research, 42-2*(12), 1473-1477.

Ishii, N., Senoo-Matsuda, N., Miyake, K., Yasuda, K., Ishii, T., Hartman, P. S., & Furukawa, S. (2004). Coenzyme Q10 can prolong C. elegans lifespan by lowering oxidative stress. *Mechanisms of Ageing and Development, 125*(1), 41–46. doi:10.1016/j.mad.2003.10.002 PMID:14706236

Jalili, T., Carlstrom, J., Kim, S., Freeman, D., Jin, H. F., Wu, T. C., & David Symons, J. et al. (2006). Quercetin-supplemented diets lower blood pressure and attenuate cardiac hypertrophy in rats with aortic constriction. *Journal of Cardiovascular Pharmacology, 47*(4), 531–541. doi:10.1097/01.fjc.0000211746.78454.50 PMID:16680066

James, P. A., Oparil, S., Carter, B. L., Cushman, W. C., Dennison-Himmelfarb, C., Handler, J., & Ortiz, E. et al. (2014). 2014 evidence-based guideline for the management of high blood pressure in adults: Report from the panel members appointed to the Eighth Joint National Committee (JNC 8). *Journal of the American Medical Association, 311*(5), 507–520. doi:10.1001/jama.2013.284427 PMID:24352797

Jenkins, D. J., Kendall, C. W., Axelsen, M., Augustin, L. S., & Vuksan, V. (2000). Viscous and nonviscous fibres, nonabsorbable and low glycaemic index carbohydrates, blood lipids and coronary heart disease. *Current Opinion in Lipidology, 11*(1), 49–56. doi:10.1097/00041433-200002000-00008 PMID:10750694

Jun, W. J., Han, B. K., Yu, K. W., Kim, M. S., Chang, I. S., & Kim, H. Y. (2001). Antioxidant effects of Origanum majorana L. on superoxide anion radicals. *Food Chemistry, 75*(4), 439–444. doi:10.1016/S0308-8146(01)00233-3

Kameda, K., Takaku, T., Okuda, H., Kimura, Y., Okuda, T., Hatano, T., & Arichi, S. et al. (1987). Inhibitory effects of various flavonoids isolated from leaves of persimmon on angiotensin-converting enzyme activity. *Journal of Natural Products, 50*(4), 680–683. doi:10.1021/np50052a017 PMID:3430165

Kameda, K., Takaku, T., Okuda, H., Kimura, Y., Okuda, T., Hatano, T., & Arichi, S. et al. (1987). Inhibitory effects of various flavonoids isolated from leaves of persimmon on angiotensin-converting enzyme activity. *Journal of Natural Products, 50*(4), 680–683. doi:10.1021/np50052a017 PMID:3430165

Kim, M. K., Sasaki, S., Sasazuki, S., Okubo, S., Hayashi, M., & Tsugane, S. (2002). Lack of long-term effect of vitamin C supplementation on blood pressure. *Hypertension, 40*(6), 797–803. doi:10.1161/01.HYP.0000038339.67450.60 PMID:12468560

Kressmann, S., Muller, W. E., & Blume, H. H. (2002). Pharmaceutical quality of different Ginkgo biloba brands. *The Journal of Pharmacy and Pharmacology, 54*(5), 661–669. doi:10.1211/0022357021778970 PMID:12005361

Kudolo, G. B. (2000). The effect of 3-month ingestion of Ginkgo biloba extract on pancreatic beta-cell function in response to glucose loading in normal glucose tolerant individuals. *Journal of Clinical Pharmacology, 40*(6), 647–654. doi:10.1002/j.1552-4604.2000.tb05991.x PMID:10868316

Kulisic, T., Krisko, A., Dragovic-Uzelac, V., Milos, M., & Pifat, G. (2007). The effects of essential oils and aqueous tea infusions of oregano (Origanum vulgare L. spp. hirtum), thyme (Thymus vulgaris L.) and wild thyme (Thymus serpyllum L.) on the copper-induced oxidation of human low-density lipoproteins. *International Journal of Food Sciences and Nutrition*, *58*(2), 87–93. doi:10.1080/09637480601108307 PMID:17469764

Kuriyama, S. (2008). The relation between green tea consumption and cardiovascular disease as evidenced by epidemiological studies. *The Journal of Nutrition*, *138*(8), 1548S–1553S. PMID:18641205

Kwak, J. S., Kim, J. Y., Paek, J. E., Lee, Y. J., Kim, H.-R., Park, D.-S., & Kwon, O. (2014). Garlic powder intake and cardiovascular risk factors: A meta-analysis of randomized controlled clinical trials. *Nutrition Research and Practice*, *8*(6), 644–654. doi:10.4162/nrp.2014.8.6.644 PMID:25489404

Langsjoen, P., Langsjoen, P., Willis, R., & Folkers, K. (1994). Treatment of essential hypertension with coenzyme Q10. *Molecular Aspects of Medicine*, *15*(Suppl), S265–S272. doi:10.1016/0098-2997(94)90037-X PMID:7752851

Larson, A. J., Symons, J. D., & Jalili, T. (2012). Therapeutic Potential of Quercetin to Decrease Blood Pressure: Review of Efficacy and Mechanisms. *Advances in Nutrition*, *3*(1), 39–46. doi:10.3945/an.111.001271 PMID:22332099

Le Bon, A.-M., Vernevaut, M.-F., Guenot, L., Kahane, R., Auger, J., Arnault, I., & Siess, M.-H. et al. (2003). Effects of garlic powders with varying alliin contents on hepatic drug metabolizing enzymes in rats. *Journal of Agricultural and Food Chemistry*, *51*(26), 7617–7623. doi:10.1021/jf0346758 PMID:14664517

Lemhadri, A., Zeggwagh, N. A., Maghrani, M., Jouad, H., & Eddouks, M. (2004). Anti-hyperglycaemic activity of the aqueous extract of Origanum vulgare growing wild in Tafilalet region. *Journal of Ethnopharmacology*, *92*(2), 251–256. doi:10.1016/j.jep.2004.02.026 PMID:15138008

Lerman, A., Burnett, J. C. Jr, Higano, S. T., McKinley, L. J., & Holmes, D. R. Jr. (1998). Long-term L-arginine supplementation improves small-vessel coronary endothelial function in humans. *Circulation*, *97*(21), 2123–2128. doi:10.1161/01.CIR.97.21.2123 PMID:9626172

Liu, Y., Chen, L.-Y., Sokolowska, M., Eberlein, M., Alsaaty, S., Martinez-Anton, A., & Shelhamer, J. H. et al. (2014). The fish oil ingredient, docosahexaenoic acid, activates cytosolic phospholipase A2 via GPR120 receptor to produce prostaglandin E2 and plays an anti-inflammatory role in macrophages. *Immunology*, *143*(1), 81–95. doi:10.1111/imm.12296 PMID:24673159

Lonnrot, K., Porsti, I., Alho, H., Wu, X., Hervonen, A., & Tolvanen, J. P. (1998). Control of arterial tone after long-term coenzyme Q10 supplementation in senescent rats. *British Journal of Pharmacology*, *124*(7), 1500–1506. doi:10.1038/sj.bjp.0701970 PMID:9723964

Macan, H., Uykimpang, R., Alconcel, M., Takasu, J., Razon, R., & Amagase, H. (2006). Aged garlic extract may be safe for patients on warfarin therapy. *The Journal of Nutrition*, *136*(3), 793S–795S. PMID:16484565

Mackraj, I., Govender, T., & Ramesar, S. (2008). The anti hypertensive effects of quercetin in a salt-sensitive model of hypertension. *Journal of Cardiovascular Pharmacology*, *51*(3), 239–245. doi:10.1097/FJC.0b013e318162011f PMID:18356687

Manohar, V., Ingram, C., Gray, J., Talpur, N. A., Echard, B. W., Bagchi, D., & Preuss, H. G. (2001). Antifungal activities of origanum oil against Candida albicans. *Molecular and Cellular Biochemistry*, *228*(1-2), 111–117. doi:10.1023/A:1013311632207 PMID:11855736

Mansour, S. M., Bahgat, A. K., El-Khatib, A. S., & Khayyal, M. T. (2011). Ginkgo biloba extract (EGb 761) normalizes hypertension in 2K, 1C hypertensive rats: Role of antioxidant mechanisms, ACE inhibiting activity and improvement of endothelial dysfunction. *Phytomedicine*, *18*(8-9), 641–647. doi:10.1016/j.phymed.2011.01.014 PMID:21353510

Martina, V., Masha, A., Gigliardi, V. R., Brocato, L., Manzato, E., Berchio, A., & Iannone, A. et al. (2008). Long-term N-acetylcysteine and L-arginine administration reduces endothelial activation and systolic blood pressure in hypertensive patients with type 2 diabetes. *Diabetes Care*, *31*(5), 940–944. doi:10.2337/dc07-2251 PMID:18268065

Mester, R., Toren, P., Mizrachi, I., Wolmer, L., Karni, N., & Weizman, A. (1995). Caffeine withdrawal increases lithium blood levels. *Biological Psychiatry*, *37*(5), 348–350. doi:10.1016/0006-3223(94)00243-V PMID:7748990

Mihailovic-Stanojevic, N., Belscak-Cvitanovic, A., Grujic-Milanovic, J., Ivanov, M., Jovovic, D., Bugarski, D., & Miloradović, Z. (2013). Antioxidant and Antihypertensive Activity of Extract from Thymus serpyllum L. in Experimental Hypertension. *Plant Foods for Human Nutrition (Dordrecht, Netherlands)*, *68*(3), 235–240. doi:10.1007/s11130-013-0368-7 PMID:23828496

Morris, C. R., Morris, S. M. Jr, Hagar, W., Van Warmerdam, J., Claster, S., Kepka-Lenhart, D., & Vichinsky, E. P. et al. (2003). Arginine therapy: A new treatment for pulmonary hypertension in sickle cell disease? *American Journal of Respiratory and Critical Care Medicine*, *168*(1), 63–69. doi:10.1164/rccm.200208-967OC PMID:12626350

Mozaffarian, D., Benjamin, E. J., Go, A. S., Arnett, D. K., Blaha, M. J., Cushman, M., & Turner, M. B. et al. (2015). Heart disease and stroke statistics-2015 update: A report from the american heart association. *Circulation*, *131*(4), e29–e322. doi:10.1161/CIR.0000000000000152 PMID:25520374

Muniyappa, R., Hall, G., Kolodziej, T. L., Karne, R. J., Crandon, S. K., & Quon, M. J. (2008). Cocoa consumption for 2 wk enhances insulin-mediated vasodilatation without improving blood pressure or insulin resistance in essential hypertension. *The American Journal of Clinical Nutrition*, *88*(6), 1685–1696. doi:10.3945/ajcn.2008.26457 PMID:19064532

Naccarato, M., Yoong, D., & Gough, K. (2012). A potential drug-herbal interaction between Ginkgo biloba and efavirenz. *J Int Assoc Physicians AIDS Care (Chic)*, *11*(2), 98–100. doi:10.1177/1545109711435364 PMID:22323244

Nagaya, N., Yamamoto, H., Uematsu, M., Itoh, T., Nakagawa, K., & Miyazawa, T. (2004). Green tea reverses endothelial dysfunction in healthy smokers. *Heart (British Cardiac Society)*, *90*(12), 1485–1486. doi:10.1136/hrt.2003.026740 PMID:15547040

Nahan, R., Barnes, P., Stussman, B., & Bloom, B. (2011). Costs of complementary and alternative medicine (CAM) and frequency of visits to CAM practitioners: United States, 2007. National Health Statistics Reports no. 18. Hyattsville, MD: National Center for Health Statistics; 2009.

Nantz, M. P., Rowe, C. A., Bukowski, J. F., & Percival, S. S. (2009). Standardized capsule of Camellia sinensis lowers cardiovascular risk factors in a randomized, double-blind, placebo-controlled study. *Nutrition (Burbank, Los Angeles County, Calif.)*, *25*(2), 147–154. doi:10.1016/j.nut.2008.07.018 PMID:18848434

Neri, I., Monari, F., Sgarbi, L., Berardi, A., Masellis, G., & Facchinetti, F. (2010). L-arginine supplementation in women with chronic hypertension: Impact on blood pressure and maternal and neonatal complications. *The Journal of Maternal-Fetal & Neonatal Medicine*, *23*(12), 1456–1460. doi:10.3109/14767051003677962 PMID:20958228

NHLBI. (2015). *Description of high blood pressure*. Retrieved from http://www.nhlbi.nih.gov/health/health-topics/topics/hbp/

Novak, J., Bitsch, C., Langbehn, J., Pank, F., Skoula, M., & Gotsiou, Y. (2000). Ratios of cis-and trans-sabinene hydrate in Origanum majorana L. and Origanum microphyllum (Bentham) Vogel. *Biochemical Systematics and Ecology*, *28*(7), 697–704. doi:10.1016/S0305-1978(99)00098-8 PMID:10854745

Pal, S., Khossousi, A., Binns, C., Dhaliwal, S., & Radavelli-Bagatini, S. (2012). The effects of 12-week psyllium fibre supplementation or healthy diet on blood pressure and arterial stiffness in overweight and obese individuals. *The British Journal of Nutrition*, *107*(5), 725–734. doi:10.1017/S0007114511003497 PMID:21787454

Palloshi, A., Fragasso, G., Piatti, P., Monti, L. D., Setola, E., Valsecchi, G., & Margonato, A. et al. (2004). Effect of oral L-arginine on blood pressure and symptoms and endothelial function in patients with systemic hypertension, positive exercise tests, and normal coronary arteries. *The American Journal of Cardiology*, *93*(7), 933–935. doi:10.1016/j.amjcard.2003.12.040 PMID:15050504

Papademetriou, V., Narayan, P., & Kokkinos, P. (2004). Angiotensin-Converting Enzyme Inhibitors and Angiotensin Receptor Blockers in African-American Patients With Hypertension. *Journal of Clinical Hypertension*, *6*(6), 310–314. doi:10.1111/j.1524-6175.2004.03446.x PMID:15187493

Parker, J. O., Parker, J. D., Caldwell, R. W., Farrell, B., & Kaesemeyer, W. H. (2002). The effect of supplemental L-arginine on tolerance development during continuous transdermal nitroglycerin therapy. *Journal of the American College of Cardiology*, *39*(7), 1199–1203. doi:10.1016/S0735-1097(02)01729-1 PMID:11923046

Pepe, S., Marasco, S. F., Haas, S. J., Sheeran, F. L., Krum, H., & Rosenfeldt, F. L. (2007). Coenzyme Q10 in cardiovascular disease. *Mitochondrion*, *7*(Suppl), S154–S167. doi:10.1016/j.mito.2007.02.005 PMID:17485243

Persson, I. A., Persson, K., Hagg, S., & Andersson, R. G. (2011). Effects of cocoa extract and dark chocolate on angiotensin-converting enzyme and nitric oxide in human endothelial cells and healthy volunteersa nutrigenomics perspective. *Journal of Cardiovascular Pharmacology*, *57*(1), 44–50. doi:10.1097/FJC.0b013e3181fe62e3 PMID:20966764

Pimple, B. P., Kadam, P. V., & Patil, M. J. (2012). Comparative antihyperglycaemic and antihyperlipidemic effect of Origanum majorana extracts in NIDDM rats. *Oriental Pharmacy and Experimental Medicine*, *12*(1), 41–50. doi:10.1007/s13596-011-0047-x

Preuss, H. G., Echard, B., Polansky, M. M., & Anderson, R. (2006). Whole cinnamon and aqueous extracts ameliorate sucrose-induced blood pressure elevations in spontaneously hypertensive rats. *Journal of the American College of Nutrition*, *25*(2), 144–150. doi:10.1080/07315724.2006.10719525 PMID:16582031

Qidwai, W., & Ashfaq, T. (2013). Role of garlic usage in cardiovascular disease prevention: An evidence-based approach. *Evidence-Based Complementary and Alternative Medicine*. PMID:23690831

Regulations. (2015). *Electronic Code of Federal Regulations. Title 21. Part 182 -- Substances Generally Recognized As Safe*. Retrieved from http://www.accessdata.fda.gov/scripts/cdrh/cfdocs/cfcfr/CFRSearch.cfm?CFRPart=182

Robaszkiewicz, A., Balcerczyk, A., & Bartosz, G. (2007). Antioxidative and prooxidative effects of quercetin on A549 cells. *Cell Biology International*, *31*(10), 1245–1250. doi:10.1016/j.cellbi.2007.04.009 PMID:17583542

Rostami, A., Khalili, M., Haghighat, N., Eghtesadi, S., Shidfar, F., & Heidari, I. (2015). High-cocoa polyphenol-rich chocolate improves blood pressure in patients with diabetes and hypertension. *ARYA Atheroscler*, *11*(1), 21–29. PMID:26089927

Rundek, T., Naini, A., Sacco, R., Coates, K., & DiMauro, S. (2004). Atorvastatin decreases the coenzyme Q10 level in the blood of patients at risk for cardiovascular disease and stroke. *Archives of Neurology*, *61*(6), 889–892. doi:10.1001/archneur.61.6.889 PMID:15210526

Sanders, T. A. B., Vickers, M., & Haines, A. P. (1981). Effect on blood lipids and haemostasis of a supplement of cod-liver oil, rich in eicosapentaenoic and docosahexaenoic acids, in healthy young men. *Clinical Science*, *61*(3), 317–324. doi:10.1042/cs0610317 PMID:6266735

Sato, K., Dohi, Y., Kojima, M., Miyagawa, K., Takase, H., & Katada, E. (2006). Effects of ascorbic acid on ambulatory blood pressure in elderly patients with refractory hypertension. *Arzneimittel-Forschung*, *56*(7), 535–540. doi:10.1055/s-0031-1296748 PMID:16927536

Shoji, N., Iwasa, A., Takemoto, T., Ishida, Y., & Ohizumi, Y. (1982). Cardiotonic principles of ginger (Zingiber officinale Roscoe). *Journal of Pharmaceutical Sciences*, *71*(10), 1174–1175. doi:10.1002/jps.2600711025 PMID:7143220

Simons, L. A., Balasubramaniam, S., Vonkonigsmark, M., Parfitt, A., Simons, J., & Peters, W. (1995). On the effect of garlic on plasma-lipids and lipoproteins in mild hypercholesterolemia. *Atherosclerosis*, *113*(2), 219–225. doi:10.1016/0021-9150(94)05449-S PMID:7605361

Simons, S., Wollersheim, H., & Thien, T. (2009). A systematic review on the influence of trial quality on the effect of garlic on blood pressure. *The Netherlands Journal of Medicine*, *67*(6), 212–219. PMID:19749390

Singh, R. B., Niaz, M. A., Rastogi, S. S., Shukla, P. K., & Thakur, A. S. (1999). Effect of hydrosoluble coenzyme Q10 on blood pressures and insulin resistance in hypertensive patients with coronary artery disease. *Journal of Human Hypertension*, *13*(3), 203–208. doi:10.1038/sj.jhh.1000778 PMID:10204818

Stabler, S. N., Tejani, A. M., Huynh, F., & Fowkes, C. (2012a). Garlic for the prevention of cardiovascular morbidity and mortality in hypertensive patients. *Cochrane Database of Systematic Reviews, 8*, CD007653–CD007653. doi:10.1002/14651858.CD007653.pub2 PMID:22895963

Stabler, S. N., Tejani, A. M., Huynh, F., & Fowkes, C. (2012b). Garlic for the prevention of cardiovascular morbidity and mortality in hypertensive patients. *Cochrane Database of Systematic Reviews,* (8). doi: 10.1002/14651858.CD007653.pub2

Stamler, J., Caggiula, A. W., & Grandits, G. A. (1997). Relation of body mass and alcohol, nutrient, fiber, and caffeine intakes to blood pressure in the special intervention and usual care groups in the Multiple Risk Factor Intervention Trial. *The American Journal of Clinical Nutrition, 65*(1Suppl), 338S–365S. PMID:8988947

Suhaj, M. (2006). Spice antioxidants isolation and their antiradical activity: A review. *Journal of Food Composition and Analysis, 19*(6), 531–537. doi:10.1016/j.jfca.2004.11.005

Tabassum, N., & Ahmad, F. (2011). Role of natural herbs in the treatment of hypertension. *Pharmacognosy Reviews, 5*(9), 30.

Tahraoui, A., El-Hilaly, J., Israili, Z. H., & Lyoussi, B. (2007). Ethnopharmacological survey of plants used in the traditional treatment of hypertension and diabetes in south-eastern Morocco (Errachidia province). *Journal of Ethnopharmacology, 110*(1), 105–117. doi:10.1016/j.jep.2006.09.011 PMID:17052873

Taubert, D., Berkels, R., Roesen, R., & Klaus, W. (2003). Chocolate and blood pressure in elderly individuals with isolated systolic hypertension. *Journal of the American Medical Association, 290*(8), 1029–1030. doi:10.1001/jama.290.8.1029 PMID:12941673

Taubert, D., Roesen, R., Lehmann, C., Jung, N., & Schomig, E. (2007). Effects of low habitual cocoa intake on blood pressure and bioactive nitric oxide: A randomized controlled trial. *Journal of the American Medical Association, 298*(1), 49–60. doi:10.1001/jama.298.1.49 PMID:17609490

Taubert, D., Roesen, R., & Schoemig, E. (2007). Effect of cocoa and tea intake on blood pressure - A meta-analysis. *Archives of Internal Medicine, 167*(7), 626–634. doi:10.1001/archinte.167.7.626 PMID:17420419

Tong, X., Taylor, A. W., Giles, L., Wittert, G. A., & Shi, Z. (2014). Tea consumption is inversely related to 5-year blood pressure change among adults in Jiangsu, China: A cross-sectional study. *Nutrition Journal, 13*(1), 98. doi:10.1186/1475-2891-13-98 PMID:25311544

Tsai, P.-J., Tsai, T.-H., Yu, C.-H., & Ho, S.-C. (2007). Evaluation of NO-suppressing activity of several Mediterranean culinary spices. *Food and Chemical Toxicology, 45*(3), 440–447. doi:10.1016/j.fct.2006.09.006 PMID:17074427

Ueshima, H., Stamler, J., Elliott, P., Chan, Q., Brown, I. J., Carnethon, M. R., & Zhou, B. et al. (2007). Food omega-3 fatty acid intake of individuals (total, linolenic acid, long-chain) and their blood pressure INTERMAP study. *Hypertension, 50*(2), 313–319. doi:10.1161/HYPERTENSIONAHA.107.090720 PMID:17548718

Ulker, S., McKeown, P. P., & Bayraktutan, U. (2003). Vitamins reverse endothelial dysfunction through regulation of eNOS and NAD(P)H oxidase activities. *Hypertension*, *41*(3), 534–539. doi:10.1161/01.HYP.0000057421.28533.37 PMID:12623955

Urivetzky, M., Kessaris, D., & Smith, A. D. (1992). Ascorbic acid overdosing: A risk factor for calcium oxalate nephrolithiasis. *The Journal of Urology*, *147*(5), 1215–1218. PMID:1569652

Varma, K. R., Jain, T. C., & Bhattacharyya, S. C. (1962). Terpenoids—XXXIV: Structure and stereochemistry of zingiberol and juniper camphor. *Tetrahedron*, *18*(8), 979–984. doi:10.1016/S0040-4020(01)92752-8

Vrolijk, M. F., Haenen, G. R., Opperhuizen, A., Jansen, E. H., Schiffers, P. M., & Bast, A. (2015). The supplement–drug interaction of quercetin with tamsulosin on vasorelaxation. *European Journal of Pharmacology*, *746*, 132–137. doi:10.1016/j.ejphar.2014.11.006 PMID:25449042

Wang, L. Y., Chan, K. W., Yuwen, Y., Shi, N. N., Han, X. J., & Lu, A. (2013). Expert consensus on the treatment of hypertension with chinese patent medicines. *Evidence-Based Complementary and Alternative Medicine*, *510146*. doi:10.1155/2013/510146 PMID:23662141

WHO. (2013). *WHO traditional medicine strategy: 2014-2023*. World Health Organization.

Williams, M. J. A., Sutherland, W. H. F., McCormick, M. P., Yeoman, D. J., & de Jong, S. A. (2005). Aged garlic extract improves endothelial function in men with coronary artery disease. *Phytotherapy Research*, *19*(4), 314–319. doi:10.1002/ptr.1663 PMID:16041725

Wu, G., & Meininger, C. J. (2000). Arginine nutrition and cardiovascular function. *The Journal of Nutrition*, *130*(11), 2626–2629. PMID:11053497

Xie, C., Xie, Z., Xu, X., & Yang, D. (2015). Persimmon (Diospyros kaki L.) leaves: A review on traditional uses, phytochemistry and pharmacological properties. *Journal of Ethnopharmacology*, *163*, 229–240. doi:10.1016/j.jep.2015.01.007 PMID:25637828

Xiong, X. J., Wang, P. Q., Li, S. J., Li, X. K., Zhang, Y. Q., & Wang, J. (2015). Garlic for hypertension: A systematic review and meta-analysis of randomized controlled trials. *Phytomedicine*, *22*(3), 352–361. doi:10.1016/j.phymed.2014.12.013 PMID:25837272

Yamamoto, Y., & Oue, E. (2006). Antihypertensive effect of quercetin in rats fed with a high-fat high-sucrose diet. *Bioscience, Biotechnology, and Biochemistry*, *70*(4), 933–939. doi:10.1271/bbb.70.933 PMID:16636461

Yang, C. S., & Pan, E. (2012). The effects of green tea polyphenols on drug metabolism. *Expert Opinion on Drug Metabolism & Toxicology*, *8*(6), 677–689. doi:10.1517/17425255.2012.681375 PMID:22509899

Yang, Y. K., Wang, L. P., Chen, L., Yao, X. P., Yang, K. Q., Gao, L. G., & Zhou, X.-L. (2015). Coenzyme Q10 treatment of cardiovascular disorders of ageing including heart failure, hypertension and endothelial dysfunction. *Clinica Chimica Acta*, *450*, 83–89. doi:10.1016/j.cca.2015.08.002 PMID:26254995

Yao, L. H., Jiang, Y. M., Shi, J., Tomas-Barberan, F. A., Datta, N., & Singanusong, R. (2004). Flavonoids in food and their health benefits. *Plant Foods for Human Nutrition (Dordrecht, Netherlands)*, *59*(3), 113–122. doi:10.1007/s11130-004-0049-7 PMID:15678717

Yashodhara, B. M., Umakanth, S., Pappachan, J. M., Bhat, S. K., Kamath, R., & Choo, B. H. (2009). Omega-3 fatty acids: A comprehensive review of their role in health and disease. *Postgraduate Medical Journal*, *85*(1000), 84–90. doi:10.1136/pgmj.2008.073338 PMID:19329703

Yazdanparast, R., & Shahriyary, L. (2008). Comparative effects of Artemisia dracunculus, Satureja hortensis and Origanum majorana on inhibition of blood platelet adhesion, aggregation and secretion. *Vascular Pharmacology*, *48*(1), 32–37. doi:10.1016/j.vph.2007.11.003 PMID:18069068

Young, J. M., Florkowski, C. M., Molyneux, S. L., McEwan, R. G., Frampton, C. M., Nicholls, M. G., & George, P. M. et al. (2012). A randomized, double-blind, placebo-controlled crossover study of coenzyme Q10 therapy in hypertensive patients with the metabolic syndrome. *American Journal of Hypertension*, *25*(2), 261–270. doi:10.1038/ajh.2011.209 PMID:22113168

Chapter 16
Resveratrol:
An Epigenetic Regulator of SIRT1 – Is It a Magic Tool to Prevent Cardiovascular Disease?

Catherine A. Powell
Texas A&M Health Science Center, USA

John D. Bowman
Texas A&M Health Science Center, USA

Jian Zhang
Texas A&M Health Science Center, USA

Mahua Choudhury
Texas A&M Health Science Center, USA

ABSTRACT

Cardiovascular disease (CVD) is the leading cause of death in both men and women and has largely been attributed to genetic makeup and lifestyle factors. However, genetic regulation does not fully explain the pathophysiology. Recently, epigenetic regulation, the regulation of the genetic code by modifications that affect the transcription and translation of target genes, has been shown to be important. Silent information regulator-2 proteins or sirtuins are an epigenetic regulator family of class III histone deacetylases (HDACs), unique in their dependency on coenzyme NAD+, that are postulated to mediate the beneficial effects of calorie restriction, thus promoting longevity by reducing the incidence of chronic diseases such as cancer, diabetes, and CVD. Emerging evidence shows that SIRT1 is ubiquitously expressed throughout the body. Resveratrol, a plant polyphenol, has cardioprotective effects and its mechanism of action is attributed to regulation of SIRT1. Incoproation of resveratrol into the diet may be a powerful therapeutic option for the prevention and treatment of CVD.

INTRODUCTION

Cardiovascular Disease

Cardiovascular diseases (CVDs) are a group of disorders of the heart and blood vessels, including coronary heart disease, cerebrovascular disease, peripheral arterial disease, rheumatic heart disease, congenital heart disease, deep vein thrombosis and pulmonary embolism (WHO, 2015). CVD is the

DOI: 10.4018/978-1-5225-2092-4.ch016

leading cause of death in most developed countries including the United States (Naghavi et al., 2015). As the leading cause of worldwide death, CVD represents nearly 30% of all deaths, and in 2008 caused 17 million deaths and led to 151 million disability-adjusted life years (Bloom, 2011). Behavioral risk factors such as physical inactivity, tobacco use, and unhealthy diet explain nearly 80% of the CVD burden. The greatest contributors to CVD mortality and morbidity are chronic heart failure, coronary heart disease, and stroke. The global cost in 2010 has been estimated at US$ 863 billion (Bloom, 2011). Even though multiple risk factors have been identified, the current approach to treatment is only to decrease modifiable risk factors through healthy lifestyle changes and the use of medications, such as statins to lower cholesterol. Despite extensive study and efforts over many years, CVD remains the leading cause of death. This is due in part to the difficulty in adhering to lifestyle changes such as weight loss, regular exercise, and dietary modification, and in part to non-modifiable risk factors such as a family history of CVD. Since modifying behavioral risk factors involves individual choices, approaches such as government regulation, advertising, and public policy statements have had limited impact on CVD incidence. Innovative approaches are needed to reduce further the negative impact of CVD.

Current treatment of cardiovascular diseases requires lifestyle changes with or without medications. Evidence-based recommendations were provided in 2013 by the American College of Cardiology and the American Heart Association (Jensen et al., 2014; Stone et al., 2014). The new guidelines refined the original Framingham risk assessments with new knowledge and involve matching individuals' CVD risk with the intensity of prevention steps (Wenger, 2014).

Two decades ago, following the discovery of the double helical structure of DNA and subsequent automation of DNA sequencing, scientists held high hopes that unraveling the human genome would uncover the genetic basis of many human diseases such as cancer, and that would lead to new and effective treatments. However, early gene linkage studies revealed only rare cases of single-gene disorders. Also, analysis of many genome-wide association studies has found little contribution to disease variation to date (Bjorkegren, Kovacic, Dudley, & Schadt, 2015). Accordingly, other explanations for disease development and expression have been sought. Recently, the interaction between genes and the environment has emerged as a new frontier for studying how networks of developmentally programmed genes may lead to several major pathologies. Epigenetic studies may identify pathologic mechanisms early enough in human development to suggest ways to alter adverse gene expression in chronic disease. Humans are particularly susceptible to epigenetic influences during fertilization, gametogenesis, and early embryo development (Martinez, Gay, & Zhang, 2015). In addition, these epigenetic marks can also accumulate during adult life to increase disease susceptibility.

Sirtuins

Histone deacetylases (HDACs) are enzymes that remove acetyl groups from histone and non-histone proteins to counterbalance the activity of histone acetyltransferases (HATs). These activities control the epigenetic regulation of gene expression through post-transcriptional modifications to proteins (Z. Y. Wang, Qin, & Yi, 2015). Four classes of HDACs have been characterized according to their homology to yeast HDACs, and a total of 18 mammalian HDACs have been identified. HDACs are divided into four classes, class I (HDAC1, 2, 3, and 8), class II (HDAC4, 5, 6, 9, and 10), and class IV comprising only HDAC11 (Z. Y. Wang et al., 2015). A unique class, class III, is made up of the sirtuin family of enzymes that are not susceptible to inhibition by classical HDAC inhibitors such as vorinostat (Chavan & Somani, 2010).

Sirtuins (silent information regulator-2 proteins) are class III histone deacetylases that can deacetylate lysine residues on histone and non-histone proteins alike. Sirtuins are unique among all HDACs due to their dependency on the coenzyme nicotinamide adenine dinucleotide (NAD+) (Winnik, Auwerx, Sinclair, & Matter, 2015). Dependency on NAD+ for deacetylase activity suggests that sirtuins are closely involved in energy metabolism (Z. Y. Wang et al., 2015). Members of the sirtuin family also possess ADP-ribosyltransferase activity (Luo et al., 2014). Sirtuins were first identified in yeast, the founding member being Sir2, which deacetylates histones and, therefore, condenses chromatin and represses transcription. Following the discovery of yeast Sir2, seven mammalian sirtuins (SIRT1-7) have been identified. Sirtuins exhibit a wide functional behavior due to their tissue- and cell-specific localization. Sirtuins are further classified into subclasses based on the homology of a 250 amino acid core domain. SIRT1 is a member of class I, along with SIRT2 and SIRT3, and is the most similar to yeast Sir2 in evolution and function. Class I possesses the strongest lysine deacetylase activity of all the SIRTs. Class II contains SIRT4, which has ADP-ribosyltransferase activity. SIRT5 is in class III with unclear enzymatic activity (Lu, Scott, Webster, & Sack, 2009). SIRT 6 and SIRT7 make up class IV (Luo et al., 2014).

SIRT1 is primarily expressed in the brain, skeletal muscle, heart, kidney, and uterus (Villalba & Alcain, 2012). It is involved in aging and lifespan regulation, age-related diseases, cell survival, metabolism, oxidative stress, and inflammation (Cencioni et al., 2015; Villalba & Alcain, 2012; Z. Y. Wang et al., 2015). SIRT1 is primarily localized in the nucleus in most cells, however along with its two nuclear localization signals, SIRT1 also possesses two nuclear exportation signals; studies have demonstrated that SIRT1 can be localized in the cytoplasm to interact with targets, and in some cell types it is primarily localized in the cytoplasm (Tanno, Sakamoto, Miura, Shimamoto, & Horio, 2007). Localization of SIRT1 can also change, for example, in fetal mouse hearts where it is nuclear, compared to adult mouse hearts where it is cytoplasmic (Tanno et al., 2007).

Mechanistically, SIRT1 deacetylates both histone proteins (H1, H3, and H4) and non-histone protein targets (Balcerczyk & Pirola, 2010; Luo et al., 2014). Non-histone targets for SIRT1 deacetylase are p53, NF-κB subunit p65, forkhead box O (FOXO) transcription factors, peroxisome proliferator-activated receptors (PPARs), peroxisome proliferator-activated receptor γ coactivator 1 alpha (PGC-1α), and p300 (Balcerczyk & Pirola, 2010; Luo et al., 2014).

SIRT1 has been shown to have both positive and negative effects on cardiovascular health (Cencioni et al., 2015; Z. Z. Chong, Wang, Shang, & Maiese, 2012; Hsu, Odewale, Alcendor, & Sadoshima, 2008; Ma & Li, 2015; Matsushima & Sadoshima, 2015; Sebastian, Satterstrom, Haigis, & Mostoslavsky, 2012; Webster, 2012). SIRT1 has also been associated with improving endothelial dysfunction and providing cellular antioxidant effects (Winnik et al., 2015). In addition, SIRT1 lowers plasma low-density lipoprotein levels and inhibits tissue factor activity which may diminish the development of arterial thrombotic events. The plant based antioxidant resveratrol has been shown to induce SIRT1 in several organs, which may lead to a potential cardioprotective effect (Figure 1).

Resveratrol

The enormous burden of cardiovascular disease (CVD) on the quality and length of life requires novel approaches in prevention and treatment. Many natural components from food or plants, such as resveratrol, piceatannol, quercetin, pyrroloindoline quinone (PQQ) (Bauerly et al., 2011), epigallocatechin gallate (EGCG), and lycopene have shown preventive and therapeutic benefits in different forms of CVD. Preclinical studies have shown that natural components, such as resveratrol, have beneficial effects in

Figure 1. SIRT1 signaling pathways in cardiovascular disease. Alteration or deregulation of SIRT1 results in a wide variety of cellular dysfunction or downstream pathways which ultimately leads to cardiovascular disease. Upregulation of SIRT1 may lead to cardioprotection. Straight (—) and dash (-----) lines indicate the factors that are found upregulated or downregulated, respectively, in specific cellular functions. In the figure, specific key events regulated by SIRT are represented

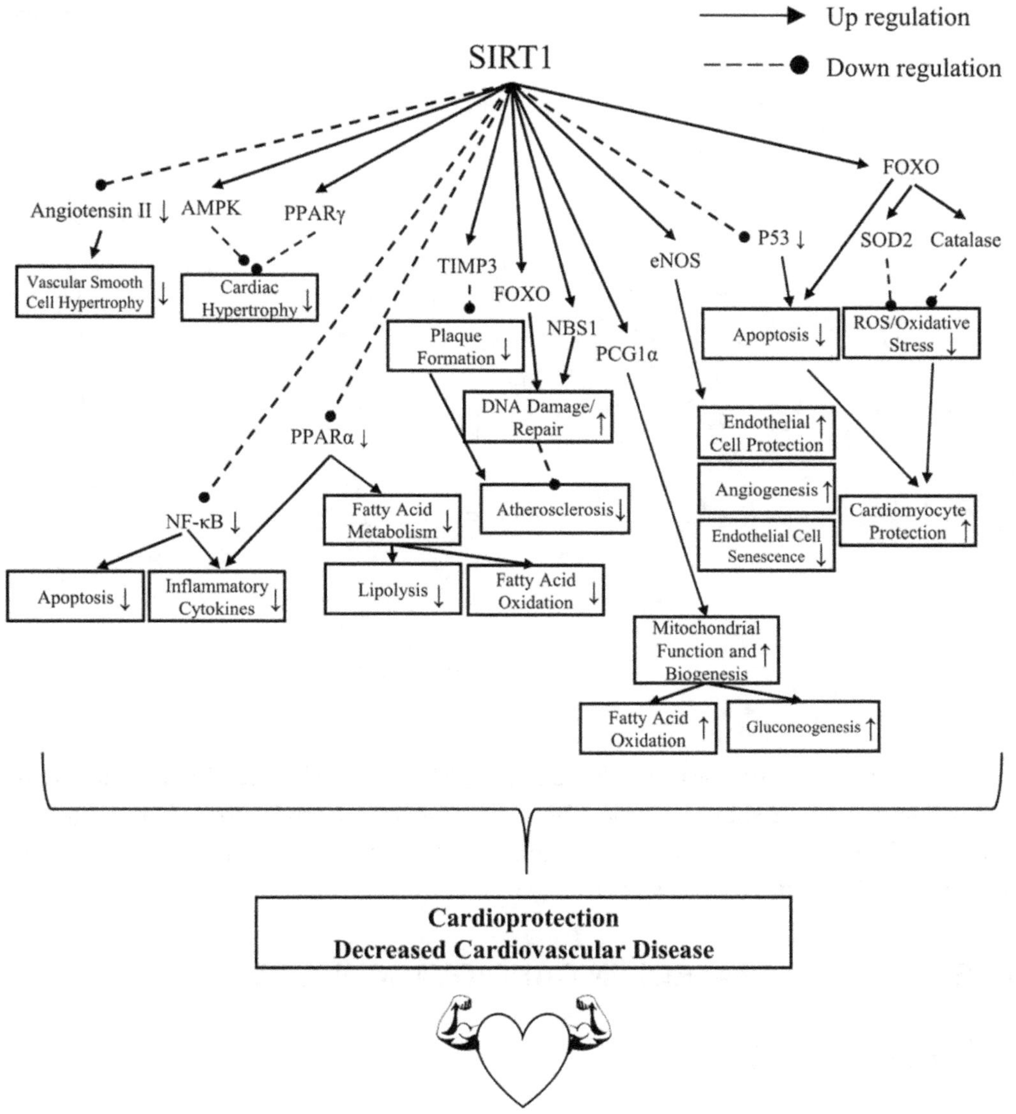

animal models of ischemic heart disease, cardiac hypertrophy, heart failure, hypertension, atherosclerosis, stroke, arrhythmia, chemotherapy-induced cardiotoxicity, and diabetic cardiomyopathy (Zordoky, Robertson, & Dyck, 2015). Resveratrol mediates some of its beneficial cardiovascular effects through regulation of SIRT, AMPK, Akt or FOXO.

Resveratrol (3,5,4′-trihydroxy-*trans*-stilbene), a phytoalexin, is produced by plants as a reaction to stresses such as infection or injury (Quarles et al., 2015). It has been shown to have cardioprotective (Hung, Su, & Chen, 2004; Lekakis et al., 2005; Z. Wang et al., 2005; Zern, West, & Fernandez, 2003),

Figure 2. Resveratrol-mediated protective effects in cardiovascular disease. Alteration or deregulation of several molecules including SIRT1 affect a wide variety of cellular functions or downstream pathways which can ultimately lead to cardioprotection. Straight (—) and dash (-----) lines indicate the factors that are upregulated or downregulated, respectively, in specific cellular functions. In the figure, specific key events regulated by resveratrol are represented

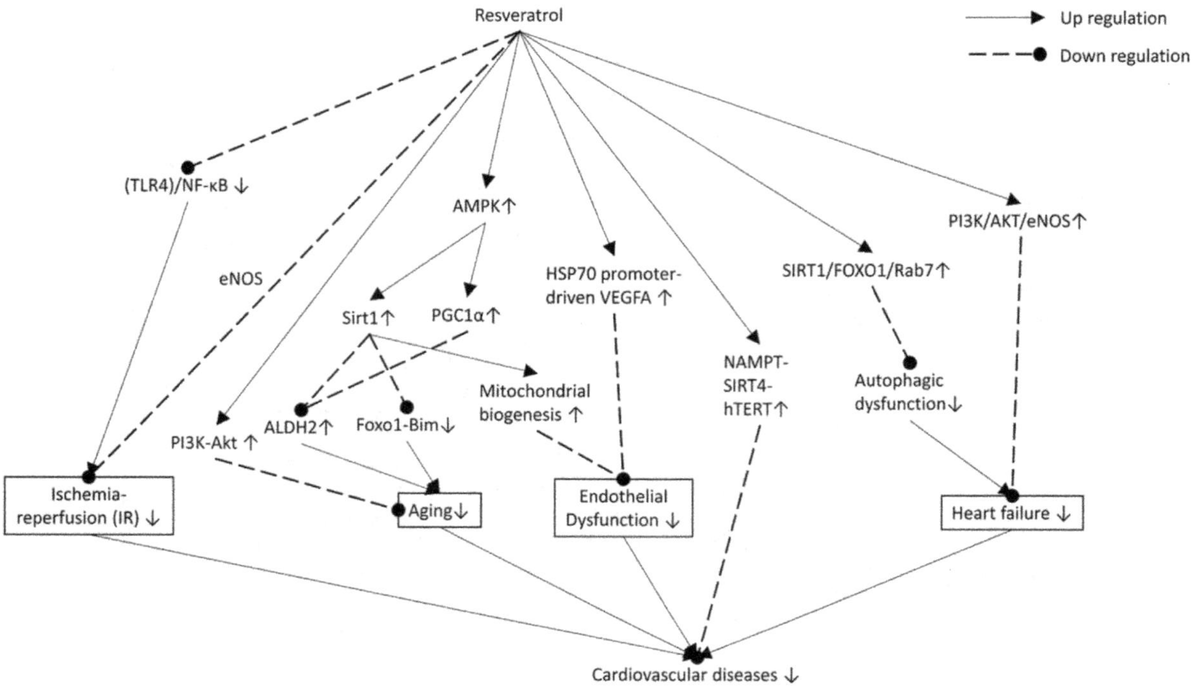

cancer chemopreventive (Kraft, Parisotto, Schempp, & Efferth, 2009; Patel, Misra, Patel, & Majumdar, 2010), anti-inflammatory (Bishayee, Barnes, Bhatia, Darvesh, & Carroll, 2010; Kang et al., 2009), anti-oxidant (Rizvi & Pandey, 2010), anti-amyloidogenic (Riviere et al., 2007) and neuroprotective (Albani, Polito, Signorini, & Forloni, 2010) effects (Figure 2).

SIRTUINS AND RESVERATROL IN CARDIOVASCULAR DISEASE

Endothelial Cell Damage

Endothelial cells form the inner lining of blood vessels and highly express SIRT1 (Ota et al., 2007). Endothelial cells undergo reactive oxygen species (ROS) damage, apoptosis, and senescence as a part of aging and disease (Alcendor et al., 2007; Cencioni et al., 2015; Chiao & Rabinovitch, 2015). SIRT1 protects the endothelial cells from ROS damage by upregulating endothelial nitric oxide synthase (eNOS) (Ota et al., 2010); this protects the angiogenic potential of endothelial cells (Winnik et al., 2015). SIRT1 also deacetylates p53 leading to decreased senescence and apoptosis (Poulose & Raju, 2015). For SIRT1 to mediate these effects, nuclear localization of SIRT1 is required. Translocation of SIRT1 from the cytoplasm of endothelial cells undergoing apoptosis to the nucleus can ameliorate the apoptotic stress (Hou, Chong, Shang, & Maiese, 2010; Hou, Wang, Shang, Chong, & Maiese, 2011).

Resveratrol promotes differentiation of endothelial cells from mesenchymal stem cell (MSC) precursors, promotes endothelial cell sprouting, and neovascularization of MSCs (Chen et al., 2015). *Cis*-resveratrol, induced MSC tube formation *in vitro* (Chen et al., 2015). Resveratrol mediates its effects, in part, through enhanced vascular endothelial growth factor A (VEGFA) expression by heat shock protein 70 (HSP70) promoter recruitment (Chen et al., 2015). Using resveratrol to enhance tube formation in MSCs though VEGFA have implications for stem cell-based gene therapies in ischemic reperfusion (IR) injury and regeneration of damaged tissues in heart disease and beyond (Chen et al., 2015).

Resveratrol's cardiovascular benefits emulate an exercise regimen of a healthy person (Handschin, 2016). Exercise-associated vascular laminar shear stress may protect the endothelial cell by affecting the mitochondria, thereby exerting atheroprotective effects in the vasculature (Kim et al., 2015a). Circulating endothelial microparticles are observed in hypertension and other cardiovascular disorders and represent endothelial dysfunction (Kim et al., 2015a). Resveratrol elicited an effect in endothelial cells similar to laminar shear stress by reducing endothelial microparticles released from the cell and activated mitochondrial biogenesis through a SIRT1-dependent mechanism (Kim et al., 2015b). Loss of SIRT1 completely abolished the protective effects of shear stress, but disruption of mitochondrial integrity significantly increased the number of total and activated endothelial microparticles back to basal levels even during shear stress (Kim et al., 2015b). These findings show that resveratrol has a potential mitochondrial structural integrity-enhancing effect which may provide a novel therapeutic option for cardiovascular disease. Moreover, aerobic exercise mitigates endothelial dysfunction by promoting mitochondrial biogenesis through systemically prolonged laminar shear stress in the vessel wall (Kim et al., 2015b).

Resveratrol protects the endothelial cell from disturbed flow–induced senescence (Warboys et al., 2014). Disrupting the flow by using either an orbital shaker or a syringe pump flow bioreactor promoted endothelial cell senescence via a p53-p21 signaling pathway compared with static conditions, whereas uninterrupted flow reduced senescence. SIRT1 activation by resveratrol treatment suppressed EC senescence that contributes to the development of atherosclerosis and promotes overall cardiovascular health (Warboys et al., 2014).

The Ageing Heart

An aging heart is characterized by cardiac hypertrophy (thickening of the heart) which decreases its function (Chiao & Rabinovitch, 2015). Even in the abscence of factors such as hypertension, or other cardiovascular diseases, the heart will age, and its function will decline. SIRT1 activity shows an age-dependent decline, so, as the heart ages, the protective function of SIRT1 decreases leaving the heart more susceptible to injury and disease (Braidy et al., 2011). Heart-specific overexpression of SIRT1 is beneficial and protective against cardiac dysfunction if expressed moderately (2.5- 2.7-fold). However, this protective effect is lost when SIRT1 overexpression was highly upregulated (12.5-fold) and induced cardiac failure in mice (Alcendor et al., 2007). This suggests that SIRT1 is acting in a protective manner in cardiac health; however, tight control of SIRT1 is necessary to achieve cardioprotection. Downregulation of SIRT1 increases damaging cardiac inflammation due to increased acetylation of NF-κB and subsequent nuclear translocation and transcriptional regulation of inflammatory genes (Costantino, Paneni, & Cosentino, 2015). SIRT1 also activates AMPK, which leads to improved glucose homeostasis and increased endothelial integrity, which aging disrupts leading to cardiac hypertrophy (Costantino et al.,

2015). Hwang et al showed that SIRT1 deacetylates p53 during oxidative stress and reduced apoptosis in the ageing heart (Hwang, Yao, Caito, Sundar, & Rahman, 2013).

SIRT1 is involved in protecting the myoblasts from ROS damage, which can contribute, to cardiac dysfunction and aging (Z. Z. Chong et al., 2012; Tanno et al., 2010). Myoblasts experience increased oxidative stress during differentiation into myocytes, which SIRT1 protect against by enhancing manganese superoxide dismutase (MnSOD, SOD2), a downstream target of FOXO, to provide resistance to oxidative stress (Z. Z. Chong et al., 2012; Tanno et al., 2010). PGC-1α, a major mitochondrial biogenesis molecule, is downregulated in ageing hearts which can lead to increased gluconeogenesis and fatty acid oxidation. SIRT1 may possess anti-ageing properties in the heart, in part, through PGC-1α and its energy metabolism properties (Matsushima & Sadoshima, 2015; Rowe & Arany, 2014).

Interestingly, resveratrol has been shown to protect the heart from functional decline due to aging, and mediates its effects largely through SIRT1 (Chung, Manganiello, & Dyck, 2012; Y. Zhang et al., 2014). Specifically, it can reverse age-induced cardiomyocyte dysfunction by regulating AMPK phosphorylation, and increase the expression of SIRT1, PGC-1α, and UCP-2 (Y. Zhang et al., 2014). Aldehyde dehydrogenase 2 (ALDH2) expression increases in aging cardiomyocytes and contributes to the functional decline of the heart as it ages (Y. Zhang et al., 2014). Resveratrol regulates the damaging effects of ALDH2 overexpression in mice (Y. Zhang et al., 2014). Additionally, resveratrol plays an essential role in regulating AMPK-SIRT1 signaling to attenuate ALDH2-enhanced cardiomyocyte dysfunction and mitochondrial injury due to cardiac aging (Y. Zhang et al., 2014).

Supplementation of resveratrol may delay or decrease the effects of ageing and functional decline of the heart. Resveratrol has been shown to decrease fibrotic collagen deposition, a common accumulation found in aging hearts and decrease oxidative damage (Sin et al., 2014). Resveratrol also dampened pro-apoptotic signaling in aging hearts via deacetylation mechanism of SIRT1 (Sin et al., 2014). Long-term supplementation of resveratrol elevated SIRT1 expression and activity in aging hearts leading to decreased FOXO1 acetylation and decreased pro-apoptotic FOXO-Bim signaling (Sin et al., 2014). Lin et al showed that resveratrol also regulates the effects of aging in the heart by SIRT1 and the PI3K-Akt signaling axis (Lin et al., 2014). While analyzing the effect of exercise or exercise and resveratrol supplementation, exercise with resveratrol supplementation enhanced SIRT1 and the PI3K-Akt pathways and prevented FOXO3 accumulation in the aging hearts of rats (Lin et al., 2014).

Resveratrol has been shown to mediate its anti-aging effects through various signaling pathways, not just SIRT1, in a number of diseases (Harikumar & Aggarwal, 2008). In the aging heart, resveratrol enhances the NAMPT-SIRT4-hTERT signaling axis which leads to stabilization of telomere length in cardiomyocites, preventing telomere shortening, a contributing factor in ageing, both *in vitro* and *in vivo* (Huang et al., 2015).

In conclusion, resveratrol protects the heart from an aging-induced decline in function by regulating a network of pathways to dampen apoptosis, oxidative damage, and accumulation of harmful proteins in the heart. With its antiaging properties, resveratrol supplementation has the potential to decrease age-induced decline in the heart leading to a longer life with fewer cardiovascular complications.

Autophagy and Cardioprotection

Autophagy is an essential process in post-mitotic cells leading to balanced energy and cell survival because loss of these cells would be detrimental (Schiattarella & Hill, 2015; Tong & Sadoshima, 2016). Cardiomyocytes utilize autophagy in times of stress, such as nutrient deprivation or ischemia in order to break down cell components and recycle them into the major building blocks (amino acids, lipids, carbohydrates) for the cell's use (Schiattarella & Hill, 2015). During fasting, SIRT1 was found to deacetylate a downstream target, FOXO, which led to autophagosome-lysosome fusion and energy homeostasis (Ng & Tang, 2013). Alterations in this pathway, such as inhibiting deacetylation of FOXO1, prevented autophagy and increased cardiac dysfunction (Ng & Tang, 2013).

Resveratrol modulates autophagic signaling in hearts during heart failure and chronic ischemia (Kanamori et al., 2013; Sabe, Elmadhun, Dalal, Robich, & Sellke, 2014). Resverartrol upregulates autophagy in heart failure by decreasing damaging post-ischemic remodeling in enlarged, aged hearts and thus providing cardioprotective benefits (Kanamori et al., 2013). In chronically ischemic hearts, supplementation of resveratrol in combination with a high cholesterol diet led to increased autophagy and decreased heart remodeling suggesting a therapeutic role for resveratrol in improving outcome post ischemia (Sabe et al., 2014). SIRT1 and resveratrol regulate autophagy and improve energy balance in the heart during heart failure.

Heart Failure

In healthy hearts, free fatty acids are the predominant molecules used to generate ATP. However, as hearts age or are subjected to stress, the source of ATP shifts from free fatty acids to glucose (An & Rodrigues, 2006; Witteles & Fowler, 2008). As heart failure (HF) progresses, insulin resistance in the heart muscle increases and leads to decreased glucose usage and an overall drop in ATP production (An & Rodrigues, 2006). In HF the shift in energy balance suggests mitochondrial dysfunction and as SIRT1 is a major mitochondrial protein deacetylase involved in energy production and oxidative stress, it is implicated in HF (Tanno, Kuno, Horio, & Miura, 2012). SIRT1 alters fatty acid uptake and usage by binding to PPARα displacing its binding partner, RXRα, and preventing fatty acid uptake that further disturbs the energy balance in failing hearts (Oka et al., 2015).

ROS production in the heart is normally high. High ROS levels can irreversibly damage the heart by cellular and mitochondrial damage that can lead to heart failure over time. SIRT1, as a cardioprotective molecule, is known to upregulate MnSOD, which functions as a detoxification molecule in the mitochondria to clear the ROS. This may prevent ROS damage to the heart which contributes to heart failure (Tanno et al., 2012). SIRT1-mediated activation of FOXO also increases antioxidants such as MnSOD and catalase increasing resistance to oxidative stress (Luo et al., 2014). SIRT1 can also regulate cardiomyocyte cell death or survival. Cardiomyocyte cell death occurs by apoptosis, necrosis, and autophagy and SIRT1 has been shown to regulate each of these processes (Tanno et al., 2012). An increase in SIRT1 has been shown to regulate cardiomyocyte apoptosis by deacetylating apoptotic proteins p53, and Ku70, and thereby preventing Bax interaction leading to apoptosis (Tanno et al., 2012). Resveratrol shows beneficial properties in cases of heart failure through direct or indirect effects in animal stuides (Tome-Carneiro et al., 2013; Zordoky et al., 2015). Resveratrol restored the levels of mitochondrial oxidative phosphorylation complexes and cardiac AMP-activated protein kinase activation leading to improved energetic myocardial status in a mouse model of heart failure (Sung et al., 2015). Also, non-cardiac symptoms of HF, such as peripheral insulin sensitivity, glucose metabolism, vascular function, and physical activity, were also improved by resveratrol treatment. As a result, resveratrol treatment significantly increased median survival of mice with HF, reduced cardiac fibrosis, decreased markers of hypertrophy and HF-related extracellular remodeling, and improved diastolic function and energy metabolism (Sung et al., 2015).

In streptozotocin (STZ) induced diabetic cardiomyopathy mice, long-term resveratrol treatment improved cardiac function, ameliorated oxidative injury and reduced apoptosis in the heart (B. Wang et al., 2014). Resveratrol reduced apoptosis by regulating dysfunctional autophagic flux through the SIRT1/FOXO1/Rab7 axis (B. Wang et al., 2014). In coronary ligation-induced HF in rabbits, resveratrol decreased left atrial fibrosis and reduced atrial fibrillation by regulating the PI3K/AKT/eNOS signaling pathway (E. Chong et al., 2015). Polydatin (PD), a resveratrol glucoside, also showed beneficial actions on cardiac hypertrophy by inhibiting ROS-dependent Rho kinase activation (Dong et al., 2015). PD attenuated phenylephrine-induced increased cell surface area and atrial natriuretic protein expression in cultured neonatal rat ventricular myocytes. PD treatment in transverse aortic constriction inhibited phenylephrine-induced oxidative stress and consequently suppressed ROCK activation in cardiomyocytes. Decreased oxidative stress and ROCK activation leads to reduced hypertrophy and improved cardiac function (Dong et al., 2015).

Ischemic-Reperfusion Injury

Ischemia-reperfusion (IR) injury occurs when cardiomyocytes experience a lack of oxygen due to angina or myocardial infarction, and once reperfusion of blood flow is established, an IR injury occurs. As the heart ages, it becomes more susceptible to IR injury and subsequent myocardial infarction leading to increased incidence of death. Ischemic preconditioning by starving the heart of oxygen for short periods of time has a protective role against IR injury (Poulose & Raju, 2015). Ischemic preconditioning, protects the heart, in part, through SIRT1 activity (Wojtovich, Nadtochiy, Brookes, & Nehrke, 2012). Moreover, inhibition of SIRT1 prevented the protective effect of ischemic preconditioning in mouse hearts. The decline of SIRT1 in aging hearts may contribute to the inability of the heart to protect against IR injury. Though the underlying mechanism by which SIRT1 mediates its effects is not yet known, mTOR and AMPK signaling have been suggested from from studies into the benefitial role of SIRT1 and calorie restriction (Ghosh, McBurney, & Robbins, 2010; Shinmura et al., 2007).

Resveratrol-supplemented high cholesterol fed Yorkshire swine that were subjected to IR injury showed 76 differentially regulated proteins (out of 669) compared to high cholesterol fed swine without resveratrol supplementation. Proteomic and pathway analyzes identified proteins downregulated in resveratrol supplemented ischemic myocardium in a number of pathways including mitochondrial dysfunction, cell death, and detrimental cardiac remodeling (Sabe et al., 2015). Resveratrol protects the cardiomyocytes and myocardium from detrimental consequences of IR injury through regulation of not only SIRT1 but inflammatory and cell death pathways.

In IR injury, resveratrol improves the outcome of cardiomyocytes through regulation of SIRT1. Resveratrol improved cardiomyocyte outcome in I/R-treated Wistar-Kyoto rats by reducing apoptosis and restoring SIRT1 activity and NAD+ levels (Cattelan et al., 2015). In another study using mice undergoing IR injury, resveratrol treatment increased SIRT1 activity and reduced infarct size (Shalwala et al., 2014).

Resveratrol decreases inflammation associated with I/R injury through a number of mechanisms. In rats subjected to I/R injury, resveratrol inhibited Toll-like receptor 4 (TLR4)/NF-κB signaling and therefore, dampening early inflammation in heart (J. Li et al., 2015). Resveratrol also reduced apoptosis, decreased the amount of lactate dehydrogenase release (a marker for necrosis), reduced inflammatory cytokine levels in cardiomyocytes of rats subjected to IR injury (C. Zhang et al., 2012).

Atherosclerosis

Atherosclerosis is a chronic inflammatory disease where immune cell infiltration and endothelial proliferation lead to the thickening of the artery wall and formation of plaques. Atherosclerosis can go undetected and asymptomatic for years before being diagnosed because of a secondary condition such as a heart attack (Lusis, 2000). SIRT1 has the potential to prevent the development of atherosclerosis in a number of ways. SIRT1 in the endothelium can decrease apoptosis by blocking oxidative stress-induced apoptosis, thereby protecting the endothelium (Z. Z. Chong et al., 2012). Also, SIRT1 improved endothelium function such as relaxation by regulating endothelial nitric oxide synthase (eNOS) and nitric oxide concentration in the cells (Mattagajasingh et al., 2007). Patients with coronary heart disease have decreased SIRT1 expression and in atherosclerosis, SIRT1 expression modulates multiple pathways including LXR, CXCR7, and NF-κB to protect against atherosclerosis (Stein & Matter, 2011).

The cellular localization of SIRT1 also plays a role in disease. In healthy human hearts, SIRT1 is expressed predominantly in the cytoplasm. However, in diseased human hearts, such as chronic heart failure, SIRT1 is localized to the nucleus in cardiomyocytes (Tanno et al., 2007). Subcellular localization of SIRT1 impacts its function in disease states as well as the targets available for deacetylation.

SIRT1 also regulates vascular smooth muscle cell hypertrophy which contributes to atherosclerosis. Angiotensin II induces vascular smooth muscle cell hypertrophy, a process that overexpression of SIRT1 inhibits (L. Li et al., 2011). SIRT1 regulates tissue inhibitor of matrix metalloproteinase 3 (TIMP3), which inhibits matrix metalloproteinase 3, an important mediator of plaque formation, and thereby reduce plaque formation leading to atherosclerosis (Cardellini et al., 2009; Stein & Matter, 2011). Through its mediation of oxidative stress and catalase through FOXO signaling, SIRT1 signaling prevents or improves atherosclerosis development (Alcendor et al., 2007; Cervelli, Borghini, Galli, & Andreassi, 2012; Q. J. Zhang et al., 2008). Furthermore, it is suggested SIRT1 is involved in DNA damage sensing and repair that may play a role in preventing atherosclerosis by targeting DNA damage repair signaling molecule Nibrin (NBS1) (Cervelli et al., 2012; Yuan & Seto, 2007).

Blood Pressure and Hypertension

Hypertension (or high blood pressure), leads to heart failure if uncontrolled. High blood pressure affects most people at some point in their life and is often the result of increased peripheral vascular resistance. The underlying cause of hypertension is not well understood and therefore, treatments target the symptoms but not the cause (Hamza & Dyck, 2014). Resveratrol has been shown to exhibit antihypertensive properties, and it is being evaluated for the treatment of hypertension. Resveratrol restored the transcription factor nuclear factor-E2-related factor-2 (Nrf2, a master regulator of numerous genes encoding antioxidant and phase II-detoxifying enzymes and molecules) function, reduced renal inflammation, and mitigated hypertension in spontaneously hypertensive rats (Javkhedkar et al., 2015). In one recent meta-analysis in humans, resveratrol consumption significantly decreased the systolic blood pressure level at the higher dose, but had no significant effects on diastolic blood pressure levels (Liu, Ma, Zhang, He, & Huang, 2015). Resveratrol works not only on the heart, but the central nervous system, the renal system, and peripheral vasculature to control ROS and directly affect the vasculature to maintain a healthy blood pressure level (Hamza & Dyck, 2014).

Calorie Restriction

Decreased caloric intake without malnutrition can increase lifespan and reduce the effects of aging. Calorie restriction has been shown to prevent cardiovascular disease by maintaining healthy metabolic parameters including decreased body weight and increased insulin sensitivity (Testa, Biasi, Poli, & Chiarpotto, 2014; Wei, 2014). Calorie restriction has also been shown to decrease ROS damage to cardiomyocytes, staving off atherosclerosis (Wei, 2014). While the full underlying mechanism of calorie restriction is unclear, it helps prevent cardiovascular diseases associated with poor metabolic health and aging (Y. Wang, 2014). SIRT1 has been long studied as a nutrient sensor related to longevity. Calorie restriction increases SIRT1 expression, along with SIRT2-4 and -7, in the heart (Wei, 2014). The Mediterranean diet is low calorie and dense in polyphenols, including resveratrol, antioxidants, and omega-3-fatty acids that come from red wine, fruits and vegetables, and fish, respectively. Those that adhere to a Mediterranean diet benefit from reduced risks for cardiovascular disease (Pallauf, Giller, Huebbe, & Rimbach, 2013).

Resveratrol has been shown to act as a calorie restriction (CR) mimetic with potential anti-aging properties (Testa et al., 2014). Resveratrol mimics CR through endothelial nitric oxide synthase (eNOS). Interestingly, without eNOS, resveratrol fails to provide cardioprotective benefits, even with the resveratrol-induced increase in SIRT1 activity (Shinmura et al., 2015). This shows that resveratrol may work independent of SIRT1 pathway.

CONCLUSION

In conclusion, resveratrol, has been lauded for its protective effects against cardiovascular disease. Resveratrol treatment in mice decreases age-related cardiac dysfunction. Resveratrol mediates its effects of cardioprotection, in part, through activation of an epigenetic regulator SIRT1. Resveratrol is available as a supplement over the counter and has been shown to be well tolerated in patients and has been used in humans for its cardioprotective effects (Raj, Zieroth, & Netticadan, 2015). Patients with cardiovascular disease are encouraged to lead a healthier, more active lifestyle. Supplementation of resveratrol into the diet through plants containing high polyphenol content such as grapes may aid in a heart healthy lifestyle and reduce the need for pharmaceutical intervention. Furthermore, after a patient suffers a heart attack, incorporating resveratrol into the treatment plan may decrease damaging remodeling and protect the heart as it heals. Targeting SIRT1 directly would be an alternative or combination strategy in the prevention and treatment of cardiovascular disease. Its cardioprotective properties can become a powerful pharmaceutical target for development in cardiovascular disease in the near future.

REFERENCES

Albani, D., Polito, L., Signorini, A., & Forloni, G. (2010). Neuroprotective properties of resveratrol in different neurodegenerative disorders. *BioFactors (Oxford, England)*, *36*(5), 370–376. doi:10.1002/biof.118 PMID:20848560

Alcendor, R. R., Gao, S., Zhai, P., Zablocki, D., Holle, E., Yu, X., & Sadoshima, J. et al. (2007). Sirt1 regulates aging and resistance to oxidative stress in the heart. *Circulation Research, 100*(10), 1512–1521. doi:10.1161/01.RES.0000267723.65696.4a PMID:17446436

An, D., & Rodrigues, B. (2006). Role of changes in cardiac metabolism in development of diabetic cardiomyopathy. *American Journal of Physiology. Heart and Circulatory Physiology, 291*(4), H1489–H1506. doi:10.1152/ajpheart.00278.2006 PMID:16751293

Balcerczyk, A., & Pirola, L. (2010). Therapeutic potential of activators and inhibitors of sirtuins. *BioFactors (Oxford, England), 36*(5), 383–393. doi:10.1002/biof.112 PMID:20848588

Bauerly, K., Harris, C., Chowanadisai, W., Graham, J., Havel, P. J., Tchaparian, E., & Rucker, R. B. et al. (2011). Altering pyrroloquinoline quinone nutritional status modulates mitochondrial, lipid, and energy metabolism in rats. *PLoS ONE, 6*(7), e21779. doi:10.1371/journal.pone.0021779 PMID:21814553

Bishayee, A., Barnes, K. F., Bhatia, D., Darvesh, A. S., & Carroll, R. T. (2010). Resveratrol suppresses oxidative stress and inflammatory response in diethylnitrosamine-initiated rat hepatocarcinogenesis. *Cancer Prevention Research (Philadelphia, Pa.), 3*(6), 753–763. doi:10.1158/1940-6207.CAPR-09-0171 PMID:20501860

Bjorkegren, J. L., Kovacic, J. C., Dudley, J. T., & Schadt, E. E. (2015). Genome-wide significant loci: How important are they? Systems genetics to understand heritability of coronary artery disease and other common complex disorders. *Journal of the American College of Cardiology, 65*(8), 830–845. doi:10.1016/j.jacc.2014.12.033 PMID:25720628

Bloom, D. E., Cafiero, E. T., Jané-Llopis, E., Abrahams-Gessel, S., Bloom, L. R., Fathima, S.,... Weinstein, C. (2011). *The Global Economic Burden of Non-communicable Diseases*. Retrieved from www.weforum.org/EconomicsOfNCD

Braidy, N., Guillemin, G. J., Mansour, H., Chan-Ling, T., Poljak, A., & Grant, R. (2011). Age related changes in NAD+ metabolism oxidative stress and Sirt1 activity in wistar rats. *PLoS ONE, 6*(4), e19194. doi:10.1371/journal.pone.0019194 PMID:21541336

Cardellini, M., Menghini, R., Martelli, E., Casagrande, V., Marino, A., Rizza, S., & Federici, M. et al. (2009). TIMP3 is reduced in atherosclerotic plaques from subjects with type 2 diabetes and increased by SirT1. *Diabetes, 58*(10), 2396–2401. doi:10.2337/db09-0280 PMID:19581416

Cattelan, A., Ceolotto, G., Bova, S., Albiero, M., Kuppusamy, M., De Martin, S., & Avogaro, A. et al. (2015). NAD(+)-dependent SIRT1 deactivation has a key role on ischemia-reperfusion-induced apoptosis. *Vascular Pharmacology, 70*, 35–44. doi:10.1016/j.vph.2015.02.004 PMID:25863291

Cencioni, C., Spallotta, F., Mai, A., Martelli, F., Farsetti, A., Zeiher, A. M., & Gaetano, C. (2015). Sirtuin function in aging heart and vessels. *Journal of Molecular and Cellular Cardiology, 83*, 55–61. doi:10.1016/j.yjmcc.2014.12.023 PMID:25579854

Cervelli, T., Borghini, A., Galli, A., & Andreassi, M. G. (2012). DNA damage and repair in atherosclerosis: Current insights and future perspectives. *International Journal of Molecular Sciences, 13*(12), 16929–16944. doi:10.3390/ijms131216929 PMID:23443128

Chavan, A. V., & Somani, R. R. (2010). HDAC inhibitors - new generation of target specific treatment. *Mini Reviews in Medicinal Chemistry*, *10*(13), 1263–1276. doi:10.2174/138955751110091263 PMID:20701588

Chen, Y. B., Lan, Y. W., Hung, T. H., Chen, L. G., Choo, K. B., Cheng, W. T., & Chong, K. Y. et al. (2015). Mesenchymal stem cell-based HSP70 promoter-driven VEGFA induction by resveratrol promotes angiogenesis in a mouse model. *Cell Stress & Chaperones*, *20*(4), 643–652. doi:10.1007/s12192-015-0588-x PMID:25860916

Chiao, Y. A., & Rabinovitch, P. S. (2015). The Aging Heart. *Cold Spring Harb Perspect Med*, *5*(9), a025148. doi:10.1101/cshperspect.a025148 PMID:26328932

Chong, E., Chang, S. L., Hsiao, Y. W., Singhal, R., Liu, S. H., Leha, T., & Chen, S. A. et al. (2015). Resveratrol, a red wine antioxidant, reduces atrial fibrillation susceptibility in the failing heart by PI3K/AKT/eNOS signaling pathway activation. *Heart Rhythm*, *12*(5), 1046–1056. doi:10.1016/j.hrthm.2015.01.044 PMID:25640634

Chong, Z. Z., Wang, S., Shang, Y. C., & Maiese, K. (2012). Targeting cardiovascular disease with novel SIRT1 pathways. *Future Cardiol*, *8*(1), 89–100. doi:10.2217/fca.11.76 PMID:22185448

Chung, J. H., Manganiello, V., & Dyck, J. R. (2012). Resveratrol as a calorie restriction mimetic: Therapeutic implications. *Trends in Cell Biology*, *22*(10), 546–554. doi:10.1016/j.tcb.2012.07.004 PMID:22885100

Costantino, S., Paneni, F., & Cosentino, F. (2015). Ageing, metabolism and cardiovascular disease. *The Journal of Physiology*. doi:10.1113/JP270538 PMID:26391109

Dong, M., Ding, W., Liao, Y., Liu, Y., Yan, D., Zhang, Y., & Liu, J. et al. (2015). Polydatin prevents hypertrophy in phenylephrine induced neonatal mouse cardiomyocytes and pressure-overload mouse models. *European Journal of Pharmacology*, *746*, 186–197. doi:10.1016/j.ejphar.2014.11.012 PMID:25449040

Ghosh, H. S., McBurney, M., & Robbins, P. D. (2010). SIRT1 negatively regulates the mammalian target of rapamycin. *PLoS ONE*, *5*(2), e9199. doi:10.1371/journal.pone.0009199 PMID:20169165

Hamza, S. M., & Dyck, J. R. (2014). Systemic and renal oxidative stress in the pathogenesis of hypertension: Modulation of long-term control of arterial blood pressure by resveratrol. *Frontiers in Physics*, *5*, 292. doi:10.3389/fphys.2014.00292 PMID:25140155

Handschin, C. (2016). Caloric restriction and exercise mimetics: Ready for prime time? *Pharmacological Research*, *103*, 158–166. doi:10.1016/j.phrs.2015.11.009 PMID:26658171

Harikumar, K. B., & Aggarwal, B. B. (2008). Resveratrol: A multitargeted agent for age-associated chronic diseases. *Cell Cycle (Georgetown, Tex.)*, *7*(8), 1020–1035. doi:10.4161/cc.7.8.5740 PMID:18414053

Hou, J., Chong, Z. Z., Shang, Y. C., & Maiese, K. (2010). Early apoptotic vascular signaling is determined by Sirt1 through nuclear shuttling, forkhead trafficking, bad, and mitochondrial caspase activation. *Current Neurovascular Research*, *7*(2), 95–112. doi:10.2174/156720210791184899 PMID:20370652

Hou, J., Wang, S., Shang, Y. C., Chong, Z. Z., & Maiese, K. (2011). Erythropoietin employs cell longevity pathways of SIRT1 to foster endothelial vascular integrity during oxidant stress. *Current Neurovascular Research*, *8*(3), 220–235. doi:10.2174/156720211796558069 PMID:21722091

Hsu, C. P., Odewale, I., Alcendor, R. R., & Sadoshima, J. (2008). Sirt1 protects the heart from aging and stress. *Biological Chemistry*, *389*(3), 221–231. doi:10.1515/BC.2008.032 PMID:18208353

Huang, P., Riordan, S. M., Heruth, D. P., Grigoryev, D. N., Zhang, L. Q., & Ye, S. Q. (2015). A critical role of nicotinamide phosphoribosyltransferase in human telomerase reverse transcriptase induction by resveratrol in aortic smooth muscle cells. *Oncotarget*, *6*(13), 10812–10824. doi:10.18632/oncotarget.3580 PMID:25926556

Hung, L. M., Su, M. J., & Chen, J. K. (2004). Resveratrol protects myocardial ischemia-reperfusion injury through both NO-dependent and NO-independent mechanisms. *Free Radical Biology & Medicine*, *36*(6), 774–781. doi:10.1016/j.freeradbiomed.2003.12.016 PMID:14990356

Hwang, J. W., Yao, H., Caito, S., Sundar, I. K., & Rahman, I. (2013). Redox regulation of SIRT1 in inflammation and cellular senescence. *Free Radical Biology & Medicine*, *61*, 95–110. doi:10.1016/j.freeradbiomed.2013.03.015 PMID:23542362

Javkhedkar, A. A., Quiroz, Y., Rodriguez-Iturbe, B., Vaziri, N. D., Lokhandwala, M. F., & Banday, A. A. (2015). Resveratrol restored Nrf2 function, reduced renal inflammation, and mitigated hypertension in spontaneously hypertensive rats. *American Journal of Physiology. Regulatory, Integrative and Comparative Physiology*, *308*(10), R840–R846. doi:10.1152/ajpregu.00308.2014 PMID:25761698

Jensen, M. D., Ryan, D. H., Apovian, C. M., Ard, J. D., Comuzzie, A. G., Donato, K. A., & Yanovski, S. Z. et al. (2014). 2013 AHA/ACC/TOS guideline for the management of overweight and obesity in adults: A report of the American College of Cardiology/American Heart Association Task Force on Practice Guidelines and The Obesity Society. *Journal of the American College of Cardiology*, *63*(2525 Pt B), 2985–3023. doi:10.1016/j.jacc.2013.11.004 PMID:24239920

Kanamori, H., Takemura, G., Goto, K., Tsujimoto, A., Ogino, A., Takeyama, T., & Minatoguchi, S. et al. (2013). Resveratrol reverses remodeling in hearts with large, old myocardial infarctions through enhanced autophagy-activating AMP kinase pathway. *American Journal of Pathology*, *182*(3), 701–713. doi:10.1016/j.ajpath.2012.11.009 PMID:23274061

Kang, O. H., Jang, H. J., Chae, H. S., Oh, Y. C., Choi, J. G., Lee, Y. S., & Kwon, D. Y. et al. (2009). Anti-inflammatory mechanisms of resveratrol in activated HMC-1 cells: Pivotal roles of NF-kappaB and MAPK. *Pharmacological Research*, *59*(5), 330–337. doi:10.1016/j.phrs.2009.01.009 PMID:19416633

Kim, J. S., Kim, B., Lee, H., Thakkar, S., Babbitt, D. M., Eguchi, S., & Park, J. Y. et al. (2015a). Shear stress-induced mitochondrial biogenesis decreases the release of microparticles from endothelial cells. *American Journal of Physiology. Heart and Circulatory Physiology*, *309*(3), H425–H433. doi:10.1152/ajpheart.00438.2014 PMID:26024684

Kim, J. S., Kim, B., Lee, H., Thakkar, S., Babbitt, D. M., Eguchi, S.,... Park, J. Y. (2015b). Shear Stress-Induced Mitochondrial Biogenesis Decreases the Release of Microparticles from Endothelial Cells. *Am J Physiol Heart Circ Physiol*. doi:10.1152/ajpheart.00438.2014

Kraft, T. E., Parisotto, D., Schempp, C., & Efferth, T. (2009). Fighting cancer with red wine? Molecular mechanisms of resveratrol. *Critical Reviews in Food Science and Nutrition*, *49*(9), 782–799. doi:10.1080/10408390802248627 PMID:20443159

Lekakis, J., Rallidis, L. S., Andreadou, I., Vamvakou, G., Kazantzoglou, G., Magiatis, P., & Kremastinos, D. T. et al. (2005). Polyphenolic compounds from red grapes acutely improve endothelial function in patients with coronary heart disease. *European Journal of Cardiovascular Prevention and Rehabilitation, 12*(6), 596–600. PMID:16319551

Li, J., Xie, C., Zhuang, J., Li, H., Yao, Y., Shao, C., & Wang, H. (2015). Resveratrol attenuates inflammation in the rat heart subjected to ischemia-reperfusion: Role of the TLR4/NF-kappaB signaling pathway. *Mol Med Rep, 11*(2), 1120–1126. doi:10.3892/mmr.2014.2955 PMID:25405531

Li, L., Gao, P., Zhang, H., Chen, H., Zheng, W., Lv, X., & Liang, C. et al. (2011). SIRT1 inhibits angiotensin II-induced vascular smooth muscle cell hypertrophy. *Acta Biochimica et Biophysica Sinica, 43*(2), 103–109. doi:10.1093/abbs/gmq104 PMID:21118843

Lin, C. H., Lin, C. C., Ting, W. J., Pai, P. Y., Kuo, C. H., Ho, T. J., & Lin, W. T. et al. (2014). Resveratrol enhanced FOXO3 phosphorylation via synergetic activation of SIRT1 and PI3K/Akt signaling to improve the effects of exercise in elderly rat hearts. *Age (Dordrecht, Netherlands), 36*(5), 9705. doi:10.1007/s11357-014-9705-5 PMID:25158994

Liu, Y., Ma, W., Zhang, P., He, S., & Huang, D. (2015). Effect of resveratrol on blood pressure: A meta-analysis of randomized controlled trials. *Clinical Nutrition (Edinburgh, Lothian), 34*(1), 27–34. doi:10.1016/j.clnu.2014.03.009 PMID:24731650

Lu, Z., Scott, I., Webster, B. R., & Sack, M. N. (2009). The emerging characterization of lysine residue deacetylation on the modulation of mitochondrial function and cardiovascular biology. *Circulation Research, 105*(9), 830–841. doi:10.1161/CIRCRESAHA.109.204974 PMID:19850949

Luo, X. Y., Qu, S. L., Tang, Z. H., Zhang, Y., Liu, M. H., Peng, J., & Jiang, Z. S. et al. (2014). SIRT1 in cardiovascular aging. *Clinica Chimica Acta, 437*, 106–114. doi:10.1016/j.cca.2014.07.019 PMID:25063737

Lusis, A. J. (2000). Atherosclerosis. *Nature, 407*(6801), 233–241. doi:10.1038/35025203 PMID:11001066

Ma, L., & Li, Y. (2015). SIRT1: Role in cardiovascular biology. *Clinica Chimica Acta, 440*, 8–15. doi:10.1016/j.cca.2014.10.036 PMID:25444742

Martinez, S. R., Gay, M. S., & Zhang, L. (2015). Epigenetic mechanisms in heart development and disease. *Drug Discovery Today, 20*(7), 799–811. doi:10.1016/j.drudis.2014.12.018 PMID:25572405

Matsushima, S., & Sadoshima, J. (2015). The role of sirtuins in cardiac disease. *American Journal of Physiology. Heart and Circulatory Physiology, 309*(9), H1375–H1389. doi:10.1152/ajpheart.00053.2015 PMID:26232232

Mattagajasingh, I., Kim, C. S., Naqvi, A., Yamamori, T., Hoffman, T. A., Jung, S. B., & Irani, K. et al. (2007). SIRT1 promotes endothelium-dependent vascular relaxation by activating endothelial nitric oxide synthase. *Proceedings of the National Academy of Sciences of the United States of America, 104*(37), 14855–14860. doi:10.1073/pnas.0704329104 PMID:17785417

Naghavi, M., Wang, H., Lozano, R., Davis, A., Liang, X., Zhou, M., & Murray, C. J. et al. (2015). Global, regional, and national age-sex specific all-cause and cause-specific mortality for 240 causes of death, 19902013: A systematic analysis for the Global Burden of Disease Study 2013. *Lancet*, *385*(9963), 117–171. doi:10.1016/S0140-6736(14)61682-2 PMID:25530442

Ng, F., & Tang, B. L. (2013). Sirtuins modulation of autophagy. *Journal of Cellular Physiology*, *228*(12), 2262–2270. doi:10.1002/jcp.24399 PMID:23696314

Oka, S., Zhai, P., Yamamoto, T., Ikeda, Y., Byun, J., Hsu, C. P., & Sadoshima, J. (2015). Peroxisome Proliferator Activated Receptor-alpha Association With Silent Information Regulator 1 Suppresses Cardiac Fatty Acid Metabolism in the Failing Heart. *Circulation: Heart Failure*, *8*(6), 1123–1132. doi:10.1161/CIRCHEARTFAILURE.115.002216 PMID:26443578

Ota, H., Akishita, M., Eto, M., Iijima, K., Kaneki, M., & Ouchi, Y. (2007). Sirt1 modulates premature senescence-like phenotype in human endothelial cells. *Journal of Molecular and Cellular Cardiology*, *43*(5), 571–579. doi:10.1016/j.yjmcc.2007.08.008 PMID:17916362

Ota, H., Eto, M., Ogawa, S., Iijima, K., Akishita, M., & Ouchi, Y. (2010). SIRT1/eNOS axis as a potential target against vascular senescence, dysfunction and atherosclerosis. *Journal of Atherosclerosis and Thrombosis*, *17*(5), 431–435. doi:10.5551/jat.3525 PMID:20215708

Pallauf, K., Giller, K., Huebbe, P., & Rimbach, G. (2013). Nutrition and healthy ageing: Calorie restriction or polyphenol-rich "MediterrAsian" diet? *Oxidative Medicine and Cellular Longevity*, *707421*. doi:10.1155/2013/707421 PMID:24069505

Patel, V. B., Misra, S., Patel, B. B., & Majumdar, A. P. (2010). Colorectal cancer: Chemopreventive role of curcumin and resveratrol. *Nutrition and Cancer*, *62*(7), 958–967. doi:10.1080/01635581.2010.510259 PMID:20924971

Poulose, N., & Raju, R. (2015). Sirtuin regulation in aging and injury. *Biochimica et Biophysica Acta*, *1852*(11), 2442–2455. doi:10.1016/j.bbadis.2015.08.017 PMID:26303641

Quarles, E. K., Dai, D. F., Tocchi, A., Basisty, N., Gitari, L., & Rabinovitch, P. S. (2015). Quality control systems in cardiac aging. *Ageing Res Rev, 23*(Pt A), 101-115. doi:10.1016/j.arr.2015.02.003

Raj, P., Zieroth, S., & Netticadan, T. (2015). An overview of the efficacy of resveratrol in the management of ischemic heart disease. *Annals of the New York Academy of Sciences*, *1348*(1), 55–67. doi:10.1111/nyas.12828 PMID:26227659

Riviere, C., Richard, T., Quentin, L., Krisa, S., Merillon, J. M., & Monti, J. P. (2007). Inhibitory activity of stilbenes on Alzheimer's beta-amyloid fibrils in vitro. *Bioorg Med Chem, 15*(2), 1160-1167. doi:S0968-0896(06)00817-0 [pii] 10.1016/j.bmc.2006.09.069

Rizvi, S. I., & Pandey, K. B. (2010). Activation of the erythrocyte plasma membrane redox system by resveratrol: A possible mechanism for antioxidant properties. *Pharmacological Reports*, *62*(4), 726–732. doi:10.1016/S1734-1140(10)70330-3 PMID:20885013

Rowe, G. C., & Arany, Z. (2014). Genetic models of PGC-1 and glucose metabolism and homeostasis. *Reviews in Endocrine & Metabolic Disorders*, *15*(1), 21–29. doi:10.1007/s11154-013-9273-5 PMID:24057597

Sabe, A. A., Elmadhun, N. Y., Dalal, R. S., Robich, M. P., & Sellke, F. W. (2014). Resveratrol regulates autophagy signaling in chronically ischemic myocardium. *The Journal of Thoracic and Cardiovascular Surgery*, *147*(2), 792–798, Discussion 798–799. doi:10.1016/j.jtcvs.2013.06.062 PMID:24267781

Sabe, A. A., Sadek, A. A., Elmadhun, N. Y., Dalal, R. S., Robich, M. P., Bianchi, C., & Sellke, F. W. (2015). Investigating the effects of resveratrol on chronically ischemic myocardium in a Swine model of metabolic syndrome: A proteomics analysis. *Journal of Medicinal Food*, *18*(1), 60–66. doi:10.1089/jmf.2014.0036 PMID:25089828

Schiattarella, G. G., & Hill, J. A. (2015). Therapeutic targeting of autophagy in cardiovascular disease. *Journal of Molecular and Cellular Cardiology*. doi:10.1016/j.yjmcc.2015.11.019 PMID:26602750

Sebastian, C., Satterstrom, F. K., Haigis, M. C., & Mostoslavsky, R. (2012). From sirtuin biology to human diseases: An update. *The Journal of Biological Chemistry*, *287*(51), 42444–42452. doi:10.1074/jbc.R112.402768 PMID:23086954

Shalwala, M., Zhu, S. G., Das, A., Salloum, F. N., Xi, L., & Kukreja, R. C. (2014). Sirtuin 1 (SIRT1) activation mediates sildenafil induced delayed cardioprotection against ischemia-reperfusion injury in mice. *PLoS ONE*, *9*(1), e86977. doi:10.1371/journal.pone.0086977 PMID:24466304

Shinmura, K., Tamaki, K., Ito, K., Yan, X., Yamamoto, T., Katsumata, Y., & Ishii, I. et al. (2015). Indispensable role of endothelial nitric oxide synthase in caloric restriction-induced cardioprotection against ischemia-reperfusion injury. *American Journal of Physiology. Heart and Circulatory Physiology*, *308*(8), H894–H903. doi:10.1152/ajpheart.00333.2014 PMID:25681423

Shinmura, K., Tamaki, K., Saito, K., Nakano, Y., Tobe, T., & Bolli, R. (2007). Cardioprotective effects of short-term caloric restriction are mediated by adiponectin via activation of AMP-activated protein kinase. *Circulation*, *116*(24), 2809–2817. doi:10.1161/CIRCULATIONAHA.107.725697 PMID:18040027

Sin, T. K., Yu, A. P., Yung, B. Y., Yip, S. P., Chan, L. W., Wong, C. S., & Siu, P. M. et al. (2014). Modulating effect of SIRT1 activation induced by resveratrol on Foxo1-associated apoptotic signalling in senescent heart. *The Journal of Physiology*, *592*(Pt 12), 2535–2548. doi:10.1113/jphysiol.2014.271387 PMID:24639483

Stein, S., & Matter, C. M. (2011). Protective roles of SIRT1 in atherosclerosis. *Cell Cycle (Georgetown, Tex.)*, *10*(4), 640–647. doi:10.4161/cc.10.4.14863 PMID:21293192

Stone, N. J., Robinson, J. G., Lichtenstein, A. H., Bairey Merz, C. N., Blum, C. B., Eckel, R. H., & Wilson, P. W. et al. (2014). 2013 ACC/AHA guideline on the treatment of blood cholesterol to reduce atherosclerotic cardiovascular risk in adults: A report of the American College of Cardiology/American Heart Association Task Force on Practice Guidelines. *Journal of the American College of Cardiology*, *63*(2525 Pt B), 2889–2934. doi:10.1016/j.jacc.2013.11.002 PMID:24239923

Sung, M. M., Das, S. K., Levasseur, J., Byrne, N. J., Fung, D., Kim, T. T., & Dyck, J. R. et al. (2015). Resveratrol treatment of mice with pressure-overload-induced heart failure improves diastolic function and cardiac energy metabolism. *Circulation: Heart Failure*, *8*(1), 128–137. doi:10.1161/CIRCHEARTFAILURE.114.001677 PMID:25394648

Tanno, M., Kuno, A., Horio, Y., & Miura, T. (2012). Emerging beneficial roles of sirtuins in heart failure. *Basic Research in Cardiology*, *107*(4), 273. doi:10.1007/s00395-012-0273-5 PMID:22622703

Tanno, M., Kuno, A., Yano, T., Miura, T., Hisahara, S., Ishikawa, S., & Horio, Y. et al. (2010). Induction of manganese superoxide dismutase by nuclear translocation and activation of SIRT1 promotes cell survival in chronic heart failure. *The Journal of Biological Chemistry*, *285*(11), 8375–8382. doi:10.1074/jbc.M109.090266 PMID:20089851

Tanno, M., Sakamoto, J., Miura, T., Shimamoto, K., & Horio, Y. (2007). Nucleocytoplasmic shuttling of the NAD+-dependent histone deacetylase SIRT1. *The Journal of Biological Chemistry*, *282*(9), 6823–6832. doi:10.1074/jbc.M609554200 PMID:17197703

Testa, G., Biasi, F., Poli, G., & Chiarpotto, E. (2014). Calorie restriction and dietary restriction mimetics: A strategy for improving healthy aging and longevity. *Current Pharmaceutical Design*, *20*(18), 2950–2977. doi:10.2174/13816128113196660699 PMID:24079773

Tome-Carneiro, J., Larrosa, M., Gonzalez-Sarrias, A., Tomas-Barberan, F. A., Garcia-Conesa, M. T., & Espin, J. C. (2013). Resveratrol and clinical trials: The crossroad from in vitro studies to human evidence. *Current Pharmaceutical Design*, *19*(34), 6064–6093. doi:10.2174/13816128113199990407 PMID:23448440

Tong, M., & Sadoshima, J. (2016). Mitochondrial autophagy in cardiomyopathy. *Current Opinion in Genetics & Development*, *38*, 8–15. doi:10.1016/j.gde.2016.02.006 PMID:27003723

Villalba, J. M., & Alcain, F. J. (2012). Sirtuin activators and inhibitors. *BioFactors (Oxford, England)*, *38*(5), 349–359. doi:10.1002/biof.1032 PMID:22730114

Wang, B., Yang, Q., Sun, Y. Y., Xing, Y. F., Wang, Y. B., Lu, X. T., & Zhao, Y. X. et al. (2014). Resveratrol-enhanced autophagic flux ameliorates myocardial oxidative stress injury in diabetic mice. *Journal of Cellular and Molecular Medicine*, *18*(8), 1599–1611. doi:10.1111/jcmm.12312 PMID:24889822

Wang, Y. (2014). Molecular Links between Caloric Restriction and Sir2/SIRT1 Activation. *Diabetes Metab J*, *38*(5), 321–329. doi:10.4093/dmj.2014.38.5.321 PMID:25349818

Wang, Z., Zou, J., Cao, K., Hsieh, T. C., Huang, Y., & Wu, J. M. (2005). Dealcoholized red wine containing known amounts of resveratrol suppresses atherosclerosis in hypercholesterolemic rabbits without affecting plasma lipid levels. *International Journal of Molecular Medicine*, *16*(4), 533–540. PMID:16142383

Wang, Z. Y., Qin, W., & Yi, F. (2015). Targeting histone deacetylases: Perspectives for epigenetic-based therapy in cardio-cerebrovascular disease. *J Geriatr Cardiol*, *12*(2), 153–164. doi:10.11909/j.issn.1671-5411.2015.02.010 PMID:25870619

Warboys, C. M., de Luca, A., Amini, N., Luong, L., Duckles, H., Hsiao, S., & Evans, P. C. et al. (2014). Disturbed flow promotes endothelial senescence via a p53-dependent pathway. *Arteriosclerosis, Thrombosis, and Vascular Biology*, *34*(5), 985–995. doi:10.1161/ATVBAHA.114.303415 PMID:24651677

Webster, K. A. (2012). A sirtuin link between metabolism and heart disease. *Nature Medicine*, *18*(11), 1617–1619. doi:10.1038/nm.2983 PMID:23135512

Wei, Y. Z. H., Lin, R., Fu, Y., & Wang, W. (2014). Short-term calorie restriction activates SIRT1-4 and -7 in cardiomyocytes in vivo and in vitro. *Molecular Medicine Reports*, *9*(4), 1218–1224. doi:10.3892/mmr.2014.1944 PMID:24535021

Wenger, N. K. (2014). Prevention of cardiovascular disease: Highlights for the clinician of the 2013 American College of Cardiology/American Heart Association guidelines. *Clinical Cardiology*, *37*(4), 239–251. doi:10.1002/clc.22264 PMID:24633723

WHO. (2015, January). *Cardiovascular diseases (CVDs)*. Retrieved from http://www.who.int/mediacentre/factsheets/fs317/en/

Winnik, S., Auwerx, J., Sinclair, D. A., & Matter, C. M. (2015). Protective effects of sirtuins in cardiovascular diseases: From bench to bedside. *European Heart Journal*, *36*(48), 3404–3412. doi:10.1093/eurheartj/ehv290 PMID:26112889

Witteles, R. M., & Fowler, M. B. (2008). Insulin-resistant cardiomyopathy clinical evidence, mechanisms, and treatment options. *Journal of the American College of Cardiology*, *51*(2), 93–102. doi:10.1016/j.jacc.2007.10.021 PMID:18191731

Wojtovich, A. P., Nadtochiy, S. M., Brookes, P. S., & Nehrke, K. (2012). Ischemic preconditioning: The role of mitochondria and aging. *Experimental Gerontology*, *47*(1), 1–7. doi:10.1016/j.exger.2011.11.001 PMID:22100642

Yuan, Z., & Seto, E. (2007). A functional link between SIRT1 deacetylase and NBS1 in DNA damage response. *Cell Cycle (Georgetown, Tex.)*, *6*(23), 2869–2871. doi:10.4161/cc.6.23.5026 PMID:18156798

Zern, T. L., West, K. L., & Fernandez, M. L. (2003). Grape polyphenols decrease plasma triglycerides and cholesterol accumulation in the aorta of ovariectomized guinea pigs. *The Journal of Nutrition*, *133*(7), 2268–2272. PMID:12840191

Zhang, C., Lin, G., Wan, W., Li, X., Zeng, B., Yang, B., & Huang, C. (2012). Resveratrol, a polyphenol phytoalexin, protects cardiomyocytes against anoxia/reoxygenation injury via the TLR4/NF-kappaB signaling pathway. *International Journal of Molecular Medicine*, *29*(4), 557–563. doi:10.3892/ijmm.2012.885 PMID:22246136

Zhang, Q. J., Wang, Z., Chen, H. Z., Zhou, S., Zheng, W., Liu, G., & Liang, C. C. et al. (2008). Endothelium-specific overexpression of class III deacetylase SIRT1 decreases atherosclerosis in apolipoprotein E-deficient mice. *Cardiovascular Research*, *80*(2), 191–199. doi:10.1093/cvr/cvn224 PMID:18689793

Zhang, Y., Mi, S. L., Hu, N., Doser, T. A., Sun, A., Ge, J., & Ren, J. (2014). Mitochondrial aldehyde dehydrogenase 2 accentuates aging-induced cardiac remodeling and contractile dysfunction: Role of AMPK, Sirt1, and mitochondrial function. *Free Radical Biology & Medicine*, *71*, 208–220. doi:10.1016/j.freeradbiomed.2014.03.018 PMID:24675227

Zordoky, B. N., Robertson, I. M., & Dyck, J. R. (2015). Preclinical and clinical evidence for the role of resveratrol in the treatment of cardiovascular diseases. *Biochimica et Biophysica Acta*, *1852*(6), 1155–1177. doi:10.1016/j.bbadis.2014.10.016 PMID:25451966

KEY TERMS AND DEFINITIONS

Cardiovascular Disease: A group of disorders affecting the heart and vasculature.

Epigenetics: The study of heritable changes to the gene expression without a change to the DNA sequence.

Histone Deacetylase (HDAC): Class of epigenetic modifiers that deacetylate histone and non-histone proteins.

Polyphenol: Metabolite of naturally occurring compounds found in the diet containing multiple phenol groups.

Sirtuin: Family of NAD+ dependent HDAC.

APPENDIX

Abbreviations

Akt Protein kinase B
ALDH2 aldehyde dehydrogenase 2
AMPK AMP-activated protein kinase α
CR calorie restriction
CVD cardiovascular disease
CXCR7 C-X-C Chemokine Receptor Type 7
EC endothelial cell
eNOS endothelial nitric oxide synthase
FOXO forkhead box O
HATs histone acetyltransferases
HDACs histone deacetylases
HF heart failure
HSP70 heat shock protein 70
hTERT telomerase reverse transcriptase
IR Ischemia-reperfusion
LXR liver X receptor
MD muscular dystrophy
MnSOD manganese superoxide dismutase
MSC mesenchymal stem cell
NAD+ nicotinamide adenine dinucleotide
NAMPT nicotinamide phosphoribosyltransferase
NF-κB nuclear factor kappa-light-chain-enhancer of activated B cells
Nrf2 nuclear factor-E2-related factor-2
NBS1 nibrin
PGC-1α Peroxisome proliferator-activated receptor gamma coactivator 1-alpha
PI3K Phosphoinositide 3-kinase
PPARs peroxisome proliferator-activated receptors
PVAT perivascular adipose tissue
ROCK Rho kinase
ROS reactive oxygen species
RXRα Retinoid X receptor alpha
TIMP3 matrix metalloproteinase 3
TLR4 Toll-like receptor 4
UCP-2 uncoupling protein 2
VEGFA vascular endothelial growth factor A
VSMCs vascular smooth muscle

Section 5

Recent Ideas in Social and Applied Cardiovascular Sciences

Chapter 17
The Effects of Social and Demographic Factors on Cardiovascular Disease

Hosik Min
University of South Alabama, USA

ABSTRACT

The chapter investigates the effects of social and demographic factors on cardiovascular disease (CVD) controlling health related factors. The data used in this study is the National Health and Nutrition Examination Survey data, and are merged the three waves, 2009-2010, 2011-2012, and 2013-2014. The logit regression analysis is used as a statistical model, and the results of this study confirm the significant associations with CVD in age, race/ethnicity, marital status, and educational attainment as expected ways. Health behaviors also show significant and strong relationships with CVD, which support the current prevention and intervention programs' strategy that focuses on changing lifestyles on an individual and a community level. The results of the social and demographic factors on CVD confirm that having CVD is not only a medical or biological process but also a social outcome. Thus, a better understanding of the social and demographic factors on CVD helps us to not only reduce the mortality rate, but also develop more effective policies and programs.

INTRODUCTION

This chapter is to examine the impact of social and demographic factors on CVD. The CVD is the leading cause of death in the U.S. for both men and women (Go et al., 2014; Mensah & Brown, 2007; Mozaffarian et al., 2015). It has been ranked the number one cause of death over the last several years as in Table 1 (Center Disease Control, 2016a, 2016b; Hoyert, 2012; Xu, Murphy, Kochanek, & Bastian, 2016), although the morality rates for CVD and other leading causes of death have been declined (see Figure 1) (Center Disease Control, 2016a, 2016b; Ma, Ward, Siegel, & Jemal, 2015). In 2010, one out of every three deaths is caused by CVD, which adds up to about 610,000 people. The direct and indirect cost of CVD totaled about $320.1 billion as of 2008, and is expected to triple by 2030 (Go et al., 2014; Mozaffarian et al., 2015), making CVD an extremely important public health issue (Mensah, 2005).

DOI: 10.4018/978-1-5225-2092-4.ch017

Table 1. The top 5 leading causes of deaths: 1980-2013

Ranking	1980	1990	2000	2010	2013
1	Heart Disease	Heart Disease	Heart Disease	Heart Disease	Heart Disease
2	Cancer	Cancer	Cancer	Cancer	Cancer
3	Stroke	Stroke	Stroke	CLRD	CLRD
4	Accidents	Accidents	CLRD	Stroke	Accidents
5	COPD	COPD	Accidents	Accidents	Stroke

Note: COPD - Chronic Obstructive Pulmonary Disease

CLRD - Chronic Lower Respiratory Disease

Figure 1. Mortality rates of the top 3 leading causes of death: 1980-2013

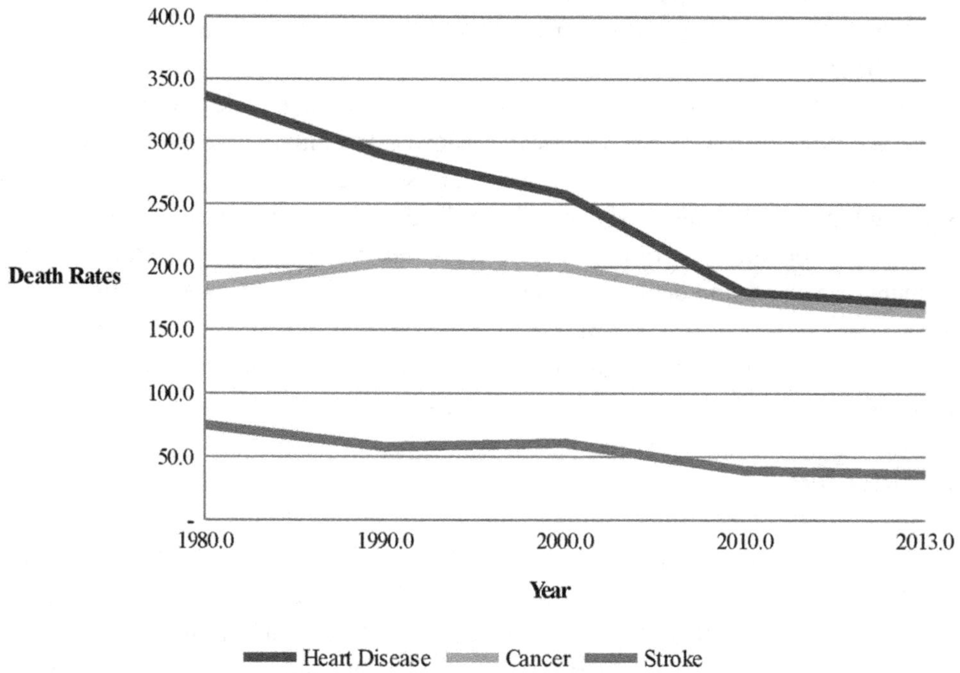

Factors Associated with CVD

Prior studies have identified health-related risk factors that make a person more likely to have CVD, including high blood pressure, high Low-density lipoprotein (LDL) cholesterol, diabetes, smoking, low physical activity, and obesity (Corella & Ordov'as, 2014; Dankel, Loenneke, & Loprinzi, 2015; Garcia-Fontana et al., 2016; Go et al., 2014; Li & Siegrist, 2012; Mozaffarian et al., 2015; Naimi et al., 2005; Ski, King-Shier, & Thompson, 2014). When someone has one or more of these conditions except physical activity, he/she is more likely to have CVD. When a person doing the physical activity regularly, the chance of having CVD is substantially low (Li & Siegrist, 2012; Stampfer, Hu, Manson, Rimm, & Willett, 2000).

The prevalence and the mortality rate of CVD, however, vary by social and demographic variables such as age, gender, race/ethnicity, and socioeconomic status (SES), which are called health disparities in CVD (Haynes, Feinleib, Levine, Scotch, & Kennel, 1980; Marshall et al., 2015; Mensah, 2005; Mensah & Brown, 2007; Mosca, Barrett-Connor, & Wenger, 2011; Rutledge et al., 2003; Ski et al., 2014). These social structures influence the health of individuals and can contribute to the identified risk factors and therefore their chance of having CVD (House, 2002; Lang, Lepage, Schieber, Lamy, & Kelley-Irving, 2012; Link, 2008; Link & Phelan, 1995; McKinlay, 1996; Phelan, Link, & Tehranifar, 2010; Williams & Jackson, 2005; Yang et al., 2015).

Many studies have found significant relationships between social and demographic factors and CVD (Cooper et al., 2000; Kanjilal et al., 2006; Mensah, 2005; Mozaffarian et al., 2015; Naimi et al., 2005; Winkleby, Jatulis, Frank, & Fortmann, 1992). Common variables for social and demographic factors are age, gender, marital status, educational attainment, and household income. The chance of having CVD increases with age (Diaz-Toro, Verdejo, & Castro, 2015). Women show a lower CVD prevalence rate than men because they tend to engage in healthier behaviors. As Mozaffarian and his colleagues (2015) reported, however, women aged 85 and over compared to men aged 85 and over had higher numbers of diagnosed as heart attacks and coronary heart disease. African Americans tend to show a higher incidence of CVD than white, while Asians and Hispanics have shown a lower prevalence of CVD. Native Americans and Native Hawaiians, meanwhile, showed the highest prevalence of all heart disease measurements with the exception of coronary heart disease (Mensah & Brown, 2007). Married couples are the most advantaged as they tend to have a higher level of social integration and a greater reinforcement of healthy behaviors and economic resources (Trovato & Lauri, 1989). Changes in marital status often lead to increased stress and depression and unhealthy outcomes (Zick & Smith, 1991). Education and income have been reported to be the important and consistent factors with a positive influence on a person's health: the higher the educational attainment and the higher the income, the lower the chance of CVD (Rutledge et al., 2003; Williams & Jackson, 2005).

Research Objective

An understanding of these social determinants of CVD is crucial in developing health policies and programs to reduce CVD. Thus, the goal of chapter is to make people more aware of the social and demographic factors. To do so, this chapter will use the National Health and Nutrition Examination Survey (NHANES) data, which collects information on CVD, the major risk factors, and social and demographic variables.

Methods

Data

The NHANES is a survey to assess the health and nutritional status of adults and children in the U. S. and examines a nationally representative sample of about 5,000 people each year. The NHANES includes demographic, socioeconomic, dietary, and health-related questions. The examination component consists of medical, dental, and physiological measurements, as well as laboratory tests administered by highly trained medical personnel. Findings from this survey will be used to determine the prevalence of major diseases and risk factors their diseases. The results will be used to assess nutritional status and its association with health promotion and disease prevention. Data from this survey will be used in epidemiological studies and health sciences research, which help develop sound public health policy, direct and design health programs and services, and expand the health knowledge across the nation (Center for Disease Control, 2015a).

Methods

This study hypothesizes that whether the social and demographic factors along with other health-related risk factors have significant associations with CVD. As the dependent variable, CVD, has a binary outcome (yes/no), this study employs a logistic regression model (Hamilton, 2013; Long & Freeze, 2005) and uses the STATA 14.1 version as statistical software. Initially two variables are considered to use CVD for the analysis. One is if a person has ever had a severe chest pain for more than half an hour, and the other is that if a person has ever had shortness of breath either when hurrying on the level ground or walking up a slight hill (Center Disease Control, 2015b). Only the latter is used for this analysis because there are not enough samples of the former to run an analysis. As these CVD variables are collected for adults aged 40 years old and over (Center Disease Control, 2015b), the sample size is significantly decreased. To obtain a high enough sample size to run the analysis, this chapter merges three NHANES datasets together: 2007-2008, 2009-2010, and 2011-2012.

The independent variables used to predict CVD as follows: Age is measured in years from ages 40 to 80. Gender is measured by whether the respondent is female (yes=1, no=0). Race is measured with four dummy variables, with white used as a reference group (yes=1, no=0), African American, Hispanics, and other. Asians and other categories are not large enough to have consistent race and ethnicity measurements in all datasets. Marital status is as follows: Married including unmarried partners (yes=1, no=0), never married, and non-married. Educational attainment is measured in four categories: less than high school, high school, some college, and college and beyond. The following health-related conditions are measured as dummy variables (yes=1, no=0): hypertension, high cholesterol, and diabetes are defined by whether a respondent has the condition or not. Physical activity is defined whether a respondent have done any kind of vigorous or moderate physical activity at work or for recreation for at least 10 minutes per day. Although this is not an ideal definition and the CDC recommends at least 60 minutes per day (U.S. Department of Health and Human Services, 2008), the definition here is used in order to have enough sample to run the analysis. Obesity is defined by whether a respondent has a BMI of 30 or greater (Center Disease Control, 2015c). Smoking is defined by whether the respondent is a current smoker. Drinking is measured by the average number of drinks per day in the past 12 months.

Results

Figure 2 demonstrates the percentage of the outcome, about one thirds of respondents who are 40 years old and older report that they have had shortness of breath either when they are hurrying on the level ground or walking up a slight hill.

Table 2 presents the descriptive statistics of CVD. The average age is 57 years old, but the average years of age in fact would be higher than this, because all adults aged 80 and over are coded as 80 years

Figure 2. The percentage of CVD: Shortness of breath

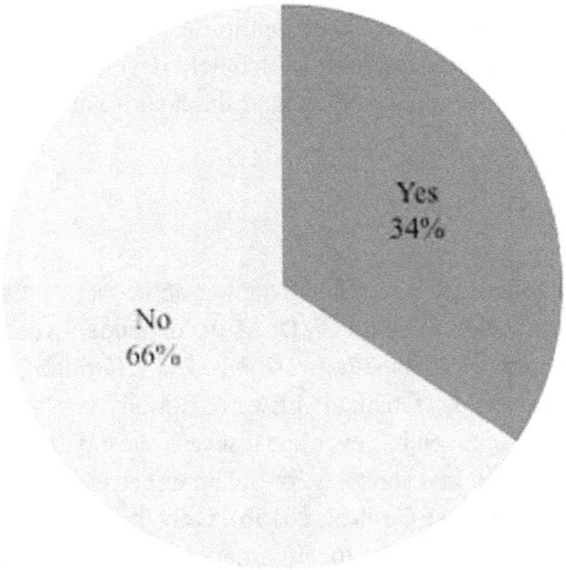

old. Forty-four percent of the respondents are female, and 81% of adults are white, 9% are black, 7% Hispanic, 4% Asian, and 6% Other. More than two third of the respondents are married including unmarried couples, 7% have never been married, and 26% have a different marital status including divorced, widowed, and separated. Educational attainment in Table 2 presents the percentages of each category for easier understanding, although this variable is used as a continuous variable in the analysis. A total of 17% of the respondents have less than high school level of education; 23% have a high school level of education; one third have some college level of education; and one fourth have been to college and beyond. About 70% of the respondents do vigorous or moderate activities at work or for recreation. More than one third of the respondents are obese, 46% of them have hypertension, and almost half of them have high cholesterol. Respondents drink 2.6 alcoholic beverages per day on average in the past 12 months, and 35% of them are current smokers.

Table 3 presents the results of the logistic regression models for CVD. The most coefficients show the expected relationships with the dependent variable. For easier understanding of logit coefficients, this paper converted the coefficients to the odds ratios (Long & Freeze, 2005; Poston & Min, 2008). Additional age increased the risk of CVD by 1% among the adults aged 40 and over in the first column in Table 3. Hispanics compared to whites are 35% less likely to have CVD. Those who were never married compared to those who are married are 53% more likely to have CVD, and those in the "other" category are 64% more likely to have CVD. Additional education decreases the likelihood of having CVD by 11%. A person who is doing any kind of vigorous or moderate physical activities at work and for recreation is 25% less likely to have CVD. Other health conditions show positive associations with CVD: those with obesity are 79% more likely to have CVD, those with hypertension are 69% more likely, those with high cholesterol are 23% more likely, those with diabetes are 71% more likely, and smokers are 81% more likely. Drinking is not significant.

Table 2. Descriptive statistics (Weighted = 110,033,053)

Variable	%	Std. Error	(95% CI)	
Age*	57.34	0.31	56.71	57.97
Female	44.05	1.44	41.16	46.94
Race/Ethnicity				
White	80.70	1.74	77.20	84.20
African American	8.53	1.13	6.26	10.81
Hispanics	6.97	0.85	5.25	8.69
Other	3.80	0.47	2.85	4.74
Marital Status				
Married	67.36	1.65	64.05	70.67
Never married	6.97	1.00	4.96	8.99
Other marital status	25.67	1.09	23.47	27.87
Educational Attainment				
Less than high school	16.81	1.27	14.27	19.36
High school	23.44	1.55	20.33	26.55
Some college	33.35	1.90	29.52	37.17
College and beyond	26.40	2.01	22.37	30.44
Health Behaviors				
Any Exercise	69.88	1.52	66.83	72.94
Alcohol consumption	2.61	0.08	2.45	2.78
Currently smoking	35.24	1.49	32.24	38.24
Health Conditions				
Obesity	35.59	1.01	33.56	37.62
Hypertension	45.79	1.15	43.48	48.10
High cholesterol	49.41	1.22	46.97	51.85
Diabetes	10.75	0.72	9.30	12.19

Note: * average

CONCLUSION AND DISCUSSION

This chapter aims to shed light on the effect of social and demographic factors on CVD. The results support the hypotheses. The overall model is significant and social and demographic factors indeed have substantial influences on CVD. There are several implications from this research. First, it is worthwhile to study CVD with social and demographic factors. This is justified not only because CVD is an important public health issue, but also because a majority of adults with CVD worsen their health conditions, and can even be fatal (Center Disease Control, 2015d). Second, since having a disease or illness is not only a medical or biological process but also a social outcome, a better understanding of the social and demographic factors on CVD helps us to reduce the mortality rate and develop more effective policies

Table 3. The results of the logit model (Weighted = 110,033,053)

Variable	Odds Ratio	Coefficient		(95% CI)	
Age 40+	1.01	0.01	***	1.00	1.02
Female	1.10	0.10		0.87	1.40
Race/Ethnicity					
African American	0.86	-0.15		0.67	1.10
Hispanics	0.65	-0.44	**	0.48	0.87
Other	0.73	-0.32		0.42	1.27
Marital Status					
Never married	1.53	0.43	***	1.01	2.32
Other marital status	1.64	0.49	**	1.20	2.23
Educational Attainment	0.89	-0.12	***	0.80	0.98
Health Behaviors					
Any Exercise	0.75	-0.29	***	0.59	0.95
Alcohol consumption	1.03	0.03		0.98	1.08
Currently smoking	1.81	0.59	*	1.41	2.33
Health Conditions					
Obesity	1.79	0.58	*	1.37	2.34
Hypertension	1.69	0.53	*	1.31	2.20
High cholesterol	1.23	0.21	***	1.01	1.49
Diabetes	1.71	0.54	*	1.33	2.20
Constant	0.16	-1.83	**	0.06	0.45

Note: * <.001; ** <.01; *** <.05

and programs (Cooper et al., 2000; Diez Roux, Link, & Northridge, 2000; Marshall et al., 2015; Pearcy & Keppel, 2002). This will contribute to achieve the one of the Healthy 2020 goals, eliminating the health disparities (Office of Disease Prevention and Health Promotion, 2015). Third, related to the second, the results have found the substantial benefits of being married; married people live healthier lives than non-married ones and have a reduced likelihood of having other major risk factors as well as CVD. In other words, policies and programs need to pay closer attention to unmarried people. Educational attainment also reduces the chance to have CVD significantly as expected. Fourth, the results present the significant relationships between CVD and the health-related risk factors such as obesity, hypertension, high cholesterol, diabetes, smoking, and physical activity. This supports the current prevention and intervention programs' strategy that focuses on changing lifestyles on an individual and a community level (Cooper et al., 2000; Diaz-Toro et al., 2015; Mensah, 2005; Stampfer et al., 2000).

Limitations

This study, however, has limitations. First of all, the results of race/ethnicity are somewhat unexpected; the African American and Other variables are not significant at all, while the Hispanic variable was significant. Two things can be discussed as plausible explanations. The African American mortality rate of CVD is higher than that of whites, but the prevalence rates for African Americans for stroke and other heart diseases are lower than those of whites (Mensah & Brown, 2007). African Americans, however, have higher prevalence rates for hypertension, obesity, and other health conditions (Mensah, 2005). In addition, minority groups including African Americans have reported that they tend to have a lower diagnosis rate of CVD than that of whites due to the barriers to diagnose (McKinlay, 1996). Further analysis on this is needed to understand why the African American variable was insignificant. Second, more detailed categories of the race/ethnicity to obtain more precise results are also necessary. This chapter does not have detailed categories such as Asian, Native American, and Native Hawaiian, because those categories are not available on all three datasets. It would be worth running the analysis with detailed racial and ethnic groups when that information is obtainable. Third, gender was not significant, because women also may tend to be under-diagnosed as described above (McKinlay, 1996). Women have a lower prevalence rate of CVD than their male counterparts, but the have a higher mortality rate due to delayed or late detection (Cooper et al., 2000; Fang, Perraillon, Ghosh, Cutler, & Rosen, 2014). Women aged 70 and over show higher prevalence rate of stroke than male counterparts (He, Campbell, & McGregor, 2012). African American women in particular have higher prevalence rate than their male counterparts. Fourth, the measurements of physical activity and drinking need to be changed in future studies. Physical activity in this survey includes vigorous or moderate physical activities for at least 10 minutes to obtain enough samples to analyze. The Center Disease Control recommends testing for positive effect at least 60 minutes of exercise per day. When that variable is available for several datasets, it would be appropriate to run that analysis.

REFERENCES

Center for Disease Control. (2015a). *National Health and Nutrition Examination Survey*. Retrieved from http://www.cdc.gov/nchs/nhanes/about_nhanes.htm

Center for Disease Control. (2015b). *Cardiovascular disease*. Retrieved from http://wwwn.cdc.gov/Nchs/Nhanes/2013-2014/CDQ_H.htm, accessed December 22, 2015

Center for Disease Control. (2015c). *About Adult Obesity*. Retrieved from http://www.cdc.gov/healthyweight/assessing/bmi/adult_bmi/index.html#Definition

Center for Disease Control. (2015d). *Heart Disease Facts*. Retrieved from http://www.cdc.gov/heartdisease/facts.htm

Center for Disease Control. (2016b). *Top 10 Leading Causes of Death: United States, 1999–2013*. Retrieved from http://blogs.cdc.gov/nchs-data-visualization/leading-causes-of-death/

Center for Disease Control. (2016a). *Leading Causes of Death: 1900-1998*. Retrieved from http://www.cdc.gov/nchs/data/dvs/lead1900_98.pdf

Cooper, R., Cutler, J., Desvigne-Nickens, P., Fortmann, S., Friedmann, L., Havlik, R., & Thom, T. et al. (2000). Trends and disparities in coronary heart disease, stroke, and other cardiovascular diseases in the United States findings of the national conference on cardiovascular disease. *Circulation*, *25*(25), 3137–3147. doi:10.1161/01.CIR.102.25.3137 PMID:11120707

Corella, D., & Ordovas, J. M. (2014). Ageing and cardiovascular diseases: The role of gene-diet interactions. *Ageing Research Reviews*, *18*, 53–73. doi:10.1016/j.arr.2014.08.002 PMID:25159268

Dankel, S. J., Loenneke, J. P., & Loprinzi, P. D. (2015). Letter to the editor. The Impact of overweight/obesity duration on the association between physical activity and cardiovascular disease risk: An application of the fat but fit program. *International Journal of Cardiology*, *201*, 88–89. doi:10.1016/j.ijcard.2015.07.070 PMID:26292271

Diaz-Toro, F., Verdejo, H. E., & Castro, P. F. (2015). Socioeconomic Inequalities in Heart Failure. *Heart Failure Clinics*, *11*(4), 507–513. doi:10.1016/j.hfc.2015.07.012 PMID:26462090

Diez Roux, A. V., Link, B. G., & Northridge, M. E. (2000). A multilevel analysis of income inequality and cardiovascular disease risk factors. *Social Science & Medicine*, *50*(5), 673–687. doi:10.1016/S0277-9536(99)00320-2 PMID:10658848

Fang, M. C., Perraillon, M. C., Ghosh, K., Cutler, D. M., & Rosen, A. B. (2014). Trends in Stroke Rates, Risk, and Outcomes in the United States, 1988 to 2008. *The American Journal of Medicine*, *127*(7), 608–615. doi:10.1016/j.amjmed.2014.03.017 PMID:24680794

Garcia-Fontana, B., Morales-Santana, S., Navarro, C. D., Rozas-Moreno, P., Genilloud, O., Perez, F. V., & Munoz-Torres, M. et al. (2016). Metabolomic profile related to cardiovascular disease in patients with type 2 diabetes mellitus: A pilot study. *Talanta*, *148*, 135–143. doi:10.1016/j.talanta.2015.10.070 PMID:26653434

Go, A. S., Mozaffarian, D., Roger, V. L., Benjamin, E. J., Berry, J. D., Blaha, M. J., & Tumer, M. B. et al. (2014). Heart Disease and Stroke Statistics2014 Update: A Report From the American Heart Association. *Circulation*, *129*(3), e28–e292. doi:10.1161/01.cir.0000441139.02102.80 PMID:24352519

Hamilton, L. C. (2013). *Statistics with STATA: Version 12*. Boston, MA: Cengage Learning

Haynes, S. G., Feinleib, M., Levine, S., Scotch, N., & Kannel, W. B. (1980). The relationship of psychosocial factors to coronary heart disease in the Framingham Study. III. Eight-year incidence of coronary heart disease. *American Journal of Epidemiology*, *107*(5), 384–402. PMID:665655

He, F. J., Campbell, N. R. C., & MacGregor, G. A. (2012). Reducing salt intake to prevent hypertension and cardiovascular disease. *Pan American Journal of Public Health*, *32*(4), 293–300. doi:10.1590/S1020-49892012001000008 PMID:23299291

House, J. S. (2002). Understanding Social Factors and Inequalities in Health: 20th Century Progress and 21st Century Prospects. *Journal of Health and Social Behavior*, *43*(2), 125–142. doi:10.2307/3090192 PMID:12096695

Hoyert, D. L. (2012). *75 years of mortality in the United States, 1935–2010. NCHS Data Brief, 88.* Hyattsville, MD: National Center for Health Statistics

Kanjilal, S., Gregg, E. W., Cheng, Y. J., Zhang, P., Nelson, D. E., Mensah, G., & Beckles, G. L. A. (2006). Socioeconomic Status and Trends in Disparities in 4 major Risk Factors for Cardiovascular Disease among US Adults, 19712002. *Archives of Internal Medicine*, *166*(21), 2348–2355. doi:10.1001/archinte.166.21.2348 PMID:17130388

Lang, T., Lepage, B., Schieber, A.-C., Lamy, S., & Kelley-Irving, M. (2012). Social Determinants of Cardiovascular Diseases. *Public Health Reviews*, *33*(2), 601–622

Li, J., & Siegrist, J. (2012). Physical Activity and Risk of Cardiovascular Disease: A Meta-Analysis of Prospective Cohort Studies. *International Journal of Environmental Research and Public Health*, *9*(12), 391–407. doi:10.3390/ijerph9020391 PMID:22470299

Link, B. G. (2008). Epidemiological Sociology and the Social Shaping of Population Health. *Journal of Health and Social Behavior*, *49*(4), 367–384. doi:10.1177/002214650804900401 PMID:19181044

Link, B. G., & Phelan, J. (1995). Social Conditions as Fundamental Causes of Disease. *Journal of Health and Social Behavior*, *35*, 80–94. doi:10.2307/2626958 PMID:7560851

Long, J. S., & Freeze, J. (2005). *Regression Models for Categorical Dependent Variables Using Stata* (2nd ed.). College Station, TX: Stata Press

Ma, J., Ward, E. M., Siegel, R. L., & Jemal, A. (2015). Temporal Trends in Mortality in the United States, 19692013. *Journal of the American Medical Association*, *314*(16), 1731–1739. doi:10.1001/jama.2015.12319 PMID:26505597

Marshall, I., Wang, Y., Crichton, S., McKevitt, C., Rudd, A. G., & Wolfe, C. D. (2015). The effects of socioeconomic status on stroke risk and outcomes. *Lancet Neurology*, *14*(12), 1206–1218. doi:10.1016/S1474-4422(15)00200-8 PMID:26581971

McKinlay, J. B. (1996). Some contributions from the social system to gender inequalities in heart disease. *Journal of Health and Social Behavior*, *37*(1), 1–26. doi:10.2307/2137228 PMID:8820308

Mensah, G. A. (2005). State of Disparities in Cardiovascular Health in the United States. *Circulation*, *111*(10), 1233–1241. doi:10.1161/01.CIR.0000158136.76824.04 PMID:15769763

Mensah, G. A., & Brown, D. W. (2007). An Overview of Cardiovascular Disease Burden in the United States. *Health Affairs*, *26*(1), 38–48. doi:10.1377/hlthaff.26.1.38 PMID:17211012

Mosca, L., Barrett-Connor, E., & Wenger, K. N. (2011). Sex/Gender Differences in Cardiovascular Disease Prevention: What a Difference a Decade Makes. *Circulation*, *124*(19), 2145–2154. doi:10.1161/CIRCULATIONAHA.110.968792 PMID:22064958

Mozaffarian, D., Benjamin, E. J., Go, A. S., Amett, D. K., Blaha, M. J., Cushman, M.,... Tumer, M. B. (2015). Heart Disease and Stroke Statistics--2015 Update: A Report From the American Heart Association. *Circulation*, *131*(4), e29-e322. Available at: http://circ.ahajournals.org/cgi/doi/10.1161/CIR.0000000000000152

Naimi, T. S., Brown, D. W., Brewer, R. D., Giles, W. H., Mensah, G., Serdula, M. K., & Stroup, D. F. et al. (2005). Cardiovascular risk factors and confounders among nondrinking and moderate-drinking U.S. adults. *American Journal of Preventive Medicine*, *28*(4), 369–373. doi:10.1016/j.amepre.2005.01.011 PMID:15831343

Office of Disease Prevention and Health Promotion. (2015). *Social Determinants of Health*. Retrieved from http://www.healthypeople.gov/2020/topics-objectives/topic/social-determinants-health

Percy, J. N., & Keppel, K. G. (2002). A Summary of Health Disparity. *Public Health Reports, 117*(3), 273–280. doi:10.1016/S0033-3549(04)50161-9 PMID:12432138

Phelan, J., Link, B. G., & Tehranifar, P. (2010). Social Conditions as Fundamental Causes of health Inequalities: Theory, Evidence, and Policy Implications. *Journal of Health and Social Behaviors, 51*(s), 28-40

Poston, D. Jr, & Min, H. (2008). Statistical Modeling for Causes of Death: Multinomial Logit Regression Model. *Journal of Modern Statistical Methods*, *7*(2), 597–606

Rutledge, T., Reis, S. E., Olson, M., Owens, J., Kelsey, S. E., Pepine, C. J., & Rogers, W. J. et al. (2003). Socioeconomic Status Variables Predict Cardiovascular Disease Risk Factors and Prospective Mortality Risk among Women with Chest Pain: The WISE Study. *Behavior Modification*, *27*(1), 54–67. doi:10.1177/0145445502238693 PMID:12587260

Ski, C. F., King-Shier, K. M., & Thompson, D. R. (2014). Gender, socioeconomic and ethnic/racial dispairties in cardiovascular disease: A time for change. *International Journal of Cardiology*, *170*(3), 255–257. doi:10.1016/j.ijcard.2013.10.082 PMID:24238906

Stampfer, M. J., Hu, F. B., Manson, J. E., Rimm, E. B., & Willett, W. C. (2000). Primary prevention of coronary heart disease in women through diet and lifestyle. *The New England Journal of Medicine*, *343*(24), 1814–1815. doi:10.1056/NEJM200012143432415 PMID:10882764

Trovato, F., & Lauris, G. (1989). Marital Status and Mortality in Canada: 1951- 1981. *Journal of Marriage and the Family*, *51*(4), 907–922. doi:10.2307/353204

U.S. Department of Health and Human Services. (2008). *2008 Physical Activity Guidelines for Americans*. Retrieved from www.health.gov/paguidelines

Williams, D. R., & Jackson, P. B. (2005). Social Sources of Racial Disparities in Health. *Health Affairs*, *24*(2), 325–334. doi:10.1377/hlthaff.24.2.325 PMID:15757915

Winkleby, M. A., Jatulis, D. E., Frank, E., & Fortmann, S. P. (1992). Socioeconomic status and health: How education, income, and occupation contribute to risk factors for cardiovascular disease. *American Journal of Public Health*, *82*(6), 816–820. doi:10.2105/AJPH.82.6.816 PMID:1585961

Xu, J. Q., Murphy, S. L., Kochanek, K. D., & Bastian, B. A. (2016). *Deaths: Final data for 2013. National Vital Statistics Reports, 64(2)*. Hyattsville, MD: National Center for Health Statistics

Yang, Q., Zhong, Y., Ritchey, M., Cobain, M., Gillespie, C., Merritt, R., & Bowman, B. A. (2015). *Vital Signs: Predicted Heart Age and Racial Disparities in Heart Age among U.S. Adults at the State Level. Morbidity and Mortality Weekly Report 64*. Hyattsville, MD: National Center for Health Statistics

Zick, C. D., & Smith, K. R. (1991). Marital Transitions, Poverty, and Gender Differences in Mortality. *Journal of Marriage and the Family*, *53*(2), 327–336. doi:10.2307/352902

KEY TERMS AND DEFINITIONS

Cardiovascular Disease (CVD): The term "heart disease" is often used interchangeably with the term "cardiovascular disease." Cardiovascular disease generally refers to conditions that involve narrowed or blocked blood vessels that can lead to a heart attack, chest pain (angina) or stroke. Other heart conditions, such as those that affect your heart's muscle, valves or rhythm, also are considered forms of heart disease.

Leading Causes of Death: Lading causes of death are defined as underlying cause of death categories or major ICD (International Cause of Death) groupings (such as Diseases of the Heart, Malignant Neoplasms, Accidents, etc.) that usually account for large numbers of deaths within a specified population group and time period.

Logistic Model: The logistic model is a regression model where the dependent variable is binary or dichotomous, i.e. it only contains data coded as 1 (TRUE, success, pregnant, etc.) or 0 (FALSE, failure, non-pregnant, etc.).

Odds Ratio: An odds ratio (OR) is a measure of association between an exposure and an outcome. The OR represents the odds that an outcome will occur given a particular exposure, compared to the odds of the outcome occurring in the absence of that exposure. If OR is 1, it means that the exposure does not affect odds of outcome; if OR is greater than 1, it means the exposure associated with higher odds of outcome; and if OR is lesser than 1, the exposure associated with lower odds of outcome.

Sociodemographic Factors: Sociodemographic factors are characterized by a combination of sociological (= related to sociology) and demographic (= relating to populations) characteristics such as age, sex, education level, income level, marital status, occupation, religion, birth rate, death rate, average size of a family, and average age at marriage.

Chapter 18
Forensic Assessment of Natural Unexpected Cardiovascular Death

Gulnaz T. Javan
Alabama State University, USA

Sheree J. Finley
Alabama State University, USA

Sait Ozsoy
Gulhane Military Medical Academy (GMMA), Turkey

ABSTRACT

In the United States, sudden unexpected deaths attributable to diseases of the cardiovascular system account for almost 50% of all natural deaths with up to 600,000 deaths per year. Over the past decade, substantial developments have been made to provide definitive determinations in the diagnosis of cardiac death for adjudication in the criminal justice system and closure for decedent's families. In order to make postmortem diagnostic determinations, coordinated multidisciplinary efforts include collaboration between clinical and forensic pathologists. Forensic protocols include examination of the heart, histological sampling, toxicology testing, and molecular analyses. Lack of alternative diagnoses generally prompts pathologists to report sudden cardiac arrest as the main cause of death in many cases even though the accuracy of this finding might be in question; therefore, a forensic pathologist should examine unexplained cases of death in more depth to avoid this possible misdiagnosis.

INTRODUCTION

Sudden cardiac death (SCD) is unexpected natural death that results within one hour of onset of known or unknown heart pathologies with or without prior complaints. According to data published by the Centers for Disease Control and Prevention (CDC), sudden cardiac death is a major health concern, constituting approximately 20% of total mortality in the United States, and affecting over 600,000 patients annually. Each year the incidence of SCD in the United States is approximately 250 to 400 thousand cases, a rate associated with advanced age and male gender (Lee et al., 2008).

DOI: 10.4018/978-1-5225-2092-4.ch018

Figure 1. Number of death SCD per sport participation of 820 students
Adopted from American Heart Association Inc, 2011 data
For a more accurate representation of this figure, please see the electronic version.

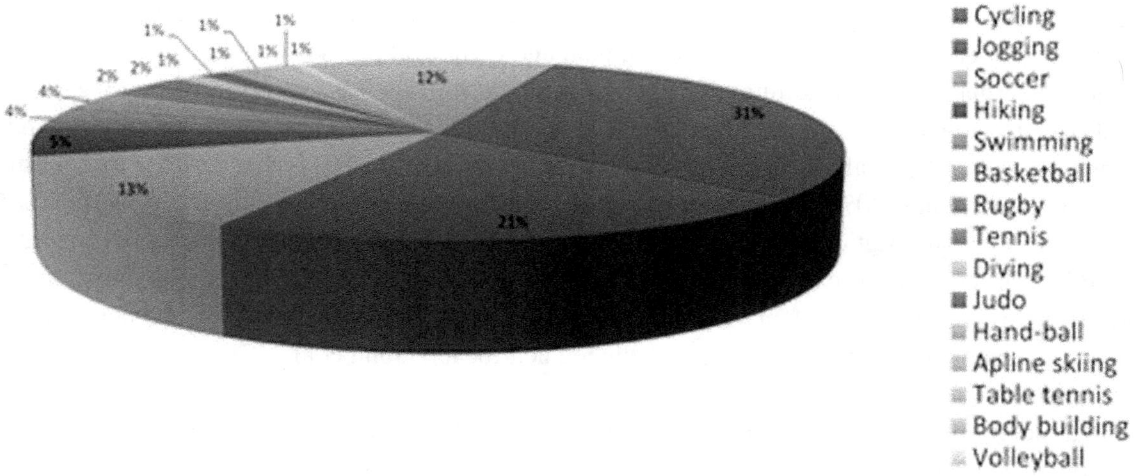

Most studies show that there is an inverse relationship between an increase in regular physical activity and sudden cardiac death. However, recent studies point to a moderate level of exercise as beneficial activity. Despite a conclusion by most studies that prove the beneficial effects of exercise on general health, there are evidences that show a direct relationship between sudden cardiac deaths and higher than normal frequency of vigorous exercise (Deo et al., 2012). Figure 1 depicts the relationship between various sports and the number of deaths associated with each one.

Pathologists are responsible for determining the cause of death in cases of sudden unexpected death. Autopsy is essential to reveal the cause of death in sudden death cases. Despite macroscopic, histological and toxicological examinations of sudden death cases, in 1-5% of these cases the cause of death cannot be explained. This phenomenon is referred to as "negative autopsy" (Koponen et al., 2003; Di Maio et al., 2001; Dowling et al., 2005).

It is important to obtain information related to the case before an autopsy in sudden death cases. This information includes some or all of the following: person's age, sex, profession, lifestyle (e.g., smoking, alcohol consumption), physical activity status, whether there was an eyewitness or not, time of death if known, place of death, medical history, and medications (Basso et al., 2008).

FORENSIC PATHOLOGY

Forensic pathology plays a crucial role in diagnosing natural cardiovascular death as the cause of death in forensic investigations. There are five terms used to clinically describe the cause of death: natural (as in sudden, unexpected cardiac deaths), accident, suicide, homicide, or undetermined (Yu et al., 2014). In the United States, postmortem examinations are performed according to practical guidelines established by the College of American Pathologists (Hutchins et al., 1999). Coroners, forensic pathologists, and criminal investigators synergistically process all available ante-, peri-, and postmortem evidence pertaining to the corpse and the death scene. The goal is to determine the precise organ system(s) involved and the manner of death, in order to derive an official diagnosis of the factors contributing to the fatality. A forensic investigation is often needed to determine if violence is the cause of death, if medical malpractice has occurred during surgery or hospital stay, and to determine if cardiac dysfunction was the cause of a traffic accident or fatality (Suarez-Mier and Aguilera, 2015). Frequently their official diagnoses are required as evidence in the adjudication of criminal and civil legal cases.

Sudden cardiac deaths constitute a substantial percentage of the casework for medico-legal professionals. A very high percentage (between 70- 90%) of all sudden unexpected deaths that require forensic autopsy are caused by fatal dysfunctions of the heart (Roberts et al., 2011; Suarez-Mier and Aguilera, 2015). In approximately 30% of sudden cardiac death cases, death occurs in structurally normal hearts, and death is the first manifestation of the disorder (Semsarian et al., 2015); therefore, an autopsy is necessary.

Sudden cardiac death is caused by unexpected cessation of cardiac activity with hemodynamic collapse, usually caused by persistent ventricular tachycardia (pulse rate greater than 100 beats per minute) or ventricular fibrillation (rapid, uncoordinated heartbeats) (John et al., 2012). Medical examiners make observations based on standard gross inspection of the pericardial cavity followed by a detailed examination of other anatomy of the heart (Basso et al., 2008). Specifically, the tests include histological sampling, toxicology testing, and molecular analyses and are performed at the request and consent of the next of kin (Molina et al., 2007) or to provide evidence to the appropriate legal authorities to be presented in a court of law (Fronczek et al., 2014). The performance of one test may actuate the need for one or more other ancillary examinations. For example, histological analysis of the heart may lead to toxicology investigations if the tissues display evidence of the presence of exogenous toxins during histological examinations (Dettmeyer, 2014).

Histological Sampling

Forensic histopathology is usually performed after an initial gross autopsy examination. Histological samples provide visual evidence that can be cross-compared with other autopsy data to confirm, clarify, or repudiate initial findings (Maeda et al., 2011). In the case of unexpected cardiac death, in which no obvious lesions are detected, histology sampling is highly recommended to substantiate the phenotype of natural cardiac death (Bailey, 2015). The postmortem investigation of the heart begins with the removal of the sternum in a cut that extends along the midline in the anterior thorax of the chest (Suarez-Mier and Aguilera, 2015). Subsequently, there is abstraction of representative cadaveric specimens from major internal organs for histopathological sampling (Dettmeyer, 2014).

Several very specific steps are performed during a standard pathological examination involving deaths relating to the cardiovascular system (Figure 2). Cardiac autopsy starts with the opening of the sternum to examine the postmortem anatomy of the heart. The heart is examined to rule out potential intrapericardial effusion of cardiac fluid and mediastinal hemorrhage caused by extrapericardial rupture (Suarez-Mier and Aguilera, 2015). The pericardial sac is then inspected to determine if gas embolism has occurred. The aorta is dissected to observe potential tears in the intima and to rule out cardiac tamponade (i.e., effusion of fluid or gas into the pericardial space) and aortic hemorrhage in the mediastina or retroperitoneum. For further inspection of the entire heart, it is completely removed by in incision that severs the inferior vena cava above the diaphragm. The heart is then washed and weighed, and a gross examination of the external anatomy (pericardium and epicardium), ventricles, valves, coronary arteries, atria, and aorta is performed (Suarez-Mier and Aguilera, 2015). Representative pieces of the anterior, lateral, and posterior right and left ventricles and the septum are also sampled (Bailey, 2015).

Furthermore, it is also suggested that these samples are obtained from both of the atria, the mid-ventricular transverse, and the right ventricular outflow tract. Additionally, any other areas of the heart that show substantial observable abnormalities are sampled (Basso et al., 2008).

Figure 2. Steps for the standard pathological examination in sudden cardiac death cases
Adapted from Basso et al., 2008

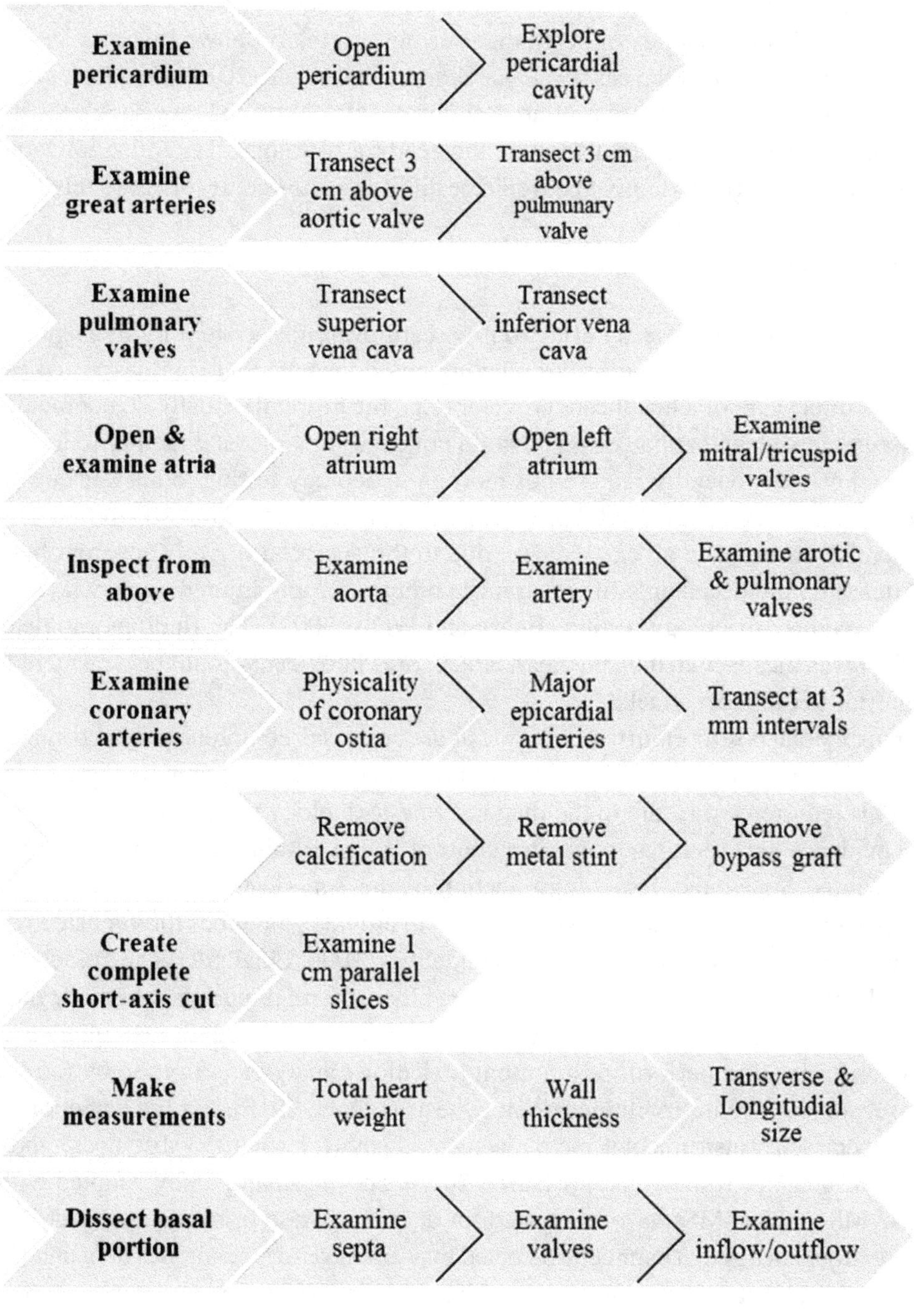

The cause of death is established by histology in only 8% of cases (De La Grandmaison et al., 2010; Fronczek et al., 2014). Therefore, there is a contingency among pathology professionals that challenges the notion that histological organ and tissue sampling is necessary as a routine practice in forensic investigations. The question was asked by Molina et al. (2007) whether or not routine histopathological examination was necessary in cases in which the cause of death is readily demonstrated during the gross autopsy. In a retrospective study of 500 cases of British adults with discrepancies in the cause and manner of death, histological examinations were performed in 287 of the cases (Fronczek et al., 2014). Of the 287 cases, only a small percentage (8%) was confirmed as the cause of death. Conversely, in support of histological sampling to determine the manner of death, a prospective study on 428 autopsy cases demonstrated that the manner of death that was not originally shown by gross anatomic findings was discovered in about 40% of the cases (De La Grandmaison et al., 2010). De-Giorgio and Vertrugno (2014) would disagree with the use of routine postmortem histology, and they suggest that permitting a forensic pathologist the discretion to determine the need for histological examination would introduce degrees of subjectivity and uncertainty that would be difficult for the courts of law to rely on the evidence.

Toxicology Testing

Exogenous, toxic substances have an effect on the cardiovascular system by damaging the integrity of blood capillaries and constricting and/or relaxing blood vessels. Sudden unexpected cardiac deaths while under the direct care of a healthcare provider (e.g., the hospital) usually do not require toxicology testing. However, in sudden cardiac deaths that do not occur in a medical facility (e.g., in the home or during a violent crime) generally require postmortem toxicology testing to answer questions whether or not toxic substances were involved. For example, if a medico-legal investigation determines that a decedent's demise occurred in an car accident due to the deceased driver's apparent heart attack, interested parties (i.e., the decedent's life insurance company or any injured party who seeks to collect damages) may require toxicology testing (Hearn and Walls, 2007). The findings can determine if the deceased driver was incapacitated by the heart attack, or if intoxicants could be considered the cause of the accident prior to the heart attack.

It is compulsory that postmortem toxicology tests are universal, comprehensive and unbiased. Further, a strong emphasis is placed on specificity and accuracy in the identification of all possible toxicants in specimens. This requirement is due to the mandate that toxicology results are reliable and accurate as unequivocal evidence for expert testimony in a court of law in criminal and civil cases (Wyman, 2012). Thus, in the United States, the Toxicology Section of the American Academy of Forensic Sciences (AAFS) and the Society of Forensic Toxicology (SOFT) provide guidelines for forensic toxicology laboratory protocols (http://www.soft-tox.org/files/Guidelines_2006_Final.pdf). The guidelines dictate that 50 g of brain, liver, and kidney tissue, 25 ml of heart blood, 15 ml of peripheral blood, and all available volumes of vitreous humor, bile, urine, and gastric contents are collected for toxicological examination.

The diagnostics used to perform postmortem toxicology analyses are generally the same methods used to test substances in ante-mortem toxicology tests (Linnet, 2013). For the detection of substances in cadaveric specimens, instrumental methods such as gas (for volatile substances) and liquid chromatography (GC and LC, respectively) (Maurer, 2013), and chromatography coupled with mass spectrometry (GC-MS and LC-MS) have been used for decades. These instruments detect the presence of common recreational drugs that cannot be detected by immunoassay techniques (Wu and French, 2013). Chromatography is a separation technique in which organic and inorganic compounds form complex, time-specific patterns of peaks and bands representing the assorted components in a mixture (e.g., cadaveric fluids and tissues). The patterns serve as chemical-specific, spectroscopic fingerprints for each compound (Bell, 2009). Forensic experts compare the patterns to calibrated standards to identify the presence of the substance (Smith et al., 2007). Modern chromatography instruments are often coupled with MS (Peters and Remane, 2012) and liquid chromatography-tandem mass spectrometry (LC–MS/MS) (Peters, 2011). As with chromatography, MS is a separation technique in which compounds are ionized and fragmented, and the charged fragments are separated into patterns that are characteristic to the specific substances. A recent study using ultra high pressure LC–MS/MS to detect and quantify 15 basic pharmaceuticals in postmortem whole blood samples demonstrated that the method was rapid, selective, and applicable for use in forensic toxicology cases (Amundsen et al., 2013).

Following death, blood ceases to circulate which allows it to settle in certain regions of the body. Therefore, certain drugs have a high propensity to be artificially increased in blood samples obtained from the heart due to a well-known phenomenon called postmortem redistribution (PMR) of toxins (Gunn, 2011). As a result, postmortem concentrations of drugs do not accurately represent the concentrations prior to and present at the time of death (Pounder and Jones, 1990; Pelissier-Alicot et al., 2003). To overcome the effects of PMR, the optimum site for sampling blood is a ligated or clamped femoral vein (Pounder and Jones, 1990). The redistribution generally involves drugs such as tricyclic antidepressants, digoxin, and amphetamines that move from solid organs (e.g., the lungs, liver, and myocardium) to the blood (Yarema et al., 2004). Digoxin is of particular interest in the diagnosis of unexpected cardiac death because it is routinely used to treat arrhythmias and heart failure (Trial et al., 1997).

Some of the drugs commonly screened in unexpected cardiac deaths are cocaine, which blocks the reuptake of norepinephrine causing intense vasoconstriction (Jorge et al. 2012) and right ventricular dysfunction which can lead to a myocardial infarction (Zhan et al., 2015). Dietary nitrates that induce the ventricular relaxation of smooth muscle (Bailey et al., 2014) are also screened. Although they represent only a small minority, several pharmaceuticals are documented as stimulators of drug-induced heart failure. Such drugs include cytostatics, immunomodulating drugs, anti-depressant drugs, calcium channel blocking agents, non-steroidal anti-inflammatory drugs, anti-arrhythmic drugs, β-adrenergic receptor blocking agents, and anesthetics (Feenstra, 1999).

Molecular Analyses

Ackerman et al. (2001) coined the term "molecular autopsy" to describe genetic studies of DNA extracted from cadaveric blood and tissue samples to establish the cause of death in autopsy-negative cases. Molecular autopsies allow the continued examination via cardiologic and/or genetic screening of relatives and postmortem genetic analysis of the deceased to elucidate the underlying causative mechanism(s) of the sudden cardiac death (Boczek et al., 2012). These studies are particularly useful in sudden cardiac deaths resulting from heart channelopathies of hearts that failed to demonstrate any structural abnormalities upon gross examination (Tester and Ackerman, 2012). The prevalence of structurally normal hearts in unexplained cardiac deaths that revealed autopsy-negative results is approximately 3% (Boczek et al., 2012). Deaths caused by long QT syndrome (LQTS), catecholaminergic polymorphic ventricular tachycardia (CPVT), and Brugada syndrome (BrS) produce no indication of heart channelopathies during autopsy.

During molecular autopsies, a blood sample is taken from the cadaver and DNA is extracted using commercially available DNA extraction kits. Sequencing of the extracted DNA is analyzed via traditional Sanger sequencing and high-throughput next-generation platforms to detect the disease-causing mutations (Boczek et al., 2012). The protein coding exons of the three major genes that cause LQTS, I_{Ks} K^+ channel α-subunit, I_{Kr} K^+ channel α-subunit, I_{Na} Na^+ channel α-subunit (*KCNQ1, KCNH2, SCN5A*, respectively), and the gene that causes CPVT, Ryanodine receptor gene (*RYR2*) are probed. The *SCN5A* gene is also probed to detect BrS. The detection rate for the aforementioned probes ranges from less than 1% to 15% (Boczek et al., 2012). Recent advances have emerged to expand the science beyond the four genes to include whole exomes and genomes that are also screened for pathogenic mutations. Cardiac gene panels containing 200 genes, along with the exomes, or all of the protein coding exons of approximately 22,000-30,000 human genes have been performed in molecular autopsies (Bagnall et al., 2014). A Loporcaro et al., (2014) whole exome next-generation sequencing study revealed a mutation R249Q-MYH7 that caused sudden death by hypertrophic cardiomyopathy for a previously healthy adolescent female.

CAUSES OF SUDDEN CARDIOVASCULAR DEATH

Sudden cardiovascular death occurs within an hour of the onset of symptoms and results in the loss of heart function without any apparent clinical heart condition (Zipes and Wellens, 1998). Clinical conditions that commonly cause unexpected cardiac death are inflammation of the membrane sac that surround the heart (pericarditis), the heart muscle (myocarditis), and the inner lining of the heart (endocarditis), or dysfunction in the myocardium (heart muscle). In the past decade, postmortem imaging has been increasingly utilized in forensic autopsy in the determination of the cause of natural deaths associated with cardiovascular illnesses.

Pericardial Disease

Pericarditis results from inflammation of the sac that surrounds the heart and the great vessels origins. The disease is a consequence of the accumulation of fluid in the pericardium, the flask- or pyramidal-shaped space surrounding the heart. The etiologic causes of pericarditis are most frequently due to nonspecific idiopathic origins or viral infection (Lange and Hillis, 2004). There are several pathological steps of pericarditis that lead to sudden cardiac death (Khandaker et al., 2010). The pericardial sac usually holds 20-50 ml of lubricating, serous fluid, pus, and fibrin; however, rapid accumulation of approximately 120 ml of extra fluid in the pericardium presses against the heart tissue and can cause dysfunction (Goyle and Walling, 2002). The added pressure prevents the heart from fully expanding also preventing blood from filling or leaving the heart leading to a decrease in blood oxygen saturation. The amount of oxygen that reaches the organs is greatly diminished. The clinical results that ensue include tachycardia, tachypnea, and decreased blood pressure. All of these steps lead to loss of consciousness, ultimately causing sudden cardiac death. A gross examination of the pericardium that reveals whitish patches, also known as Soldier's patches, is indicative of mechanical trauma to the heart (Suarez-Mier and Aguilera, 2015).

The incidence of postmortem diagnosis, or confirmation of the diagnosis, ranges from 1-6% of patients using conventional histological and autopsy methods (Lange and Hillis, 2004). Modern diagnostic imagining techniques are gaining popularity in forensic medicine particularly for the diagnostic determination of traumatic cardiac ruptures (Leth, 2015). Because of their minimally invasive nature, postmortem coronary computed tomography (PMCT) angiography combined with image-guided biopsy, has demonstrated the potential use in the diagnosis of the cause of death after acute chest pain (Ross et al., 2012; Roberts et al, 2011). This technique was able to reveal the complete opacification of the lumens of the major coronary along with the side branches into their distal parts in all cases (Ross et al., 2012). The best way to access the vascular system by postmortem CT is via unilateral intravenous cannulation of the femoral vessels. These vessels are selected due to their large diameters and quick access (approximately 10 minutes) (Ross et al, 2014). Other possible vessels are located in the neck (jugular vein, carotid artery) and the upper extremities (brachial vein and artery); however, the leg is preferred because it is less invasive and in an area not normally visualized at a funeral. Further, postmortem multislice computed tomography (MSCT) scanners have also been employed to confirm the cause of death in a traumatic cardiac rupture (Zhou et al., 2015). In the Zhou et al. (2015) study, a biopsy needle was used as guided by the MSCT scanner. Another forensic study established that MSCT scanners can be used in the postmortem diagnosis of an acute pericardial tamponade (most commonly as result of traumatic cardiac ruptures caused by falls, automobile collisions, sporting activities, and rare complication from cardiopulmonary resuscitation (CPR) (Huang et al., 2012). In the absence of an autopsy, Huang et al. (2012), using whole-body MSCT and complete health records, determined the cause of death as acute pericardial tamponade as a result of blunt trauma to the chest.

Myocardial Diseases

Myocardial diseases are dysfunctions of the heart caused by inflammation of the myocardium, the middle layer of muscle in heart wall (Thygesen et al., 2012). The myocardium is responsible for constricting and enlarging the heart muscles to pump blood to the rest of the body. Three of the major types of myocardial diseases that lead to natural cardiac deaths are coronary artery disease, myocarditis, and heart hypertrophy.

Coronary Artery Disease

As the leading cause of death in America, coronary artery (or heart) disease affects more than 13 million Americans (Thom et al., 2006). The long-standing description of the disease (also known as atherosclerosis) by the World Health Organization (WHO) is the variations in the intima of arteries entailing the accumulation of lipids, carbohydrates, blood products, fibrous tissue, and calcium deposits forming artery-narrowing plaque (WHO, 1958). The formation of plaque consists of the induction of inflammatory cells and is mediated by cellular adhesion molecules that are expressed in response to inflammatory activation (Blankenberg et al., 2003). The disease primarily damages the aorta and its main branches as well as the coronaries, cerebral arteries, and renal arteries. There has been a steady decrease in cardiovascular deaths during the late 20th and early 21st centuries that correlate with major advances in cardiovascular medicine (Nabel & Braunwald, 2012).

Kumar et al. (2012) provides a histopathothological study on how to determine the degree of atherosclerosis in cadavers. To start, the postmortem heart is fixed in 10% formalin solution for 2–5 days. Specific segments of the coronary arteries (e.g. left anterior descending coronary artery, left circumflex artery, and right coronary artery) are commonly sectioned into 3-mm samples. The specimens are stained with hematoxylin and eosin (H&E) and examined microscopically at 40x magnification. The percentage of luminal narrowing is determined (Kumar et al., 2012). At the conclusion of the autopsy, if there is an incidence of greater than 90% occlusion in one or more of the blood vessels, the finding is adequate to determine constriction or obstruction in the cardiovascular system as the cause of death (Bailey, 2015).

In recent years, postmortem computer topography and magnetic imaging have been used to detect coronary heart disease, and the applicability of radiology for diagnosis and/or confirmation of atherosclerosis-related deaths (Michaud et al., 2014). A recent study investigating postmortem use of multi-detector computed tomography (MDCT) and MDCT-angiography for unexpected cardiac deaths pertaining to atherosclerosis that caused ischemic heart disease was evaluated. The findings of the conventional autopsy of 23 cadavers were compared to the results of MDCT-angiography (Michaud et al., 2012). These radiological techniques visualized the calcification of the coronary arteries in approximately 80% of the cases, which were not reported in the initial autopsies. Thus, visualization of the coronary arteries via MDCT coupled with angiography was more enhanced than with MDCT alone and permitted the assessment of narrowing and occlusions of the arteries.

Myocarditis

Myocarditis is a rare, but life-threatening inflammatory dysfunction of the heart that is not subsequent to ischemia involving the myocardium, the middle muscular layer of the heart. The prevalence of myocarditis leading to sudden cardiac death among certain populations has been shown to be difficult to ascertain by postmortem investigations with reports of variability in diagnosis ranging from 2-42% (Caforio et al., 2013). It is most commonly caused by viral infection, but other heterogeneous etiologies exist. Some etiologies include microbial (bacterial and protozoal) infections, endogenous toxins, drug (prescription and illicit) reactions, post-viral immune responses, giant cell myocarditis, and cardiac sarcoidosis (Morentin et al., 2015; Blauwet and Cooper, 2010). While viral infection is the major cause of myocarditis in advanced countries, in developing countries, rheumatic carditis, and infections caused by the parasite *Trypanosoma cruzi*, and *Corynebacterium diphtheriae* are significant contributors to the disease (Sagar et al., 2012). Microbial and non-infectious (e.g. drugs, toxins, sarcoidosis, et al.) pathogens cause direct damage to myocytes (Caforio et al., 2013). Viral infections induce several effects that can cause significant damage to the heart. After viral invasion through specific receptors on the surface of myocytes, acute damage to the cells is caused by viral replication which induces myocyte necrosis, exposure of cardiac-specific antigens, and host autoimmune responses. The immune responses are primarily constituted by the initial invasion of natural killer cells and macrophages then T lymphocytes (Kindermann et al., 2012). The acute phase of myocarditis takes only a few days. The subacute and chronic phases cover a few weeks to several months. Upon the death of myocytes, chemokines and cytokines are released that subsequently activate the immune system, leading to inflammation. Contractile dysfunction is due to prolonged activation of tumor necrosis factor-alpha (TNF-α), interleukin (IL)-1 and -6, and antibodies that not only target viral but also cardiac proteins that lead to cardiac damage (Kindermann et al., 2012).

Myocardial infarction is defined as myocardial cell death due to prolonged ischemia. Histological examination is used to assess damage to the myocardial tissue using H&E staining (Figure 3 and 4). This assay is only feasible if the patient's demise had occurred within six hours after the start of the ischemic injury (Campobasso et al., 2008). H&E staining is necessary because in some cases a minimum of six hours must transpire antemortem before myocardial necrosis can be determined by the usual postmortem macroscopic or microscopic examinations and is contingent upon the reactivity of the sampled myocytes.

To identify location of myocardial infarction, determining the location of the coronary artery blockage, and its circulation anatomy are important. The most common place for blockage is the first 2-cm region of the descending front branch of the left coronary artery followed by the middle region of the right coronary artery.

Figure 3. Chronic myocardial infarction findings show hypertrophic fibers (arrowhead), multi foci fibrosis areas (star) and mononuclear inflammation cell (arrow)
With permission from Dr. Teke, H.Y.)

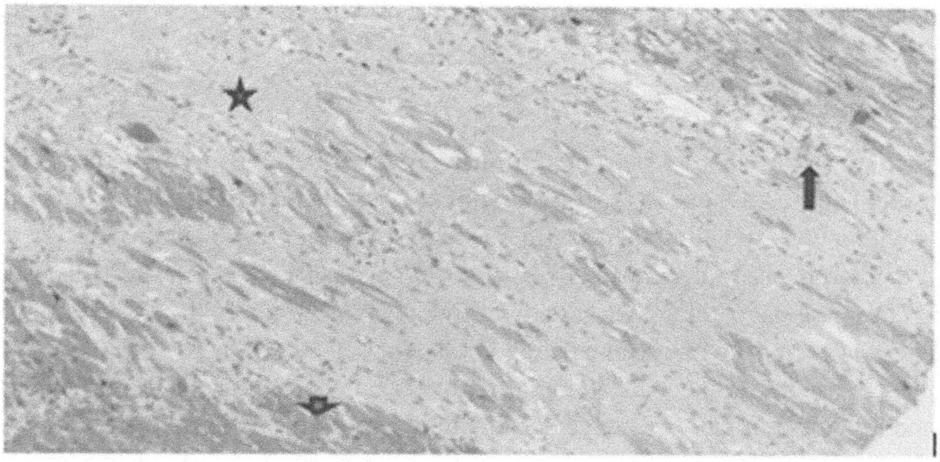

Figure 4. Rupture of the back wall of the left ventricular of neighboring area to myocardial infarction findings (arrow)
With permission from Dr. Teke H.Y.)

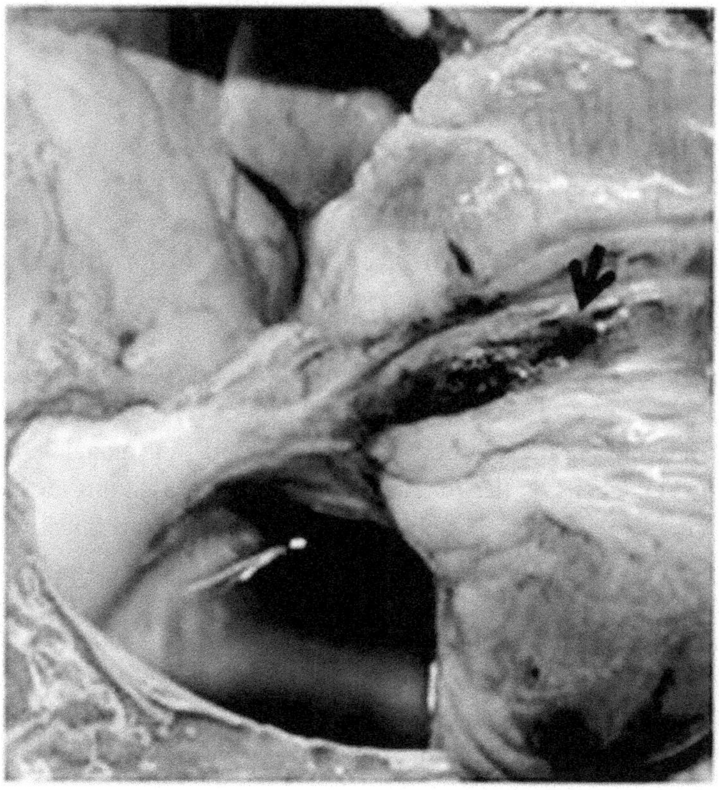

Coronary artery abnormalities can result in sudden death when their anatomical placement is not normal. For instance, in patients where the left main coronary artery is on the right or in the non-coronary Valsalva sinus, the risk of sudden death is higher.

Heart rupture is the major complication of acute myocardial infarction (6%) (Benton et al., 2007).

Heart Hypertrophy

Cardiac hypertrophy is an adaptive, morphologic increase in cardiac mass resulting from enlargement of the heart muscle. The increase due to pressure or volume stress on the heart (Frey et al., 2004). The heart compensates with a corresponding increase in the capacity of the heart chambers (Dorn et al., 2003). Pathological cardiac hypertrophy causes interstitial fibrosis and myocyte death that leads to cardiac dysfunction. Physiological cardiac hypertrophy, also known as athlete's heart, is heart growth caused by chronic physical exercise with no congenital or valvular defects (Bernardo et al., 2010). In response to the chronic increase in cardiac load, an initial growth occurs in cardiac muscle to stabilize the added wall stress and to allow normal cardiovascular function. Unfortunately, if the increase in wall stress is not abated, the hypertrophic expansion of cardiac tissue can eventually lead to heart failure.

Postmortem diagnosis of heart hypertrophy is determined by direct measurements of gravimetric weight of the heart (Diwan and Dorn, 2007). A recent study using the heart weight of 27,645 autopsy cases were used to determine equations to calculate the predicted heart weight in relations to age, sex, body weight and height (Wingren and Ottosson, 2015). The piecewise linear regression model produced an online heart weight calculator. During the gross examination of the cadaver heart during autopsy, the observation of valves larger that 10-15 mm in thickness of the septum and LV, and 3-4 mm for the RV, is indicative of cardiac hypertrophy (Suarez-Mier and Aguilera, 2015)

Endocarditis

Endocarditis is defined as inflammation of the inner layer of the heart (endocardium), especially the valvular endothelium, chordae tendinae and mural endocardium (Geller, 2013). The disease is better described by the terms infective or infectious endocarditis (IE). It occurs as a result of a microbial infection that enters the bloodstream, travels to the heart, and lodges on abnormal heart valves or damaged heart tissues. The disease is characterized by abnormal lesions, or vegetations, which form in the heart at the site of the infection (Mylonakis and Calderwood, 2001). The lesions contain platelets, fibrin, inflammatory cells, and microorganisms; however, due to the wide use of antibiotics, the presence of microorganisms on Gram stain of vegetations is often undetected (Fernandez et al., 2012). Staphylococci and streptococci, respectively, are the etiological pathogens that are responsible for approximately 80% of the cases of infective endocarditis (Hoen and Duval, 2013). Individuals most predisposed to endocarditis are patients with prosthetic cardiac valves, patients with previous infective endocarditis, cardiac transplant patients who have structurally abnormal valves that cause valve regurgitation, congenital heart disease (Nishimura et al., 2014).

Two-dimensional echocardiograms, particularly transesophageal echocardiogram (TEE), are often used to visualize morphological changes caused by valve vegetations to determine antemortem cardiovascular infection (Ker et al., 2010; Fernandez et al., 2012). During autopsy, the occurrence of vegetations in cardiac valves or mural endocardium composed of fibrin, platelets, leukocytes, or histiocytes are determined (Fernandez et al., 2012). Isolated and/or combined mitral or aortic valves are the most common sites of infective endocarditis discovered during autopsy.

Cardiac Tumors

Any abnormal growth of cells is called a "tumor." The heart is not any different from other organs in the body. Primary tumors, originating in the heart, are less common by 30-40 fold than secondary tumors, which originate in other tissues such as lungs, skin, breast etc. They are difficult to diagnose and are most often found incidentally during an examination and imaging of the heart for an unrelated indication. Symptoms are very similar to many other heart conditions. More than half of all cardiac tumors are myxomas, which are gelatinous, irregular, and non-cancerous tumors, and often require emergency surgery. Myxomas are predominantly located in the left atrium and the heart chamber where oxygenated blood from the lungs enters the heart (Roever et al., 2014).

Cardiac Conduction Disorders

A significant portion of unexplained sudden cardiac deaths is attributable to defects in the cardiac conduction system. Cardiac conduction system disorders related to sudden cardiac deaths are less common in the elderly. The most common heart related death in this group is from atherosclerotic coronary artery disease.

Sudden cardiac cases, where ventricular hypertrophy with coronary artery lesion is detected, are primarily reported as hypertrophic cardiomyopathies and/or atherosclerotic diseases. When there are not enough findings to explain the death, the lack of examination of cardiac conduction system is detected. The unexplained sudden deaths after exercise may accompany the existing pathological changes in heart conduction system disorders (Song et al., 2001; Lie et al., 1975).

CONCLUSION

Forensic pathologists are not only concerned with trauma induced deaths. Traumatic deaths compared to non-traumatic death offer more information to a forensic pathologist. Sudden and unexpected deaths have a special importance in forensic medicine because of their suspicious nature. Despite cardiovascular diseases being the number one cause of death in the world, sudden unexpected deaths have an important place in science because of the amount of the information they provide and immense expertise that is required in determining the cause of death in some of the cases.

ACKNOWLEDGMENT

This work was supported by the National Science Foundation (NSF) grant HRD 1401075 and Forensic Sciences Foundation Lucas Research Grant.

REFERENCES

Ackerman, M. J., Tester, D. J., & Driscoll, D. J. (2001). Molecular autopsy of sudden unexplained death in the young. *The American Journal of Forensic Medicine and Pathology*, *22*(2), 105–111. doi:10.1097/00000433-200106000-00001 PMID:11394742

Alpert, J. S., Thygesen, K., Antman, E., & Bassand, J. P. (2000). Myocardial infarction redefined—a consensus document of the Joint European Society of Cardiology/American College of Cardiology committee for the redefinition of myocardial infarction: The Joint European Society of Cardiology/American College of Cardiology Committee. *Journal of the American College of Cardiology*, *36*(3), 959–969. doi:10.1016/S0735-1097(00)00804-4 PMID:10987628

Amundsen, I., Øiestad, Å. M., Ekeberg, D., & Kristoffersen, L. (2013). Quantitative determination of fifteen basic pharmaceuticals in ante-and post-mortem whole blood by high pH mobile phase reversed phase ultrahigh performance liquid chromatography–tandem mass spectrometry. *Journal of Chromatography. B, Analytical Technologies in the Biomedical and Life Sciences*, *927*, 112–123. doi:10.1016/j.jchromb.2012.12.039 PMID:23380540

Bagnall, R. D., Das, J., Duflou, J., & Semsarian, C. (2014). Exome analysis–based molecular autopsy in cases of sudden unexplained death in the young. *Heart Rhythm*, *11*(4), 655–662. doi:10.1016/j.hrthm.2014.01.017 PMID:24440382

Bailey, D. (2015). *Guidelines on autopsy practice: Sudden death with likely cardiac pathology*. Retrieved from http://www.rcpath.org/NR/rdonlyres/98390BBB-BEF4-4459-A0AE-EE34366D327C/0/G145_DRAFT_GAPCardiacDeath_Apr15.pdf

Bailey, J. C., Feelisch, M., Horowitz, J. D., Frenneaux, M. P., & Madhani, M. (2014). Pharmacology and therapeutic role of inorganic nitrite and nitrate in vasodilatation. *Pharmacology & Therapeutics*, *144*(3), 303–320. doi:10.1016/j.pharmthera.2014.06.009 PMID:24992304

Basso, C., Burke, M., Fornes, P., Gallagher, P. J., de Gouveia, R. H., Sheppard, M., & van der Wal, A. et al. (2008). Guidelines for autopsy investigation of sudden cardiac death. *Virchows Archiv*, *452*(1), 11–18. doi:10.1007/s00428-007-0505-5 PMID:17952460

Basso, C., Burke, M., Fornes, P., Gallagher, P. J., De Gouveia, R. H., Sheppard, M., & Van Der Wal, A. et al. (2010). Association for European Cardiovascular Pathology. Guidelines for autopsy investigation of sudden cardiac death. *Pathologica*, *102*(5), 391–404. PMID:21361120

Bell, S. (2009). Forensic chemistry. *Annual Review of Analytical Chemistry*, *2*(1), 297–319. doi:10.1146/annurev-anchem-060908-155251 PMID:20636064

Benton, N. G., & Maginot, K. R. (2007). Sudden Cardiac Death in Young Athletes: Trying to Find the Needle in the Haystack. *WMJ: Official Publication of the State Medical Society of Wisconsin*, *106*(6), 335–342. PMID:17970016

Bernardo, B. C., Weeks, K. L., Pretorius, L., & McMullen, J. R. (2010). Molecular distinction between physiological and pathological cardiac hypertrophy: Experimental findings and therapeutic strategies. *Pharmacology & Therapeutics*, *128*(1), 191–227. doi:10.1016/j.pharmthera.2010.04.005 PMID:20438756

Blankenberg, S., Barbaux, S., & Tiret, L. (2003). Adhesion molecules and atherosclerosis. *Atherosclerosis, 170*(2), 191–203. doi:10.1016/S0021-9150(03)00097-2 PMID:14612198

Blauwet, L. A., & Cooper, L. T. (2010). Myocarditis. *Progress in Cardiovascular Diseases, 52*(4), 274–288. doi:10.1016/j.pcad.2009.11.006 PMID:20109598

Boczek, N. J., Tester, D. J., & Ackerman, M. J. (2012). The molecular autopsy: an indispensable step following sudden cardiac death in the young? *Herzschrittmachertherapie & Elektrophysiologie, 23*(3). doi:10.1007/s00399-012-0222-x

Caforio, A. L., Pankuweit, S., Arbustini, E., Basso, C., Gimeno-Blanes, J., Felix, S. B., & Elliott, P. M. et al. (2013). Current state of knowledge on aetiology, diagnosis, management, and therapy of myocarditis: A position statement of the European Society of Cardiology Working Group on Myocardial and Pericardial Diseases. *European Heart Journal, 34*(33), 2636–2648. doi:10.1093/eurheartj/eht210 PMID:23824828

Campobasso, C. P., DellErba, A. S., Addante, A., Zotti, F., Marzullo, A., & Colonna, M. F. (2008). Sudden cardiac death and myocardial ischemia indicators: A comparative study of four immunohistochemical markers. *The American Journal of Forensic Medicine and Pathology, 29*(2), 154–161. doi:10.1097/PAF.0b013e318177eab7 PMID:18520484

Chugh, S. S., Kelly, K. L., & Titus, J. L. (2000). Sudden cardiac death with apparently normal heart. *Circulation, 102*(6), 649–654. doi:10.1161/01.CIR.102.6.649 PMID:10931805

De-Giorgio, F., & Vetrugno, G. (2014). Is histological examination always necessary to determine a cause of death? Of course it is! *Forensic Science, Medicine, and Pathology, 10*(3), 477–478. doi:10.1007/s12024-014-9543-x PMID:24577851

De La Grandmaison, G. L., Charlier, P., & Durigon, M. (2010). Usefulness of Systematic Histological Examination in Routine Forensic Autopsy*. *Journal of Forensic Sciences, 55*(1), 85–88. doi:10.1111/j.1556-4029.2009.01240.x PMID:20002264

Deo, R., & Albert, C. M. (2012). Epidemiology and genetics of sudden cardiac death. *Circulation, 125*(4), 620–637. doi:10.1161/CIRCULATIONAHA.111.023838 PMID:22294707

Di Maio, D. J., & Di Maio, V. J. M. (2001). *Forensic Pathology* (2nd ed.). CRC Press.

Diwan, A., & Dorn, G. W. (2007). Decompensation of cardiac hypertrophy: Cellular mechanisms and novel therapeutic targets. *Physiology (Bethesda, MD), 22*(1), 56–64. doi:10.1152/physiol.00033.2006 PMID:17289931

Dorn, G. W., Robbins, J., & Sugden, P. H. (2003). Phenotyping Hypertrophy Eschew Obfuscation. *Circulation Research, 92*(11), 1171–1175. doi:10.1161/01.RES.0000077012.11088.BC PMID:12805233

Dowling, G. (2005). Sudden Natural Death. In D. Dolinak & E. Matshes (Eds.), *W, & Lew, E.O. Forensic Pathology: Principles and Practise* (pp. 71–119). Elseiver Academic Press.

Feenstra, J., Grobbee, D., Remme, W., & Stricker, B. (1999). Drug-induced heart failure. *Journal of the American College of Cardiology, 33*(5), 1152–1162. doi:10.1016/S0735-1097(99)00006-6 PMID:10193711

Fernández, G. M., Álvarez, B., Manzarbeitia, F., & Renedo, G. (2012). Infective endocarditis at autopsy: A review of pathologic manifestations and clinical correlates. *Medicine*, *91*(3), 152–164. doi:10.1097/MD.0b013e31825631ea PMID:22543628

Frey, N., Katus, H. A., Olson, E. N., & Hill, J. A. (2004). Hypertrophy of the heart a new therapeutic target? *Circulation*, *109*(13), 1580–1589. doi:10.1161/01.CIR.0000120390.68287.BB PMID:15066961

Geller, S. A. (2013). Infective endocarditis: A history of the development of its understanding. *Autopsy and Case Reports*, *3*(4), 5–12. doi:10.4322/acr.2013.033

Goyle, K. K., & Walling, A. D. (2002). Diagnosing pericarditis. *American Family Physician*, *66*(9), 1695–1704. PMID:12449268

Gunn, A. (2011). *Essential forensic biology*. John Wiley & Sons.

Hearn and Walls. (2007). Introduction to Postmortem Toxicology. In B. Karch Steven (Ed.), *Postmortem toxicology of abused drugs*. CRC Press.

Hoen, B., & Duval, X. (2013). Infective endocarditis. *The New England Journal of Medicine*, *368*(15), 1425–1433. doi:10.1056/NEJMcp1206782 PMID:23574121

Huang, P., Wan, L., Qin, Z., Zhang, J., Liu, N., Zou, D., & Chen, Y. (2012). Post-mortem MSCT diagnosis of acute pericardial tamponade caused by blunt trauma to the chest in a motor-vehicle collision. *Romanian Journal of Legal Medicine*, *20*(2), 117–122. doi:10.4323/rjlm.2012.117

Hutchins, G. M., Berman, J. J., Moore, G. W., & Hanzlick, R. (1999). Practice guidelines for autopsy pathology: Autopsy reporting. *Archives of Pathology & Laboratory Medicine*, *123*(11), 1085. PMID:10539932

John, R. M., Tedrow, U. B., Koplan, B. A., Albert, C. M., Epstein, L. M., Sweeney, M. O., & Stevenson, W. G. et al. (2012). Ventricular arrhythmias and sudden cardiac death. *Lancet*, *380*(9852), 1520–1529. doi:10.1016/S0140-6736(12)61413-5 PMID:23101719

Jorge Dinis-Oliveira, R., Carvalho, F., Alberto Duarte, J., Brandao Proenca, J., Santos, A., & Magalhães, T. (2012). Clinical and forensic signs related to cocaine abuse. *Current Drug Abuse Reviews*, *5*(1), 64–83. doi:10.2174/1874473711205010064 PMID:22280333

Ker, J., Toit-Prinsloo, L. D., Van Heerden, W., & Saayman, G. (2010). Post-Mortem Echocardiography as a Guide to Cardiac Autopsy—A Worthwhile Concept? Clinical Medicine Insights. *Cardiology*, *4*, 59–61. PMID:20859531

Khandaker, M. H., Espinosa, R. E., Nishimura, R. A., Sinak, L. J., Hayes, S. N., Melduni, R. M., & Oh, J. K. (2010). Pericardial disease: Diagnosis and management. *Mayo Clinic Proceedings*, *85*(6), 572–593. doi:10.4065/mcp.2010.0046 PMID:20511488

Koponen, M. A., & Lantz, P. E. (2003). Sudden Unexpected Adult Deaths. In R. C. Froede (Ed.), *Handbook of Forensic Pathology* (2nd ed.; pp. 89–92). CAP.

Kumar, S., Kumar, V. A., Kumar, N., Baranwal, R. K., Kumar, V. R., & Singh, M. (2011). Coronary atherosclerosis--a postmortem histopathological study. *Bratislavske lekarske listy*, *113*(4), 217-219.

Lange, R. A., & Hillis, L. D. (2004). Acute pericarditis. *The New England Journal of Medicine*, *351*(21), 2195–2202. doi:10.1056/NEJMcp041997 PMID:15548780

Lee, K. K., Al-Ahmad, A., Wang, P. J., & Myerburg, R. J. (2008). Epidemiology and Etiologies of Sudden Cardiac Death. In P. J. Wang, A. Al-Ahmad, H. H. Hsia, & P. C. Zei (Eds.), *Ventricular Arrhythmias and Sudden Cardiac Death* (pp. 199–212). Blackwell Publishing. doi:10.1002/9781444300307.ch17

Leth, P. M. (2015). Computed Tomography in Forensic Medicine. *Danish Medical Journal*, *62*(6), 1–26. PMID:26036889

Lie, J. T. (1975). Histopathology of the conduction system in sudden death from coronary heart disease. *Circulation*, *51*(3), 446–452. doi:10.1161/01.CIR.51.3.446 PMID:1139756

Linnet, K. (2013). Toxicological Screening and Quantitation Using Liquid Chromatography/Time-of-Flight Mass Spectrometry. *Journal of Forensic Science & Criminology*, *1*(1), e101. doi:10.15744/2348-9804.1.e101

Lloyd-Jones, D., Adams, R. J., Brown, T. M., Carnethon, M., Dai, S., De Simone, G., & Wylie-Rosett, J. et al. (2010). Heart disease and stroke statistics–2010 update: A report from the American Heart Association. *Circulation*, *121*(7), e46–e215. doi:10.1161/CIRCULATIONAHA.109.192667 PMID:20019324

Loporcaro, C. G., Tester, D. J., Maleszewski, J. J., Kruisselbrink, T., & Ackerman, M. J. (2014). Confirmation of cause and manner of death via a comprehensive cardiac autopsy including whole exome next-generation sequencing. *Archives of Pathology & Laboratory Medicine*, *138*(8), 1083–1089. doi:10.5858/arpa.2013-0479-SA PMID:24298987

Maeda, H., Ishikawa, T., & Michiue, T. (2011). Forensic biochemistry for functional investigation of death: Concept and practical application. *Legal Medicine (Tokyo)*, *13*(2), 55–67. doi:10.1016/j.legalmed.2010.12.005 PMID:21269863

Maurer, H. H. (2013). What is the future of (ultra) high performance liquid chromatography coupled to low and high resolution mass spectrometry for toxicological drug screening? *Journal of Chromatography. A*, *1292*, 19–24. doi:10.1016/j.chroma.2012.08.069 PMID:22964051

Michaud, K., Grabherr, S., Doenz, F., & Mangin, P. (2012). Evaluation of postmortem MDCT and MDCT-angiography for the investigation of sudden cardiac death related to atherosclerotic coronary artery disease. *The International Journal of Cardiovascular Imaging*, *28*(7), 1807–1822. doi:10.1007/s10554-012-0012-x PMID:22238022

Michaud, K., Grabherr, S., Jackowski, C., Bollmann, M. D., Doenz, F., & Mangin, P. (2014). Postmortem imaging of sudden cardiac death. *International Journal of Legal Medicine*, *128*(1), 127–137. doi:10.1007/s00414-013-0819-6 PMID:23322013

Molina, D. K., Wood, L. E., & Frost, R. E. (2007). Is routine histopathologic examination beneficial in all medicolegal autopsies? *The American Journal of Forensic Medicine and Pathology*, *28*(1), 1–3. doi:10.1097/01.paf.0000257388.83605.0a PMID:17325455

Morentin, B., Aguilera, B., Carmena, M. D. G. C., & Alonso-Pulpón, L. A. (2015). Myocarditis. In *Clinico-Pathological Atlas of Cardiovascular Diseases* (pp. 233–263). Springer International Publishing.

Mylonakis, E., & Calderwood, S. B. (2001). Infective endocarditis in adults. *The New England Journal of Medicine*, *345*(18), 1318–1330. doi:10.1056/NEJMra010082 PMID:11794152

Nabel, E. G., & Braunwald, E. (2012). A tale of coronary artery disease and myocardial infarction. *The New England Journal of Medicine*, *366*(1), 54–63. doi:10.1056/NEJMra1112570 PMID:22216842

Nishimura, R. A., Otto, C. M., Bonow, R. O., Carabello, B. A., Erwin, J. P. III, Guyton, R. A., & Thomas, J. D. et al. (2014). 2014 AHA/ACC guideline for the management of patients with valvular heart disease: executive summary: a report of the American College of Cardiology/American Heart Association Task Force on Practice Guidelines. *Circulation*, *129*(23), 2440–2492. doi:10.1161/CIR.0000000000000029 PMID:24589852

Pélissier-Alicot, A. L., Gaulier, J. M., Champsaur, P., & Marquet, P. (2003). Mechanisms underlying postmortem redistribution of drugs: A review. *Journal of Analytic Toxicolology*, *27*(8), 533–544. doi:10.1093/jat/27.8.533 PMID:14670131

Peters, F. T., & Remane, D. (2012). Aspects of matrix effects in applications of liquid chromatography-mass spectrometry to forensic and clinical toxicologya review. *Analytical and Bioanalytical Chemistry*, *403*(8), 2155–2172. doi:10.1007/s00216-012-6035-2 PMID:22549818

Pounder, D. J., & Jones, G. R. (1990). Post-mortem drug redistributiona toxicological nightmare. *Forensic Science International*, *45*(3), 253–263. doi:10.1016/0379-0738(90)90182-X PMID:2361648

Roberts, I. S. D., Benamore, R. E., Peebles, C., Roobottom, C., & Traill, Z. C. (2011). Diagnosis of coronary artery disease using minimally invasive autopsy: Evaluation of a novel method of post-mortem coronary CT angiography. *Clinical Radiology*, *66*(7), 645–650. doi:10.1016/j.crad.2011.01.007 PMID:21377145

Roever, L., Casella-Filho, A., Dourado, P. M., Resende, E. S., & Chagas, A. C. (2014). Cardiac tumors: A brief commentary. *Front Public Health*, *2*, 264. doi:10.3389/fpubh.2014.00264 PMID:25538934

Ross, S. G., Bolliger, S. A., Ampanozi, G., Oesterhelweg, L., Thali, M. J., & Flach, P. M. (2014). Post-mortem CT angiography: Capabilities and limitations in traumatic and natural causes of death. *Radiographics*, *34*(3), 830–846. doi:10.1148/rg.343115169 PMID:24819799

Ross, S. G., Thali, M. J., Bolliger, S., Germerott, T., Ruder, T. D., & Flach, P. M. (2012). Sudden death after chest pain: Feasibility of virtual autopsy with postmortem CT angiography and biopsy. *Radiology*, *264*(1), 250–259. doi:10.1148/radiol.12092415 PMID:22570504

Sagar, S., Liu, P. P., & Cooper, L. T. Jr. (2012). Myocarditis. *Lancet*, *379*(9817), 738–747. doi:10.1016/S0140-6736(11)60648-X PMID:22185868

Semsarian, C., Ingles, J., & Wilde, A. A. (2015). Sudden cardiac death in the young: The molecular autopsy and a practical approach to surviving relatives. *European Heart Journal*. PMID:25765769

Smith, M. L., Vorce, S. P., Holler, J. M., Shimomura, E., Magluilo, J., Jacobs, A. J., & Huestis, M. A. (2007). Modern Instrumental Methods in Forensic Toxicology. *Journal of Analytical Toxicology*, *31*(5), 237–9A. doi:10.1093/jat/31.5.237 PMID:17579968

Society of Forensic Toxicologists/American Academy of Forensic Sciences. SOFT/AAFS forensic laboratory guidelines. (2006). Available at: http://www.soft-tox.org/files/Guidelines_2006_Final.pdf Accessed June 19, 2015.

Song, Y., Laaksonen, H., Saukko, S., Toivonen, S., & Zhu, J. (2001). Histopathological findings of cardiac conduction system of 150 Finns. *Forensic Science International*, *119*(3), 310–317. doi:10.1016/S0379-0738(00)00457-6 PMID:11390145

Suarez-Mier, M. P., & Aguiler, B. (2014). Methodological Approach to Cardiac Autopsy. In Clinico-Pathological Atlas of Cardiovascular Diseases. Springer.

Tester, D. J., & Ackerman, M. J. (2012). The Molecular Autopsy: Should the Evaluation Continue After the Funeral? *Pediatric Cardiology*, *33*(3), 461–470. doi:10.1007/s00246-012-0160-8 PMID:22307399

Thygesen, K., Alpert, J. S., Jaffe, A. S., Simoons, M. L., Chaitman, B. R., White, H. D., & Mendis, S et al.. (2012). Third Universal Definition of Myocardial Infarction. *Journal of the American College of Cardiology*, *60*(16), 1581–1598. doi:10.1016/j.jacc.2012.08.001 PMID:22958960

Trial, M. (1997). The effect of digoxin on mortality and morbidity in patients with heart failure. *The New England Journal of Medicine*, *336*(8), 525–533. doi:10.1056/NEJM199702203360801 PMID:9036306

Wingren, C. J., & Ottosson, A. (2015). Postmortem heart weight modelled using piecewise linear regression in 27,645 medicolegal autopsy cases. *Forensic Science International*, *252*, 157–162. doi:10.1016/j.forsciint.2015.04.036 PMID:26004078

Wu, A. H., & French, D. (2013). Implementation of liquid chromatography/mass spectrometry into the clinical laboratory. *Clinica Chimica Acta*, *420*, 4–10. doi:10.1016/j.cca.2012.10.026 PMID:23085380

Wyman, J. F. (2012). Principles and procedures in forensic toxicology. *Clinics in Laboratory Medicine*, *32*(3), 493–507. doi:10.1016/j.cll.2012.06.005 PMID:22939304

Yarema, M. C., & Becker, C. E. (2005). Key concepts in postmortem drug redistribution. *Clinical Toxicology (Philadelphia, PA)*, *43*(4), 235–241. doi:10.1081/CLT-58950 PMID:16035199

Yu, X., Wang, H., Feng, L., & Zhu, J. (2014). Quantitative Research in Modern Forensic Analysis of Death Cause: New Classification of Death Cause, Degree of Contribution, and Determination of Manner of Death. *Journal of Forensic Research*, *5*(2), 1.

Zhan, Z. Q., Nikus, K. C., & Wang, C. Q. (2015). Cocaine-induced right ventricular dysfunction: Right ventricular infarction or afterload elevation? *The American Journal of Emergency Medicine*, *33*(9), 1318–1319. doi:10.1016/j.ajem.2015.05.016 PMID:26027888

Zhou, S., Wan, L., Shao, Y., Ying, C., Wang, Y., Zou, D., & Chen, Y. et al. (2015). Detection of aortic rupture using post-mortem computed tomography and post-mortem computed tomography angiography by cardiac puncture. *International Journal of Legal Medicine*, 1–6. PMID:25773916

Zipes, D. P., & Wellens, H. J. (1998). Sudden cardiac death. *Circulation*, *98*(21), 2334–2351. doi:10.1161/01.CIR.98.21.2334 PMID:9826323

Compilation of References

Abbas, A. (2003). Transplantation Immunology. *Cellular & Molecular Immunology*, 359–381.

Abbasi, T., & Garcia, J. G. (2013). Sphingolipids in lung endothelial biology and regulation of vascular integrity. *Handb Exp Pharmacol,* (216), 201-226. doi: 10.1007/978-3-7091-1511-4_10

Abbasi, F., Hayat, T., & Alsaedi, A. (2015). Peristaltic transport of magneto-nanoparticles submerged in water: Model for drug delivery system. *Physica E, Low-Dimensional Systems and Nanostructures*, *123*. doi:10.1016/j.physe.2014.12.026

Acharya, G., & Park, K. (2006). Mechanisms of controlled drug release from drug-eluting stents. *Advanced Drug Delivery Reviews, 58*, 387-401. doi:10.1016/j.addr.2006.01.016

Ackerman, M. J., Tester, D. J., & Driscoll, D. J. (2001). Molecular autopsy of sudden unexplained death in the young. *The American Journal of Forensic Medicine and Pathology*, *22*(2), 105–111. doi:10.1097/00000433-200106000-00001 PMID:11394742

Actis-Goretta, L., Ottaviani, J. I., & Fraga, C. G. (2006). Inhibition of angiotensin converting enzyme activity by flavanol-rich foods. *Journal of Agricultural and Food Chemistry*, *54*(1), 229–234. doi:10.1021/jf052263o PMID:16390204

Adler, D. H., Cogan, J. D., Phillips, J. A. III, Schnetz-Boutaud, N., & Milne, G. L. et al.. (2008). Inherited human cPLA(2alpha) deficiency is associated with impaired eicosanoid biosynthesis, small intestinal ulceration, and platelet dysfunction. *The Journal of Clinical Investigation*, *118*, 2121–2131. PMID:18451993

Aggarwal, S., & Pittenger, M. F. (2005). Human mesenchymal stem cells modulate allogeneic immune cell responses. *Blood*, *105*(4), 1815–1822. doi:10.1182/blood-2004-04-1559 PMID:15494428

Aggeli, C., Felekos, I., Kastellanos, S., Panagopoulou, V., Oikonomou, E., Tsiamis, E., & Tousoulis, D. (2015). Real-time three-dimensional echocardiography: Never before clinical efficacy looked so picturesque. *International Journal of Cardiology*, *198*, 15–21. doi:10.1016/j.ijcard.2015.06.052 PMID:26149331

Ahmed, R. M., Mohamed, E.-H. A., Ashraf, M., Maithili, S., Nabil, F., Rami, R., & Mohamed, T. I. (2013). Effect of remote ischemic preconditioning on serum troponin T level following elective percutaneous coronary intervention. *Catheterization and Cardiovascular Interventions*, *82*(5), E647–E653. doi:10.1002/ccd.24825 PMID:23404916

Ahmmed, G. U., Mehta, D., Vogel, S., Holinstat, M., Paria, B. C., Tiruppathi, C., & Malik, A. B. (2004). Protein kinase Calpha phosphorylates the TRPC1 channel and regulates store-operated Ca2+ entry in endothelial cells. *The Journal of Biological Chemistry*, *279*(20), 20941–20949. doi:10.1074/jbc.M313975200 PMID:15016832

Aird, W. C. (2012). Endothelial cell heterogeneity. *Cold Spring Harb Perspect Med*, *2*(1), a006429. doi:10.1101/cshperspect.a006429 PMID:22315715

Akilen, R., Tsiami, A., Devendra, D., & Robinson, N. (2010). Glycated haemoglobin and blood pressure-lowering effect of cinnamon in multi-ethnic Type 2 diabetic patients in the UK: A randomized, placebo-controlled, double-blind clinical trial. *Diabetic Medicine*, *27*(10), 1159–1167. doi:10.1111/j.1464-5491.2010.03079.x PMID:20854384

Al Hawas, R., Ren, Q., Ye, S., Karim, Z. A., Filipovich, A. H., & Whiteheart, S. W. (2012). Munc18b/STXBP2 is required for platelet secretion. *Blood*, *120*(12), 2493–2500. doi:10.1182/blood-2012-05-430629 PMID:22791290

Alaghband-Zadeh, J., Das, I., Hanson, M. R., MacGregor, C. A., de Wardener, H. E., & Laycock, J. F.AlaghbandZadeh. (1996). Hypothalamic and plasma total nitrate/nitrite concentrations in spontaneously hypertensive rats. *Experimental Physiology*, *81*(5), 881–883. doi:10.1113/expphysiol.1996.sp003984 PMID:8889485

Albani, D., Polito, L., Signorini, A., & Forloni, G. (2010). Neuroprotective properties of resveratrol in different neurodegenerative disorders. *BioFactors (Oxford, England)*, *36*(5), 370–376. doi:10.1002/biof.118 PMID:20848560

Albers, C. A., Cvejic, A., Favier, R., Bouwmans, E. E., Alessi, M. C., Bertone, P., & Ouwehand, W. H. et al. (2011). Exome sequencing identifies NBEAL2 as the causative gene for gray platelet syndrome. *Nature Genetics*, *43*(8), 735–737. doi:10.1038/ng.885 PMID:21765411

Albinsson, S., Skoura, A., Yu, J., DiLorenzo, A., Fernandez-Hernando, C., Offermanns, S., & Sessa, W. C. et al. (2011). Smooth muscle miRNAs are critical for post-natal regulation of blood pressure and vascular function. *PLoS ONE*, *6*(4), e18869. doi:10.1371/journal.pone.0018869 PMID:21526127

Albinsson, S., Suarez, Y., Skoura, A., Offermanns, S., Miano, J. M., & Sessa, W. C. (2010). MicroRNAs are necessary for vascular smooth muscle growth, differentiation, and function. *Arteriosclerosis, Thrombosis, and Vascular Biology*, *30*(6), 1118–1126. doi:10.1161/ATVBAHA.109.200873 PMID:20378849

Alcendor, R. R., Gao, S., Zhai, P., Zablocki, D., Holle, E., Yu, X., & Sadoshima, J. et al. (2007). Sirt1 regulates aging and resistance to oxidative stress in the heart. *Circulation Research*, *100*(10), 1512–1521. doi:10.1161/01.RES.0000267723.65696.4a PMID:17446436

AlGhatrif, M., & Lindsay, J. (2012). A brief review: History to understand fundamentals of electrocardiography. *J Community Hosp Intern Med Perspect*, *2*(1). doi:10.3402/jchimp.v2i1.14383 PMID:23882360

Ali, Z. A., Callaghan, C. J., Lim, E., Ali, A. A., Nouraei, S. A., Akthar, A. M., & Gaunt, M. E. et al. (2007). Remote ischemic preconditioning reduces myocardial and renal injury after elective abdominal aortic aneurysm repair: A randomized controlled trial. *Circulation*, *116*(11Suppl), I98–I105. doi:10.1161/circulationaha.106.679167 PMID:17846333

Allen, B. S., Barth, M. J., & Ilbawi, M. N. (2001). Pediatric myocardial protection: An overview. *Seminars in Thoracic and Cardiovascular Surgery*, *13*(1), 56–72. doi:10.1053/stcs.2001.22738 PMID:11309728

Alpert, J. S., Thygesen, K., Antman, E., & Bassand, J. P. (2000). Myocardial infarction redefined—a consensus document of the Joint European Society of Cardiology/American College of Cardiology committee for the redefinition of myocardial infarction: The Joint European Society of Cardiology/American College of Cardiology Committee. *Journal of the American College of Cardiology*, *36*(3), 959–969. doi:10.1016/S0735-1097(00)00804-4 PMID:10987628

Al-Qattan, K. K., Khan, I., Alnaqeeb, M. A., & Ali, M. (2001). Thromboxane-B2, prostaglandin-E2 and hypertension in the rat 2-kidney 1-clip model: A possible mechanism of the garlic induced hypotension. *Prostaglandins, Leukotrienes, and Essential Fatty Acids*, *64*(1), 5–10. doi:10.1054/plef.2000.0232 PMID:11161580

Al-Qattan, K. K., Thomson, M., Al-Mutawa'a, S., Al-Hajeri, D., Drobiova, H., & Ali, M. (2006). Nitric oxide mediates the blood-pressure lowering effect of garlic in the rat two-kidney, one-clip model of hypertension. *The Journal of Nutrition*, *136*(3), 774S–776S. PMID:16484561

Alraies, M. C., & Eckman, P. (2014). Adult heart transplant: Indications and outcomes. *Journal of Thoracic Disease*, *6*(8), 1120. PMID:25132979

Alshbool, F. Z., Karim, Z. A., Vemana, H. P., Conlon, C., Lin, O. A., & Khasawneh, F. T. (2015). The regulator of G-protein signaling 18 regulates platelet aggregation, hemostasis and thrombosis. *Biochemical and Biophysical Research Communications*, *462*(4), 378–382. doi:10.1016/j.bbrc.2015.04.143 PMID:25969426

Altemeier, W. A., & Sinclair, S. E. (2007). Hyperoxia in the intensive care unit: Why more is not always better. *Current Opinion in Critical Care*, *13*(1), 73–78. doi:10.1097/MCC.0b013e32801162cb PMID:17198052

Althaus, K., Najm, J., & Greinacher, A. (2011). MYH9 related platelet disorders - often unknown and misdiagnosed. *Klinische Padiatrie*, *223*(03), 120–125. doi:10.1055/s-0031-1275664 PMID:21567368

Altman, R. B. (2011). Pharmacogenomics: Noninferiority Is Sufficient for Initial Implementation. *Clinical Pharmacology and Therapeutics*, *89*(3), 248–350. doi:10.1038/clpt.2010.310 PMID:21326263

Amat, R., Planavila, A., Chen, S. L., Iglesias, R., Giralt, M., & Villarroya, F. (2009). SIRT1 Controls the Transcription of the Peroxisome Proliferator-activated Receptor-γ Co-activator-1α (PGC-1α) Gene in Skeletal Muscle through the PGC-1α Autoregulatory Loop and Interaction with MyoD. *The Journal of Biological Chemistry*, *284*(33), 21872–21880. doi:10.1074/jbc.M109.022749 PMID:19553684

Ambrose, J. A., & Barua, R. S. (2004). The pathophysiology of cigarette smoking and cardiovascular diseaseAn update. *Journal of the American College of Cardiology*, *43*(10), 1731–1737. doi:10.1016/j.jacc.2003.12.047 PMID:15145091

Amundsen, I., Øiestad, Å. M., Ekeberg, D., & Kristoffersen, L. (2013). Quantitative determination of fifteen basic pharmaceuticals in ante-and post-mortem whole blood by high pH mobile phase reversed phase ultrahigh performance liquid chromatography–tandem mass spectrometry. *Journal of Chromatography. B, Analytical Technologies in the Biomedical and Life Sciences*, *927*, 112–123. doi:10.1016/j.jchromb.2012.12.039 PMID:23380540

An, D., & Rodrigues, B. (2006). Role of changes in cardiac metabolism in development of diabetic cardiomyopathy. *American Journal of Physiology. Heart and Circulatory Physiology*, *291*(4), H1489–H1506. doi:10.1152/ajpheart.00278.2006 PMID:16751293

Anderson, J. L., Adams, C. D., Antman, E. M., Bridges, C. R., Califf, R. M., Casey, D. E. Jr, & Riegel, B. et al. (2007). ACC/AHA 2007 guidelines for the management of patients with unstable angina/non-ST-elevation myocardial infarction: A report of the American College of Cardiology/American Heart Association task force on practice guidelines (writing committee to revise the 2002 guidelines for the management of patients with unstable angina/non-ST-elevation myocardial infarction) developed in collaboration with the American College of Emergency Physicians, the Society for Cardiovascular Angiography and Interventions, and the Society of Thoracic Surgeons endorsed by the American Association of Cardiovascular and Pulmonary Rehabilitation and the Society for Academic Emergency Medicine. *Journal of the American College of Cardiology*, *50*(7), e1–e157. doi:10.1016/j.jacc.2007.02.013 PMID:17692738

Anderson, J. W., Zeigler, J. A., Deakins, D. A., Floore, T. L., Dillon, D. W., & Wood, C. L. (1991). Metabolic effects of high-carbohydrate, high-fiber diets for insulin-dependent diabetic individuals. *The American Journal of Clinical Nutrition*, *54*(5), 936–943. PMID:1659172

Andreou, I., Tousoulis, D., Miliou, A., Tentolouris, C., Zisimos, K., Gounari, P., & Stefanadis, C. et al. (2010). Effects of rosuvastatin on myeloperoxidase levels in patients with chronic heart failure: A randomized placebo-controlled study. *Atherosclerosis*, *210*(1), 194–198. doi:10.1016/j.atherosclerosis.2009.10.046 PMID:19962701

Andrés, A., Satrústegui, J., & Machado, A. (1980). Development of NADPH-producing pathways in rat heart. *The Biochemical Journal*, *186*(3), 799–803. doi:10.1042/bj1860799 PMID:7396838

Andrew Taylor, R., Oliva, I., Van Tonder, R., Elefteriades, J., Dziura, J., & Moore, C. L. (2012). Point-of-care Focused Cardiac Ultrasound for the Assessment of Thoracic Aortic Dimensions, Dilation, and Aneurysmal Disease. *Academic Emergency Medicine*, *19*(2), 244–247. doi:10.1111/j.1553-2712.2011.01279.x PMID:22288871

Andrews, R. K., & Berndt, M. C. (2013). Bernard-Soulier syndrome: An update. *Seminars in Thrombosis and Hemostasis*, *39*(06), 656–662. doi:10.1055/s-0033-1353390 PMID:23929303

An, H. S., Bae, E. J., Kim, G. B., Kwon, B. S., Beak, J. S., Kim, E. K., & Yun, Y. S. et al. (2010). Pulmonary Hypertension in Preterm Infants With Bronchopulmonary Dysplasia. *Korean Circ J*, *40*(3), 131–136. doi:10.4070/kcj.2010.40.3.131 PMID:20339498

Anker, S. D., Ponikowski, P., Mitrovic, V., Peacock, W. F., & Filippatos, G. (2015). Ularitide for the treatment of acute decompensated heart failure: From preclinical to clinical studies. *European Heart Journal*, *36*(12), 715–723. doi:10.1093/eurheartj/ehu484 PMID:25670819

Annapragada, A. (2015). Advances in nanoparticle imaging technology for vascular pathologies. *Annual Review of Medicine*, *66*(1), 177–193. doi:10.1146/annurev-med-042513-125551 PMID:25587649

Anthony, D., George, P., & Eaton, C. B. (2014). Cardiac risk factors: biomarkers and genetic tests to determine cardiovascular risk. *FP Essent, 421*, 11-15. Retrieved from http://www.ncbi.nlm.nih.gov/pubmed/24936714

Antzelevitch, C., Sicouri, S., Litovsky, S. H., Lukas, A., Krishnan, S. C., Di Diego, J. M., & Liu, D. W. et al. (1991). Heterogeneity within the ventricular wall. Electrophysiology and pharmacology of epicardial, endocardial, and M cells. *Circulation Research*, *69*(6), 1427–1449. doi:10.1161/01.RES.69.6.1427 PMID:1659499

Anusha, N. (2007, November). Seneviratne, Bawani Sivagurunathan, Claudia Monaco.Toll-like receptors and macrophage activation in atherosclerosis. *Trends in Molecular Medicine*, *13*(11), 460–469. PMID:18029230

Aon, M. A., Cortassa, S., & ORourke, B. (2010). Redox-optimized ROS balance: A unifying hypothesis. *Biochimica et Biophysica Acta (BBA) -. Bioenergetics*, *1797*(6–7), 865–877. doi:10.1016/j.bbabio.2010.02.016

Aoshima, M., Yokota, M., Shiraishi, Y., Kyoku, I., Kitano, M., Shimada, I., & Mizuhara, S. (1988). Prolonged aortic cross-clamping in early infancy and method of myocardial preservation. *The Journal of Cardiovascular Surgery*, *29*(5), 591–595. PMID:3182928

Asdaq, S. M., & Inamdar, M. N. (2010). Potential of garlic and its active constituent, S-allyl cysteine, as antihypertensive and cardioprotective in presence of captopril. *Phytomedicine*, *17*(13), 1016–1026. doi:10.1016/j.phymed.2010.07.012 PMID:20739164

Ashina, K., Tsubosaka, Y., Nakamura, T., Omori, K., Kobayashi, K., Hori, M., & Murata, T. et al. (2015). Histamine Induces Vascular Hyperpermeability by Increasing Blood Flow and Endothelial Barrier Disruption In Vivo. *PLoS ONE*, *10*(7), e0132367. doi:10.1371/journal.pone.0132367 PMID:26158531

Ashrafian, H., Docherty, L., Leo, V., Towlson, C., Neilan, M., Steeples, V., & Dear, T. N. et al. (2010). A mutation in the mitochondrial fission gene Dnm1l leads to cardiomyopathy. *PLOS Genetics*, *6*(6), e1001000. doi:10.1371/journal.pgen.1001000 PMID:20585624

Aspden, P., Wolcott, J., Bootman, J. L., & Cronenwett, L. R. (Eds.). (2007). Committee on Identifying and Preventing Medication Errors. Board on Health Care Services; Institute of Medicine. Preventing Medication Errors. Washington, DC: National Academies Press.

Assimes, T. L., Knowles, J. W., Basu, A., Iribarren, C., Southwick, A., Tang, H., & Quertermous, T. et al. (2008). Susceptibility locus for clinical and subclinical coronary artery disease at chromosome 9p21 in the multi-ethnic ADVANCE study. *Human Molecular Genetics*, *17*(15), 2320–2328. doi:10.1093/hmg/ddn132 PMID:18443000

Ast, J., Jablecka, A., Bogdanski, P., Smolarek, I., Krauss, H., & Chmara, E. (2010). Evaluation of the antihypertensive effect of L-arginine supplementation in patients with mild hypertension assessed with ambulatory blood pressure monitoring. *Medical Science Monitor*, *16*(5), CR266–CR271. PMID:20424555

Aussel, C., Marhaba, R., Pelassy, C., & Breittmayer, J. P. (1996). Submicromolar La3+ concentrations block the calcium release-activated channel, and impair CD69 and CD25 expression in CD3- or thapsigargin-activated Jurkat cells. *The Biochemical Journal*, *313*(Pt 3), 909–913. doi:10.1042/bj3130909 PMID:8611174

Autiero, M., Luttun, A., Tjwa, M., & Carmeliet, P. (2003). Placental growth factor and its receptor, vascular endothelial growth factor receptor-1: Novel targets for stimulation of ischemic tissue revascularization and inhibition of angiogenic and inflammatory disorders. *Journal of Thrombosis and Haemostasis*, *1*(7), 1356–1370. doi:10.1046/j.1538-7836.2003.00263.x PMID:12871269

Azzam HA, Goneim HR, El-Saddik AM, Azmy E, Hassan M, El-Sharawy S. 2012. The condensed MCMDM-1 VWD bleeding questionnaire as a predictor of bleeding disorders in women with unexplained menorrhagia. *Blood Coagulation & Fibrinolysis: An International Journal in Haemostasis and Thrombosis, 23*, 311-5.

Baber, U., Brener, S., Sergie, Z., Yu, J., Xu, K., Dangas, G., & Stone, G. et al. (2012). Impact of bivalirudin on access and non-access related bleeding in patients undergoing balloon aortic valvuloplasty: Results from A 2 center registry. *Journal of the American College of Cardiology*, *59*, E42.

Baddour, L. M., Wilson, W. R., Bayer, A. S., Fowler, V. G. Jr, Tleyjeh, I. M., Rybak, M. J., & Taubert, K. A. et al. (2015). Infective Endocarditis in Adults: Diagnosis, Antimicrobial Therapy, and Management of Complications: A Scientific Statement for Healthcare Professionals From the American Heart Association. *Circulation*, *132*(15), 1435–1486. doi:10.1161/CIR.0000000000000296 PMID:26373316

Baeuerle, P. A. (1998). IkB–NF-kB Structures: At the interface of inflammation control. *Cell*, *95*, 729–731. doi:10.1016/S0092-8674(00)81694-3 PMID:9865689

Bagnall, R. D., Das, J., Duflou, J., & Semsarian, C. (2014). Exome analysis–based molecular autopsy in cases of sudden unexplained death in the young. *Heart Rhythm*, *11*(4), 655–662. doi:10.1016/j.hrthm.2014.01.017 PMID:24440382

Bahrami, H., Kronmal, R., Bluemke, D. A., Olson, J., Shea, S., Liu, K., & Lima, J. A. et al. (2008). Differences in the incidence of congestive heart failure by ethnicity: The Multi-Ethnic Study of Atherosclerosis. *Archives of Internal Medicine*, *168*(19), 2138–2145. doi:10.1001/archinte.168.19.2138 PMID:18955644

Bailey, D. (2015). *Guidelines on autopsy practice: Sudden death with likely cardiac pathology*. Retrieved from http://www.rcpath.org/NR/rdonlyres/98390BBB-BEF4-4459-A0AE-EE34366D327C/0/G145_DRAFT_GAPCardiacDeath_Apr15.pdf

Bailey, J. C., Feelisch, M., Horowitz, J. D., Frenneaux, M. P., & Madhani, M. (2014). Pharmacology and therapeutic role of inorganic nitrite and nitrate in vasodilatation. *Pharmacology & Therapeutics*, *144*(3), 303–320. doi:10.1016/j.pharmthera.2014.06.009 PMID:24992304

Baker, C. D., Abman, S. H., & Mourani, P. M. (2014). Pulmonary Hypertension in Preterm Infants with Bronchopulmonary Dysplasia. *Pediatric Allergy, Immunology, and Pulmonology*, *27*(1), 8–16. doi:10.1089/ped.2013.0323 PMID:24669351

Bak, Z., Sjoberg, F., Rousseau, A., Steinvall, I., & Janerot-Sjoberg, B. (2007). Human cardiovascular dose-response to supplemental oxygen. *Acta Physiologica (Oxford, England), 191*(1), 15–24. doi:10.1111/j.1748-1716.2007.01710.x PMID:17506865

Balasubramaniam, V., Mervis, C. F., Maxey, A. M., Markham, N. E., & Abman, S. H. (2007). Hyperoxia reduces bone marrow, circulating, and lung endothelial progenitor cells in the developing lung: Implications for the pathogenesis of bronchopulmonary dysplasia. *American Journal of Physiology. Lung Cellular and Molecular Physiology, 292*(5), L1073–L1084. doi:10.1152/ajplung.00347.2006 PMID:17209139

Balcerczyk, A., & Pirola, L. (2010). Therapeutic potential of activators and inhibitors of sirtuins. *BioFactors (Oxford, England), 36*(5), 383–393. doi:10.1002/biof.112 PMID:20848588

Baldini, M. G. (1969). Platelet defect in Wiskott-Aldrich syndrome. *The New England Journal of Medicine, 281*(2), 107. doi:10.1056/NEJM196907102810224 PMID:5784770

Baldwin, A. S. Jr. (1996). The NF-kB and IkB proteins: New discoveries and insights. *Annual Review of Immunology, 14*(1), 649–681. doi:10.1146/annurev.immunol.14.1.649 PMID:8717528

Bandali, K. S., Belanger, M. P., & Wittnich, C. (2004). Hyperoxia causes oxygen free radical-mediated membrane injury and alters myocardial function and hemodynamics in the newborn. *American Journal of Physiology. Heart and Circulatory Physiology, 287*(2), H553–H559. doi:10.1152/ajpheart.00657.2003 PMID:15277198

Bandyk, D. F., & Armstrong, P. A. (2009). Use of intravascular ultrasound as a "Quality Control" technique during carotid stent-angioplasty: Are there risks to its use? *The Journal of Cardiovascular Surgery, 50*(6), 727–733. PMID:19935603

Baron, E. J., Scott, J. D., & Tompkins, L. S. (2005). Prolonged Incubation and Extensive Subculturing Do Not Increase Recovery of Clinically Significant Microorganisms from Standard Automated Blood Cultures. *Clinical Infectious Diseases, 41*(11), 1677–1680. doi:10.1086/497595 PMID:16267743

Barry, J., Campbell, S., Nabel, E. G., Mead, K., & Selwyn, A. P. (1987). Ambulatory monitoring of the digitized electrocardiogram for detection and early warning of transient myocardial ischemia in angina pectoris. *The American Journal of Cardiology, 60*(7), 483–488. doi:10.1016/0002-9149(87)90290-6 PMID:3115078

Basile & Bloch. (2015). *Overview of hypertension in adults*. Retrieved from http://www.uptodate.com/contents/overview-of-hypertension-in-adults?source=search_result&search=hypertension+overview&selectedTitle=1~150

Basso, C., Burke, M., Fornes, P., Gallagher, P. J., de Gouveia, R. H., Sheppard, M., & van der Wal, A. et al. (2008). Guidelines for autopsy investigation of sudden cardiac death. *Virchows Archiv, 452*(1), 11–18. doi:10.1007/s00428-007-0505-5 PMID:17952460

Basso, C., Burke, M., Fornes, P., Gallagher, P. J., De Gouveia, R. H., Sheppard, M., & Van Der Wal, A. et al. (2010). Association for European Cardiovascular Pathology. Guidelines for autopsy investigation of sudden cardiac death. *Pathologica, 102*(5), 391–404. PMID:21361120

Bates, D. O., & Harper, S. J. (2002). Regulation of vascular permeability by vascular endothelial growth factors. *Vascular Pharmacology, 39*(4-5), 225–237. doi:10.1016/S1537-1891(03)00011-9 PMID:12747962

Battelli, M. G., Polito, L., Bortolotti, M., & Bolognesi, A. (2016). Xanthine Oxidoreductase-Derived Reactive Species: Physiological and Pathological Effects. *Oxidative Medicine and Cellular Longevity, 3527579*. doi:10.1155/2016/3527579 PMID:26823950

Baudhuin, L. M., Miller, W. L., Train, L., Bryant, S., Hartman, K. A., Phelps, M., & Jaffe, A. S. et al. (2010). Relation of ADRB1, CYP2D6, and UGT1A1 polymorphisms with dose of, and response to, carvedilol or metoprolol therapy in patients with chronic heart failure. *The American Journal of Cardiology*, *106*(3), 402–408. doi:10.1016/j.amjcard.2010.03.041 PMID:20643254

Bauerly, K., Harris, C., Chowanadisai, W., Graham, J., Havel, P. J., Tchaparian, E., & Rucker, R. B. et al. (2011). Altering pyrroloquinoline quinone nutritional status modulates mitochondrial, lipid, and energy metabolism in rats. *PLoS ONE*, *6*(7), e21779. doi:10.1371/journal.pone.0021779 PMID:21814553

Beckers, C. M., Knezevic, N., Valent, E. T., Tauseef, M., Krishnan, R., Rajendran, K., & van Nieuw Amerongen, G. P. et al. (2015). ROCK2 primes the endothelium for vascular hyperpermeability responses by raising baseline junctional tension. *Vascular Pharmacology*, *70*, 45–54. doi:10.1016/j.vph.2015.03.017 PMID:25869521

Bell, S. (2009). Forensic chemistry. *Annual Review of Analytical Chemistry*, *2*(1), 297–319. doi:10.1146/annurev-anchem-060908-155251 PMID:20636064

Belmont, P. J., Chen, W. J., San Pedro, M. N., Thuerauf, D. J., Gellings Lowe, N., Gude, N., & Glembotski, C. C. et al. (2010). Roles for endoplasmic reticulum-associated degradation and the novel endoplasmic reticulum stress response gene Derlin-3 in the ischemic heart. *Circulation Research*, *106*(2), 307–316. doi:10.1161/CIRCRESAHA.109.203901 PMID:19940266

Benard, G., Bellance, N., James, D., Parrone, P., Fernandez, H., Letellier, T., & Rossignol, R. (2007). Mitochondrial bioenergetics and structural network organization. *Journal of Cell Science*, *120*(Pt 5), 838–848. doi:10.1242/jcs.03381 PMID:17298981

Benden, C., Edwards, L. B., Kucheryavaya, A. Y., Christie, J. D., Dipchand, A. I., Dobbels, F., & Hertz, M. I. et al. (2012). The Registry of the International Society for Heart and Lung Transplantation: Fifteenth pediatric lung and heart-lung transplantation report2012. *The Journal of Heart and Lung Transplantation*, *31*(10), 1087–1095. doi:10.1016/j.healun.2012.08.005 PMID:22975098

Benton, N. G., & Maginot, K. R. (2007). Sudden Cardiac Death in Young Athletes: Trying to Find the Needle in the Haystack. *WMJ: Official Publication of the State Medical Society of Wisconsin*, *106*(6), 335–342. PMID:17970016

Benvenuto, M., Benziger, D. P., Yankelev, S., & Vigliani, G. (2006). Pharmacokinetics and tolerability of daptomycin at doses up to 12 milligrams per kilogram of body weight once daily in healthy volunteers. *Antimicrobial Agents and Chemotherapy*, *50*(10), 3245–3249. doi:10.1128/AAC.00247-06 PMID:17005801

Berenson, G. S., Wattigney, W. A., Bao, W., Srinivasan, S. R., & Radhakrishnamurthy, B. (1995). Rationale to Study the Early Natural History of Heart Disease: The Bogalusa Heart Study. *The American Journal of the Medical Sciences*, *310*, S22–S28. doi:10.1097/00000441-199512000-00005 PMID:7503119

Bernardo, B. C., Weeks, K. L., Pretorius, L., & McMullen, J. R. (2010). Molecular distinction between physiological and pathological cardiac hypertrophy: Experimental findings and therapeutic strategies. *Pharmacology & Therapeutics*, *128*(1), 191–227. doi:10.1016/j.pharmthera.2010.04.005 PMID:20438756

Berridge, M. J. (1993). Inositol trisphosphate and calcium signalling. *Nature*, *361*(6410), 315–325. doi:10.1038/361315a0 PMID:8381210

Berridge, M. J., Bootman, M. D., & Roderick, H. L. (2003). Calcium signalling: Dynamics, homeostasis and remodelling. *Nature Reviews. Molecular Cell Biology*, *4*(7), 517–529. doi:10.1038/nrm1155 PMID:12838335

Bers, D. M. (2002). Cardiac excitation-contraction coupling. *Nature*, *415*(6868), 198–205. doi:10.1038/415198a PMID:11805843

Bers, D. M. (2008). Calcium cycling and signaling in cardiac myocytes. *Annual Review of Physiology*, *70*(1), 23–49. doi:10.1146/annurev.physiol.70.113006.100455 PMID:17988210

Bhatnagar, S., Panguluri, S. K., Gupta, S. K., Dahiya, S., Lundy, R. F., & Kumar, A. (2010). Tumor necrosis factor-alpha regulates distinct molecular pathways and gene networks in cultured skeletal muscle cells. *PLoS ONE*, *5*(10), e13262. doi:10.1371/journal.pone.0013262 PMID:20967264

Bijani, F. M. (2012). Toll-like receptor signaling pathways in cardiovascular diseases: Challenges and opportunities. *International Reviews of Immunology*, *31*(5), 379–395. doi:10.3109/08830185.2012.706761 PMID:23083347

Binder, A., & Aledort, L. (2015). Glanzmann's thrombasthenia: meeting the anticoagulation challenge. *Haemophilia: The Official Journal of the World Federation of Hemophilia.*

Birben, E., Sahiner, U. M., Sackesen, C., Erzurum, S., & Kalayci, O. (2012). Oxidative Stress and Antioxidant Defense. *The World Allergy Organization Journal, 5*(1), 9-19. doi: 10.1097/WOX.0b013e3182439613

Bird, G. S., Hwang, S. Y., Smyth, J. T., Fukushima, M., Boyles, R. R., & Putney, J. W. Jr. (2009). STIM1 is a calcium sensor specialized for digital signaling. *Current Biology*, *19*(20), 1724–1729. doi:10.1016/j.cub.2009.08.022 PMID:19765994

Birnbaumer, L. (2009). The TRPC class of ion channels: A critical review of their roles in slow, sustained increases in intracellular Ca(2+) concentrations. *Annual Review of Pharmacology and Toxicology*, *49*(1), 395–426. doi:10.1146/annurev.pharmtox.48.113006.094928 PMID:19281310

Birukova, A. A., Smurova, K., Birukov, K. G., Kaibuchi, K., Garcia, J. G., & Verin, A. D. (2004). Role of Rho GTPases in thrombin-induced lung vascular endothelial cells barrier dysfunction. *Microvascular Research*, *67*(1), 64–77. doi:10.1016/j.mvr.2003.09.007 PMID:14709404

Bishayee, A., Barnes, K. F., Bhatia, D., Darvesh, A. S., & Carroll, R. T. (2010). Resveratrol suppresses oxidative stress and inflammatory response in diethylnitrosamine-initiated rat hepatocarcinogenesis. *Cancer Prevention Research (Philadelphia, Pa.)*, *3*(6), 753–763. doi:10.1158/1940-6207.CAPR-09-0171 PMID:20501860

Bjorkegren, J. L., Kovacic, J. C., Dudley, J. T., & Schadt, E. E. (2015). Genome-wide significant loci: How important are they? Systems genetics to understand heritability of coronary artery disease and other common complex disorders. *Journal of the American College of Cardiology*, *65*(8), 830–845. doi:10.1016/j.jacc.2014.12.033 PMID:25720628

Black, B. L., & Olson, E. N. (1998). Transcriptional control of muscle development by myocyte enhancer factor-2 (mef2) proteins. *Annual Review of Cell and Developmental Biology*, *14*(1), 167–196. doi:10.1146/annurev.cellbio.14.1.167 PMID:9891782

Blaho, V. A., Galvani, S., Engelbrecht, E., Liu, C., Swendeman, S. L., Kono, M., & Hla, T. et al. (2015). HDL-bound sphingosine-1-phosphate restrains lymphopoiesis and neuroinflammation. *Nature*, *523*(7560), 342–346. doi:10.1038/nature14462 PMID:26053123

Blankenberg, S., Barbaux, S., & Tiret, L. (2003). Adhesion molecules and atherosclerosis. *Atherosclerosis*, *170*(2), 191–203. doi:10.1016/S0021-9150(03)00097-2 PMID:14612198

Blasig, I. E., Ebert, B., Hennig, C., Pali, T., & Tosaki, A. (1990). Inverse relationship between ESR spin trapping of oxyradicals and degree of functional recovery during myocardial reperfusion in isolated working rat heart. *Cardiovascular Research*, *24*(4), 263–270. doi:10.1093/cvr/24.4.263 PMID:2161288

Blauwet, L. A., & Cooper, L. T. (2010). Myocarditis. *Progress in Cardiovascular Diseases*, *52*(4), 274–288. doi:10.1016/j.pcad.2009.11.006 PMID:20109598

Blavignac, J., Bunimov, N., Rivard, G. E., & Hayward, C. P. (2011). Quebec platelet disorder: Update on pathogenesis, diagnosis, and treatment. *Seminars in Thrombosis and Hemostasis*, *37*(06), 713–720. doi:10.1055/s-0031-1291382 PMID:22102275

Block, G., Mangels, A. R., Norkus, E. P., Patterson, B. H., Levander, O. A., & Taylor, P. R. (2001). Ascorbic acid status and subsequent diastolic and systolic blood pressure. *Hypertension*, *37*(2), 261–267. doi:10.1161/01.HYP.37.2.261 PMID:11230282

Bloom, D. E., Cafiero, E. T., Jané-Llopis, E., Abrahams-Gessel, S., Bloom, L. R., Fathima, S., . . . Weinstein, C. (2011). *The Global Economic Burden of Non-communicable Diseases*. Retrieved from www.weforum.org/EconomicsOfNCD

Boczek, N. J., Tester, D. J., & Ackerman, M. J. (2012). The molecular autopsy: an indispensable step following sudden cardiac death in the young? *Herzschrittmachertherapie & Elektrophysiologie*, *23*(3). doi:10.1007/s00399-012-0222-x

Bogaard, H. J., Abe, K., Vonk Noordegraaf, A., & Voelkel, N. F. (2009). The right ventricle under pressure: Cellular and molecular mechanisms of right-heart failure in pulmonary hypertension. *Chest*, *135*(3), 794–804. doi:10.1378/chest.08-0492 PMID:19265089

Boleracki, M., Farkas, F., Meszely, A., Szikszai, Z., & Sik Lanyi, C. (2015). Developing an Animal Counting Game in Second Life for a Young Adult with Down Syndrome. *Studies in Health Technology and Informatics*, *217*, 71–77. PMID:26294455

Bolli, R., Jeroudi, M. O., Patel, B. S., DuBose, C. M., Lai, E. K., Roberts, R., & McCay, P. B. (1989a). Direct evidence that oxygen-derived free radicals contribute to postischemic myocardial dysfunction in the intact dog. *Proceedings of the National Academy of Sciences of the United States of America*, *86*(12), 4695–4699. doi:10.1073/pnas.86.12.4695 PMID:2543984

Boros, P., Ochando, J. C., Chen, S. H., & Bromberg, J. S. (2010). Myeloid-derived suppressor cells: Natural regulators for transplant tolerance. *Human Immunology*, *71*(11), 1061–1066. doi:10.1016/j.humimm.2010.08.001 PMID:20705113

Bøtker, H. E., Kharbanda, R., Schmidt, M. R., Bøttcher, M., Kaltoft, A. K., Terkelsen, C. J., & Nielsen, T. T. et al. (2010). Remote ischaemic conditioning before hospital admission, as a complement to angioplasty, and effect on myocardial salvage in patients with acute myocardial infarction: A randomised trial. *Lancet*, *375*(9716), 727–734. doi:10.1016/S0140-6736(09)62001-8 PMID:20189026

Bottega, R., Pecci, A., De Candia, E., Pujol-Moix, N., Heller, P. G., Noris, P., & Savoia, A. et al. (2013). Correlation between platelet phenotype and NBEAL2 genotype in patients with congenital thrombocytopenia and alpha-granule deficiency. *Haematologica*, *98*(6), 868–874. doi:10.3324/haematol.2012.075861 PMID:23100277

Bottillo, I., Castori, M., De Bernardo, C., Fabbri, R., Grammatico, B., Preziosi, N., & Grammatico, P. et al. (2013). Prenatal diagnosis and post-mortem examination in a fetus with thrombocytopenia-absent radius (TAR) syndrome due to compound heterozygosity for a 1q21.1 microdeletion and a RBM8A hypomorphic allele: A case report. *BMC Research Notes*, *6*(1), 376. doi:10.1186/1756-0500-6-376 PMID:24053387

Brady, N. R., Elmore, S. P., van Beek, J. J., Krab, K., Courtoy, P. J., Hue, L., & Westerhoff, H. V. (2004). Coordinated behavior of mitochondria in both space and time: A reactive oxygen species-activated wave of mitochondrial depolarization. *Biophysical Journal*, *87*(3), 2022–2034. doi:10.1529/biophysj.103.035097 PMID:15345578

Bragadottir, G., Birgisdottir, E. R., Gudmundsdottir, B. R., Hilmarsdottir, B., Vidarsson, B., Magnusson, M. K., & Onundarson, P. T. et al. (2015). Clinical phenotype in heterozygote and biallelic Bernard-Soulier syndromea case control study. *American Journal of Hematology*, *90*(2), 149–155. doi:10.1002/ajh.23891 PMID:25370924

Braidy, N., Guillemin, G. J., Mansour, H., Chan-Ling, T., Poljak, A., & Grant, R. (2011). Age related changes in NAD+ metabolism oxidative stress and Sirt1 activity in wistar rats. *PLoS ONE*, *6*(4), e19194. doi:10.1371/journal.pone.0019194 PMID:21541336

Brand, K., Page, S., Rogler, G., Bartsch, A., Brandl, R., Knuechel, R., & Neumeier, D. et al. (1996, April1). Activated transcription factor nuclear factor-kappa B is present in the atherosclerotic lesion. *The Journal of Clinical Investigation*, *97*(7), 1715–1722. doi:10.1172/JCI118598 PMID:8601637

Brandman, O., Liou, J., Park, W. S., & Meyer, T. (2007). STIM2 is a feedback regulator that stabilizes basal cytosolic and endoplasmic reticulum Ca2+ levels. *Cell*, *131*(7), 1327–1339. doi:10.1016/j.cell.2007.11.039 PMID:18160041

Braunersreuther, V., Montecucco, F., Asrih, M., Pelli, G., Galan, K., Frias, M., & Jaquet, V. et al. (2013). Role of NADPH oxidase isoforms NOX1, NOX2 and NOX4 in myocardial ischemia/reperfusion injury. *Journal of Molecular and Cellular Cardiology*, *64*, 99–107. doi:10.1016/j.yjmcc.2013.09.007 PMID:24051369

Brenner, J. S., & Dolmetsch, R. E. (2007). TrpC3 regulates hypertrophy-associated gene expression without affecting myocyte beating or cell size. *PLoS ONE*, *2*(8), e802. doi:10.1371/journal.pone.0000802 PMID:17726532

Brinkley, T. E., Lovato, J. F., Arnold, A. M., Furberg, C. D., Kuller, L. H., Burke, G. L., & Williamson, J. D. et al. (2010). Effect of Ginkgo biloba on blood pressure and incidence of hypertension in elderly men and women. *American Journal of Hypertension*, *23*(5), 528–533. doi:10.1038/ajh.2010.14 PMID:20168306

Britt, N. S., Potter, E. M., Patel, N., & Steed, M. E. (2015). Comparison of the Effectiveness and Safety of Linezolid and Daptomycin in Vancomycin-Resistant Enterococcal Bloodstream Infection: A National Cohort Study of Veterans Affairs Patients. *Clinical Infectious Diseases*, *61*(6), 871–878. doi:10.1093/cid/civ444 PMID:26063715

Broadbent, H. M., Peden, J. F., Lorkowski, S., Goel, A., Ongen, H., Green, F., & Watkins, H. et al. (2008). Susceptibility to coronary artery disease and diabetes is encoded by distinct, tightly linked SNPs in the ANRIL locus on chromosome 9p. *Human Molecular Genetics*, *17*(6), 806–814. doi:10.1093/hmg/ddm352 PMID:18048406

Brock, T. G., & Giulio, C. D. (2006). Prolonged Exposure to Hyperoxia Increases Perivascular Mast Cells in Rat Lungs. *The Journal of Histochemistry and Cytochemistry*, *54*(11), 1239–1246. doi:10.1369/jhc.6A7007.2006 PMID:16899761

Bronze-da-Rocha, E. (2014). MicroRNAs expression profiles in cardiovascular diseases. *Biomed Res Int*, *985408*. doi:10.1155/2014/985408 PMID:25013816

Bronze-da-Rocha, E., Novoa, A., Teixeira, N., Vasconcelos, C. S., Cerveira, C., Castro e Melo, J., & Carvalho, M. C. (2012). Evaluation of the reactivity of sera from patients with systemic lupus erythematosus against the human MCP1. *Journal of Clinical Immunology*, *32*(4), 721–728. doi:10.1007/s10875-012-9665-4 PMID:22371290

Brook, R. D., Appel, L. J., Rubenfire, M., Ogedegbe, G., Bisognano, J. D., Elliott, W. J., & Rajagopalan, S. et al. (2013). Beyond medications and diet: Alternative approaches to lowering blood pressure a scientific statement from the American heart association. *Hypertension*, *61*(6), 1360–1383. doi:10.1161/HYP.0b013e318293645f PMID:23608661

Brooks, A. C., Guo, Y., Singh, M., McCracken, J., Xuan, Y. T., Srivastava, S., & Bhatnagar, A. et al. (2014). Endoplasmic reticulum stress-dependent activation of ATF3 mediates the late phase of ischemic preconditioning. *Journal of Molecular and Cellular Cardiology*, *76*, 138–147. doi:10.1016/j.yjmcc.2014.08.011 PMID:25151953

Brown, J. M., White, C. W., Terada, L. S., Grosso, M. A., Shanley, P. F., Mulvin, D. W., & Repine, J. E. et al. (1990). Interleukin 1 pretreatment decreases ischemia/reperfusion injury. *Proceedings of the National Academy of Sciences of the United States of America*, *87*(13), 5026–5030. doi:10.1073/pnas.87.13.5026 PMID:2367521

Brunet, S., Aimond, F., Li, H., Guo, W., Eldstrom, J., Fedida, D., & Nerbonne, J. M. et al. (2004). Heterogeneous expression of repolarizing, voltage-gated K+ currents in adult mouse ventricles. *The Journal of Physiology*, *559*(Pt 1), 103–120. doi:10.1113/jphysiol.2004.063347 PMID:15194740

Brusin, J. H. (2008). Osteogenesis imperfecta. *Radiologic Technology*, *79*, 535–548, quiz 49–51. PMID:18650529

Budnitz, D. S., Lovegrove, M. C., Shehab, N., & Richards, C. L. (2011). Emergency Hospitalizations for Adverse Drug Events in Older Americans. *The New England Journal of Medicine*, *365*(21), 2002–2012. doi:10.1056/NEJMsa1103053 PMID:22111719

Buitrago, L., Rendon, A., Liang, Y., Simeoni, I., Negri, A., Filizola, M., & Coller, B. S. et al. (2015). alphaIIbbeta3 variants defined by next-generation sequencing: Predicting variants likely to cause Glanzmann thrombasthenia. *Proceedings of the National Academy of Sciences of the United States of America*, *112*(15), E1898–E1907. doi:10.1073/pnas.1422238112 PMID:25827233

Burke, B. E., Neuenschwander, R., & Olson, R. D. (2001). Randomized, double-blind, placebo-controlled trial of coenzyme Q10 in isolated systolic hypertension. *Southern Medical Journal*, *94*(11), 1112–1117. doi:10.1097/00007611-200111000-00015 PMID:11780680

Burke, V., Hodgson, J. M., Beilin, L. J., Giangiulioi, N., Rogers, P., & Puddey, I. B. (2001). Dietary protein and soluble fiber reduce ambulatory blood pressure in treated hypertensives. *Hypertension*, *38*(4), 821–826. doi:10.1161/hy1001.092614 PMID:11641293

Bush, E. W., Hood, D. B., Papst, P. J., Chapo, J. A., Minobe, W., Bristow, M. R., & McKinsey, T. A. et al. (2006). Canonical transient receptor potential channels promote cardiomyocyte hypertrophy through activation of calcineurin signaling. *The Journal of Biological Chemistry*, *281*(44), 33487–33496. doi:10.1074/jbc.M605536200 PMID:16950785

Buxton, D. B. (2009). Nanomedicine for the management of lung and blood diseases. *Nanomedicine (London)*, *4*(3), 331–339. doi:10.2217/nnm.09.8 PMID:19331540

Cacciuttolo, M. A., Trinh, L., Lumpkin, J. A., & Rao, G. (1993). Hyperoxia induces DNA damage in mammalian cells. *Free Radical Biology & Medicine*, *14*(3), 267–276. doi:10.1016/0891-5849(93)90023-N PMID:8458584

Caforio, A. L., Pankuweit, S., Arbustini, E., Basso, C., Gimeno-Blanes, J., Felix, S. B., & Elliott, P. M. et al. (2013). Current state of knowledge on aetiology, diagnosis, management, and therapy of myocarditis: A position statement of the European Society of Cardiology Working Group on Myocardial and Pericardial Diseases. *European Heart Journal*, *34*(33), 2636–2648. doi:10.1093/eurheartj/eht210 PMID:23824828

Cahalan, M. D. (2009). STIMulating store-operated Ca(2+) entry. *Nature Cell Biology*, *11*(6), 669–677. doi:10.1038/ncb0609-669 PMID:19488056

Cahill, T. J., Leo, V., Kelly, M., Stockenhuber, A., Kennedy, N. W., Bao, L., & Ashrafian, H. et al. (2015). Resistance of dynamin-related protein 1 oligomers to disassembly impairs mitophagy, resulting in myocardial inflammation and heart failure. *The Journal of Biological Chemistry*, *290*(43), 25907–25919. doi:10.1074/jbc.M115.665695 PMID:26370078

Cai, Z. P., Parajuli, N., Zheng, X., & Becker, L. (2012). Remote ischemic preconditioning confers late protection against myocardial ischemia-reperfusion injury in mice by upregulating interleukin-10. *Basic Research in Cardiology*, *107*(4), 277–277. doi:10.1007/s00395-012-0277-1 PMID:22752341

Campobasso, C. P., DellErba, A. S., Addante, A., Zotti, F., Marzullo, A., & Colonna, M. F. (2008). Sudden cardiac death and myocardial ischemia indicators: A comparative study of four immunohistochemical markers. *The American Journal of Forensic Medicine and Pathology*, *29*(2), 154–161. doi:10.1097/PAF.0b013e318177eab7 PMID:18520484

Cao, S., Liu, Y., Wang, H., Mao, X., Chen, J., Liu, J., . . . Yu, T. (2016). Ischemic postconditioning influences electron transport chain protein turnover in Langendorff-perfused rat hearts. *PeerJ, 4*, e1706. doi: 10.7717/peerj.1706

Cao, X., Choi, S., Maleth, J. J., Park, S., Ahuja, M., & Muallem, S. (2015). The ER/PM microdomain, PI(4,5)P(2) and the regulation of STIM1-Orai1 channel function. *Cell Calcium*, *58*(4), 342–348. doi:10.1016/j.ceca.2015.03.003 PMID:25843208

Cardellini, M., Menghini, R., Martelli, E., Casagrande, V., Marino, A., Rizza, S., & Federici, M. et al. (2009). TIMP3 is reduced in atherosclerotic plaques from subjects with type 2 diabetes and increased by SirT1. *Diabetes*, *58*(10), 2396–2401. doi:10.2337/db09-0280 PMID:19581416

Carlsson, M., Andersson, R., Bloch, K. M., Steding-Ehrenborg, K., Mosen, H., Stahlberg, F., & Arheden, H. et al. (2012). Cardiac output and cardiac index measured with cardiovascular magnetic resonance in healthy subjects, elite athletes and patients with congestive heart failure. *Journal of Cardiovascular Magnetic Resonance*, *14*(1), 51. doi:10.1186/1532-429X-14-51 PMID:22839436

Casapao, A. M., Kullar, R., Davis, S. L., Levine, D. P., Zhao, J. J., Potoski, B. A., & Rybak, M. J. et al. (2013). Multicenter study of high-dose daptomycin for treatment of enterococcal infections. *Antimicrobial Agents and Chemotherapy*, *57*(9), 4190–4196. doi:10.1128/AAC.00526-13 PMID:23774437

Caslake, M. J., Packard, C. J., Suckling, K. E., Holmes, S. D., Chamberlain, P., & Macphee, C. H. (2000). Lipoprotein-associated phospholipase A(2), platelet-activating factor acetylhydrolase: A potential new risk factor for coronary artery disease. *Atherosclerosis*, *150*(2), 413–419. Retrieved from http://www.ncbi.nlm.nih.gov/pubmed/10856534 doi:10.1016/S0021-9150(99)00406-2 PMID:10856534

Castro, C., Gil Lorenzo, A., Gonzalez, A., & Cruzado, M. (2010). Garlic components inhibit angiotensin II-induced cell-cycle progression and migration: Involvement of cell-cycle inhibitor p27(Kip1) and mitogen-activated protein kinase. *Molecular Nutrition & Food Research*, *54*(6), 781–787. doi:10.1002/mnfr.200900108 PMID:19904760

Cattelan, A., Ceolotto, G., Bova, S., Albiero, M., Kuppusamy, M., De Martin, S., & Avogaro, A. et al. (2015). NAD(+)-dependent SIRT1 deactivation has a key role on ischemia-reperfusion-induced apoptosis. *Vascular Pharmacology*, *70*, 35–44. doi:10.1016/j.vph.2015.02.004 PMID:25863291

Ceconi, C., Bernocchi, P., Boraso, A., Cargnoni, A., Pepi, P., Curello, S., & Ferrari, R. (2000). New insights on myocardial pyridine nucleotides and thiol redox state in ischemia and reperfusion damage. *Cardiovascular Research*, *47*(3), 586–594. doi:10.1016/S0008-6363(00)00104-8 PMID:10963731

Cencioni, C., Spallotta, F., Mai, A., Martelli, F., Farsetti, A., Zeiher, A. M., & Gaetano, C. (2015). Sirtuin function in aging heart and vessels. *Journal of Molecular and Cellular Cardiology*, *83*, 55–61. doi:10.1016/j.yjmcc.2014.12.023 PMID:25579854

Center for Disease Control. (2015a). *National Health and Nutrition Examination Survey*. Retrieved from http://www.cdc.gov/nchs/nhanes/about_nhanes.htm

Center for Disease Control. (2015b). *Cardiovascular disease*. Retrieved from http://wwwn.cdc.gov/Nchs/Nhanes/2013-2014/CDQ_H.htm, accessed December 22, 2015

Center for Disease Control. (2015c). *About Adult Obesity*. Retrieved from http://www.cdc.gov/healthyweight/assessing/bmi/adult_bmi/index.html#Definition

Center for Disease Control. (2015d). *Heart Disease Facts*. Retrieved from http://www.cdc.gov/heartdisease/facts.htm

Center for Disease Control. (2016a). *Leading Causes of Death: 1900-1998*. Retrieved from http://www.cdc.gov/nchs/data/dvs/lead1900_98.pdf

Center for Disease Control. (2016b). *Top 10 Leading Causes of Death: United States, 1999–2013*. Retrieved from http://blogs.cdc.gov/nchs-data-visualization/leading-causes-of-death/

Cervelli, T., Borghini, A., Galli, A., & Andreassi, M. G. (2012). DNA damage and repair in atherosclerosis: Current insights and future perspectives. *International Journal of Molecular Sciences*, *13*(12), 16929–16944. doi:10.3390/ijms131216929 PMID:23443128

Chaggar, P. S., Malkin, C. J., Shaw, S. M., Williams, S. G., & Channer, K. S. (2009). Neuroendocrine effects on the heart and targets for therapeutic manipulation in heart failure. *Cardiovascular Therapeutics*, *27*(3), 187–193. doi:10.1111/j.1755-5922.2009.00094.x PMID:19689618

Chai, J. G., Ratnasothy, K., Bucy, R. P., Noelle, R. J., Lechler, R., & Lombardi, G. (2015). Allospecific CD4(+) T cells retain effector function and are actively regulated by Treg cells in the context of transplantation tolerance. *European Journal of Immunology*, *45*(7), 2017–2027. doi:10.1002/eji.201545455 PMID:25944401

Chambers, D. E., Parks, D. A., Patterson, G., Roy, R., McCord, J. M., Yoshida, S., & Downey, J. M. et al. (1985). Xanthine oxidase as a source of free radical damage in myocardial ischemia. *Journal of Molecular and Cellular Cardiology*, *17*(2), 145–152. doi:10.1016/S0022-2828(85)80017-1 PMID:3839024

Chambers, H. F. (2001). The changing epidemiology of Staphylococcus aureus? *Emerging Infectious Diseases*, *7*(2), 178–182. doi:10.3201/eid0702.010204 PMID:11294701

Chan, J., Rhee, J., & Farokhzad, O. (2011). In vivo prevention of arterial restenosis with paclitaxel-encapsulated targeted lipid—polymeric nanoparticles. *Proceedings of the National Academy of Sciences of the United States of America.*

Chang, T. C., & Mendell, J. T. (2007). microRNAs in vertebrate physiology and human disease. *Annual Review of Genomics and Human Genetics*, *8*(1), 215–239. doi:10.1146/annurev.genom.8.080706.092351 PMID:17506656

Chapalamadugu, K. C., Panguluri, S. K., Bennett, E. S., Kolliputi, N., & Tipparaju, S. M. (2015). High level of oxygen treatment causes cardiotoxicity with arrhythmias and redox modulation. *Toxicology and Applied Pharmacology*, *282*(1), 100–107. doi:10.1016/j.taap.2014.10.019 PMID:25447406

Chava, K. R., Tauseef, M., Sharma, T., & Mehta, D. (2012). Cyclic AMP response element-binding protein prevents endothelial permeability increase through transcriptional controlling p190RhoGAP expression. *Blood*, *119*(1), 308–319. doi:10.1182/blood-2011-02-339473 PMID:22049513

Chavan, A. V., & Somani, R. R. (2010). HDAC inhibitors - new generation of target specific treatment. *Mini Reviews in Medicinal Chemistry*, *10*(13), 1263–1276. doi:10.2174/138955751100091263 PMID:20701588

Chavez, A., Schmidt, T. T., Yazbeck, P., Rajput, C., Desai, B., Sukriti, S., & Mehta, D. et al. (2015). S1PR1 Tyr143 phosphorylation downregulates endothelial cell surface S1PR1 expression and responsiveness. *Journal of Cell Science*, *128*(5), 878–887. doi:10.1242/jcs.154476 PMID:25588843

Chavez, A., Smith, M., & Mehta, D. (2011). New insights into the regulation of vascular permeability. *Int Rev Cell Mol Biol*, *290*, 205–248. doi:10.1016/B978-0-12-386037-8.00001-6 PMID:21875566

Check, J., Gotteiner, N., Liu, X., Su, E., Porta, N., Steinhorn, R., & Mestan, K. K. (2013). Fetal growth restriction and pulmonary hypertension in premature infants with bronchopulmonary dysplasia. *Journal of Perinatology*, *33*(7), 553–557. doi:10.1038/jp.2012.164 PMID:23328924

Che, H., Li, G., Sun, H. Y., Xiao, G. S., Wang, Y., & Li, G. R. (2015). Roles of store-operated Ca2+ channels in regulating cell cycling and migration of human cardiac c-kit+ progenitor cells. *American Journal of Physiology. Heart and Circulatory Physiology*, *309*(10), H1772–H1781. PMID:26453325

Cheng, A., & Owens, D. (2015). Marfan syndrome, inherited aortopathies and exercise: What is the right answer? *Heart (British Cardiac Society)*, *101*(10), 752–757. doi:10.1136/heartjnl-2014-306440 PMID:25911666

Cheng, H. L., Mostoslavsky, R., Saito, S., Manis, J. P., Gu, Y., Patel, P., & Chua, K. F. et al. (2003). Developmental defects and p53 hyperacetylation in Sir2 homolog (SIRT1)-deficient mice. *Proceedings of the National Academy of Sciences of the United States of America*, *100*(19), 10794–10799. doi:10.1073/pnas.1934713100 PMID:12960381

Cheng, K. T., Ong, H. L., Liu, X., & Ambudkar, I. S. (2013). Contribution and regulation of TRPC channels in store-operated Ca2+ entry. *Curr Top Membr*, *71*, 149–179. doi:10.1016/B978-0-12-407870-3.00007-X PMID:23890115

Chen, H., Chomyn, A., & Chan, D. C. (2005). Disruption of fusion results in mitochondrial heterogeneity and dysfunction. *The Journal of Biological Chemistry*, *280*(28), 26185–26192. doi:10.1074/jbc.M503062200 PMID:15899901

Chen, H., Detmer, S. A., Ewald, A. J., Griffin, E. E., Fraser, S. E., & Chan, D. C. (2003). Mitofusins Mfn1 and Mfn2 coordinately regulate mitochondrial fusion and are essential for embryonic development. *The Journal of Cell Biology*, *160*(2), 189–200. doi:10.1083/jcb.200211046 PMID:12527753

Chen, L., Gong, Q., Stice, J. P., & Knowlton, A. A. (2009). Mitochondrial OPA1, apoptosis, and heart failure. *Cardiovascular Research*, *84*(1), 91–99. doi:10.1093/cvr/cvp181 PMID:19493956

Chen, Q., Moghaddas, S., Hoppel, C. L., & Lesnefsky, E. J. (2008). Ischemic defects in the electron transport chain increase the production of reactive oxygen species from isolated rat heart mitochondria. *American Journal of Physiology. Cell Physiology*, *294*(2), C460–C466. doi:10.1152/ajpcell.00211.2007 PMID:18077608

Chen, X., Yang, X., Liu, T., Guan, M., Feng, X., Dong, W., & Sun, Z. et al. (2012, October). Xiaojun Chen Kaempferol regulates MAPKs and NF-κB signaling pathways to attenuate LPS-induced acute lung injury in mice. *International Immunopharmacology*, *14*(2), 209–216. doi:10.1016/j.intimp.2012.07.007 PMID:22835426

Chen, Y. B., Lan, Y. W., Hung, T. H., Chen, L. G., Choo, K. B., Cheng, W. T., & Chong, K. Y. et al. (2015). Mesenchymal stem cell-based HSP70 promoter-driven VEGFA induction by resveratrol promotes angiogenesis in a mouse model. *Cell Stress & Chaperones*, *20*(4), 643–652. doi:10.1007/s12192-015-0588-x PMID:25860916

Chen, Y. H., Wu, X. D., Yao, S. T., Sun, S., & Liu, X. H. (2011). Calcineurin is involved in cardioprotection induced by ischemic postconditioning through attenuating endoplasmic reticulum stress. *Chinese Medical Journal*, *124*(20), 3334–3340. PMID:22088531

Chiao, Y. A., & Rabinovitch, P. S. (2015). The Aging Heart. *Cold Spring Harb Perspect Med*, *5*(9), a025148. doi:10.1101/cshperspect.a025148 PMID:26328932

Chinnadurai, G. (2003). CtBP family proteins: more than transcriptional corepressors. *BioEssays: News and Reviews in Molecular, Cellular and Developmental Biology*, *25*(1), 9-12. doi: 10.1002/bies.10212

Choi, E. J., Chee, K. M., & Lee, B. H. (2003). Anti- and prooxidant effects of chronic quercetin administration in rats. *European Journal of Pharmacology*, *482*(1-3), 281–285. doi:10.1016/j.ejphar.2003.09.067 PMID:14660033

Choi, W., Karim, Z. A., & Whiteheart, S. W. (2010). Protein expression in platelets from six species that differ in their open canalicular system. *Platelets*, *21*(3), 167–175. doi:10.3109/09537101003611385 PMID:20196629

Chong, E., Chang, S. L., Hsiao, Y. W., Singhal, R., Liu, S. H., Leha, T., & Chen, S. A. et al. (2015). Resveratrol, a red wine antioxidant, reduces atrial fibrillation susceptibility in the failing heart by PI3K/AKT/eNOS signaling pathway activation. *Heart Rhythm*, *12*(5), 1046–1056. doi:10.1016/j.hrthm.2015.01.044 PMID:25640634

Chong, Z. Z., Wang, S., Shang, Y. C., & Maiese, K. (2012). Targeting cardiovascular disease with novel SIRT1 pathways. *Future Cardiol*, *8*(1), 89–100. doi:10.2217/fca.11.76 PMID:22185448

Christensen, P. M., Liu, C. H., Swendeman, S. L., Obinata, H., Qvortrup, K., Nielsen, L. B., & Christoffersen, C. et al. (2016). Impaired endothelial barrier function in apolipoprotein M-deficient mice is dependent on sphingosine-1-phosphate receptor 1. *The FASEB Journal*, *30*(6), 2351–2359. doi:10.1096/fj.201500064 PMID:26956418

Chugh, S. S., Kelly, K. L., & Titus, J. L. (2000). Sudden cardiac death with apparently normal heart. *Circulation*, *102*(6), 649–654. doi:10.1161/01.CIR.102.6.649 PMID:10931805

Chung, J. H., Manganiello, V., & Dyck, J. R. (2012). Resveratrol as a calorie restriction mimetic: Therapeutic implications. *Trends in Cell Biology*, *22*(10), 546–554. doi:10.1016/j.tcb.2012.07.004 PMID:22885100

Chun, S.-S., Vattem, D. A., Lin, Y.-T., & Shetty, K. (2005). Phenolic antioxidants from clonal oregano (Origanum vulgare) with antimicrobial activity against Helicobacter pylori. *Process Biochemistry*, *40*(2), 809–816. doi:10.1016/j.procbio.2004.02.018

Cicero, A. F., Derosa, G., Manca, M., Bove, M., Borghi, C., & Gaddi, A. V. (2007). Different effect of psyllium and guar dietary supplementation on blood pressure control in hypertensive overweight patients: A six-month, randomized clinical trial. *Clinical and Experimental Hypertension (New York, N.Y.)*, *29*(6), 383–394. doi:10.1080/10641960701578378 PMID:17729055

Cífková, R. (2008). Epidemiology and risk of hypertension. *Archives of Medical Science*, *5*(2A), S199–S211.

Cioffi, D. L., Barry, C., & Stevens, T. (2010). Store-operated calcium entry channels in pulmonary endothelium: The emerging story of TRPCS and Orai1. *Advances in Experimental Medicine and Biology*, *661*, 137–154. doi:10.1007/978-1-60761-500-2_9 PMID:20204728

Circu, M. L., Maloney, R. E., & Aw, T. Y. (2011). Disruption of pyridine nucleotide redox status during oxidative challenge at normal and low-glucose states: Implications for cellular adenosine triphosphate, mitochondrial respiratory activity, and reducing capacity in colon epithelial cells. *Antioxidants & Redox Signalling*, *14*(11), 2151–2162. doi:10.1089/ars.2010.3489 PMID:21083422

Clarke, T. C., Black, L. I., Stussman, B. J., Barnes, P. M., & Nahin, R. L. (2015). Trends in the use of complementary health approaches among adults: United States, 2002–2012. *National Health Statistics Reports*, (79): 1–16. PMID:25671660

Clement, Y. (2009). Can green tea do that? A literature review of the clinical evidence. *Preventive Medicine*, *49*(2-3), 83–87. doi:10.1016/j.ypmed.2009.05.005 PMID:19465043

Clinical Annotation Levels of Evidence. (n.d.). Retrieved from https://www.pharmgkb.org/page/clinAnnLevels

Collins, H. E., Zhu-Mauldin, X., Marchase, R. B., & Chatham, J. C. (2013). STIM1/Orai1-mediated SOCE: Current perspectives and potential roles in cardiac function and pathology. *American Journal of Physiology. Heart and Circulatory Physiology*, *305*(4), H446–H458. doi:10.1152/ajpheart.00104.2013 PMID:23792674

Collins, T., Read, M. A., Neish, A. S., Whitley, M. Z., Thanos, D., & Maniatis, T. (1995). Transcriptional regulation of endothelial cell adhesion molecules: NF-kappa-B and cytokine-inducible enhancers. *The FASEB Journal*, *9*, 899–909. PMID:7542214

Colucci, W. S. (2015). *Pathophysiology of heart failure: Neurohormonal adaptations*. UpToDate®. Retrieved March 6, 2016 from http://www.uptodate.com/contents/pathophysiology-of-heart-failure-neurohumoral-adaptations

Connell, D. W., & McLachlan, R. (1972). Natural pungent compounds: IV. Examination of the gingerols, shogaols, paradols and related compounds by thin-layer and gas chromatography. *Journal of Chromatography. A*, *67*(1), 29–35. doi:10.1016/S0021-9673(01)97144-4

Consortium, C. P. I. Prioritization of Genes/Drugs. (n.d.). Retrieved from https://cpicpgx.org/prioritization/-cpicLevels

Cooper, R., Cutler, J., Desvigne-Nickens, P., Fortmann, S., Friedmann, L., Havlik, R., & Thom, T. et al. (2000). Trends and disparities in coronary heart disease, stroke, and other cardiovascular diseases in the United States findings of the national conference on cardiovascular disease. *Circulation*, *25*(25), 3137–3147. doi:10.1161/01.CIR.102.25.3137 PMID:11120707

Copstead, L.-E., & Banasik, J. L. (2010). Determinants of cardiac output. In *Pathophysiology* (pp. 419–421). St. Louis, MO: Saunders Elsevier.

Corella, D., & Ordovas, J. M. (2014). Ageing and cardiovascular diseases: The role of gene-diet interactions. *Ageing Research Reviews*, *18*, 53–73. doi:10.1016/j.arr.2014.08.002 PMID:25159268

Cosentino, S., Tuberoso, C. I. G., Pisano, B., Satta, M., Mascia, V., Arzedi, E., & Palmas, F. (1999). In-vitro antimicrobial activity and chemical composition of Sardinian Thymus essential oils. *Letters in Applied Microbiology*, *29*(2), 130–135. doi:10.1046/j.1472-765X.1999.00605.x PMID:10499301

Costantini, D. L., Arruda, E. P., Agarwal, P., Kim, K. H., Zhu, Y., Zhu, W., & Bruneau, B. G. et al. (2005b). The homeodomain transcription factor Irx5 establishes the mouse cardiac ventricular repolarization gradient. *Cell*, *123*(2), 347–358. doi:10.1016/j.cell.2005.08.004 PMID:16239150

Costantino, S., Paneni, F., & Cosentino, F. (2015). Ageing, metabolism and cardiovascular disease. *The Journal of Physiology*. doi:10.1113/JP270538 PMID:26391109

Covington, E. D., Wu, M. M., & Lewis, R. S. (2010). Essential role for the CRAC activation domain in store-dependent oligomerization of STIM1. *Molecular Biology of the Cell*, *21*(11), 1897–1907. doi:10.1091/mbc.E10-02-0145 PMID:20375143

Crow, R. S., Hannan, P. J., & Folsom, A. R. (2003). Prognostic Significance of Corrected QT and Corrected JT Interval for Incident Coronary Heart Disease in a General Population Sample Stratified by Presence or Absence of Wide QRS Complex: The ARIC Study With 13 Years of Follow-Up. *Circulation*, *108*(16), 1985–1989. doi:10.1161/01.CIR.0000095027.28753.9D PMID:14517173

Cubicin®: FDA Briefing Document for Anti-Infective Drugs Advisory Committee Meeting. (2006). Retrieved on 2/23/2016 from http://www.fda.gov/ohrms/dockets/ac/06/briefing/2006-4209B1_02_01-FDA-Background.pdf

Cui, L., Tominaga, E., Neoh, H., & Hiramatsu, K. (2006). Correlation Between Reduced Daptomycin Susceptibilities and Vancomycin Resistance in Vancomycin-Intermediated *Staphylococcus aureus*. *Antimicrobial Agents and Chemotherapy*, *50*(3), 1079–1082. doi:10.1128/AAC.50.3.1079-1082.2006 PMID:16495273

Curry, C. W., Nelson, G. S., Wyman, B. T., Declerck, J., Talbot, M., Berger, R. D., & Kass, D. A. et al. (2000). Mechanical dyssynchrony in dilated cardiomyopathy with intraventricular conduction delay as depicted by 3D tagged magnetic resonance imaging. *Circulation*, *101*(1), E2. doi:10.1161/01.CIR.101.1.e2 PMID:10618315

Cutlip, D. (n.d.). *Comparison of drug-eluting intracoronary stents*. Retrieved from http://www.uptodate.com/contents/drug-eluting-compared-to-bare-metal-intracoronary-stents?source=see_link

Dahl, A., Rasmussen, R. V., Bundgaard, H., Hassager, C., Bruun, L. E., Lauridsen, T. K., & Bruun, N. E. et al. (2013). Enterococcus faecalis infective endocarditis: A pilot study of the relationship between duration of gentamicin treatment and outcome. *Circulation*, *127*(17), 1810–1817. doi:10.1161/CIRCULATIONAHA.112.001170 PMID:23543002

Dallongeville, J., Yarnell, J., Ducimetiere, P., Arveiler, D., Ferrieres, J., & Montaye, M. (2003). Fish consumption is associated with lower heart rates. *Circulation*, *108*(7), 820–825. doi:10.1161/01.CIR.0000084542.64687.97 PMID:12912821

Damiani, E., Adrario, E., Girardis, M., Romano, R., Pelaia, P., Singer, M., & Donati, A. (2014). Arterial hyperoxia and mortality in critically ill patients: A systematic review and meta-analysis. *Critical Care (London, England)*, *18*(6), 711. doi:10.1186/s13054-014-0711-x PMID:25532567

Daneshjou, N., Sieracki, N., van Nieuw Amerongen, G. P., Conway, D. E., Schwartz, M. A., Komarova, Y. A., & Malik, A. B. (2015). Rac1 functions as a reversible tension modulator to stabilize VE-cadherin trans-interaction. *The Journal of Cell Biology*, *209*(1), 181. doi:10.1083/jcb.20140910803202015c PMID:25847538

Dangas, G., & Kuepper, F. (2002). Restenosis: Repeat Narrowing of a Coronary Artery. *Circulation*, *220*(105), 2586–2587. doi:10.1161/01.CIR.0000019122.00032.DF PMID:12045160

Dankel, S. J., Loenneke, J. P., & Loprinzi, P. D. (2015). Letter to the editor. The Impact of overweight/obesity duration on the association between physical activity and cardiovascular disease risk: An application of the fat but fit program. *International Journal of Cardiology*, *201*, 88–89. doi:10.1016/j.ijcard.2015.07.070 PMID:26292271

Darst, C. K. Jr, & Miyamoto, S. D. (2012). Cardiovascular Diseases. *CURRENT Diagnosis & Treatment. Pediatrics*, *21e*, 20.

Darwish, R. M., & Aburjai, T. A. (2010). Effect of ethnomedicinal plants used in folklore medicine in Jordan as antibiotic resistant inhibitors on Escherichia coli. *BMC Complementary and Alternative Medicine*, *10*(1), 9. doi:10.1186/1472-6882-10-9 PMID:20187978

Dastidar, A. G., Rodrigues, J. C. L., Ahmed, N., Baritussio, A., & Bucciarelli-Ducci, C. (2015). The Role of Cardiac MRI in Patients with Troponin-Positive Chest Pain and Unobstructed Coronary Arteries. *Current Cardiovascular Imaging Reports*, *8*(8), 28. doi:10.1007/s12410-015-9345-x PMID:26146527

Dauger, S., Ferkdadji, L., Saumon, G., Vardon, G., Peuchmaur, M., Gaultier, C., & Gallego, J. (2003). Neonatal Exposure to 65% Oxygen Durably Impairs Lung Architecture and Breathing Pattern in Adult Mice*. *Chest*, *123*(2), 530–538. doi:10.1378/chest.123.2.530 PMID:12576377

Dawood, B. B., Lowe, G. C., Lordkipanidze, M., Bem, D., Daly, M. E., Makris, M., & Watson, S. P. et al. (2012). Evaluation of participants with suspected heritable platelet function disorders including recommendation and validation of a streamlined agonist panel. *Blood*, *120*(25), 5041–5049. doi:10.1182/blood-2012-07-444281 PMID:23002116

de Korte, C. L., & van der Steen, A. F. W. (2002). Intravascular ultrasound elastography: an overview. *Ultrasonics, 40*(1-8), 859-865. doi:10.1016/s0041-624x(02)00227-5

de Korte, C. L., Pasterkamp, G., van der Steen, A. F. W., Woutman, H. A., & Bom, N. (2000). Characterization of Plaque Components With Intravascular Ultrasound Elastography in Human Femoral and Coronary Arteries In Vitro. *Circulation*, *102*(6), 617–623. doi:10.1161/01.CIR.102.6.617 PMID:10931800

De Korte, C. L., Schaar, J. A., Mastik, F., Serruys, P. W., & Van Der Der Steen, A. F. W. (2003). Intravascular Elastography. From Bench to Bedside. *Journal of Interventional Cardiology*, *16*(3), 253–259. doi:10.1034/j.1600-0854.2003.8049.x PMID:12800404

De La Grandmaison, G. L., Charlier, P., & Durigon, M. (2010). Usefulness of Systematic Histological Examination in Routine Forensic Autopsy*. *Journal of Forensic Sciences*, *55*(1), 85–88. doi:10.1111/j.1556-4029.2009.01240.x PMID:20002264

de Moerloose, P., Casini, A., & Neerman-Arbez, M. (2013). Congenital fibrinogen disorders: An update. *Seminars in Thrombosis and Hemostasis*, *39*(06), 585–595. doi:10.1055/s-0033-1349222 PMID:23852822

de Sa, D. D., & Chen, H. H. (2008). The role of natriuretic peptides in heart failure. *Current Cardiology Reports*, *10*(3), 182–189. doi:10.1007/s11886-008-0032-2 PMID:18489861

Deanfield, J. E. et al.. (2007). Contemporary Reviews in Cardiovascular Medicine Endothelial Function and Dysfunction Testing and Clinical Relevance. *Circulation*, *115*, 1285–1295. PMID:17353456

DebRoy, A., Vogel, S. M., Soni, D., Sundivakkam, P. C., Malik, A. B., & Tiruppathi, C.DebRoy. (2014). Cooperative signaling via transcription factors NF-kappaB and AP1/c-Fos mediates endothelial cell STIM1 expression and hyper-permeability in response to endotoxin. *The Journal of Biological Chemistry*, *289*(35), 24188–24201. doi:10.1074/jbc.M114.570051 PMID:25016017

De-Giorgio, F., & Vetrugno, G. (2014). Is histological examination always necessary to determine a cause of death? Of course it is! *Forensic Science, Medicine, and Pathology*, *10*(3), 477–478. doi:10.1007/s12024-014-9543-x PMID:24577851

DeHaven, W. I., Smyth, J. T., Boyles, R. R., & Putney, J. W. Jr. (2007). Calcium inhibition and calcium potentiation of Orai1, Orai2, and Orai3 calcium release-activated calcium channels. *The Journal of Biological Chemistry*, *282*(24), 17548–17556. doi:10.1074/jbc.M611374200 PMID:17452328

Dejana, E., Orsenigo, F., Molendini, C., Baluk, P., & McDonald, D. M. (2009). Organization and signaling of endothelial cell-to-cell junctions in various regions of the blood and lymphatic vascular trees. *Cell and Tissue Research*, *335*(1), 17–25. doi:10.1007/s00441-008-0694-5 PMID:18855014

Dejana, E., Tournier-Lasserve, E., & Weinstein, B. M. (2009). The control of vascular integrity by endothelial cell junctions: Molecular basis and pathological implications. *Developmental Cell*, *16*(2), 209–221. doi:10.1016/j.devcel.2009.01.004 PMID:19217423

Delettre, C., Griffoin, J.-M., Kaplan, J., Dollfus, H., Lorenz, B., Faivre, L., & Hamel, C. P. et al. (2001). Mutation spectrum and splicing variants in the OPA1gene. *Human Genetics*, *109*(6), 584–591. doi:10.1007/s00439-001-0633-y PMID:11810270

Demling, R., Lalonde, C., Youn, Y. K., & Picard, L. (1995). Effect of graded increases in smoke inhalation injury on the early systemic response to a body burn. *Critical Care Medicine*, *23*(1), 171–178. doi:10.1097/00003246-199501000-00027 PMID:8001368

Deng, M. C. (2002). Cardiac transplantation. *Heart (British Cardiac Society)*, *87*(2), 177–184. doi:10.1136/heart.87.2.177 PMID:11796563

Deo, R., & Albert, C. M. (2012). Epidemiology and genetics of sudden cardiac death. *Circulation*, *125*(4), 620–637. doi:10.1161/CIRCULATIONAHA.111.023838 PMID:22294707

Desbiolles, N., Piroth, L., Lequeu, C., Neuwirth, C., Portier, H., & Chavanet, P. (2001). Fractional maximal effect method for in vitro synergy between amoxicillin and ceftriaxone and between vancomycin and ceftriaxone against Enterococcus faecalis and penicillin-resistant Streptococcus pneumoniae. *Antimicrobial Agents and Chemotherapy*, *45*(12), 3328–3333. doi:10.1128/AAC.45.12.3328-3333.2001 PMID:11709304

Dewald, O., Ren, G., Duerr, G. D., Zoerlein, M., Klemm, C., Gersch, C., & Frangogiannis, N. G. et al. (2004). Of Mice and Dogs: Species-Specific Differences in the Inflammatory Response Following Myocardial Infarction. *American Journal of Pathology*, *164*(2), 665–677. doi:10.1016/S0002-9440(10)63154-9 PMID:14742270

Dhand, A., Bayer, A. S., Pogliano, J., Yang, S. J., Bolaris, M., Nizet, V., & Sakoulas, G. et al. (2011). Use of antistaphylococcal beta-lactams to increase daptomycin activity in eradicating persistent bacteremia due to methicillin-resistant Staphylococcus aureus: Role of enhanced daptomycin binding. *Clinical Infectious Diseases*, *53*(2), 158–163. doi:10.1093/cid/cir340 PMID:21690622

Dhawan, V., & Jain, S. (2005). Garlic supplementation prevents oxidative DNA damage in essential hypertension. *Molecular and Cellular Biochemistry*, *275*(1-2), 85–94. doi:10.1007/s11010-005-0824-2 PMID:16335787

Di Maio, D. J., & Di Maio, V. J. M. (2001). *Forensic Pathology* (2nd ed.). CRC Press.

Di, A., Kawamura, T., Gao, X. P., Tang, H., Berdyshev, E., Vogel, S. M., & Malik, A. B. et al. (2010). A novel function of sphingosine kinase 1 suppression of JNK activity in preventing inflammation and injury. *The Journal of Biological Chemistry*, *285*(21), 15848–15857. doi:10.1074/jbc.M109.075549 PMID:20299461

Di, A., Mehta, D., & Malik, A. B. (2016). ROS-activated calcium signaling mechanisms regulating endothelial barrier function. *Cell Calcium*, *60*(3), 163–171. doi:10.1016/j.ceca.2016.02.002 PMID:26905827

Diaz-Toro, F., Verdejo, H. E., & Castro, P. F. (2015). Socioeconomic Inequalities in Heart Failure. *Heart Failure Clinics*, *11*(4), 507–513. doi:10.1016/j.hfc.2015.07.012 PMID:26462090

Dickstein, K., Cohen-Solal, A., Filippatos, G., McMurray, J. J., Ponikowski, P., Poole-Wilson, P. A., & Tendera, M. et al. (2008). ESC guidelines for the diagnosis and treatment of acute and chronic heart failure 2008: The task force for the diagnosis and treatment of acute and chronic heart failure 2008 of the European Society of Cardiology. Developed in collaboration with the heart failure association of the ESC (HFA) and endorsed by the European Society of Intensive Care Medicine (ESICM). *European Heart Journal*, *29*(19), 2388–2442. doi:10.1093/eurheartj/ehn309 PMID:18799522

Diet, nutrition and the prevention of chronic diseases. (2003). *World Health Organ Tech Rep Ser*, *916*, i-viii, 1-149.

Dietrich, A., & Gudermann, T. (2011). TRP channels in the cardiopulmonary vasculature. *Advances in Experimental Medicine and Biology*, *704*, 781–810. doi:10.1007/978-94-007-0265-3_41 PMID:21290327

Diez Roux, A. V., Link, B. G., & Northridge, M. E. (2000). A multilevel analysis of income inequality and cardiovascular disease risk factors. *Social Science & Medicine*, *50*(5), 673–687. doi:10.1016/S0277-9536(99)00320-2 PMID:10658848

Digiesi, V., Cantini, F., Oradei, A., Bisi, G., Guarino, G. C., Brocchi, A., & Littarru, G. P. et al. (1994). Coenzyme Q10 in essential hypertension. *Molecular Aspects of Medicine*, *15*(Suppl), s257–s263. doi:10.1016/0098-2997(94)90036-1 PMID:7752838

Dillmann, W. (2010). Cardiac hypertrophy and thyroid hormone signaling. *Heart Failure Reviews*, *15*(2), 125–132. doi:10.1007/s10741-008-9125-7 PMID:19125327

Din, S., Mason, M., Völkers, M., Johnson, B., Cottage, C. T., Wang, Z., & Sussman, M. A. et al. (2013). Pim-1 preserves mitochondrial morphology by inhibiting dynamin-related protein 1 translocation. *Proceedings of the National Academy of Sciences of the United States of America*, *110*(15), 5969–5974. doi:10.1073/pnas.1213294110 PMID:23530233

Disatnik, M., Ferreira, J. C. B., Campos, J. C., Gomes, K. S., Dourado, P. M. M., Qi, X., & Mochly-Rosen, D. (2013). Acute inhibition of excessive mitochondrial fission after myocardial infarction prevents long-term cardiac dysfunction. *Journal of the American Heart Association: Cardiovascular and Cerebrovascular Disease*, *2*(5), e000461. doi:10.1161/JAHA.113.000461 PMID:24103571

Diwan, A., & Dorn, G. W. (2007). Decompensation of cardiac hypertrophy: Cellular mechanisms and novel therapeutic targets. *Physiology (Bethesda, MD)*, *22*(1), 56–64. doi:10.1152/physiol.00033.2006 PMID:17289931

Doggrell, S. A., & Brown, L. (1998). Rat models of hypertension, cardiac hypertrophy and failure. *Cardiovascular Research*, *39*(1), 89–105. doi:10.1016/S0008-6363(98)00076-5 PMID:9764192

Dolci, A., & Panteghini, M. (2006). The exciting story of cardiac biomarkers: From retrospective detection to gold diagnostic standard for acute myocardial infarction and more. *Clinica Chimica Acta*, *369*(2), 179–187. doi:10.1016/j.cca.2006.02.042 PMID:16698005

Doll, J. A., Neely, M. L., Roe, M. T., Armstrong, P. W., White, H. D., Prabhakaran, D., & Fox, K. A. et al. (2016). Impact of CYP2C19 Metabolizer Status on Patients With ACS Treated With Prasugrel Versus Clopidogrel. *Journal of the American College of Cardiology*, *67*(8), 936–947. doi:10.1016/j.jacc.2015.12.036 PMID:26916483

Dong, M., Ding, W., Liao, Y., Liu, Y., Yan, D., Zhang, Y., & Liu, J. et al. (2015). Polydatin prevents hypertrophy in phenylephrine induced neonatal mouse cardiomyocytes and pressure-overload mouse models. *European Journal of Pharmacology*, *746*, 186–197. doi:10.1016/j.ejphar.2014.11.012 PMID:25449040

Dorge, H., Schulz, R., Belosjorow, S., Post, H., van de Sand, A., Konietzka, I., & Heusch, G. et al. (2002). Coronary microembolization: The role of TNF-alpha in contractile dysfunction. *Journal of Molecular and Cellular Cardiology*, *34*(1), 51–62. doi:10.1006/jmcc.2001.1489 PMID:11812164

Dorn, G. W., Robbins, J., & Sugden, P. H. (2003). Phenotyping Hypertrophy Eschew Obfuscation. *Circulation Research*, *92*(11), 1171–1175. doi:10.1161/01.RES.0000077012.11088.BC PMID:12805233

Doroudgar, S., Thuerauf, D. J., Marcinko, M. C., Belmont, P. J., & Glembotski, C. C. (2009). Ischemia Activates the ATF6 Branch of the Endoplasmic Reticulum Stress Response. *The Journal of Biological Chemistry*, *284*(43), 29735–29745. doi:10.1074/jbc.M109.018036 PMID:19622751

Dostalek, M., Hardy, K. D., Milne, G. L., Morrow, J. D., Chen, C., Gonzalez, F. J., & Guengerich, F. P. et al. (2008). Development of Oxidative Stress by Cytochrome P450 Induction in Rodents Is Selective for Barbiturates and Related to Loss of Pyridine Nucleotide-dependent Protective Systems. *The Journal of Biological Chemistry*, *283*(25), 17147–17157. doi:10.1074/jbc.M802447200 PMID:18442974

Dowling, G. (2005). Sudden Natural Death. In D. Dolinak & E. Matshes (Eds.), *W, & Lew, E.O. Forensic Pathology: Principles and Practise* (pp. 71–119). Elseiver Academic Press.

Duarte, J., Jimenez, R., OValle, F., Galisteo, M., Perez-Palencia, R., Vargas, F., & Tamargo, J. et al. (2002). Protective effects of the flavonoid quercetin in chronic nitric oxide deficient rats. *Journal of Hypertension*, *20*(9), 1843–1854. doi:10.1097/00004872-200209000-00031 PMID:12195128

Duda, G., Suliburska, J., & Pupek-Musialik, D. (2008). Effects of short-term garlic supplementation on lipid metabolism and antioxidant status in hypertensive adults. *Pharmacological Reports*, *60*(2), 163–170. PMID:18443377

Duffy, S. J., Gokce, N., Holbrook, M., Huang, A., Frei, B., Keaney, J. F. Jr, & Vita, J. A. (1999). Treatment of hypertension with ascorbic acid. *Lancet*, *354*(9195), 2048–2049. doi:10.1016/S0140-6736(99)04410-4 PMID:10636373

Dunning, K., & Safo, A. O. (2011). The ultimate Wright-Giemsa stain: 60 years in the making. *Biotechnic & Histochemistry*, *86*(2), 69–75. doi:10.3109/10520295.2010.515496 PMID:21395491

Durack, D. T., & Beeson, P. B. (1972). Experimental bacterial endocarditis. I. Colonization of a sterile vegetation. *British Journal of Experimental Pathology*, *53*, 44–49. PMID:5014243

Durack, D. T., Beeson, P. B., & Petersdorf, R. G. (1972). Experimental endocarditis. 3. Production and progress of the disease in rabbits. *British Journal of Experimental Pathology*, *54*, 142–151. PMID:4700697

Durak, I., Kavutcu, M., Aytac, B., Avci, A., Devrim, E., Ozbek, H., & Öztürk, H. S. (2004). Effects of garlic extract consumption on blood lipid and oxidant/antioxidant parameters in humans with high blood cholesterol. *The Journal of Nutritional Biochemistry*, *15*(6), 373–377. doi:10.1016/j.jnutbio.2004.01.005 PMID:15157944

Earley, S., & Brayden, J. E. (2015). Transient receptor potential channels in the vasculature. *Physiological Reviews*, *95*(2), 645–690. doi:10.1152/physrev.00026.2014 PMID:25834234

Early Communication about an Ongoing Safety Review of clopidogrel bisulfate (marketed as Plavix). (2009). Retrieved from http://www.fda.gov/Drugs/DrugSafety/PostmarketDrugSafetyInformationforPatientsandProviders/DrugSafetyInformationforHeathcareProfessionals/ucm079520.htm

Ed Rainger, G., Chimen, M., Harrison, M. J., Yates, C. M., Harrison, P., Watson, S. P., & Nash, G. B. et al. (2015). The role of platelets in the recruitment of leukocytes during vascular disease. *Platelets*, *26*(6), 507–520. doi:10.3109/09537104.2015.1064881 PMID:26196409

Edfeldt, K. (2002, March12). Expression of Toll-Like Receptors in Human Atherosclerotic Lesions: A Possible Pathway for Plaque Activation.Circulation. *Journal of the American Heart Association Issue*, *105*(10), 1158–116.

Egido, J. et al.. (1997). Angiotensin-Converting Enzyme Inhibition Prevents Arterial Nuclear Factor-κB Activation, Monocyte Chemoattractant Protein-1 Expression, and Macrophage Infiltration in a Rabbit Model of Early Accelerated Atherosclerosis. *Circulation*, *95*(6), 1532–1541. doi:10.1161/01.CIR.95.6.1532 PMID:9118522

Eid, S.S., Kamal, N.R., Shubeilat, T.S., & Wael, A.G. (2008). Inherited bleeding disorders: a 14-year retrospective study. *Clinical Laboratory Science: Journal of the American Society for Medical Technology, 21*, 210-4.

Elahi, M. M., Yii, M., & Matata, B. M. (2008). Significance of oxidants and inflammatory mediators in blood of patients undergoing cardiac surgery. *J Cardiothorac Vasc Anesth, 22*(3), 455-467. doi: 10.1053/j.jvca.2007.12.022

El-Ashmawy, I. M., El-Nahas, A. F., & Salama, O. M. (2005). Protective effect of volatile oil, alcoholic and aqueous extracts of Origanum majorana on lead acetate toxicity in mice. *Basic & Clinical Pharmacology & Toxicology*, *97*(4), 238–243. doi:10.1111/j.1742-7843.2005.pto_136.x PMID:16176560

Engler, M. B., Engler, M. M., Chen, C. Y., Malloy, M. J., Browne, A., Chiu, E. Y., & Mietus-Snyder, M. L. et al. (2004). Flavonoid-rich dark chocolate improves endothelial function and increases plasma epicatechin concentrations in healthy adults. *Journal of the American College of Nutrition*, *23*(3), 197–204. doi:10.1080/07315724.2004.10719361 PMID:15190043

English, M. A., & Mastrean, M. B. (1995). Congestive heart failure: Public and private burden. *Critical Care Nursing Quarterly*, *18*, 1–6. PMID:7719944

Erbel, R., Rohmann, S., Drexler, M., Mohr-Kahaly, S., Gerharz, C. D., Iversen, S., & Meyer, J. et al. (1988). Improved diagnostic value of echocardiography in patients with infective endocarditis by transesophageal approach: A prospective study. *European Heart Journal*, *9*, 43–53. PMID:3345769

Ernst, E. (2012). Complementary and alternative medicine (CAM) for disease prevention. *Preventive Medicine*, *55*(6), 558–559. doi:10.1016/j.ypmed.2012.06.027 PMID:22809872

Fabre, L. F. Jr, Banks, R. C., McIsaac, W. M., & Farrell, G. (1965). Effects of Ubiquinone and Related Substances on Secretion of Aldosterone and Cortisol. *The American Journal of Physiology*, *208*, 1275–1280. PMID:14301392

Faggian, G., Forni, A., Milano, A. D., Chiominto, B., Walpoth, B. H., Scarabelli, T., & Mazzucco, A. (2010). Antithymocyte globulin induction therapy in heart transplantation: Prospective randomized study of high vs standard dosage. *Transplantation Proceedings*, *42*(9), 3679–3687. doi:10.1016/j.transproceed.2010.06.036 PMID:21094838

Fahrner, M., Derler, I., Jardin, I., & Romanin, C. (2013). The STIM1/Orai signaling machinery. *Channels (Austin, Tex.)*, *7*(5), 330–343. doi:10.4161/chan.26742 PMID:24107921

Falagas, M. E., Manta, K. G., Ntziora, F., & Vardakas, K. Z. (2006). Linezolid for the treatment of patients with endocarditis: A systematic review of the published evidence. *The Journal of Antimicrobial Chemotherapy*, *58*(2), 273–280. doi:10.1093/jac/dkl219 PMID:16735427

Fanaroff, A. A., Wright, L. L., Stevenson, D. K., Shankaran, S., Donovan, E. F., Ehrenkranz, R. A., & Verter, J. et al. (1995). Very-low-birth-weight outcomes of the National Institute of Child Health and Human Development Neonatal Research Network, May 1991 through December 1992. *American Journal of Obstetrics and Gynecology*, *173*(5), 1423–1431. doi:10.1016/0002-9378(95)90628-2 PMID:7503180

Fandrich, F. (2010). Cell therapy approaches aiming at minimization of immunosuppression in solid organ transplantation. *Current Opinion in Organ Transplantation*, *15*(6), 703–708. doi:10.1097/MOT.0b013e328340669a PMID:20930635

Fang, F., Chen, D., Yu, L., Dai, X., Yang, Y., Tian, W., & Xu, Y. et al. (2013). Proinflammatory Stimuli Engage Brahma Related Gene 1 and Brahma in Endothelial Injury. *Circulation Research*, *113*(8), 986–996. doi:10.1161/CIRCRESAHA.113.301296 PMID:23963727

Fang, M. C., Perraillon, M. C., Ghosh, K., Cutler, D. M., & Rosen, A. B. (2014). Trends in Stroke Rates, Risk, and Outcomes in the United States, 1988 to 2008. *The American Journal of Medicine*, *127*(7), 608–615. doi:10.1016/j.amjmed.2014.03.017 PMID:24680794

Farquhar, H., Weatherall, M., Wijesinghe, M., Perrin, K., Ranchord, A., Simmonds, M., & Beasley, R. (2009). Systematic review of studies of the effect of hyperoxia on coronary blood flow. *American Heart Journal*, *158*(3), 371–377. doi:10.1016/j.ahj.2009.05.037 PMID:19699859

Farrell, M. H., Micale-Foody, J., & Krumholz, H. M. (2002). β-blockers in heart failure. *Journal of the American Medical Association*, *287*(7), 890–897. doi:10.1001/jama.287.7.890 PMID:11851583

FDA Drug Safety Communication. New restrictions, contraindications, and dose limitations for Zocor (simvastatin) to reduce risk of muscle injury. (2011). Retrieved from http://www.fda.gov/Drugs/DrugSafety/ucm256581.htm

FDA Drug Safety Communication. Reduced effectiveness of Plavix (clopidogrel) in patients who are poor metabolizers of the drug. (2010). Retrieved from http://www.fda.gov/Drugs/DrugSafety/PostmarketDrugSafetyInformationforPatientsandProviders/ucm203888.htm

FDA/Center for Drug Evaluation and Research. (2016). *FDA Approved Drug Products: Natrecor*. Retrieved on March 11, 2016, from http://www.accessdata.fda.gov/scripts/cder/drugsatfda/index.cfm?fuseaction=Search.DrugDetails

Feenstra, J., Grobbee, D., Remme, W., & Stricker, B. (1999). Drug-induced heart failure. *Journal of the American College of Cardiology*, *33*(5), 1152–1162. doi:10.1016/S0735-1097(99)00006-6 PMID:10193711

Fenning, R. S., & Wilensky, R. L. (2014). New Insights into the Vulnerable Plaque from Imaging Studies. *Current Atherosclerosis Reports*, *16*(3), 397. doi:10.1007/s11883-014-0397-1 PMID:24477795

Fernández, G. M., Álvarez, B., Manzarbeitia, F., & Renedo, G. (2012). Infective endocarditis at autopsy: A review of pathologic manifestations and clinical correlates. *Medicine*, *91*(3), 152–164. doi:10.1097/MD.0b013e31825631ea PMID:22543628

Fernández-Hidalgo, N., Almirante, B., Gavaldà, J., Gurgui, M., Peña, C., de Alarcón, A., & Pahissa, A. et al. (2013). Ampicillin plus ceftriaxone is as effective as ampicillin plus gentamicin for treating enterococcus faecalis infective endocarditis. *Clinical Infectious Diseases*, *56*(9), 1261–1268. doi:10.1093/cid/cit052 PMID:23392394

Fernandez, R. A., Wan, J., Song, S., Smith, K. A., Gu, Y., Tauseef, M., & Yuan, J. X.-J. et al. (2015). Upregulated expression of STIM2, TRPC6, and Orai2 contributes to the transition of pulmonary arterial smooth muscle cells from a contractile to proliferative phenotype. *American Journal of Physiology. Cell Physiology*, *308*(8), C581–C593. doi:10.1152/ajpcell.00202.2014 PMID:25673771

Ferrannini, E., Buzzigoli, G., Bonadonna, R., Giorico, M. A., Oleggini, M., Graziadei, L., & Bevilacqua, S. et al. (1987). Insulin resistance in essential hypertension. *The New England Journal of Medicine*, *317*(6), 350–357. doi:10.1056/NEJM198708063170605 PMID:3299096

Feske, S., Giltnane, J., Dolmetsch, R., Staudt, L. M., & Rao, A. (2001). Gene regulation mediated by calcium signals in T lymphocytes. *Nature Immunology*, *2*(4), 316–324. doi:10.1038/86318 PMID:11276202

Feske, S., Gwack, Y., Prakriya, M., Srikanth, S., Puppel, S. H., Tanasa, B., & Rao, A. et al. (2006). A mutation in Orai1 causes immune deficiency by abrogating CRAC channel function. *Nature*, *441*(7090), 179–185. doi:10.1038/nature04702 PMID:16582901

Fibrin-targeted perfluorocarbon nanoparticles for targeted thrombolysis. (n.d.). Retrieved May 20, 2013, from http://www.ncbi.nlm.nih.gov/pubmed/17716136

Finkel, T., Deng, C. X., & Mostoslavsky, R. (2009). Recent progress in the biology and physiology of sirtuins. *Nature*, *460*(7255), 587–591. doi:10.1038/nature08197 PMID:19641587

Fiset, C., Clark, R. B., Larsen, T. S., & Giles, W. R. (1997). A rapidly activating sustained K+ current modulates repolarization and excitation-contraction coupling in adult mouse ventricle. *The Journal of Physiology*, *504*(Pt 3), 557–563. doi:10.1111/j.1469-7793.1997.557bd.x PMID:9401964

Fiset, C., Clark, R. B., Shimoni, Y., & Giles, W. R. (1997). Shal-type channels contribute to the Ca2+-independent transient outward K+ current in rat ventricle. *The Journal of Physiology*, *500*(Pt 1), 51–64. doi:10.1113/jphysiol.1997.sp021998 PMID:9097932

Fish, R. M. M. M. G. (2011). The Transplant Patient. Tintinalli's Emergency Medicine: A Comprehensive Study Guide. Academic Press.

Flaherty, M. P., Guo, Y., Tiwari, S., Rezazadeh, A., Hunt, G., Sanganalmath, S. K., & Dawn, B. et al. (2008). The role of TNF-α receptors p55 and p75 in acute myocardial ischemia/reperfusion injury and late preconditioning. *Journal of Molecular and Cellular Cardiology*, *45*(6), 735–741. doi:10.1016/j.yjmcc.2008.08.014 PMID:18824172

Folkers, K., Drzewoski, J., Richardson, P. C., Ellis, J., Shizukuishi, S., & Baker, L. (1981). Bioenergetics in clinical medicine. XVI. Reduction of hypertension in patients by therapy with coenzyme Q10. *Research Communications in Chemical Pathology and Pharmacology*, *31*(1), 129–140. PMID:7255868

Fotherby, M. D., Williams, J. C., Forster, L. A., Craner, P., & Ferns, G. A. (2000). Effect of vitamin C on ambulatory blood pressure and plasma lipids in older persons. *Journal of Hypertension*, *18*(4), 411–415. doi:10.1097/00004872-200018040-00009 PMID:10779091

Fowler, V. G. Jr, Scheld, W. M., & Bayer, A. S. (2015). Endocarditis and Intravascular Infections. In J. E. Bennett, R. Dolin, & M. J. Blaser (Eds.), *Mandell, Douglas, and Bennett's Principles and Practices of Infectious Diseases* (pp. 990–1028). Philadelphia, PA: Elsevier Saunders.

Frangogiannis, N. G. (2008). The immune system and cardiac repair. *Pharmacological Research*, *58*(2), 88–111. doi:10.1016/j.phrs.2008.06.007 PMID:18620057

Frey, N., Katus, H. A., Olson, E. N., & Hill, J. A. (2004). Hypertrophy of the heart a new therapeutic target? *Circulation*, *109*(13), 1580–1589. doi:10.1161/01.CIR.0000120390.68287.BB PMID:15066961

Frohlich, G. M., Meier, P., White, S. K., Yellon, D. M., & Hausenloy, D. J. (2013). Myocardial reperfusion injury: Looking beyond primary PCI. *European Heart Journal*, *34*(23), 1714–1722. doi:10.1093/eurheartj/eht090 PMID:23536610

Frontera, J. A., & Gradon, J. D. (2000). Right-sided endocarditis in injection drug users: Review of proposed mechanisms of pathogenesis. *Clinical Infectious Diseases*, *30*(2), 374–379. doi:10.1086/313664 PMID:10671344

Fuchs, A., Csajka, C., Thoma, Y., Buclin, T., & Widmer, N. (2013). Benchmarking therapeutic drug monitoring software: A review of available computer tools. *Clinical Pharmacokinetics*, *52*(1), 9–22. doi:10.1007/s40262-012-0020-y PMID:23196713

Fugh-Berman, A. (2000). Herbs and dietary supplements in the prevention and treatment of cardiovascular disease. *Preventive Cardiology*, *3*(1), 24–32. doi:10.1111/j.1520-037X.2000.80355.x PMID:11834913

Fukagawa, N. K., Anderson, J. W., Hageman, G., Young, V. R., & Minaker, K. L. (1990). High-carbohydrate, high-fiber diets increase peripheral insulin sensitivity in healthy young and old adults. *The American Journal of Clinical Nutrition*, *52*(3), 524–528. PMID:2168124

Furukawa, T., Myerburg, R. J., Furukawa, N., Bassett, A. L., & Kimura, S. (1990). Differences in transient outward currents of feline endocardial and epicardial myocytes. *Circulation Research*, *67*(5), 1287–1291. doi:10.1161/01.RES.67.5.1287 PMID:2225360

Gajardo, T., Morales, R. A., Campos-Mora, M., Campos-Acuna, J., & Pino-Lagos, K. (2015). Exogenous interleukin-33 targets myeloid-derived suppressor cells and generates periphery-induced Foxp3(+) regulatory T cells in skin-transplanted mice. *Immunology*, *146*(1), 81–88. doi:10.1111/imm.12483 PMID:25988395

Galagudza, M., Korolev, D., Postnov, V., Naumisheva, E., Grigorova, Y., Uskov, I., & Shlyakhto, E. (2012). Passive targeting of ischemic-reperfused myocardium with adenosine-loaded silica nanoparticles. *International Journal of Nanomedicine*, *71671*. doi:10.2147/IJN.S29511 PMID:22619519

Galehdar, Z., Swan, P., Fuerth, B., Callaghan, S. M., Park, D. S., & Cregan, S. P. (2010). Neuronal apoptosis induced by endoplasmic reticulum stress is regulated by ATF4-CHOP-mediated induction of the Bcl-2 homology 3-only member PUMA. *The Journal of Neuroscience*, *30*(50), 16938–16948. doi:10.1523/JNEUROSCI.1598-10.2010 PMID:21159964

Gallino, A., Eugster, W., Schneider, K., Furrer, M., & Turina, M. (1988). Indications and contra-indications for heart transplantation. *Schweizerische Medizinische Wochenschrift*, *118*(14), 522–524. PMID:3287606

Gandhirajan, R. K., Meng, S., Chandramoorthy, H. C., Mallilankaraman, K., Mancarella, S., Gao, H., & Madesh, M. et al. (2013). Blockade of NOX2 and STIM1 signaling limits lipopolysaccharide-induced vascular inflammation. *The Journal of Clinical Investigation*, *123*(2), 887–902. doi:10.1172/JCI65647 PMID:23348743

Ganji, V., & Kies, C. V. (1994). Psyllium husk fibre supplementation to soybean and coconut oil diets of humans: Effect on fat digestibility and faecal fatty acid excretion. *European Journal of Clinical Nutrition*, *48*(8), 595–597. PMID:7957006

Ganz, W., Donoso, R., Marcus, H., & Swan, H. J. (1972). Coronary hemodynamics and myocardial oxygen metabolism during oxygen breathing in patients with and without coronary artery disease. *Circulation*, *45*(4), 763–768. doi:10.1161/01.CIR.45.4.763 PMID:5016013

Gao, D., Zhang, L., Dhillon, R., Hong. T. T., Shaw, R. M., Zhu, J. (2013). Dynasore protects mitochondria and improves cardiac lusitropy in Langendorff perfused mouse heart. *PLoS One, 15*(4), e60967.

Gao, J., Luo, J., Liu, F., Zheng, Y., Chen, B., Chen, Q., & Yang, Y. (2015). Short-and long-term effects of ischemic postconditioning in STEMI patients: A meta-analysis. *Lipids in Health and Disease*, *14*(1), 147. doi:10.1186/s12944-015-0151-x PMID:26573572

Garcia-Fontana, B., Morales-Santana, S., Navarro, C. D., Rozas-Moreno, P., Genilloud, O., Perez, F. V., & Munoz-Torres, M. et al. (2016). Metabolomic profile related to cardiovascular disease in patients with type 2 diabetes mellitus: A pilot study. *Talanta*, *148*, 135–143. doi:10.1016/j.talanta.2015.10.070 PMID:26653434

Garcia, J. G., Davis, H. W., & Patterson, C. E. (1995). Regulation of endothelial cell gap formation and barrier dysfunction: Role of myosin light chain phosphorylation. *Journal of Cellular Physiology*, *163*(3), 510–522. doi:10.1002/jcp.1041630311 PMID:7775594

Gareus, R., Kotsaki, E., Xanthoulea, S., van der Made, I., Gijbels, M. J. J., Kardakaris, R., & Pasparakis, M. et al. (2008, November). Endothelial cell-specific NF-kappaB inhibition protects mice from atherosclerosis. *Cell Metabolism*, *8*(5), 372–383. doi:10.1016/j.cmet.2008.08.016 PMID:19046569

Gavaldà, J., Len, O., Miró, J. M., Muñoz, P., Montejo, M., Alarcón, A., & Pahissa, A. et al. (2007). Brief communication: Treatment of Enterococcus faecalis endocarditis with ampicillin plus ceftriaxone. *Annals of Internal Medicine*, *146*(8), 574–579. doi:10.7326/0003-4819-146-8-200704170-00008 PMID:17438316

Gavaldá, J., Onrubia, P. L., Gómez, M. T., Gomis, X., Ramírez, J. L., Len, O., & Pahissa, A. et al. (2003). Efficacy of ampicillin combined with ceftriaxone and gentamicin in the treatment of experimental endocarditis due to Enterococcus faecalis with no high-level resistance to aminoglycosides. *The Journal of Antimicrobial Chemotherapy*, *52*(3), 514–517. doi:10.1093/jac/dkg360 PMID:12917251

Gavaldà, J., Torres, C., Tenorio, C., López, P., Zaragoza, M., Capdevila, J. A., & Pahissa, A. et al. (1999). Efficacy of ampicillin plus ceftriaxone in treatment of experimental endocarditis due to Enterococcus faecalis strains highly resistant to aminoglycosides. *Antimicrobial Agents and Chemotherapy*, *43*, 639–646. PMID:10049280

GBD 2013 Mortality and Causes of Death Collaborators. (2015). Global, regional, and national age–sex specific all-cause and cause-specific mortality for 240 causes of death, 1990–2013: a systematic analysis for the Global Burden of Disease Study 2013. *The Lancet, 385*(9963), 117-171. doi: 10.1016/s0140-6736(14)61682-2

Geleijnse, J. M., Giltay, E. J., Grobbee, D. E., Donders, A. R. T., & Kok, F. J. (2002). Blood pressure response to fish oil supplementation: Metaregression analysis of randomized trials. *Journal of Hypertension*, *20*(8), 1493–1499. doi:10.1097/00004872-200208000-00010 PMID:12172309

Geller, S. A. (2013). Infective endocarditis: A history of the development of its understanding. *Autopsy and Case Reports*, *3*(4), 5–12. doi:10.4322/acr.2013.033

Genevieve, D., Proulle, V., Isidor, B., Bellais, S., Serre, V., Djouadi, F., & Cormier-Daire, V. et al. (2008). Thromboxane synthase mutations in an increased bone density disorder (Ghosal syndrome). *Nature Genetics*, *40*(3), 284–286. doi:10.1038/ng.2007.66 PMID:18264100

Gershlick, A., Kandzari, D. E., Leon, M. B., Wijns, W., Meredith, I. T., Fajadet, J., & Kuntz, R. E. et al. (2007). InvestigatorsZotarolimus-eluting stents in patients with native coronary artery disease: Clinical and angiographic outcomes in 1,317 patients. *The American Journal of Cardiology*, *100*(8), 45M–55M. doi:10.1016/j.amjcard.2007.08.021 PMID:17950832

Gey, K. F., Stahelin, H. B., & Eichholzer, M. (1993). Poor plasma status of carotene and vitamin C is associated with higher mortality from ischemic heart disease and stroke: Basel Prospective Study. *The Clinical Investigator*, *71*(1), 3–6. doi:10.1007/BF00210955 PMID:8453256

Ghayur, M. N., & Gilani, A. H. (2005). Ginger lowers blood pressure through blockade of voltage-dependent calcium channels. *Journal of Cardiovascular Pharmacology*, *45*(1), 74–80. doi:10.1097/00005344-200501000-00013 PMID:15613983

Ghosh, H. S., McBurney, M., & Robbins, P. D. (2010). SIRT1 negatively regulates the mammalian target of rapamycin. *PLoS ONE*, *5*(2), e9199. doi:10.1371/journal.pone.0009199 PMID:20169165

Ghosh, S., & Rao, A. K. (1993). Lack of effect of 1-desamino-8-D-arginine vasopressin on direct adhesion of platelets to collagen. *Thrombosis Research*, *70*(5), 417–422. doi:10.1016/0049-3848(93)90083-Z PMID:7690994

Giada, F., & Bartoletti, A. (2015). Value of Ambulatory Electrocardiographic Monitoring in Syncope. *Cardiology Clinics*, *33*(3), 361–366. doi:10.1016/j.ccl.2015.04.004 PMID:26115822

Giada, F., Bertaglia, E., Reimers, B., Noventa, D., & Raviele, A. (2012). Current and Emerging Indications for Implantable Cardiac Monitors. *Pacing and Clinical Electrophysiology*, *35*(9), 1169–1178. doi:10.1111/j.1540-8159.2012.03411.x PMID:22530875

Giannotta, M., Trani, M., & Dejana, E. (2013). VE-cadherin and endothelial adherens junctions: Active guardians of vascular integrity. *Developmental Cell*, *26*(5), 441–454. doi:10.1016/j.devcel.2013.08.020 PMID:24044891

Gien, J., Seedorf, G. J., Balasubramaniam, V., Markham, N., & Abman, S. H. (2007). Intrauterine pulmonary hypertension impairs angiogenesis in vitro: Role of vascular endothelial growth factor nitric oxide signaling. *American Journal of Respiratory and Critical Care Medicine*, *176*(11), 1146–1153. doi:10.1164/rccm.200705-750OC PMID:17823355

Giricz, Z., Varga, Z. V., Baranyai, T., Sipos, P., Pálóczi, K., Kittel, Á., & Ferdinandy, P. et al. (2014). Cardioprotection by remote ischemic preconditioning of the rat heart is mediated by extracellular vesicles. *Journal of Molecular and Cellular Cardiology*, *68*, 75–78. doi:10.1016/j.yjmcc.2014.01.004 PMID:24440457

Global Lipids Genetics, C., Willer, C. J., Schmidt, E. M., Sengupta, S., Peloso, G. M., Gustafsson, S., & Abecasis, G. R. et al. (2013). Discovery and refinement of loci associated with lipid levels. *Nature Genetics*, *45*(11), 1274–1283. doi:10.1038/ng.2797 PMID:24097068

Go, A. S., Mozaffarian, D., Roger, V. L., Benjamin, E. J., Berry, J. D., Blaha, M. J., & Turner, M. B. et al. (2014). Heart Disease and Stroke Statistics2014 Update: A Report From the American Heart Association. *Circulation*, *129*(3), e28–e292. doi:10.1161/01.cir.0000441139.02102.80 PMID:24352519

Golan, D. E., Tashjian, A. H., Armstrong, E. J., & Armstrong, A. W. (2012). Integrative cardiovascular pharmacology: hypertension, ischemic heart disease, and heart failure. In *Principles of Pharmacology* (pp. 437–463). Philadelphia, PA: Lippincott Williams & Wilkins.

Gole, Y., Gargne, O., Coulange, M., Steinberg, J. G., Bouhaddi, M., Jammes, Y., & Boussuges, A. et al. (2011). Hyperoxia-induced alterations in cardiovascular function and autonomic control during return to normoxic breathing. *European Journal of Applied Physiology*, *111*(6), 937–946. doi:10.1007/s00421-010-1711-4 PMID:21069379

Gong, H., Gao, X., Feng, S., Siddiqui, M. R., Garcia, A., Bonini, M. G., & Malik, A. B. et al. (2014). Evidence of a common mechanism of disassembly of adherens junctions through Galpha13 targeting of VE-cadherin. *The Journal of Experimental Medicine*, *211*(3), 579–591. doi:10.1084/jem.20131190 PMID:24590762

Gong, H., Rehman, J., Tang, H., Wary, K., Mittal, M., Chaturvedi, P., & Malik, A. B. et al. (2015). Corrigendum. HI-F2alpha signaling inhibits adherens junctional disruption in acute lung injury. *The Journal of Clinical Investigation, 125*(3), 1364. doi:10.1172/JCI81377 PMID:25729855

Gorenoi, V., Schonermark, M. P., & Hagen, A. (2012). CT coronary angiography vs. invasive coronary angiography in CHD. *GMS Health Technol Assess, 8*, Doc02. doi:10.3205/hta000100 PMID:22536300

Goto, J., Suzuki, A. Z., Ozaki, S., Matsumoto, N., Nakamura, T., Ebisui, E., & Mikoshiba, K. et al. (2010). Two novel 2-aminoethyl diphenylborinate (2-APB) analogues differentially activate and inhibit store-operated Ca(2+) entry via STIM proteins. *Cell Calcium, 47*(1), 1–10. doi:10.1016/j.ceca.2009.10.004 PMID:19945161

Gottlieb, S. S., Stebbins, A., Voors, A. A., Hasselblad, V., Ezekowitz, J. A., Califf, R. M., & Hernandez, A. F. et al. (2013). Effects of nesiritide and predictors of urine output in acute decompensated heart failure: Results from the ASCEND-HF (acute study of clinical effectiveness of nesiritide and decompensated heart failure). *Journal of the American College of Cardiology, 62*(13), 1177–1183. doi:10.1016/j.jacc.2013.04.073 PMID:23747790

Goyle, K. K., & Walling, A. D. (2002). Diagnosing pericarditis. *American Family Physician, 66*(9), 1695–1704. PMID:12449268

Grassi, D., Necozione, S., Lippi, C., Croce, G., Valeri, L., Pasqualetti, P., & Ferri, C. et al. (2005). Cocoa reduces blood pressure and insulin resistance and improves endothelium-dependent vasodilation in hypertensives. *Hypertension, 46*(2), 398–405. doi:10.1161/01.HYP.0000174990.46027.70 PMID:16027246

Grauhan, O., Müller, J., Volk, H., Fietze, E., Cohnert, T., Meyer, R., . . . Warnecke, H. (1998). Treatment of humoral rejection after heart transplantation. *The Journal of Heart and Lung Transplantation: The Official Publication of the International Society for Heart Transplantation, 17*(12), 1184-1194.

Grewal, J., Chandavimol, M., & Ignaszewski, A. (2004). B-type natriuretic peptide: A new marker for congestive heart failure. *BCMJ, 46*(1), 24–29.

Griffiths, E. J., & Halestrap, A. P. (1995). Mitochondrial non-specific pores remain closed during cardiac ischaemia, but open upon reperfusion. *The Biochemical Journal, 307*(Pt 1), 93–98. doi:10.1042/bj3070093 PMID:7717999

Grisafi, D., Pozzobon, M., Dedja, A., Vanzo, V., Tomanin, R., Porzionato, A., & Zaramella, P. et al. (2013). Human amniotic fluid stem cells protect rat lungs exposed to moderate hyperoxia. *Pediatric Pulmonology, 48*(11), 1070–1080. doi:10.1002/ppul.22791 PMID:23533160

Grisafi, D., Tassone, E., Dedja, A., Oselladore, B., Masola, V., Guzzardo, V., & Zaramella, P. et al. (2012). L-citrulline Prevents Alveolar and Vascular Derangement in a Rat Model of Moderate Hyperoxia-induced Lung Injury. *Lung, 190*(4), 419–430. doi:10.1007/s00408-012-9382-z PMID:22430123

Gross, C., Hoffmann, A., Bassell, G. J., & Berry-Kravis, E. M. (2015). Therapeutic Strategies in Fragile X Syndrome: From Bench to Bedside and Back. *Neurotherapeutics; the Journal of the American Society for Experimental Neuro-Therapeutics, 12*(3), 584–608. doi:10.1007/s13311-015-0355-9 PMID:25986746

Grottum, K. A., Hovig, T., Holmsen, H., Abrahamsen, A. F., Jeremic, M., & Seip, M. (1969). Wiskott-Aldrich syndrome: Qualitative platelet defects and short platelet survival. *British Journal of Haematology, 17*(4), 373–388. doi:10.1111/j.1365-2141.1969.tb01383.x PMID:5346410

Group, S. R. (2015). A randomized trial of intensive versus standard blood-pressure control. *The New England Journal of Medicine, 373*(22), 2103–2116. doi:10.1056/NEJMoa1511939 PMID:26551272

Gudermann, T., & Steinritz, D. (2013). STIMulating stress fibers in endothelial cells. *Science Signaling*, *6*(267), pe8. doi:10.1126/scisignal.2004051 PMID:23512987

Gunay-Aygun, M., Falik-Zaccai, T. C., Vilboux, T., Zivony-Elboum, Y., Gumruk, F., Cetin, M., & Gahl, W. A. et al. (2011). NBEAL2 is mutated in gray platelet syndrome and is required for biogenesis of platelet alpha-granules. *Nature Genetics*, *43*(8), 732–734. doi:10.1038/ng.883 PMID:21765412

Gunay-Aygun, M., Huizing, M., & Gahl, W. A. (2004). Molecular defects that affect platelet dense granules. *Seminars in Thrombosis and Hemostasis*, *30*(5), 537–547. doi:10.1055/s-2004-835674 PMID:15497096

Gunay-Aygun, M., Zivony-Elboum, Y., Gumruk, F., Geiger, D., Cetin, M., Khayat, M., & Falik-Zaccai, T. et al. (2010). Gray platelet syndrome: Natural history of a large patient cohort and locus assignment to chromosome 3p. *Blood*, *116*(23), 4990–5001. doi:10.1182/blood-2010-05-286534 PMID:20709904

Gunn, A. (2011). *Essential forensic biology*. John Wiley & Sons.

Gupta, S., Young, D., Maitra, R. K., Gupta, A., Popovic, Z. B., Yong, S. L., & Sen, S. et al. (2008). Prevention of cardiac hypertrophy and heart failure by silencing of NF-kappaB. *Journal of Molecular Biology*, *375*(3), 637–649. doi:10.1016/j.jmb.2007.10.006 PMID:18037434

Gupta, S., Young, D., & Sen, S. (2005). Inhibition of NF-kappaB induces regression of cardiac hypertrophy, independent of blood pressure control, in spontaneously hypertensive rats. *American Journal of Physiology. Heart and Circulatory Physiology*, *289*(1), H20–H29. doi:10.1152/ajpheart.00082.2005 PMID:15749748

Gupte, S. A., Levine, R. J., Gupte, R. S., Young, M. E., Lionetti, V., Labinskyy, V., & Recchia, F. A. et al. (2006). Glucose-6-phosphate dehydrogenase-derived NADPH fuels superoxide production in the failing heart. *Journal of Molecular and Cellular Cardiology*, *41*(2), 340–349. doi:10.1016/j.yjmcc.2006.05.003 PMID:16828794

Gustafson, T. A., Bahl, J. J., Markham, B. E., Roeske, W. R., & Morkin, E. (1987). Hormonal regulation of myosin heavy chain and alpha-actin gene expression in cultured fetal rat heart myocytes. *The Journal of Biological Chemistry*, *262*(27), 13316–13322. PMID:2888758

Guyatt, G. H., Akl, E. A., Crowther, M., Gutterman, D. D., & Schuünemann, H. J. (2012). Executive summary: Antithrombotic therapy and prevention of thrombosis, 9th ed: american college of chest physicians evidence-based clinical practice guidelines. Chest, 141(2), 7S-47S. doi:10.1378/chest.1412S3

Habib, G., Lancellotti, P., Antunes, M. J., Bongiorni, M. G., Casalta, J. P., Del Zotti, F., & Zamorano, J. L. et al. (2015). 2015 ESC Guidelines for the management of infective endocarditis: The Task Force for the Management of Infective Endocarditis of the European Society of Cardiology (ESC). Endorsed by: European Association for Cardio-Thoracic Surgery (EACTS), the European Association of Nuclear Medicine (EANM). *European Heart Journal*, *36*(44), 3075–3128. doi:10.1093/eurheartj/ehv319 PMID:26320109

Häckl, L. P. N., Cuttle, G., Dovichi, S. S., Lima-Landman, M. T., & Nicolau, M. (2002). Inhibition of angiotensin-converting enzyme by quercetin alters the vascular response to bradykinin and angiotensin I. *Pharmacology*, *65*(4), 182–186. doi:10.1159/000064341 PMID:12174832

Hajra, L., Evans, A. I., Chen, M., Hyduk, S. J., Collins, T., & Cybulsky, M. I. (2000). The NF-kappa B signal transduction pathway in aortic endothelial cells is primed for activation in regions predisposed to atherosclerotic lesion formation. *Proceedings of the National Academy of Sciences of the United States of America*, *97*(16), 9052–9057. doi:10.1073/pnas.97.16.9052 PMID:10922059

Hales, K. G., & Fuller, M. T. (1997). Developmentally regulated mitochondrial fusion mediated by a conserved, novel, predicted GTPase. *Cell*, *90*(1), 121–129. doi:10.1016/S0092-8674(00)80319-0 PMID:9230308

Hamadeh, I. S., Langaee, T. Y., Dwivedi, R., Garcia, S., Burkley, B. M., Skaar, T. C., & Johnson, J. A. et al. (2014). Impact of CYP2D6 polymorphisms on clinical efficacy and tolerability of metoprolol tartrate. *Clinical Pharmacology and Therapeutics*, *96*(2), 175–181. doi:10.1038/clpt.2014.62 PMID:24637943

Hamilton, L. C. (2013). *Statistics with STATA: Version 12*. Boston, MA: Cengage Learning

Hamza, S. M., & Dyck, J. R. (2014). Systemic and renal oxidative stress in the pathogenesis of hypertension: Modulation of long-term control of arterial blood pressure by resveratrol. *Frontiers in Physics*, *5*, 292. doi:10.3389/fphys.2014.00292 PMID:25140155

Han, C. Y., Umemoto, T., Omer, M., Den Hartigh, L. J., Chiba, T., LeBoeuf, R., & Chait, A. et al. (2012). NADPH Oxidase-derived Reactive Oxygen Species Increases Expression of Monocyte Chemotactic Factor Genes in Cultured Adipocytes. *The Journal of Biological Chemistry*, *287*(13), 10379–10393. doi:10.1074/jbc.M111.304998 PMID:22287546

Handschin, C. (2016). Caloric restriction and exercise mimetics: Ready for prime time? *Pharmacological Research*, *103*, 158–166. doi:10.1016/j.phrs.2015.11.009 PMID:26658171

Haque, W. A., Boehmer, J., Clemson, B. S., Leuenberger, U. A., Silber, D. H., & Sinoway, L. I. (1996). Hemodynamic effects of supplemental oxygen administration in congestive heart failure. *Journal of the American College of Cardiology*, *27*(2), 353–357. doi:10.1016/0735-1097(95)00474-2 PMID:8557905

Haramaki, N., Assadnazari, H., Zimmer, G., Schepkin, V., & Packer, L. (1995). The influence of vitamin E and dihydrolipoic acid on cardiac energy and glutathione status under hypoxia-reoxygenation. *Biochemistry and Molecular Biology International*, *37*(3), 591–597. PMID:8595400

Harikumar, K. B., & Aggarwal, B. B. (2008). Resveratrol: A multitargeted agent for age-associated chronic diseases. *Cell Cycle (Georgetown, Tex.)*, *7*(8), 1020–1035. doi:10.4161/cc.7.8.5740 PMID:18414053

Harisseh, R., Chatelier, A., Magaud, C., Deliot, N., & Constantin, B. (2013). Involvement of TRPV2 and SOCE in calcium influx disorder in DMD primary human myotubes with a specific contribution of alpha1-syntrophin and PLC/PKC in SOCE regulation. *American Journal of Physiology. Cell Physiology*, *304*(9), C881–C894. doi:10.1152/ajpcell.00182.2012 PMID:23426965

Hartmann, J., Karl, R. M., Alexander, R. P., Adelsberger, H., Brill, M. S., Ruhlmann, C., & Konnerth, A. et al. (2014). STIM1 controls neuronal Ca(2)(+) signaling, mGluR1-dependent synaptic transmission, and cerebellar motor behavior. *Neuron*, *82*(3), 635–644. doi:10.1016/j.neuron.2014.03.027 PMID:24811382

Hartner, W., Verma, D., Levchenko, T., Bernstein, E., & Torchilin, V. (n.d). ATP-loaded liposomes for treatment of myocardial ischemia. *Wiley Interdisciplinary Reviews-Nanomedicine And Nanobiotechnology, 1*(5), 530-539.

Hausenloy, D. J., Mwamure, P. K., Venugopal, V., Harris, J., Barnard, M., Grundy, E., & Yellon, D. M. et al. (2007). Effect of remote ischaemic preconditioning on myocardial injury in patients undergoing coronary artery bypass graft surgery: A randomised controlled trial. *Lancet*, *370*(9587), 575–579. doi:10.1016/S0140-6736(07)61296-3 PMID:17707752

Hawkins, B. J., Irrinki, K. M., Mallilankaraman, K., Lien, Y. C., Wang, Y., Bhanumathy, C. D., & Madesh, M. et al. (2010). S-glutathionylation activates STIM1 and alters mitochondrial homeostasis. *The Journal of Cell Biology*, *190*(3), 391–405. doi:10.1083/jcb.201004152 PMID:20679432

Hayden, M. S., & Ghosh, S. (2004). Signaling to NF-kB. *Genes & Development*, *18*(18), 2195–2224. doi:10.1101/gad.1228704 PMID:15371334

Haynes, S. G., Feinleib, M., Levine, S., Scotch, N., & Kannel, W. B. (1980). The relationship of psychosocial factors to coronary heart disease in the Framingham Study. III. Eight-year incidence of coronary heart disease. *American Journal of Epidemiology*, *107*(5), 384–402. PMID:665655

Hazini, A., Cemek, M., Isildak, I., Alpdagtas, S., Onul, A., Senel, U., & Uyarel, H. et al. (2015). Investigation of ischemia modified albumin, oxidant and antioxidant markers in acute myocardial infarction. *Postepy Kardiol Interwencyjnej*, *11*(4), 298–303. doi:10.5114/pwki.2015.55600 PMID:26677379

Hearn and Walls. (2007). Introduction to Postmortem Toxicology. In B. Karch Steven (Ed.), *Postmortem toxicology of abused drugs*. CRC Press.

Heather, L. C., & Clarke, K. (2011). Metabolism, hypoxia and the diabetic heart. *Journal of Molecular and Cellular Cardiology*, *50*(4), 598–605. doi:10.1016/j.yjmcc.2011.01.007 PMID:21262230

Heeschen, C., Dimmeler, S., Fichtlscherer, S., Hamm, C. W., Berger, J., Simoons, M. L., & Investigators, C. et al. (2004). Prognostic value of placental growth factor in patients with acute chest pain. *Journal of the American Medical Association*, *291*(4), 435–441. doi:10.1001/jama.291.4.435 PMID:14747500

He, F. J., Campbell, N. R. C., & MacGregor, G. A. (2012). Reducing salt intake to prevent hypertension and cardiovascular disease. *Pan American Journal of Public Health*, *32*(4), 293–300. doi:10.1590/S1020-49892012001000008 PMID:23299291

Heidenreich, P. A., Albert, N. M., Allen, L. A., Bluemke, D. A., Butler, J., Fonarow, G. C., & Trogdon, J. G. et al. (2013). Forecasting the impact of heart failure in the United States: A policy statement from the American Heart Association. *Circulation: Heart Failure*, *6*(3), 606–619. doi:10.1161/HHF.0b013e318291329a PMID:23616602

Heiss, C., Kleinbongard, P., Dejam, A., Perre, S., Schroeter, H., Sies, H., & Kelm, M. (2005). Acute consumption of flavanol-rich cocoa and the reversal of endothelial dysfunction in smokers. *Journal of the American College of Cardiology*, *46*(7), 1276–1283. doi:10.1016/j.jacc.2005.06.055 PMID:16198843

He, J., Ogden, L. G., Bazzano, L. A., Vupputuri, S., Loria, C., & Whelton, P. K. (2001). Risk factors for congestive heart failure in US men and women: NHANES I epidemiologic follow-up study. *Archives of Internal Medicine*, *161*(7), 996–1002. doi:10.1001/archinte.161.7.996 PMID:11295963

He, J., Ogden, L. G., Bazzano, L. A., Vupputuri, S., Loria, C., & Whelton, P. K. (2002). Dietary sodium intake and incidence of congestive heart failure in overweight US men and women: First national health and nutrition examination survey epidemiologic follow-up study. *Archives of Internal Medicine*, *162*(14), 1619–162. doi:10.1001/archinte.162.14.1619 PMID:12123406

Helgadottir, A., Thorleifsson, G., Magnusson, K. P., Gretarsdottir, S., Steinthorsdottir, V., Manolescu, A., & Stefansson, K. et al. (2008). The same sequence variant on 9p21 associates with myocardial infarction, abdominal aortic aneurysm and intracranial aneurysm. *Nature Genetics*, *40*(2), 217–224. doi:10.1038/ng.72 PMID:18176561

Helgadottir, A., Thorleifsson, G., Manolescu, A., Gretarsdottir, S., Blondal, T., Jonasdottir, A., & Stefansson, K. et al. (2007). A common variant on chromosome 9p21 affects the risk of myocardial infarction. *Science*, *316*(5830), 1491–1493. doi:10.1126/science.1142842 PMID:17478679

Helmerhorst, H., Schultz, M., van der Voort, P., Bosman, R., Juffermans, N., de Jonge, E., & van Westerloo, D. (2014). Self-reported attitudes versus actual practice of oxygen therapy by ICU physicians and nurses. *Annals of Intensive Care*, *4*(1), 23. doi:10.1186/s13613-014-0023-y PMID:25512878

Herba thymi. (1999). In *WHO monographs on selected medicinal plants* (Vol. 1). Geneva: WHO.

Heslop, C. L., Frohlich, J. J., & Hill, J. S. (2010). Myeloperoxidase and C-reactive protein have combined utility for long-term prediction of cardiovascular mortality after coronary angiography. *Journal of the American College of Cardiology*, *55*(11), 1102–1109. doi:10.1016/j.jacc.2009.11.050 PMID:20223364

He, W., Jia, Y., & Takimoto, K. (2009). Interaction between transcription factors Iroquois proteins 4 and 5 controls cardiac potassium channel Kv4.2 gene transcription. *Cardiovascular Research*, *81*(1), 64–71. doi:10.1093/cvr/cvn259 PMID:18815185

Higuchi, Y., Otsu, K., Nishida, K., Hirotani, S., Nakayama, H., Yamaguchi, O., & Hori, M. et al. (2002). Involvement of reactive oxygen species-mediated NF-kappa B activation in TNF-alpha-induced cardiomyocyte hypertrophy. *Journal of Molecular and Cellular Cardiology*, *34*(2), 233–240. doi:10.1006/jmcc.2001.1505 PMID:11851362

Hillebrands, J.-L., Klatter, F. A., van den Hurk, B. M., Popa, E. R., Nieuwenhuis, P., & Rozing, J. (2001). Origin of neointimal endothelium and α-actin–positive smooth muscle cells in transplant arteriosclerosis. *The Journal of Clinical Investigation*, *107*(11), 1411–1422. doi:10.1172/JCI10233 PMID:11390423

Hindricks, G., Pokushalov, E., Urban, L., Taborsky, M., Kuck, K. H., Lebedev, D., & Purerfellner, H. et al. (2010). Performance of a New Leadless Implantable Cardiac Monitor in Detecting and Quantifying Atrial Fibrillation Results of the XPECT Trial. *Circulation: Arrhythmia and Electrophysiology*, *3*(2), 141–147. doi:10.1161/CIRCEP.109.877852 PMID:20160169

Hinohara, K., Nakajima, T., Takahashi, M., Hohda, S., Sasaoka, T., Nakahara, K., & Kimura, A. et al. (2008). Replication of the association between a chromosome 9p21 polymorphism and coronary artery disease in Japanese and Korean populations. *Journal of Human Genetics*, *53*(4), 357–359. doi:10.1007/s10038-008-0248-4 PMID:18264662

Hoen, B., & Duval, X. (2013). Infective endocarditis. *The New England Journal of Medicine*, *368*(15), 1425–1433. doi:10.1056/NEJMcp1206782 PMID:23574121

Hoffmeyer, M. R., Jones, S. P., Ross, C. R., Sharp, B., Grisham, M. B., Laroux, F. S., & Lefer, D. J. et al. (2000). Myocardial Ischemia/Reperfusion Injury in NADPH Oxidase–Deficient Mice. *Circulation Research*, *87*(9), 812–817. doi:10.1161/01.RES.87.9.812 PMID:11055986

Hogan, P. G., Lewis, R. S., & Rao, A. (2010). Molecular basis of calcium signaling in lymphocytes: STIM and ORAI. *Annual Review of Immunology*, *28*(1), 491–533. doi:10.1146/annurev.immunol.021908.132550 PMID:20307213

Holinstat, M., Knezevic, N., Broman, M., Samarel, A. M., Malik, A. B., & Mehta, D. (2006). Suppression of RhoA activity by focal adhesion kinase-induced activation of p190RhoGAP: Role in regulation of endothelial permeability. *The Journal of Biological Chemistry*, *281*(4), 2296–2305. doi:10.1074/jbc.M511248200 PMID:16308318

Holland, T. L., Arnold, C., & Fowler, V. G. Jr. (2014). Clinical management of Staphylococcus aureus bacteremia: A review. *Journal of the American Medical Association*, *312*(13), 1330–1341. doi:10.1001/jama.2014.9743 PMID:25268440

Hollestelle, S. C., De Vries, M. R., Van Keulen, J. K., Schoneveld, A. H., Vink, A., Strijder, C. F., & De Kleijn, D. P. et al. (2004). Toll-like receptor 4 is involved in outward arterial remodeling. *Circulation*, *109*(3), 393–398. doi:10.1161/01.CIR.0000109140.51366.72 PMID:14699006

Holmes, M. V., Perel, P., Shah, T., Hingorani, A. D., & Casas, J. P. (2011). CYP2C19 genotype, clopidogrel metabolism, platelet function, and cardiovascular events: A systematic review and meta-analysis. *Journal of the American Medical Association*, *306*(24), 2704–2714. doi:10.1001/jama.2011.1880 PMID:22203539

Holmes, N. E., Turnidge, J. D., Munckhof, W. J., Robinson, J. O., Korman, T. M., OSullivan, M. V., & Johnson, P. D. et al. (2013). Vancomycin AUC/MIC ratio and 30-day mortality in patients with Staphylococcus aureus bacteremia. *Antimicrobial Agents and Chemotherapy*, *57*(4), 1654–1663. doi:10.1128/AAC.01485-12 PMID:23335735

Holzgartner, H., Schmidt, U., & Kuhn, U. (1992). Comparison of the efficacy and tolerance of a garlic preparation vs bezafibrate. *Arzneimittel-Forschung/Drug Research, 42-2*(12), 1473-1477.

Hongeng, S., Benjaponpitak, S., Tardtong, P., Varavithya, W., Chuansumrit, A., et al. (2001). Successful allogeneic peripheral blood stem cell transplantation in Wiskott-Aldrich Syndrome Patients: first report in Thailand. *Asian Pacific Journal of Allergy and Immunology, 19*, 191-5.

Hoole, S. P., Heck, P. M., Sharples, L., Khan, S. N., Duehmke, R., Densem, C. G., & Dutka, D. P. et al. (2009). Cardiac Remote Ischemic Preconditioning in Coronary Stenting (CRISP Stent) Study: A prospective, randomized control trial. *Circulation*, *119*(6), 820–827. doi:10.1161/CIRCULATIONAHA.108.809723 PMID:19188504

Ho, T. T., Cadena, J., Childs, L. M., Gonzalez-Velez, M., & Lewis, J. S. II. (2012). Methicillin-resistant Staphylococcus aureus bacteraemia and endocarditis treated with ceftaroline salvage therapy. *The Journal of Antimicrobial Chemotherapy*, *67*(5), 1267–1270. doi:10.1093/jac/dks006 PMID:22311935

Hoth, M. (1995). Calcium and barium permeation through calcium release-activated calcium (CRAC) channels. *Pflugers Archiv*, *430*(3), 315–322. doi:10.1007/BF00373905 PMID:7491254

Hoth, M., & Penner, R. (1992). Depletion of intracellular calcium stores activates a calcium current in mast cells. *Nature*, *355*(6358), 353–356. doi:10.1038/355353a0 PMID:1309940

Hou, J., Chong, Z. Z., Shang, Y. C., & Maiese, K. (2010). Early apoptotic vascular signaling is determined by Sirt1 through nuclear shuttling, forkhead trafficking, bad, and mitochondrial caspase activation. *Current Neurovascular Research*, *7*(2), 95–112. doi:10.2174/156720210791184899 PMID:20370652

Hou, J., Wang, S., Shang, Y. C., Chong, Z. Z., & Maiese, K. (2011). Erythropoietin employs cell longevity pathways of SIRT1 to foster endothelial vascular integrity during oxidant stress. *Current Neurovascular Research*, *8*(3), 220–235. doi:10.2174/156720211796558069 PMID:21722091

Hou, L., Xie, K., Qin, M., Peng, D., Ma, S., Shang, L., & Xiong, L. et al. (2010). Effects of reactive oxygen species scavenger on the protective action of 100% oxygen treatment against sterile inflammation in mice.[doi]. *Shock (Augusta, Ga.)*, *33*(6), 646–654. doi:10.1097/SHK.0b013e3181c1b5d4 PMID:19789462

House, J. S. (2002). Understanding Social Factors and Inequalities in Health: 20th Century Progress and 21st Century Prospects. *Journal of Health and Social Behavior*, *43*(2), 125–142. doi:10.2307/3090192 PMID:12096695

Hou, X., Pedi, L., Diver, M. M., & Long, S. B. (2012). Crystal structure of the calcium release-activated calcium channel Orai. *Science*, *338*(6112), 1308–1313. doi:10.1126/science.1228757 PMID:23180775

Howden, R., Cho, H. Y., Miller-DeGraff, L., Walker, C., Clark, J. A., Myers, P. H., & Kleeberger, S. R. et al. (2012a). Cardiac physiologic and genetic predictors of hyperoxia-induced acute lung injury in mice. *American Journal of Respiratory Cell and Molecular Biology*, *46*(4), 470–478. doi:10.1165/rcmb.2011-0204OC PMID:22052878

How, O. J., Aasum, E., Severson, D. L., Chan, W. Y., Essop, M. F., & Larsen, T. S. (2006). Increased myocardial oxygen consumption reduces cardiac efficiency in diabetic mice. *Diabetes*, *55*(2), 466–473. doi:10.2337/diabetes.55.02.06.db05-1164 PMID:16443782

Hoyert, D. L. (2012). *75 years of mortality in the United States, 1935–2010. NCHS Data Brief, 88.* Hyattsville, MD: National Center for Health Statistics

Hsu, C. P., Odewale, I., Alcendor, R. R., & Sadoshima, J. (2008). Sirt1 protects the heart from aging and stress. *Biological Chemistry*, *389*(3), 221–231. doi:10.1515/BC.2008.032 PMID:18208353

Hsu, C.-P., Oka, S., Shao, D., Hariharan, N., & Sadoshima, J. (2009). Nicotinamide Phosphoribosyltransferase Regulates Cell Survival Through NAD+ Synthesis in Cardiac Myocytes. *Circulation Research*, *105*(5), 481–491. doi:10.1161/CIRCRESAHA.109.203703 PMID:19661458

Huang, A. M., Newton, D., Kunapuli, A., Gandhi, T. N., Washer, L. L., Isip, J., & Nagel, J. L. et al. (2013). Impact of rapid organism identification via matrix-assisted laser desorption/ionization time-of-flight combined with antimicrobial stewardship team intervention in adult patients with bacteremia and candidemia. *Clinical Infectious Diseases*, *57*(9), 1237–1245. doi:10.1093/cid/cit498 PMID:23899684

Huang, D., Swanson, E., Lin, C., Schuman, J., Stinson, W., Chang, W., & et, et al.. (1991). Optical coherence tomography. *Science*, *254*(5035), 1178–1181. doi:10.1126/science.1957169 PMID:1957169

Huang, L. S., Berdyshev, E., Mathew, B., Fu, P., Gorshkova, I. A., He, D., & Natarajan, V. et al. (2013). Targeting sphingosine kinase 1 attenuates bleomycin-induced pulmonary fibrosis. *The FASEB Journal*, *27*(4), 1749–1760. doi:10.1096/fj.12-219634 PMID:23315259

Huang, P., Riordan, S. M., Heruth, D. P., Grigoryev, D. N., Zhang, L. Q., & Ye, S. Q. (2015). A critical role of nicotinamide phosphoribosyltransferase in human telomerase reverse transcriptase induction by resveratrol in aortic smooth muscle cells. *Oncotarget*, *6*(13), 10812–10824. doi:10.18632/oncotarget.3580 PMID:25926556

Huang, P., Wan, L., Qin, Z., Zhang, J., Liu, N., Zou, D., & Chen, Y. (2012). Post-mortem MSCT diagnosis of acute pericardial tamponade caused by blunt trauma to the chest in a motor-vehicle collision. *Romanian Journal of Legal Medicine*, *20*(2), 117–122. doi:10.4323/rjlm.2012.117

Huang, Y., & Whiteheart, S. W. (2015). Platelet secretion paves the way. *Blood*, *126*(4), 433–434. doi:10.1182/blood-2015-05-646687 PMID:26206945

Hui, H. P., Li, X. Y., Liu, X. H., Sun, S., Lu, X. C., Liu, T., & Yang, W. (2006). Adeno-associated viral gene transfer of SERCA2a improves heart function in chronic congestive heart failure rats. *Zhonghua Xin Xue Guan Bing Za Zhi*, *34*(4), 357–362. PMID:16776934

Huizing, M., Helip-Wooley, A., Westbroek, W., Gunay-Aygun, M., & Gahl, W. A. (2008). Disorders of lysosome-related organelle biogenesis: Clinical and molecular genetics. *Annual Review of Genomics and Human Genetics*, *9*(1), 359–386. doi:10.1146/annurev.genom.9.081307.164303 PMID:18544035

Hulot, J. S., Bura, A., Villard, E., Azizi, M., Remones, V., Goyenvalle, C., & Gaussem, P. et al. (2006). Cytochrome P450 2C19 loss-of-function polymorphism is a major determinant of clopidogrel responsiveness in healthy subjects. *Blood*, *108*(7), 2244–2247. doi:10.1182/blood-2006-04-013052 PMID:16772608

Hulot, J. S., Fauconnier, J., Ramanujam, D., Chaanine, A., Aubart, F., Sassi, Y., & Engelhardt, S. et al. (2011). Critical role for stromal interaction molecule 1 in cardiac hypertrophy. *Circulation*, *124*(7), 796–805. doi:10.1161/CIRCULATIONAHA.111.031229 PMID:21810664

Hung, L. M., Su, M. J., & Chen, J. K. (2004). Resveratrol protects myocardial ischemia-reperfusion injury through both NO-dependent and NO-independent mechanisms. *Free Radical Biology & Medicine*, *36*(6), 774–781. doi:10.1016/j.freeradbiomed.2003.12.016 PMID:14990356

Hunton, D. L., Lucchesi, P. A., Pang, Y., Cheng, X., DellItalia, L. J., & Marchase, R. B. (2002). Capacitative calcium entry contributes to nuclear factor of activated T-cells nuclear translocation and hypertrophy in cardiomyocytes. *The Journal of Biological Chemistry*, *277*(16), 14266–14273. doi:10.1074/jbc.M107167200 PMID:11827959

Hunton, D. L., Zou, L., Pang, Y., & Marchase, R. B. (2004). Adult rat cardiomyocytes exhibit capacitative calcium entry. *American Journal of Physiology. Heart and Circulatory Physiology*, *286*(3), H1124–H1132. doi:10.1152/ajpheart.00162.2003 PMID:14630640

Hunt, S., Abraham, W. T., & Chin, M. H. (2009). Focused update incorporated into the ACC/AHA 2005 guidelines for the diagnosis and management of heart failure in adults: A report of the american college of cardiology foundation/american heart association task force on practice guidelines developed in collaboration with the international society for heart and lung transplantation. *Journal of the American College of Cardiology*, *53*(15), e1–e90. doi:10.1016/j.jacc.2008.11.013 PMID:19358937

Hutchins, G. M., Berman, J. J., Moore, G. W., & Hanzlick, R. (1999). Practice guidelines for autopsy pathology: Autopsy reporting. *Archives of Pathology & Laboratory Medicine*, *123*(11), 1085. PMID:10539932

Hwang, J. W., Yao, H., Caito, S., Sundar, I. K., & Rahman, I. (2013). Redox regulation of SIRT1 in inflammation and cellular senescence. *Free Radical Biology & Medicine*, *61*, 95–110. doi:10.1016/j.freeradbiomed.2013.03.015 PMID:23542362

Idahosa, C., Berardi, T. R., Shkolnikov, R., & Stoopler, E. T. (2014). Thrombocytopenia absent radius (TAR) syndrome: A case report and review for oral health care providers. *Special Care in Dentistry*, *34*(5), 251–258. doi:10.1111/scd.12060 PMID:25346959

Ido, Y. (2007). Pyridine nucleotide redox abnormalities in diabetes. *Antioxidants & Redox Signalling*, *9*(7), 931–942. doi:10.1089/ars.2007.1630 PMID:17508915

Igarashi, J., Bernier, S. G., & Michel, T. (2001). Sphingosine 1-phosphate and activation of endothelial nitric-oxide synthase. differential regulation of Akt and MAP kinase pathways by EDG and bradykinin receptors in vascular endothelial cells. *The Journal of Biological Chemistry*, *276*(15), 12420–12426. doi:10.1074/jbc.M008375200 PMID:11278407

Imberti, B., Monti, M., & Casiraghi, F. (2015). Pluripotent stem cells and tolerance induction in organ transplantation. *Current Opinion in Organ Transplantation*, *20*(1), 86–93. doi:10.1097/MOT.0000000000000144 PMID:25522138

Isaacs, A., Willems, S. M., Bos, D., Dehghan, A., Hofman, A., Ikram, M. A., & van Duijn, C. M. et al. (2013). Risk scores of common genetic variants for lipid levels influence atherosclerosis and incident coronary heart disease. *Arteriosclerosis, Thrombosis, and Vascular Biology*, *33*(9), 2233–2239. doi:10.1161/ATVBAHA.113.301236 PMID:23766260

Ishii, N., Senoo-Matsuda, N., Miyake, K., Yasuda, K., Ishii, T., Hartman, P. S., & Furukawa, S. (2004). Coenzyme Q10 can prolong C. elegans lifespan by lowering oxidative stress. *Mechanisms of Ageing and Development*, *125*(1), 41–46. doi:10.1016/j.mad.2003.10.002 PMID:14706236

Ismail, R., & Teh, L. K. (2006). The relevance of CYP2D6 genetic polymorphism on chronic metoprolol therapy in cardiovascular patients. *Journal of Clinical Pharmacy and Therapeutics*, *31*(1), 99–109. doi:10.1111/j.1365-2710.2006.00699.x PMID:16476126

Ito, K., Bick, A. G., Flannick, J., Friedman, D. J., Genovese, G., Parfenov, M. G., & Seidman, C. et al. (2014). Increased burden of cardiovascular disease in carriers of APOL1 genetic variants. *Circulation Research*, *114*(5), 845–850. doi:10.1161/CIRCRESAHA.114.302347 PMID:24379297

Iwamoto, T. a. Acoustical Imaging. http://link.springer.com/chapter/10.1007/978-1-4020-8823-0_21, 5.

Jain, K. (2008). Drug Delivery Systems. In *Drug Delivery Systems* (p. 16). Totowa, NJ: Humana. doi:10.1007/978-1-59745-210-6_1

Jalili, T., Carlstrom, J., Kim, S., Freeman, D., Jin, H. F., Wu, T. C., & David Symons, J. et al. (2006). Quercetin-supplemented diets lower blood pressure and attenuate cardiac hypertrophy in rats with aortic constriction. *Journal of Cardiovascular Pharmacology*, *47*(4), 531–541. doi:10.1097/01.fjc.0000211746.78454.50 PMID:16680066

James, P. A., Oparil, S., Carter, B. L., Cushman, W. C., Dennison-Himmelfarb, C., Handler, J., & Ortiz, E. et al. (2014). 2014 evidence-based guideline for the management of high blood pressure in adults: Report from the panel members appointed to the Eighth Joint National Committee (JNC 8). *Journal of the American Medical Association*, *311*(5), 507–520. doi:10.1001/jama.2013.284427 PMID:24352797

January, C. T., Wann, L. S., Alpert, J. S., Calkins, H., Cigarroa, J. E., Cleveland, J. C. Jr, & Yancy, C. W. et al. (2014). 2014 AHA/ACC/HRS guideline for the management of patients with atrial fibrillation: A report of the American College of Cardiology/American Heart Association Task Force on practice guidelines and the Heart Rhythm Society. *Circulation*, *130*(23), e199–e267. doi:10.1161/CIR.0000000000000041 PMID:24682347

Javkhedkar, A. A., Quiroz, Y., Rodriguez-Iturbe, B., Vaziri, N. D., Lokhandwala, M. F., & Banday, A. A. (2015). Resveratrol restored Nrf2 function, reduced renal inflammation, and mitigated hypertension in spontaneously hypertensive rats. *American Journal of Physiology. Regulatory, Integrative and Comparative Physiology*, *308*(10), R840–R846. doi:10.1152/ajpregu.00308.2014 PMID:25761698

Jenkins, D. J., Kendall, C. W., Axelsen, M., Augustin, L. S., & Vuksan, V. (2000). Viscous and nonviscous fibres, nonabsorbable and low glycaemic index carbohydrates, blood lipids and coronary heart disease. *Current Opinion in Lipidology*, *11*(1), 49–56. doi:10.1097/00041433-200002000-00008 PMID:10750694

Jensen, M. D., Ryan, D. H., Apovian, C. M., Ard, J. D., Comuzzie, A. G., Donato, K. A., & Yanovski, S. Z. et al. (2014). 2013 AHA/ACC/TOS guideline for the management of overweight and obesity in adults: A report of the American College of Cardiology/American Heart Association Task Force on Practice Guidelines and The Obesity Society. *Journal of the American College of Cardiology*, *63*(2525 Pt B), 2985–3023. doi:10.1016/j.jacc.2013.11.004 PMID:24239920

Jessup, M., Abraham, W. T., Casey, D. E., Feldman, A. M., Francis, G. S., Ganiats, T. G., & Silver, M. A. et al. (2009). 2009 focused update: ACCF/AHA guidelines for the diagnosis and management of heart failure in adults: a report of the American College of Cardiology Foundation/American Heart Association Task Force on Practice Guidelines developed in collaboration with the International Society for Heart and Lung Transplantation. *Journal of the American College of Cardiology*, *53*(15), 1343–1382. doi:10.1016/j.jacc.2008.11.009 PMID:19324967

Jho, D., Mehta, D., Ahmmed, G., Gao, X. P., Tiruppathi, C., Broman, M., & Malik, A. B. (2005). Angiopoietin-1 opposes VEGF-induced increase in endothelial permeability by inhibiting TRPC1-dependent Ca2 influx. *Circulation Research*, *96*(12), 1282–1290. doi:10.1161/01.RES.0000171894.03801.03 PMID:15920022

Jia, Y., & Takimoto, K. (2003). GATA and FOG2 transcription factors differentially regulate the promoter for Kv4.2 K+ channel gene in cardiac myocytes and PC12 cells. *Cardiovascular Research*, *60*(2), 278–287. doi:10.1016/S0008-6363(03)00528-5 PMID:14613857

Jin, H., Hadri, L., Palomeque, J., Morel, C., Karakikes, I., Kaprielian, R., & Lebeche, D. et al. (2010). KChIP2 attenuates cardiac hypertrophy through regulation of Ito and intracellular calcium signaling. *Journal of Molecular and Cellular Cardiology*, *48*(6), 1169–1179. doi:10.1016/j.yjmcc.2009.12.019 PMID:20051248

John, R. M., Tedrow, U. B., Koplan, B. A., Albert, C. M., Epstein, L. M., Sweeney, M. O., & Stevenson, W. G. et al. (2012). Ventricular arrhythmias and sudden cardiac death. *Lancet*, *380*(9852), 1520–1529. doi:10.1016/S0140-6736(12)61413-5 PMID:23101719

Johns, D. C., Nuss, H. B., & Marban, E. (1997). Suppression of neuronal and cardiac transient outward currents by viral gene transfer of dominant-negative Kv4.2 constructs. *The Journal of Biological Chemistry*, *272*(50), 31598–31603. doi:10.1074/jbc.272.50.31598 PMID:9395498

Johnson, J. A., & Cavallari, L. H. (2013). Pharmacogenetics and Cardiovascular Disease—Implications for Personalized Medicine. *Pharmacological Reviews*, *65*(3), 987–1009. doi:10.1124/pr.112.007252 PMID:23686351

Jones, R. H. (1984). Must Enlightened Mystics Be Moral? *Philosophy East & West*, *34*(3), 273–293. doi:10.2307/1398629

Jonnalagadda, D., Izu, L. T., & Whiteheart, S. W. (2012). Platelet secretion is kinetically heterogeneous in an agonist-responsive manner. *Blood*, *120*(26), 5209–5216. doi:10.1182/blood-2012-07-445080 PMID:23086755

Jorge Dinis-Oliveira, R., Carvalho, F., Alberto Duarte, J., Brandao Proenca, J., Santos, A., & Magalhães, T. (2012). Clinical and forensic signs related to cocaine abuse. *Current Drug Abuse Reviews*, *5*(1), 64–83. doi:10.2174/1874473711205010064 PMID:22280333

Jung, S.-H., Kim, J. J., Choo, S. J., Yun, T.-J., Chung, C. H., & Lee, J. W. (2011). Long-term mortality in adult orthotopic heart transplant recipients. *Journal of Korean Medical Science*, *26*(5), 599–603. doi:10.3346/jkms.2011.26.5.599 PMID:21532848

Jun, W. J., Han, B. K., Yu, K. W., Kim, M. S., Chang, I. S., & Kim, H. Y. (2001). Antioxidant effects of Origanum majorana L. on superoxide anion radicals. *Food Chemistry*, *75*(4), 439–444. doi:10.1016/S0308-8146(01)00233-3

Ju, Y. K., Chu, Y., Chaulet, H., Lai, D., Gervasio, O. L., Graham, R. M., & Allen, D. G. et al. (2007). Store-operated Ca2+ influx and expression of TRPC genes in mouse sinoatrial node. *Circulation Research*, *100*(11), 1605–1614. doi:10.1161/CIRCRESAHA.107.152181 PMID:17478725

Kahr, W. H., Hinckley, J., Li, L., Schwertz, H., Christensen, H., Rowley, J. W., & Di Paola, J. et al. (2011). Mutations in NBEAL2, encoding a BEACH protein, cause gray platelet syndrome. *Nature Genetics*, *43*(8), 738–740. doi:10.1038/ng.884 PMID:21765413

Kaiser, C., Galatius, S., Erne, P., Eberli, F., Alber, H., Rickli, H., & Pfisterer, M. et al. (2010). Drug-Eluting versus Bare-Metal Stents in Large Coronary Arteries. *The New England Journal of Medicine*, *363*(24), 2310–2319. doi:10.1056/NEJMoa1009406 PMID:21080780

Kajstura, J., Cheng, W., Reiss, K., Clark, W. A., Sonnenblick, E. H., Krajewski, S., & Anversa, P. et al. (1996). Apoptotic and necrotic myocyte cell deaths are independent contributing variables of infarct size in rats. *Laboratory Investigation*, *74*(1), 86–107. PMID:8569201

Kalil, A. C., Van Schooneveld, T. C., Fey, P. D., & Rupp, M. E. (2014). Association between vancomycin minimum inhibitory concentration and mortality among patients with Staphylococcus aureus bloodstream infections: A systematic review and meta-analysis. *Journal of the American Medical Association*, *312*(15), 1552–1564. doi:10.1001/jama.2014.6364 PMID:25321910

Kallet, R. H., & Matthay, M. A. (2013). Hyperoxic Acute Lung Injury. *Respiratory Care*, *58*(1), 123–141. doi:10.4187/respcare.01963 PMID:23271823

Kameda, K., Takaku, T., Okuda, H., Kimura, Y., Okuda, T., Hatano, T., & Arichi, S. et al. (1987). Inhibitory effects of various flavonoids isolated from leaves of persimmon on angiotensin-converting enzyme activity. *Journal of Natural Products*, *50*(4), 680–683. doi:10.1021/np50052a017 PMID:3430165

Kanafani, Z. A., Federspiel, J. J., & Fowler, V. G. Jr. (2007). Infective endocarditis caused by daptomycin-resistant Enterococcus faecalis: A case report. *Scandinavian Journal of Infectious Diseases*, *39*(1), 75–77. doi:10.1080/00365540600786465 PMID:17366018

Kanamori, H., Takemura, G., Goto, K., Tsujimoto, A., Ogino, A., Takeyama, T., & Minatoguchi, S. et al. (2013). Resveratrol reverses remodeling in hearts with large, old myocardial infarctions through enhanced autophagy-activating AMP kinase pathway. *American Journal of Pathology*, *182*(3), 701–713. doi:10.1016/j.ajpath.2012.11.009 PMID:23274061

Kang, O. H., Jang, H. J., Chae, H. S., Oh, Y. C., Choi, J. G., Lee, Y. S., & Kwon, D. Y. et al. (2009). Anti-inflammatory mechanisms of resveratrol in activated HMC-1 cells: Pivotal roles of NF-kappaB and MAPK. *Pharmacological Research*, *59*(5), 330–337. doi:10.1016/j.phrs.2009.01.009 PMID:19416633

Kang, S. M., Lim, S., Song, H., Chang, W., Lee, S., Bae, S. M., & Hwang, K. C. et al. (2006). Allopurinol modulates reactive oxygen species generation and Ca2+ overload in ischemia-reperfused heart and hypoxia-reoxygenated cardiomyocytes. *European Journal of Pharmacology*, *535*(1-3), 212–219. doi:10.1016/j.ejphar.2006.01.013 PMID:16516885

Kanjilal, S., Gregg, E. W., Cheng, Y. J., Zhang, P., Nelson, D. E., Mensah, G., & Beckles, G. L. A. (2006). Socioeconomic Status and Trends in Disparities in 4 major Risk Factors for Cardiovascular Disease among US Adults, 19712002. *Archives of Internal Medicine*, *166*(21), 2348–2355. doi:10.1001/archinte.166.21.2348 PMID:17130388

Kara, K., Lehmann, N., Neumann, T., Kalsch, H., Mohlenkamp, S., Dykun, I., & Mahabadi, A. A. et al. (2015). NT-proBNP is superior to BNP for predicting first cardiovascular events in the general population: The Heinz Nixdorf Recall Study. *International Journal of Cardiology*, *183*, 155–161. doi:10.1016/j.ijcard.2015.01.082 PMID:25666125

Karin, M., & Ben-Neriah, Y. (2000). Phosphorylation meets ubiquitination: The control of NF-kB activity. *Annual Review of Immunology*, *18*(1), 621–663. doi:10.1146/annurev.immunol.18.1.621 PMID:10837071

Karlstad, J., Sun, Y., & Singh, B. B. (2012). Ca(2+) signaling: An outlook on the characterization of Ca(2+) channels and their importance in cellular functions. *Advances in Experimental Medicine and Biology*, *740*, 143–157. doi:10.1007/978-94-007-2888-2_6 PMID:22453941

Kasahara, A., Cipolat, S., Chen, Y., Dorn, G. W. II, & Scorrano, L. (2013). Mitochondrial fusion directs cardiomyocyte differentiation via calcineurin and Notch signaling. *Science*, *342*(6159), 734–737. doi:10.1126/science.1241359 PMID:24091702

Kathiresan, S., & Srivastava, D. (2012). Genetics of human cardiovascular disease. *Cell*, *148*(6), 1242–1257. doi:10.1016/j.cell.2012.03.001 PMID:22424232

Katz, B., Rosenberg, A., & Frishman, W. H. (1995). Controlled-release drug delivery systems in cardiovascular medicine. *American Heart Journal*, *129*(2), 359–368. doi:10.1016/0002-8703(95)90019-5 PMID:7832110

Kaufman, A. L., Spitz, J., Jacobs, M., Sorrentino, M., Yuen, S., Danahey, K., & ODonnell, P. H. (2015). Evidence for Clinical Implementation of Pharmacogenomics in Cardiac Drugs. *Mayo Clinic Proceedings*, *90*(6), 716–729. doi:10.1016/j.mayocp.2015.03.016 PMID:26046407

Kaufman, R. J. (2002). Orchestrating the unfolded protein response in health and disease. *The Journal of Clinical Investigation*, *110*(10), 1389–1398. doi:10.1172/JCI0216886 PMID:12438434

Kawada, H., Niwano, S., Niwano, H., Yumoto, Y., Wakisaka, Y., Yuge, M., . . . Izumi, T. (2006). Tumor necrosis factor-alpha downregulates the voltage gated outward K+ current in cultured neonatal rat cardiomyocytes: a possible cause of electrical remodeling in diseased hearts. *Circulation Journal: Official Journal of the Japanese Circulation Society*, *70*(5), 605-609.

Kawasaki, T., Ueyama, T., Lange, I., Feske, S., & Saito, N. (2010). Protein kinase C-induced phosphorylation of Orai1 regulates the intracellular Ca2+ level via the store-operated Ca2+ channel. *The Journal of Biological Chemistry*, *285*(33), 25720–25730. doi:10.1074/jbc.M109.022996 PMID:20534587

Kearon, C., Akl, E. A., Ornelas, J., Blaivas, A., Jimenez, D., Bounameaux, H., & Moores, L. et al. (2016). Antithrombotic therapy for vte disease: Chest guideline and expert panel report. *Chest*, *149*(2), 315–352. doi:10.1016/j.chest.2015.11.026 PMID:26867832

Kemp, C. D., & Conte, J. V. (2013). The pathophysiology of heart failure. *Cardiovascular Pathology*, *21*(5), 365–371. doi:10.1016/j.carpath.2011.11.007 PMID:22227365

Ker, J., Toit-Prinsloo, L. D., Van Heerden, W., & Saayman, G. (2010). Post-Mortem Echocardiography as a Guide to Cardiac Autopsy—A Worthwhile Concept? Clinical Medicine Insights. *Cardiology*, *4*, 59–61. PMID:20859531

Khan, A. R., Binabdulhak, A. A., Alastal, Y., Khan, S., Faricy-Beredo, B. M., Luni, F. K., . . . Tinkel, J. (2014). Cardioprotective role of ischemic postconditioning in acute myocardial infarction: a systematic review and meta-analysis. *Am Heart J, 168*(4), 512-521 e514. doi: 10.1016/j.ahj.2014.06.021

Khandaker, M. H., Espinosa, R. E., Nishimura, R. A., Sinak, L. J., Hayes, S. N., Melduni, R. M., & Oh, J. K. (2010). Pericardial disease: Diagnosis and management. *Mayo Clinic Proceedings*, *85*(6), 572–593. doi:10.4065/mcp.2010.0046 PMID:20511488

Khanna, V. K. (2012). Targeted Delivery of Nanomedicines. *ISRN Pharmacology*, *2012*, 1–9. doi:10.5402/2012/571394

Khemani, E., McElhinney, D. B., Rhein, L., Andrade, O., Lacro, R. V., Thomas, K. C., & Mullen, M. P. (2007). Pulmonary artery hypertension in formerly premature infants with bronchopulmonary dysplasia: Clinical features and outcomes in the surfactant era. *Pediatrics*, *120*(6), 1260–1269. doi:10.1542/peds.2007-0971 PMID:18055675

Khimji, I. A., Kazmerski, T. M., & Webber, S. A. (2008). Immunosuppressive Agents in Pediatric Heart Transplantation. In Handbook of Pediatric Cardiovascular Drugs (pp. 190-214). Springer Science + Business Media.

Kile, B. T. (2014). The role of apoptosis in megakaryocytes and platelets. *British Journal of Haematology*, *165*(2), 217–226. doi:10.1111/bjh.12757 PMID:24467740

Kilgannon, J. H., Jones, A. E., Shapiro, N. I., Angelos, M. G., Milcarek, B., & Hunter, K.Emergency Medicine Shock Research Network, Investigators. (2010). Association between arterial hyperoxia following resuscitation from cardiac arrest and in-hospital mortality. *Journal of the American Medical Association*, *303*(21), 2165–2171. doi:10.1001/jama.2010.707 PMID:20516417

Kim, E. S., Ahn, E. H., Dvir, T., & Kim, D. H. (2014). Emerging nanotechnology approaches in tissue engineering and regenerative medicine. *International Journal of Nanomedicine*, *9*(Suppl 1), 1–5. doi:10.2147/IJN.S61212 PMID:24872698

Kim, J. S., Kim, B., Lee, H., Thakkar, S., Babbitt, D. M., Eguchi, S., & Park, J. Y. et al. (2015a). Shear stress-induced mitochondrial biogenesis decreases the release of microparticles from endothelial cells. *American Journal of Physiology. Heart and Circulatory Physiology*, *309*(3), H425–H433. doi:10.1152/ajpheart.00438.2014 PMID:26024684

Kim, M. K., Sasaki, S., Sasazuki, S., Okubo, S., Hayashi, M., & Tsugane, S. (2002). Lack of long-term effect of vitamin C supplementation on blood pressure. *Hypertension*, *40*(6), 797–803. doi:10.1161/01.HYP.0000038339.67450.60 PMID:12468560

Kingwell, K. (2011). Cardiovascular disease: microRNA protects the heart. *Nature Reviews. Drug Discovery*, *10*(2), 98. doi:10.1038/nrd3380 PMID:21283101

Kin, H., Zhao, Z.-Q., Sun, H.-Y., Wang, N.-P., Corvera, J. S., Halkos, M. E., & Vinten-Johansen, J. et al. (2004). Postconditioning attenuates myocardial ischemia–reperfusion injury by inhibiting events in the early minutes of reperfusion. *Cardiovascular Research*, *62*(1), 74–85. doi:10.1016/j.cardiores.2004.01.006 PMID:15023554

Kini, V., Chavez, A., & Mehta, D. (2010). A new role for PTEN in regulating transient receptor potential canonical channel 6-mediated Ca2+ entry, endothelial permeability, and angiogenesis. *The Journal of Biological Chemistry*, *285*(43), 33082–33091. doi:10.1074/jbc.M110.142034 PMID:20705603

Kinoshita, H., Kuwahara, K., Nishida, M., Jian, Z., Rong, X., Kiyonaka, S., & Nakao, K. et al. (2010). Inhibition of TRPC6 channel activity contributes to the antihypertrophic effects of natriuretic peptides-guanylyl cyclase-A signaling in the heart. *Circulation Research*, *106*(12), 1849–1860. doi:10.1161/CIRCRESAHA.109.208314 PMID:20448219

Kitsios, G. D., & Kent, D. M. (2012). Personalised medicine: Not just in our genes. *BMJ (Clinical Research Ed.)*, *344*, e2161. PMID:22491484

Klein, T. E., Chang, J. T., Cho, M. K., Easton, K. L., Fergerson, R., Hewett, M., & Altman, R. B. et al. (2001). Integrating Genotype and Phenotype Information: An Overview of the PharmGKB Project. *The Pharmacogenomics Journal*, *1*(3), 167–170. doi:10.1038/sj.tpj.6500035 PMID:11908751

Knezevic, N., Roy, A., Timblin, B., Konstantoulaki, M., Sharma, T., Malik, A. B., & Mehta, D. (2007). GDI-1 phosphorylation switch at serine 96 induces RhoA activation and increased endothelial permeability. *Molecular and Cellular Biology*, *27*(18), 6323–6333. doi:10.1128/MCB.00523-07 PMID:17636025

Knezevic, N., Tauseef, M., Thennes, T., & Mehta, D. (2009). The G protein betagamma subunit mediates reannealing of adherens junctions to reverse endothelial permeability increase by thrombin. *The Journal of Experimental Medicine*, *206*(12), 2761–2777. doi:10.1084/jem.20090652 PMID:19917775

Kojima, A., Kitagawa, H., Omatsu-Kanbe, M., Matsuura, H., & Nosaka, S. (2012). Presence of store-operated Ca2+ entry in C57BL/6J mouse ventricular myocytes and its suppression by sevoflurane. *British Journal of Anaesthesia*, *109*(3), 352–360. doi:10.1093/bja/aes212 PMID:22777657

Komarova, Y. A., Huang, F., Geyer, M., Daneshjou, N., Garcia, A., Idalino, L., & Malik, A. B. et al. (2012). VE-cadherin signaling induces EB3 phosphorylation to suppress microtubule growth and assemble adherens junctions. *Molecular Cell*, *48*(6), 914–925. doi:10.1016/j.molcel.2012.10.011 PMID:23159740

Komarova, Y. A., Mehta, D., & Malik, A. B. (2007). Dual regulation of endothelial junctional permeability. *Science's STKE*, *re8*(412), •••. doi:10.1126/stke.4122007re8 PMID:18000237

Konstantinov, I. E., Arab, S., Kharbanda, R. K., Li, J., Cheung, M. M. H., Cherepanov, V., & Redington, A. N. et al. (2004). The remote ischemic preconditioning stimulus modifies inflammatory gene expression in humans. *Physiological Genomics*, *19*(1), 143–150. doi:10.1152/physiolgenomics.00046.2004 PMID:15304621

Koponen, M. A., & Lantz, P. E. (2003). Sudden Unexpected Adult Deaths. In R. C. Froede (Ed.), *Handbook of Forensic Pathology* (2nd ed.; pp. 89–92). CAP.

Koppel, R., Han, R. N. N., Cox, D., Tanswell, A. K., & Rabinovitch, M. (1994). [alpha]1-Antitrypsin Protects Neonatal Rats from Pulmonary Vascular and Parenchymal Effects of Oxygen Toxicity. *Pediatric Research*, *36*(6), 763–770. doi:10.1203/00006450-199412000-00014 PMID:7898985

Kotani, K., Fujiwara, S., Tsuzaki, K., Sano, Y., Matsuoka, Y., Hamada, T., & Sakane, N. (2009). An association between angiotensin II type 2 receptor gene A/C3123 polymorphism and glycemic control marker in a general Japanese population. *Molecular Biology Reports*, *36*(5), 917–920. doi:10.1007/s11033-008-9263-y PMID:18437528

Kouklis, P., Konstantoulaki, M., Vogel, S., Broman, M., & Malik, A. B. (2004). Cdc42 regulates the restoration of endothelial barrier function. *Circulation Research*, *94*(2), 159–166. doi:10.1161/01.RES.0000110418.38500.31 PMID:14656933

Kowata, S., Isogai, S., Murai, K., Ito, S., Tohyama, K., Ema, M., & Ishida, Y. et al. (2014). Platelet demand modulates the type of intravascular protrusion of megakaryocytes in bone marrow. *Thrombosis and Haemostasis*, *112*(4), 743–756. doi:10.1160/TH14-02-0123 PMID:24965909

Kozak, J. A., Kerschbaum, H. H., & Cahalan, M. D. (2002). Distinct properties of CRAC and MIC channels in RBL cells. *The Journal of General Physiology*, *120*(2), 221–235. doi:10.1085/jgp.20028601 PMID:12149283

Kraft, T. E., Parisotto, D., Schempp, C., & Efferth, T. (2009). Fighting cancer with red wine? Molecular mechanisms of resveratrol. *Critical Reviews in Food Science and Nutrition*, *49*(9), 782–799. doi:10.1080/10408390802248627 PMID:20443159

Kressmann, S., Muller, W. E., & Blume, H. H. (2002). Pharmaceutical quality of different Ginkgo biloba brands. *The Journal of Pharmacy and Pharmacology*, *54*(5), 661–669. doi:10.1211/0022357021778970 PMID:12005361

Kudolo, G. B. (2000). The effect of 3-month ingestion of Ginkgo biloba extract on pancreatic beta-cell function in response to glucose loading in normal glucose tolerant individuals. *Journal of Clinical Pharmacology*, *40*(6), 647–654. doi:10.1002/j.1552-4604.2000.tb05991.x PMID:10868316

Kukielka, G. L., Hawkins, H. K., Michael, L., Manning, A. M., Youker, K., Lane, C., & Anderson, D. C. et al. (1993). Regulation of intercellular adhesion molecule-1 (ICAM-1) in ischemic and reperfused canine myocardium. *The Journal of Clinical Investigation*, *92*(3), 1504–1516. doi:10.1172/JCI116729 PMID:8104198

Kulisic, T., Krisko, A., Dragovic-Uzelac, V., Milos, M., & Pifat, G. (2007). The effects of essential oils and aqueous tea infusions of oregano (Origanum vulgare L. spp. hirtum), thyme (Thymus vulgaris L.) and wild thyme (Thymus serpyllum L.) on the copper-induced oxidation of human low-density lipoproteins. *International Journal of Food Sciences and Nutrition*, *58*(2), 87–93. doi:10.1080/09637480601108307 PMID:17469764

Kullar, R., Casapao, A. M., Davis, S. L., Levine, D. P., Zhao, J. J., Crank, C. W., & Rybak, M. J. et al. (2013). A multicentre evaluation of the effectiveness and safety of high-dose daptomycin for the treatment of infective endocarditis. *The Journal of Antimicrobial Chemotherapy*, *68*(12), 2921–2926. doi:10.1093/jac/dkt294 PMID:23928022

Kullar, R., Davis, S. L., Levine, D. P., & Rybak, M. J. (2011). Impact of vancomycin exposure on outcomes in patients with methicillin-resistant Staphylococcus aureus bacteremia: Support for consensus guidelines suggested targets. *Clinical Infectious Diseases*, *52*(8), 975–981. doi:10.1093/cid/cir124 PMID:21460309

Kullar, R., McKinnell, J. A., & Sakoulas, G. (2014). Avoiding the perfect storm: The biologic and clinical case for reevaluating the 7-day expectation for methicillin-resistant Staphylococcus aureus bacteremia before switching therapy. *Clinical Infectious Diseases*, *59*(10), 1455–1461. doi:10.1093/cid/ciu583 PMID:25048852

Kullar, R., Sakoulas, G., Deresinski, S., & van Hal, S. J. (2016). When sepsis persists: A review of MRSA bacteraemia salvage therapy. *The Journal of Antimicrobial Chemotherapy*, *71*(3), 576–586. doi:10.1093/jac/dkv368 PMID:26565015

Kumar, S., Kumar, V. A., Kumar, N., Baranwal, R. K., Kumar, V. R., & Singh, M. (2011). Coronary atherosclerosis--a postmortem histopathological study. *Bratislavske lekarske listy*, *113*(4), 217-219.

Kumar, A. G., Ballantyne, C. M., Michael, L. H., Kukielka, G. L., Youker, K. A., Lindsey, M. L., & Entman, M. L. et al. (1997). Induction of Monocyte Chemoattractant Protein-1 in the Small Veins of the Ischemic and Reperfused Canine Myocardium. *Circulation*, *95*(3), 693–700. doi:10.1161/01.CIR.95.3.693 PMID:9024159

Kumar, A., Lin, Z., SenBanerjee, S., & Jain, M. K. (2005). Tumor necrosis factor alpha-mediated reduction of KLF2 is due to inhibition of MEF2 by NF-kappaB and histone deacetylases. *Molecular and Cellular Biology*, *25*(14), 5893–5899. doi:10.1128/MCB.25.14.5893-5903.2005 PMID:15988006

Kuo, H. C., Cheng, C. F., Clark, R. B., Lin, J. J., Lin, J. L., Hoshijima, M., & Chien, K. R. et al. (2001). A defect in the Kv channel-interacting protein 2 (KChIP2) gene leads to a complete loss of I(to) and confers susceptibility to ventricular tachycardia. *Cell*, *107*(6), 801–813. doi:10.1016/S0092-8674(01)00588-8 PMID:11747815

Kuriyama, S. (2008). The relation between green tea consumption and cardiovascular disease as evidenced by epidemiological studies. *The Journal of Nutrition*, *138*(8), 1548S–1553S. PMID:18641205

Kuroda, J., Ago, T., Matsushima, S., Zhai, P., Schneider, M. D., & Sadoshima, J. (2010). NADPH oxidase 4 (Nox4) is a major source of oxidative stress in the failing heart. *Proceedings of the National Academy of Sciences of the United States of America*, *107*(35), 15565–15570. doi:10.1073/pnas.1002178107 PMID:20713697

Kurrelmeyer, K. M., Michael, L. H., Baumgarten, G., Taffet, G. E., Peschon, J. J., Sivasubramanian, N., & Mann, D. L. et al. (2000). Endogenous tumor necrosis factor protects the adult cardiac myocyte against ischemic-induced apoptosis in a murine model of acute myocardial infarction. *Proceedings of the National Academy of Sciences of the United States of America*, *97*(10), 5456–5461. doi:10.1073/pnas.070036297 PMID:10779546

Kuwahara, K., Wang, Y., McAnally, J., Richardson, J. A., Bassel-Duby, R., Hill, J. A., & Olson, E. N. (2006). TRPC6 fulfills a calcineurin signaling circuit during pathologic cardiac remodeling. *The Journal of Clinical Investigation*, *116*(12), 3114–3126. doi:10.1172/JCI27702 PMID:17099778

Kwak, J. S., Kim, J. Y., Paek, J. E., Lee, Y. J., Kim, H.-R., Park, D.-S., & Kwon, O. (2014). Garlic powder intake and cardiovascular risk factors: A meta-analysis of randomized controlled clinical trials. *Nutrition Research and Practice*, *8*(6), 644–654. doi:10.4162/nrp.2014.8.6.644 PMID:25489404

Kwong, J. C., McCallum, N., Sintchenko, V., & Howden, B. P. (2015). Whole genome sequencing in clinical and public health microbiology. *Pathology*, *47*(3), 199–210. doi:10.1097/PAT.0000000000000235 PMID:25730631

Labhasetwar, V., Song, C., & Levy, R. J. (1997, February 15). *Nanoparticle drug delivery system for restenosis*. Retrieved from http://ac.els-cdn.com/S0169409X96004838/1-s2.0-S0169409X96004838-main.pdf?_tid=6f3e82c6-0f13-11e5-a92a-00000aab0f6c&acdnat=1433901365_efc2bb3176ba31c69419d1000d79c27f

Lai, C. C., Sheng, W. H., Wang, J. T., Cheng, A., Chuang, Y. C., Chen, Y. C., & Chang, S. C. (2013). Safety and efficacy of high-dose daptomycin as salvage therapy for severe gram-positive bacterial sepsis in hospitalized adult patients. *BMC Infectious Diseases*, *13*(1), 66. doi:10.1186/1471-2334-13-66 PMID:23379510

Lamas, C. C., & Eykyn, S. J. (2000). Bicuspid aortic valveA silent danger: Analysis of 50 cases of infective endocarditis. *Clinical Infectious Diseases*, *30*(2), 336–341. doi:10.1086/313646 PMID:10671338

Lange, R. A., & Hillis, L. D. (2004). Acute pericarditis. *The New England Journal of Medicine*, *351*(21), 2195–2202. doi:10.1056/NEJMcp041997 PMID:15548780

Langsjoen, P., Langsjoen, P., Willis, R., & Folkers, K. (1994). Treatment of essential hypertension with coenzyme Q10. *Molecular Aspects of Medicine*, *15*(Suppl), S265–S272. doi:10.1016/0098-2997(94)90037-X PMID:7752851

Lang, T., Lepage, B., Schieber, A.-C., Lamy, S., & Kelley-Irving, M. (2012). Social Determinants of Cardiovascular Diseases. *Public Health Reviews*, *33*(2), 601–622

Larson, A. J., Symons, J. D., & Jalili, T. (2012). Therapeutic Potential of Quercetin to Decrease Blood Pressure: Review of Efficacy and Mechanisms. *Advances in Nutrition*, *3*(1), 39–46. doi:10.3945/an.111.001271 PMID:22332099

Lassègue, B., San Martín, A., & Griendling, K. K. (2012). Biochemistry, Physiology, and Pathophysiology of NADPH Oxidases in the Cardiovascular System. *Circulation Research, 110*(10), 1364–1390. doi:10.1161/CIRCRESAHA.111.243972 PMID:22581922

Laverriere, A. C., MacNeill, C., Mueller, C., Poelmann, R. E., Burch, J. B., & Evans, T. (1994). GATA-4/5/6, a subfamily of three transcription factors transcribed in developing heart and gut. *The Journal of Biological Chemistry, 269*(37), 23177–23184. PMID:8083222

Le Bon, A.-M., Vernevaut, M.-F., Guenot, L., Kahane, R., Auger, J., Arnault, I., & Siess, M.-H. et al. (2003). Effects of garlic powders with varying alliin contents on hepatic drug metabolizing enzymes in rats. *Journal of Agricultural and Food Chemistry, 51*(26), 7617–7623. doi:10.1021/jf0346758 PMID:14664517

Leclercq, C. (2007). New guidelines for cardiac resynchronisation therapy: Simplicity or complexity for the doctor? *Heart (British Cardiac Society), 93*(9), 1017–1019. doi:10.1136/hrt.2007.122267 PMID:17699167

Lee, B. K., Yun, Y. H., & Park, K. (2015). Smart nanoparticles for drug delivery: Boundaries and opportunities. *Chemical Engineering Science, 125*, 158-164. doi:10.1016/j.ces.2014.06.042

Lee, A. S. (1992). Mammalian stress response: Induction of the glucose-regulated protein family. *Current Opinion in Cell Biology, 4*(2), 267–273. doi:10.1016/0955-0674(92)90042-B PMID:1599691

Lee, H.-L., Chen, C.-L., Yeh, S. T., Zweier, J. L., & Chen, Y.-R. (2012). Biphasic modulation of the mitochondrial electron transport chain in myocardial ischemia and reperfusion. *American Journal of Physiology. Heart and Circulatory Physiology, 302*(7), H1410–H1422. doi:10.1152/ajpheart.00731.2011 PMID:22268109

Lee, K. K., Al-Ahmad, A., Wang, P. J., & Myerburg, R. J. (2008). Epidemiology and Etiologies of Sudden Cardiac Death. In P. J. Wang, A. Al-Ahmad, H. H. Hsia, & P. C. Zei (Eds.), *Ventricular Arrhythmias and Sudden Cardiac Death* (pp. 199–212). Blackwell Publishing. doi:10.1002/9781444300307.ch17

Lee, K. P., Yuan, J. P., Hong, J. H., So, I., Worley, P. F., & Muallem, S. (2010). An endoplasmic reticulum/plasma membrane junction: STIM1/Orai1/TRPCs. *FEBS Letters, 584*(10), 2022–2027. doi:10.1016/j.febslet.2009.11.078 PMID:19944100

Lee, P. J., & Choi, A. M. K. (2003). Pathways of cell signaling in hyperoxia. *Free Radical Biology & Medicine, 35*(4), 341–350. doi:10.1016/S0891-5849(03)00279-X PMID:12899937

Lee, S., Choe, P. G., Song, K. H., Park, S. W., Kim, H. B., Kim, N. J., & Oh, M. D. et al. (2011). Is cefazolin inferior to nafcillin for treatment of methicillin-susceptible Staphylococcus aureus bacteremia? *Antimicrobial Agents and Chemotherapy, 55*(11), 5122–5126. doi:10.1128/AAC.00485-11 PMID:21825299

Lekakis, J., Rallidis, L. S., Andreadou, I., Vamvakou, G., Kazantzoglou, G., Magiatis, P., & Kremastinos, D. T. et al. (2005). Polyphenolic compounds from red grapes acutely improve endothelial function in patients with coronary heart disease. *European Journal of Cardiovascular Prevention and Rehabilitation, 12*(6), 596–600. PMID:16319551

Lek, M., Karczewski, K. J., Minikel, E. V., Samocha, K. E., Banks, E., Fennell, T., & MacArthur, D. G. et al. (2016). Analysis of protein-coding genetic variation in 60,706 humans. *Nature, 536*(7616), 285–291. doi:10.1038/nature19057 PMID:27535533

Lemhadri, A., Zeggwagh, N. A., Maghrani, M., Jouad, H., & Eddouks, M. (2004). Anti-hyperglycaemic activity of the aqueous extract of Origanum vulgare growing wild in Tafilalet region. *Journal of Ethnopharmacology, 92*(2), 251–256. doi:10.1016/j.jep.2004.02.026 PMID:15138008

Lennard, M. S., Silas, J. H., Freestone, S., Ramsay, L. E., Tucker, G. T., & Woods, H. F. (1982). Oxidation phenotypea major determinant of metoprolol metabolism and response. *The New England Journal of Medicine*, *307*(25), 1558–1560. doi:10.1056/NEJM198212163072505 PMID:7144837

Lerman, A., Burnett, J. C. Jr, Higano, S. T., McKinley, L. J., & Holmes, D. R. Jr. (1998). Long-term L-arginine supplementation improves small-vessel coronary endothelial function in humans. *Circulation*, *97*(21), 2123–2128. doi:10.1161/01.CIR.97.21.2123 PMID:9626172

Lesko, L. J., Zineh, I., & Huang, S.-M. (2010). What Is Clinical Utility and Why Should We Care? *Clinical Pharmacology and Therapeutics*, *88*(6), 729–733. doi:10.1038/clpt.2010.229 PMID:21081937

Leth, P. M. (2015). Computed Tomography in Forensic Medicine. *Danish Medical Journal*, *62*(6), 1–26. PMID:26036889

Levine, D. P., & Lamp, K. C. (2007). Daptomycin in the treatment of patients with infective endocarditis: Experience from a registry. *The American Journal of Medicine*, *120*(10), S28–S33. doi:10.1016/j.amjmed.2007.07.011 PMID:17904948

Levine, G. N. (2011). *ACCF/AHA/SCAI Guideline for Percutaneous Coronary Intervention (*2011). *Circulation*, *12*, e574–e651. PMID:22064601

Levine, G. N., Bates, E. R., Bittl, J. A., Brindis, R. G., Fihn, S. D., Fleisher, L. A., & Smith, S. C. Jr et al.. (2016). 2016 ACC/AHA Guideline Focused Update on Duration of Dual Antiplatelet Therapy in Patients With Coronary Artery Disease: A Report of the American College of Cardiology/American Heart Association Task Force on Clinical Practice Guidelines. *Journal of the American College of Cardiology*, *68*(10), 1082–1115. doi:10.1016/j.jacc.2016.03.513 PMID:27036918

Lhermusier, T., Chap, H., & Payrastre, B. (2011). Platelet membrane phospholipid asymmetry: From the characterization of a scramblase activity to the identification of an essential protein mutated in Scott syndrome. *Journal of thrombosis and haemostasis. JTH*, *9*, 1883–1891. PMID:21958383

Liang, Q., De Windt, L. J., Witt, S. A., Kimball, T. R., Markham, B. E., & Molkentin, J. D. (2001). The transcription factors GATA4 and GATA6 regulate cardiomyocyte hypertrophy in vitro and in vivo. *The Journal of Biological Chemistry*, *276*(32), 30245–30253. doi:10.1074/jbc.M102174200 PMID:11356841

Libby, P., & Theroux, P. (2005). Pathophysiology of Coronary Artery Disease. *Circulation*, *111*(25), 3481–3488. doi:10.1161/CIRCULATIONAHA.105.537878 PMID:15983262

Li, C., Fang, Z., Jiang, T., Zhang, Q., Liu, C., Zhang, C., & Xiang, Y. (2013). Serum microRNAs profile from genome-wide serves as a fingerprint for diagnosis of acute myocardial infarction and angina pectoris. *BMC Medical Genomics*, *6*(1), 16. doi:10.1186/1755-8794-6-16 PMID:23641832

Lie, J. T. (1975). Histopathology of the conduction system in sudden death from coronary heart disease. *Circulation*, *51*(3), 446–452. doi:10.1161/01.CIR.51.3.446 PMID:1139756

Liesa, M., Palacin, M., & Zorzano, A. (2009). Mitochondrial dynamics in mammalian health and disease. *Physiological Reviews*, *89*(3), 799–845. doi:10.1152/physrev.00030.2008 PMID:19584314

Li, J., Cubbon, R. M., Wilson, L. A., Amer, M. S., McKeown, L., Hou, B., & Beech, D. J. et al. (2011). Orai1 and CRAC channel dependence of VEGF-activated Ca2+ entry and endothelial tube formation. *Circulation Research*, *108*(10), 1190–1198. doi:10.1161/CIRCRESAHA.111.243352 PMID:21441136

Li, J., Dai, K., Wang, Z., Cao, L., Bai, X., & Ruan, C. (2015). Platelet functional alterations in a Bernard-Soulier syndrome patient with filamin A mutation. *J Hematol Oncol*, *8*(1), 79. doi:10.1186/s13045-015-0171-z PMID:26133172

Li, J., & Siegrist, J. (2012). Physical Activity and Risk of Cardiovascular Disease: A Meta-Analysis of Prospective Cohort Studies. *International Journal of Environmental Research and Public Health*, *9*(12), 391–407. doi:10.3390/ijerph9020391 PMID:22470299

Li, J., Xie, C., Zhuang, J., Li, H., Yao, Y., Shao, C., & Wang, H. (2015). Resveratrol attenuates inflammation in the rat heart subjected to ischemia-reperfusion: Role of the TLR4/NF-kappaB signaling pathway. *Mol Med Rep*, *11*(2), 1120–1126. doi:10.3892/mmr.2014.2955 PMID:25405531

Li, L., Gao, P., Zhang, H., Chen, H., Zheng, W., Lv, X., & Liang, C. et al. (2011). SIRT1 inhibits angiotensin II-induced vascular smooth muscle cell hypertrophy. *Acta Biochimica et Biophysica Sinica*, *43*(2), 103–109. doi:10.1093/abbs/gmq104 PMID:21118843

Li, L., Zhao, L., Yi-Ming, W., Yu, Y. S., Xia, C. Y., Duan, J. L., & Su, D. F. (2009). Sirt1 hyperexpression in SHR heart related to left ventricular hypertrophy. *Canadian Journal of Physiology and Pharmacology*, *87*(1), 56–62. doi:10.1139/Y08-099 PMID:19142216

Lilly, L. S. (2012). *Pathophysiology of heart disease: a collaborative project of medical students and faculty*. Lippincott Williams & Wilkins.

Lim, W. H., Seo, W. W., Choe, W., Kang, C.-K., Park, J., Cho, H.-J., & Kim, H.-S. et al. (2011). Stent Coated With Antibody Against Vascular Endothelial-Cadherin Captures Endothelial Progenitor Cells, Accelerates Re-Endothelialization, and Reduces Neointimal Formation. *Arteriosclerosis, Thrombosis, and Vascular Biology*, *31*(12), 2798–2805. doi:10.1161/ATVBAHA.111.226134 PMID:22015656

Lin, C. H., Lin, C. C., Ting, W. J., Pai, P. Y., Kuo, C. H., Ho, T. J., & Lin, W. T. et al. (2014). Resveratrol enhanced FOXO3 phosphorylation via synergetic activation of SIRT1 and PI3K/Akt signaling to improve the effects of exercise in elderly rat hearts. *Age (Dordrecht, Netherlands)*, *36*(5), 9705. doi:10.1007/s11357-014-9705-5 PMID:25158994

Linda, K. (2009). Curtiss and Peter S. Tobias.Emerging role of Toll-like receptors in atherosclerosis. *Journal of Lipid Research*, *50*(Supplement), S340–S345. PMID:18980945

Lindenfeld, J. M. G., Shakar, S. F., Zolty, R., Lowes, B. D., Wolfel, E. E., Mestroni, L., & Kobashigawa, J. et al. (2004). Drug therapy in the heart transplant recipient–Part II: Immunosuppressive drugs. *Circulation*, *110*, 7. PMID:15611389

Lindenfeld, J., Miller, G. G., Shakar, S. F., Zolty, R., Lowes, B. D., Wolfel, E. E., & Kobashigawa, J. et al. (2004). Drug therapy in the heart transplant recipient: part I: cardiac rejection and immunosuppressive drugs. *Circulation*, *110*(24), 3734–3740. doi:10.1161/01.CIR.0000149745.83186.89 PMID:15596559

Link, B. G. (2008). Epidemiological Sociology and the Social Shaping of Population Health. *Journal of Health and Social Behavior*, *49*(4), 367–384. doi:10.1177/002214650804900401 PMID:19181044

Link, B. G., & Phelan, J. (1995). Social Conditions as Fundamental Causes of Disease. *Journal of Health and Social Behavior*, *35*, 80–94. doi:10.2307/2626958 PMID:7560851

Link, E., Parish, S., Armitage, J., Bowman, L., Heath, S., Matsuda, F., & Collins, R. et al. (2008). SLCO1B1 variants and statin-induced myopathya genomewide study. *The New England Journal of Medicine*, *359*(8), 789–799. doi:10.1056/NEJMoa0801936 PMID:18650507

Linnet, K. (2013). Toxicological Screening and Quantitation Using Liquid Chromatography/Time-of-Flight Mass Spectrometry. *Journal of Forensic Science & Criminology*, *1*(1), e101. doi:10.15744/2348-9804.1.e101

Lin, Q., Schwarz, J., Bucana, C., & Olson, N. (1997). Control of Mouse Cardiac Morphogenesis and Myogenesis by Transcription Factor MEF2C. *Science*, *276*(5317), 1404–1407. doi:10.1126/science.276.5317.1404 PMID:9162005

Lin, S. J., Ford, E., Haigis, M., Liszt, G., & Guarente, L. (2004). Calorie restriction extends yeast life span by lowering the level of NADH. *Genes & Development*, *18*(1), 12–16. doi:10.1101/gad.1164804 PMID:14724176

Liou, J., Kim, M. L., Heo, W. D., Jones, J. T., Myers, J. W., & Ferrell, J. E. Jr et al.. (2005). STIM is a Ca2+ sensor essential for Ca2+-store-depletion-triggered Ca2+ influx. *Current Biology*, *15*(13), 1235–1241. doi:10.1016/j.cub.2005.05.055 PMID:16005298

Lis, A., Peinelt, C., Beck, A., Parvez, S., Monteilh-Zoller, M., Fleig, A., & Penner, R. (2007). CRACM1, CRACM2, and CRACM3 are store-operated Ca2+ channels with distinct functional properties. *Current Biology*, *17*(9), 794–800. doi:10.1016/j.cub.2007.03.065 PMID:17442569

Liu, D. W., Gintant, G. A., & Antzelevitch, C. (1993). Ionic bases for electrophysiological distinctions among epicardial, midmyocardial, and endocardial myocytes from the free wall of the canine left ventricle. *Circulation Research*, *72*(3), 671–687. doi:10.1161/01.RES.72.3.671 PMID:8431990

Liu, H., Yu, X., Yu, S., & Kou, J. (2015). Molecular mechanisms in lipopolysaccharide-induced pulmonary endothelial barrier dysfunction. *International Immunopharmacology*, *29*(2), 937–946. doi:10.1016/j.intimp.2015.10.010 PMID:26462590

Liu, J., Xin, L., Benson, V. L., Allen, D. G., & Ju, Y. K. (2015). Store-operated calcium entry and the localization of STIM1 and Orai1 proteins in isolated mouse sinoatrial node cells. *Frontiers in Physics*, *6*, 69. PMID:25806000

Liu, X. H., Zhang, Z. Y., Sun, S., & Wu, X. D. (2008). Ischemic postconditioning protects myocardium from ischemia/reperfusion injury through attenuating endoplasmic reticulum stress. *Shock (Augusta, Ga.)*, *30*(4), 422–427. doi:10.1097/SHK.0b013e318164ca29 PMID:18323739

Liu, Y., Chen, L.-Y., Sokolowska, M., Eberlein, M., Alsaaty, S., Martinez-Anton, A., & Shelhamer, J. H. et al. (2014). The fish oil ingredient, docosahexaenoic acid, activates cytosolic phospholipase A2 via GPR120 receptor to produce prostaglandin E2 and plays an anti-inflammatory role in macrophages. *Immunology*, *143*(1), 81–95. doi:10.1111/imm.12296 PMID:24673159

Liu, Y., Ma, W., Zhang, P., He, S., & Huang, D. (2015). Effect of resveratrol on blood pressure: A meta-analysis of randomized controlled trials. *Clinical Nutrition (Edinburgh, Lothian)*, *34*(1), 27–34. doi:10.1016/j.clnu.2014.03.009 PMID:24731650

Li, Y., Cai, M., Cao, L., Qin, X., Zheng, T., Xu, X., & He, G. et al. (2014). Endurance exercise accelerates myocardial tissue oxygenation recovery and reduces ischemia reperfusion injury in mice. *PLoS ONE*, *9*(12), e114205. doi:10.1371/journal.pone.0114205 PMID:25474642

Lloyd-Jones, D. M., Larson, M. G., Leip, E. P., Beiser, A., DAgostino, R. B., Kannel, W. B., & Levy, D. et al. (2002). Lifetime risk for developing congestive heart failure: The Framingham Heart Study. *Circulation*, *106*(24), 3068–3072. doi:10.1161/01.CIR.0000039105.49749.6F PMID:12473553

Lloyd-Jones, D. M., Nam, B. H., DAgostino, R. B. Sr, Levy, D., Murabito, J. M., Wang, T. J., & ODonnell, C. J. et al. (2004). Parental cardiovascular disease as a risk factor for cardiovascular disease in middle-aged adults: A prospective study of parents and offspring. *Journal of the American Medical Association*, *291*(18), 2204–2211. doi:10.1001/jama.291.18.2204 PMID:15138242

Lloyd-Jones, D., Adams, R. J., Brown, T. M., Carnethon, M., Dai, S., De Simone, G., & Wylie-Rosett, J. et al. (2010). Heart disease and stroke statistics–2010 update: A report from the American Heart Association. *Circulation*, *121*(7), e46–e215. doi:10.1161/CIRCULATIONAHA.109.192667 PMID:20019324

Lodise, T. P. Jr, Lomaestro, B., & Drusano, G. L. (2007). Piperacillin-tazobactam for Pseudomonas aeruginosa infection: Clinical implications of an extended-infusion dosing strategy. *Clinical Infectious Diseases*, *44*(3), 357–363. doi:10.1086/510590 PMID:17205441

Loftus, J. C., Choate, J., & Albrecht, R. M. (1984). Platelet activation and cytoskeletal reorganization: High voltage electron microscopic examination of intact and Triton-extracted whole mounts. *The Journal of Cell Biology*, *98*(6), 2019–2025. doi:10.1083/jcb.98.6.2019 PMID:6539337

Lomivorotov, V. V., Shmyrev, V. A., Nepomnyaschih, V. A., Ponomarev, D. N., Knyazkova, L. G., Lomivorotov, V. N., & Karaskov, A. M. (2012). Remote ischaemic preconditioning does not protect the heart in patients undergoing coronary artery bypass grafting. *Interactive Cardiovascular and Thoracic Surgery*, *15*(1), 18–22. doi:10.1093/icvts/ivs118 PMID:22493101

Long, J. S., & Freeze, J. (2005). *Regression Models for Categorical Dependent Variables Using Stata* (2nd ed.). College Station, TX: Stata Press

Lonnrot, K., Porsti, I., Alho, H., Wu, X., Hervonen, A., & Tolvanen, J. P. (1998). Control of arterial tone after long-term coenzyme Q10 supplementation in senescent rats. *British Journal of Pharmacology*, *124*(7), 1500–1506. doi:10.1038/sj.bjp.0701970 PMID:9723964

Lopaschuk, G. D., Ussher, J. R., Folmes, C. D. L., Jaswal, J. S., & Stanley, W. C. (2010). Myocardial Fatty Acid Metabolism in Health and Disease. *Physiological Reviews*, *90*(1), 207–258. doi:10.1152/physrev.00015.2009 PMID:20086077

Lopez, B., Gonzalez, A., Lindner, D., Westermann, D., Ravassa, S., Beaumont, J., & Diez, J. et al. (2013). Osteopontin-mediated myocardial fibrosis in heart failure: A role for lysyl oxidase? *Cardiovascular Research*, *99*(1), 111–120. doi:10.1093/cvr/cvt100 PMID:23619422

Loporcaro, C. G., Tester, D. J., Maleszewski, J. J., Kruisselbrink, T., & Ackerman, M. J. (2014). Confirmation of cause and manner of death via a comprehensive cardiac autopsy including whole exome next-generation sequencing. *Archives of Pathology & Laboratory Medicine*, *138*(8), 1083–1089. doi:10.5858/arpa.2013-0479-SA PMID:24298987

Louwette, S., Van Geet, C., & Freson, K. (2012). Regulators of G protein signaling: Role in hematopoiesis, megakaryopoiesis and platelet function. *Journal of thrombosis and haemostasis. JTH*, *10*, 2215–2222. PMID:22908964

Lu, J. R., McKinsey, T. A., Xu, H., Wang, D. Z., Richardson, J. A., & Olson, E. N. (1999). FOG-2, a heart- and brain-enriched cofactor for GATA transcription factors. *Molecular and Cellular Biology*, *19*(6), 4495–4502. doi:10.1128/MCB.19.6.4495 PMID:10330188

Lund, L. H., Edwards, L. B., Kucheryavaya, A. Y., Benden, C., Christie, J. D., Dipchand, A. I., & Meiser, B. et al. (2014). The registry of the International Society for Heart and Lung Transplantation: thirty-first official adult heart transplant report—2014; focus theme: retransplantation. *The Journal of Heart and Lung Transplantation*, *33*(10), 996–1008. doi:10.1016/j.healun.2014.08.003 PMID:25242124

Lund, V. E., Kentala, E., Scheinin, H., Klossner, J., Helenius, H., Sariola-Heinonen, K., & Jalonen, J. (1999). Heart rate variability in healthy volunteers during normobaric and hyperbaric hyperoxia. *Acta Physiologica Scandinavica*, *167*(1), 29–35. doi:10.1046/j.1365-201x.1999.00581.x PMID:10519974

Luo, S. J., Zhou, Y. J., Shi, D. M., Ge, H. L., Wang, J. L., & Liu, R. F. (2013). Remote ischemic preconditioning reduces myocardial injury in patients undergoing coronary stent implantation. *The Canadian Journal of Cardiology*, *29*(9), 1084–1089. doi:10.1016/j.cjca.2012.11.022 PMID:23414904

Luo, X. Y., Qu, S. L., Tang, Z. H., Zhang, Y., Liu, M. H., Peng, J., & Jiang, Z. S. et al. (2014). SIRT1 in cardiovascular aging. *Clinica Chimica Acta*, *437*, 106–114. doi:10.1016/j.cca.2014.07.019 PMID:25063737

Luscher, T. F., Steffel, J., Eberli, F. R., Joner, M., Nakazawa, G., Tanner, F. C., & Virmani, R. (2007). Drug-Eluting Stent and Coronary Thrombosis Biological Mechanisms and Clinical Implications. *Circulation*, *115*(8), 1051–1058. doi:10.1161/CIRCULATIONAHA.106.675934 PMID:17325255

Lusis, A. J. (2000). Atherosclerosis. *Nature*, *407*(6801), 233–241. doi:10.1038/35025203 PMID:11001066

Lu, X., Yang, X., Zhou, Q., Wang, Y., Feng, S., Jin, J., & Chen, J. et al. (2014). Cardiac allograft tolerance induced by isogeneic CD4+CD25+ regulatory T cells. *Experimental and Clinical Transplantation*, *12*(2), 133–138. Retrieved from http://www.ncbi.nlm.nih.gov/pubmed/24702146 PMID:24702146

Lu, Z., Scott, I., Webster, B. R., & Sack, M. N. (2009). The emerging characterization of lysine residue deacetylation on the modulation of mitochondrial function and cardiovascular biology. *Circulation Research*, *105*(9), 830–841. doi:10.1161/CIRCRESAHA.109.204974 PMID:19850949

Macan, H., Uykimpang, R., Alconcel, M., Takasu, J., Razon, R., & Amagase, H. (2006). Aged garlic extract may be safe for patients on warfarin therapy. *The Journal of Nutrition*, *136*(3), 793S–795S. PMID:16484565

Mackraj, I., Govender, T., & Ramesar, S. (2008). The anti hypertensive effects of quercetin in a salt-sensitive model of hypertension. *Journal of Cardiovascular Pharmacology*, *51*(3), 239–245. doi:10.1097/FJC.0b013e318162011f PMID:18356687

Maeda, H., Ishikawa, T., & Michiue, T. (2011). Forensic biochemistry for functional investigation of death: Concept and practical application. *Legal Medicine (Tokyo)*, *13*(2), 55–67. doi:10.1016/j.legalmed.2010.12.005 PMID:21269863

Maekawa, N., Wada, H., Kanda, T., Niwa, T., Yamada, Y., Saito, K., & Seishima, M. et al. (2002). Improved myocardial ischemia/reperfusion injury in mice lacking tumor necrosis factor-α. *Journal of the American College of Cardiology*, *39*(7), 1229–1235. doi:10.1016/S0735-1097(02)01738-2 PMID:11923051

Ma, J., Ward, E. M., Siegel, R. L., & Jemal, A. (2015). Temporal Trends in Mortality in the United States, 19692013. *Journal of the American Medical Association*, *314*(16), 1731–1739. doi:10.1001/jama.2015.12319 PMID:26505597

Majewski, L., & Kuznicki, J. (2015). SOCE in neurons: Signaling or just refilling? *Biochimica et Biophysica Acta*, *1853*(9), 1940–1952. doi:10.1016/j.bbamcr.2015.01.019 PMID:25646572

Mak, S., Azevedo, E. R., Liu, P. P., & Newton, G. E. (2001). Effect of hyperoxia on left ventricular function and filling pressures in patients with and without congestive heart failure. *Chest*, *120*(2), 467–473. doi:10.1378/chest.120.2.467 PMID:11502645

Ma, L., & Li, Y. (2015). SIRT1: Role in cardiovascular biology. *Clinica Chimica Acta*, *440*, 8–15. doi:10.1016/j.cca.2014.10.036 PMID:25444742

Malfait, F., & De Paepe, A. (2014). The Ehlers-Danlos syndrome. *Advances in Experimental Medicine and Biology*, *802*, 129–143. doi:10.1007/978-94-007-7893-1_9 PMID:24443025

Malloy, M., & Kane, J. (2015). Agents used in dyslipidemia. In B. Katzung & A. Trevor (Eds.), Basic & Clinical Pharmacology. New York, NY: McGraw-Hill.

Mancarella, S., Wang, Y., Deng, X., Landesberg, G., Scalia, R., Panettieri, R. A., & Gill, D. L. et al. (2011). Hypoxia-induced acidosis uncouples the STIM-Orai calcium signaling complex. *The Journal of Biological Chemistry*, *286*(52), 44788–44798. doi:10.1074/jbc.M111.303081 PMID:22084246

Maniatis, N. A., Shinin, V., Schraufnagel, D. E., Okada, S., Vogel, S. M., Malik, A. B., & Minshall, R. D. (2008). Increased pulmonary vascular resistance and defective pulmonary artery filling in caveolin-1-/- mice. *American Journal of Physiology. Lung Cellular and Molecular Physiology*, *294*(5), L865–L873. doi:10.1152/ajplung.00079.2007 PMID:18192592

Manohar, V., Ingram, C., Gray, J., Talpur, N. A., Echard, B. W., Bagchi, D., & Preuss, H. G. (2001). Antifungal activities of origanum oil against Candida albicans. *Molecular and Cellular Biochemistry*, *228*(1-2), 111–117. doi:10.1023/A:1013311632207 PMID:11855736

Mansour, S. M., Bahgat, A. K., El-Khatib, A. S., & Khayyal, M. T. (2011). Ginkgo biloba extract (EGb 761) normalizes hypertension in 2K, 1C hypertensive rats: Role of antioxidant mechanisms, ACE inhibiting activity and improvement of endothelial dysfunction. *Phytomedicine*, *18*(8-9), 641–647. doi:10.1016/j.phymed.2011.01.014 PMID:21353510

Mantell, L. L., & Lee, P. J. (2000). Signal transduction pathways in hyperoxia-induced lung cell death. *Molecular Genetics and Metabolism*, *71*(1-2), 359–370. doi:10.1006/mgme.2000.3046 PMID:11001828

Marieb, E. N., & Hoehn, K. (2013). The cardiovascular system: the heart. In *Human anatomy and physiology* (pp. 658–691). Boston, MA: Pearson.

Marshall, I., Wang, Y., Crichton, S., McKevitt, C., Rudd, A. G., & Wolfe, C. D. (2015). The effects of socioeconomic status on stroke risk and outcomes. *Lancet Neurology*, *14*(12), 1206–1218. doi:10.1016/S1474-4422(15)00200-8 PMID:26581971

Martina, V., Masha, A., Gigliardi, V. R., Brocato, L., Manzato, E., Berchio, A., & Iannone, A. et al. (2008). Long-term N-acetylcysteine and L-arginine administration reduces endothelial activation and systolic blood pressure in hypertensive patients with type 2 diabetes. *Diabetes Care*, *31*(5), 940–944. doi:10.2337/dc07-2251 PMID:18268065

Martindale, J. J., Fernandez, R., Thuerauf, D., Whittaker, R., Gude, N., Sussman, M. A., & Glembotski, C. C. (2006). Endoplasmic Reticulum Stress Gene Induction and Protection From Ischemia/Reperfusion Injury in the Hearts of Transgenic Mice With a Tamoxifen-Regulated Form of ATF6. *Circulation Research*, *98*(9), 1186–1193. doi:10.1161/01.RES.0000220643.65941.8d PMID:16601230

Martinez, S. R., Gay, M. S., & Zhang, L. (2015). Epigenetic mechanisms in heart development and disease. *Drug Discovery Today*, *20*(7), 799–811. doi:10.1016/j.drudis.2014.12.018 PMID:25572405

Marwick, T. H., Cho, I., ó Hartaigh, B., & Min, J. K. (2015). Finding the Gatekeeper to the Cardiac Catheterization Laboratory. *Journal of the American College of Cardiology*, *65*(25), 2747–2756. doi:10.1016/j.jacc.2015.04.060 PMID:26112200

Masliah-Planchon, J., Darnige, L., & Bellucci, S. (2013). Molecular determinants of platelet delta storage pool deficiencies: An update. *British Journal of Haematology*, *160*(1), 5–11. doi:10.1111/bjh.12064 PMID:23025459

Massie, B. M., & Shah, N. B. (1997). Evolving trends in the epidemiologic factors of heart failure: Rationale for preventive strategies and comprehensive disease management. *American Heart Journal*, *133*(6), 703–712. doi:10.1016/S0002-8703(97)70173-X PMID:9200399

Masugata, H., Senda, S., Inukai, M., Himoto, T., Murao, K., Hosomi, N., & Goda, F. et al. (2011). Seasonal variation in estimated glomerular filtration rate based on serum creatinine levels in hypertensive patients. *The Tohoku Journal of Experimental Medicine*, *224*(2), 137–142. Retrieved from http://www.ncbi.nlm.nih.gov/pubmed/21617334 doi:10.1620/tjem.224.137 PMID:21617334

Matoba, T., & Egashira, K. (2014). Nanoparticle-Mediated Drug Delivery System for Cardiovascular Disease. *International Heart Journal*, *55*(4), 281–286. doi:10.1536/ihj.14-150 PMID:24942639

Matsuda, N., Hattori, Y., Jesmin, S., & Gando, S. (2005). Nuclear factor-κB decoy oligodeoxynucleotides prevent acute lung injury in mice with cecal ligation and puncture-induced sepsis. *Molecular Pharmacology*, *67*(4), 1018–1025. doi:10.1124/mol.104.005926 PMID:15576632

Matsui, H., Sugimoto, M., Mizuno, T., Tsuji, S., & Miyata, S. et al.. (2002). Distinct and concerted functions of von Willebrand factor and fibrinogen in mural thrombus growth under high shear flow. *Blood*, *100*(10), 3604–3610. doi:10.1182/blood-2002-02-0508 PMID:12393609

Matsushima, S., & Sadoshima, J. (2015). The role of sirtuins in cardiac disease. *American Journal of Physiology. Heart and Circulatory Physiology*, *309*(9), H1375–H1389. doi:10.1152/ajpheart.00053.2015 PMID:26232232

Mattagajasingh, I., Kim, C. S., Naqvi, A., Yamamori, T., Hoffman, T. A., Jung, S. B., & Irani, K. et al. (2007). SIRT1 promotes endothelium-dependent vascular relaxation by activating endothelial nitric oxide synthase. *Proceedings of the National Academy of Sciences of the United States of America*, *104*(37), 14855–14860. doi:10.1073/pnas.0704329104 PMID:17785417

Maurer, H. H. (2013). What is the future of (ultra) high performance liquid chromatography coupled to low and high resolution mass spectrometry for toxicological drug screening? *Journal of Chromatography. A*, *1292*, 19–24. doi:10.1016/j.chroma.2012.08.069 PMID:22964051

Ma, Y., Brewer, J. W., Alan Diehl, J., & Hendershot, L. M. (2002). Two Distinct Stress Signaling Pathways Converge Upon the CHOP Promoter During the Mammalian Unfolded Protein Response. *Journal of Molecular Biology*, *318*(5), 1351–1365. doi:10.1016/S0022-2836(02)00234-6 PMID:12083523

Mayer, C. R., & Bekeredjian, R. (2008). Ultrasonic gene and drug delivery to the cardiovascular system. *Advanced Drug Delivery Reviews, 60*, 1177-1192. doi:10.1016/j.addr.2008.03.004

McAreavey, D., Vidal, J. S., Aspelund, T., Eiriksdottir, G., Schelbert, E. B., Kjartansson, O., & Arai, A. E. et al. (2016). Midlife Cardiovascular Risk Factors and Late-Life Unrecognized and Recognized Myocardial Infarction Detect by Cardiac Magnetic Resonance: ICELAND-MI, the AGES-Reykjavik Study. *J Am Heart Assoc*, *5*(2). doi:10.1161/jaha.115.002420 PMID:26873683

McBurney, M. W., Yang, X., Jardine, K., Hixon, M., Boekelheide, K., Webb, J. R., & Lemieux, M. et al. (2003). The mammalian SIR2alpha protein has a role in embryogenesis and gametogenesis. *Molecular and Cellular Biology*, *23*(1), 38–54. doi:10.1128/MCB.23.1.38-54.2003 PMID:12482959

McKinlay, J. B. (1996). Some contributions from the social system to gender inequalities in heart disease. *Journal of Health and Social Behavior*, *37*(1), 1–26. doi:10.2307/2137228 PMID:8820308

McMurray, J. J., Packer, M., Desai, A. S., Gong, J., Lefkowitz, M. P., Rizkala, A. R., & Zile, M. R. et al. (2014). Angiotensin-neprilysin inhibition versus enalapril in heart failure. *The New England Journal of Medicine*, *371*(11), 993–1004. doi:10.1056/NEJMoa1409077 PMID:25176015

McNulty, P. H., Robertson, B. J., Tulli, M. A., Hess, J., Harach, L. A., Scott, S., & Sinoway, L. I. (2007). Effect of hyperoxia and vitamin C on coronary blood flow in patients with ischemic heart disease. *J Appl Physiol (1985), 102*(5), 2040-2045. doi: 10.1152/japplphysiol.00595.2006

McNulty, P. H., King, N., Scott, S., Hartman, G., McCann, J., Kozak, M., & Sinoway, L. I. et al. (2005). Effects of supplemental oxygen administration on coronary blood flow in patients undergoing cardiac catheterization. *American Journal of Physiology. Heart and Circulatory Physiology*, *288*(3), H1057–H1062. doi:10.1152/ajpheart.00625.2004 PMID:15706043

McPherson, R., Pertsemlidis, A., Kavaslar, N., Stewart, A., Roberts, R., Cox, D. R., & Cohen, J. C. et al. (2007). A common allele on chromosome 9 associated with coronary heart disease. *Science*, *316*(5830), 1488–1491. doi:10.1126/science.1142447 PMID:17478681

Medzhitov, R., & Janeway, C. A. Jr. (1997). Innate immunity: The virtues of a nonclonal system of recognition. *Cell*, *91*(3), 295–298. doi:10.1016/S0092-8674(00)80412-2 PMID:9363937

Mega, J. L., Close, S. L., Wiviott, S. D., Shen, L., Walker, J. R., Simon, T., & Sabatine, M. S. et al. (2010). Genetic variants in ABCB1 and CYP2C19 and cardiovascular outcomes after treatment with clopidogrel and prasugrel in the TRITON-TIMI 38 trial: A pharmacogenetic analysis. *Lancet*, *376*(9749), 1312–1319. doi:10.1016/S0140-6736(10)61273-1 PMID:20801494

Mehra, M. R., Uber, P. A., & Kaplan, B. (2006). Immunosuppression in cardiac transplantation: Science, common sense and the heart of the matter. *American Journal of Transplantation*, *6*(6), 1243–1245. doi:10.1111/j.1600-6143.2006.01326.x PMID:16686745

Mehta, D. (2012). Focal adhesion kinase regulation of endothelial barrier function, apoptosis, and neovascularization. *Microvascular Research*, *83*(1), 1–2. doi:10.1016/j.mvr.2011.10.001 PMID:22036672

Mehta, D., Ahmmed, G. U., Paria, B. C., Holinstat, M., Voyno-Yasenetskaya, T., Tiruppathi, C., & Malik, A. B. et al. (2003). RhoA interaction with inositol 1,4,5-trisphosphate receptor and transient receptor potential channel-1 regulates Ca2+ entry. Role in signaling increased endothelial permeability. *The Journal of Biological Chemistry*, *278*(35), 33492–33500. doi:10.1074/jbc.M302401200 PMID:12766172

Mehta, D., Konstantoulaki, M., Ahmmed, G. U., & Malik, A. B. (2005). Sphingosine 1-phosphate-induced mobilization of intracellular Ca2+ mediates rac activation and adherens junction assembly in endothelial cells. *The Journal of Biological Chemistry*, *280*(17), 17320–17328. doi:10.1074/jbc.M411674200 PMID:15728185

Mehta, D., & Malik, A. B. (2006). Signaling mechanisms regulating endothelial permeability. *Physiological Reviews*, *86*(1), 279–367. doi:10.1152/physrev.00012.2005 PMID:16371600

Mehta, D., Ravindran, K., & Kuebler, W. M. (2014). Novel regulators of endothelial barrier function. *American Journal of Physiology. Lung Cellular and Molecular Physiology*, *307*(12), L924–L935. doi:10.1152/ajplung.00318.2014 PMID:25381026

Mellor, R., & Woollard, M. (2010). Skill acquisition by health care workers in the Resuscitation Council (UK) 2005 Guidelines for Adult Basic Life Support. *International Emergency Nursing*, *18*(2), 61–66. doi:10.1016/j.ienj.2009.08.003 PMID:20382366

Mendell, J. T., & Olson, E. N. (2012). MicroRNAs in stress signaling and human disease. *Cell*, *148*(6), 1172–1187. doi:10.1016/j.cell.2012.02.005 PMID:22424228

Mensah, G. A. (2005). State of Disparities in Cardiovascular Health in the United States. *Circulation*, *111*(10), 1233–1241. doi:10.1161/01.CIR.0000158136.76824.04 PMID:15769763

Mensah, G. A., & Brown, D. W. (2007). An Overview of Cardiovascular Disease Burden in the United States. *Health Affairs*, *26*(1), 38–48. doi:10.1377/hlthaff.26.1.38 PMID:17211012

Mester, R., Toren, P., Mizrachi, I., Wolmer, L., Karni, N., & Weizman, A. (1995). Caffeine withdrawal increases lithium blood levels. *Biological Psychiatry*, *37*(5), 348–350. doi:10.1016/0006-3223(94)00243-V PMID:7748990

Meybohm, P., Bein, B., Brosteanu, O., Cremer, J., Gruenewald, M., Stoppe, C., & Zacharowski, K. et al. (2015). A Multicenter Trial of Remote Ischemic Preconditioning for Heart Surgery. *The New England Journal of Medicine*, *373*(15), 1397–1407. doi:10.1056/NEJMoa1413579 PMID:26436208

Michaud, K., Grabherr, S., Doenz, F., & Mangin, P. (2012). Evaluation of postmortem MDCT and MDCT-angiography for the investigation of sudden cardiac death related to atherosclerotic coronary artery disease. *The International Journal of Cardiovascular Imaging*, *28*(7), 1807–1822. doi:10.1007/s10554-012-0012-x PMID:22238022

Michaud, K., Grabherr, S., Jackowski, C., Bollmann, M. D., Doenz, F., & Mangin, P. (2014). Postmortem imaging of sudden cardiac death. *International Journal of Legal Medicine*, *128*(1), 127–137. doi:10.1007/s00414-013-0819-6 PMID:23322013

Mihailovic-Stanojevic, N., Belscak-Cvitanovic, A., Grujic-Milanovic, J., Ivanov, M., Jovovic, D., Bugarski, D., & Miloradović, Z. (2013). Antioxidant and Antihypertensive Activity of Extract from Thymus serpyllum L. in Experimental Hypertension. *Plant Foods for Human Nutrition (Dordrecht, Netherlands)*, *68*(3), 235–240. doi:10.1007/s11130-013-0368-7 PMID:23828496

Mihalov, J., & Timarova, G. (2014). A Seeming Paradox: Ischemic Stroke in the Context of Idiopathic Thrombocytopenic Purpura. *Clinical and Applied Thrombosis/Hemostasis*. PMID:25115760

Milla, F., Pinney, S. P., & Anyanwu, A. C. (2012). Indications for heart transplantation in current era of left ventricular assist devices. *Mount Sinai Journal of Medicine: A Journal of Translational and Personalized Medicine*, *79*(3), 305-316.

Milstein, M. L., Musa, H., Balbuena, D. P., Anumonwo, J. M. B., Auerbach, D. S., Furspan, P. B., & Jalife, J. et al. (2012). Dynamic reciprocity of sodium and potassium channel expression in a macromolecular complex controls cardiac excitability and arrhythmia.*Proceedings of the National Academy of Sciences*. doi:10.1073/pnas.1109370109

Minshall, R. D., Vandenbroucke, E. E., Holinstat, M., Place, A. T., Tiruppathi, C., Vogel, S. M., & Malik, A. B. et al. (2010). Role of protein kinase Czeta in thrombin-induced RhoA activation and inter-endothelial gap formation of human dermal microvessel endothelial cell monolayers. *Microvascular Research*, *80*(2), 240–249. doi:10.1016/j.mvr.2010.04.007 PMID:20417648

Mirzapoiazova, T., Moitra, J., Moreno-Vinasco, L., Sammani, S., Turner, J. R., Chiang, E. T., & Garcia, J. G. et al. (2011). Non-muscle myosin light chain kinase isoform is a viable molecular target in acute inflammatory lung injury. *American Journal of Respiratory Cell and Molecular Biology*, *44*(1), 40–52. doi:10.1165/rcmb.2009-0197OC PMID:20139351

Misra, A., Haudek, S. B., Knuefermann, P., Vallejo, J. G., Chen, Z. J., Michael, L. H., & Mann, D. L. et al. (2003). Nuclear Factor-κB Protects the Adult Cardiac Myocyte Against Ischemia-Induced Apoptosis in a Murine Model of Acute Myocardial Infarction. *Circulation*, *108*(25), 3075–3078. doi:10.1161/01.CIR.0000108929.93074.0B PMID:14676146

Mitrovic, M., Elezovic, I., Miljic, P., & Suvajdzic, N. (2014). Acquired von Willebrand syndrome in patients with Gaucher disease. *Blood Cells, Molecules & Diseases*, *52*(4), 205–207. doi:10.1016/j.bcmd.2013.11.001 PMID:24275154

Mitrovic, V., Luss, H., Nitsche, K., Forssmann, K., Maronde, E., Fricke, K., & Meyer, M. et al. (2005). Effects of the renal natiuretic peptide urodilantin (ularitide) in patients with decompensated chronic heart failure: A double-blind, placebo-controlled, ascending-dose trial. *American Heart Journal*, *150*(6), 1239.e1–1239.e8. doi:10.1016/j.ahj.2005.01.022 PMID:16338265

Mitrovic, V., Seferovic, P. M., Simeunovic, D., Ristic, A. D., Miric, M., Moiseyev, V. S., & Meyer, M. et al. (2006). Haemodynamic and clinical effects of ularitide in decompensated heart failure. *European Heart Journal*, *27*(23), 2823–2832. doi:10.1093/eurheartj/ehl337 PMID:17074775

Miyazaki, Y., Kaikita, K., Endo, M., Horio, E., Miura, M., Tsujita, K., & Oike, Y. et al. (2011). C/EBP Homologous Protein Deficiency Attenuates Myocardial Reperfusion Injury by Inhibiting Myocardial Apoptosis and Inflammation. *Arteriosclerosis, Thrombosis, and Vascular Biology*, *31*(5), 1124–1132. doi:10.1161/ATVBAHA.111.224519 PMID:21330607

Mizugishi, K., Yamashita, T., Olivera, A., Miller, G. F., Spiegel, S., & Proia, R. L. (2005). Essential role for sphingosine kinases in neural and vascular development. *Molecular and Cellular Biology*, *25*(24), 11113–11121. doi:10.1128/MCB.25.24.11113-11121.2005 PMID:16314531

Moine, P., McIntyre, R., Schwartz, M. D., Kaneko, D., Shenkar, R., Tulzo, Y. L., & Abraham, E. et al. (2000, February). NF-kappaB regulatory mechanisms in alveolar macrophages from patients with acute respiratory distress syndrome. *Shock (Augusta, Ga.)*, *13*(2), 85–91. doi:10.1097/00024382-200013020-00001 PMID:10670837

Moise, P. A., Culshaw, D. L., Wong-Beringer, A., Bensman, J., Lamp, K. C., Smith, W. J., & Zervos, M. J. et al. (2016). Comparative Effectiveness of Vancomycin Versus Daptomycin for MRSA Bacteremia With Vancomycin MIC >1 mg/L: A Multicenter Evaluation. *Clinical Therapeutics*, *38*(1), 16–30. doi:10.1016/j.clinthera.2015.09.017 PMID:26585355

Molina, D. K., Wood, L. E., & Frost, R. E. (2007). Is routine histopathologic examination beneficial in all medicolegal autopsies? *The American Journal of Forensic Medicine and Pathology*, *28*(1), 1–3. doi:10.1097/01.paf.0000257388.83605.0a PMID:17325455

Montgomery, R. A., Cozzi, E., West, L. J., & Warren, D. S. (2011). Humoral immunity and antibody-mediated rejection in solid organ transplantation. *Seminars in Immunology*, *23*(4), 224–234. doi:10.1016/j.smim.2011.08.021 PMID:21958960

Morentin, B., Aguilera, B., Carmena, M. D. G. C., & Alonso-Pulpón, L. A. (2015). Myocarditis. In *Clinico-Pathological Atlas of Cardiovascular Diseases* (pp. 233–263). Springer International Publishing.

Morgan, M. J., & Liu, Z. (2011, January). Crosstalk of reactive oxygen species and NF-κB signaling. *Cell Research*, *21*(1), 103–115. doi:10.1038/cr.2010.178 PMID:21187859

Morris, C. R., Morris, S. M. Jr, Hagar, W., Van Warmerdam, J., Claster, S., Kepka-Lenhart, D., & Vichinsky, E. P. et al. (2003). Arginine therapy: A new treatment for pulmonary hypertension in sickle cell disease? *American Journal of Respiratory and Critical Care Medicine*, *168*(1), 63–69. doi:10.1164/rccm.200208-967OC PMID:12626350

Mosca, L., Barrett-Connor, E., & Wenger, K. N. (2011). Sex/Gender Differences in Cardiovascular Disease Prevention: What a Difference a Decade Makes. *Circulation*, *124*(19), 2145–2154. doi:10.1161/CIRCULATIONAHA.110.968792 PMID:22064958

Moss, R., & Munt, B. (2003). Infection drug use and right sided endocarditis. *Heart (British Cardiac Society)*, *89*(5), 577–581. doi:10.1136/heart.89.5.577 PMID:12695478

Mottaghitalab, F., Farokhi, M., Shokrgozar, M. A., Atyabi, F., & Hosseinkhani, H. (2015). Review: Silk fibroin nanoparticle as a novel drug delivery system. *Journal of Controlled Release*, 206161–206176. doi:10.1016/j.jconrel.2015.03.020

Mozaffarian, D., Benjamin, E. J., Go, A. S., Amett, D. K., Blaha, M. J., Cushman, M., . . . Tumer, M. B. (2015). Heart Disease and Stroke Statistics--2015 Update: A Report From the American Heart Association. *Circulation, 131*(4), e29-e322. Available at: http://circ.ahajournals.org/cgi/doi/10.1161/CIR.0000000000000152

Mozaffarian, D., Benjamin, E. J., Go, A. S., Arnett, D. K., Blaha, M. J., Cushman, M., & Turner, M. B. et al. (2015). Heart Disease and Stroke Statistics—2016 Update: A Report From the American Heart Association. *Circulation*. doi:10.1161/CIR.0000000000000152 PMID:26673558

Mozaffarian, D., Benjamin, E. J., Go, A. S., Arnett, D. K., Blaha, M. J., Cushman, M., & Turner, M. B. et al. (2016). Heart disease and stroke statistics—2016 update: A report from the American Heart Association. *Circulation, 133*(4), e1–e324. doi:10.1161/CIR.0000000000000366 PMID:26673558

Mozaffarian, D., Benjamin, E. J., Go, A. S., Arnett, D. K., Blaha, M. J., Cushman, M., & Turner, M. B. et al. (2016). Heart Disease and Stroke Statistics-2016 Update: A Report From the American Heart Association. *Circulation*, *133*(4), e38–e360. doi:10.1161/CIR.0000000000000350 PMID:26673558

Mozaffari, M. S., Liu, J. Y., Abebe, W., & Baban, B. (2013). Mechanisms of load dependency of myocardial ischemia reperfusion injury. *Am J Cardiovasc Dis*, *3*(4), 180–196. PMID:24224132

Mudge, G. H. (2007). Sirolimus and Cardiac Transplantation: Is It the Magic Bullet? *Circulation*, *116*(23), 2666–2668. doi:10.1161/CIRCULATIONAHA.107.737965 PMID:18056538

Muller, F., Mutch, N. J., Schenk, W. A., Smith, S. A., Esterl, L., Spronk, H. M., & Renné, T. et al. (2009). Platelet polyphosphates are proinflammatory and procoagulant mediators in vivo. *Cell*, *139*(6), 1143–1156. doi:10.1016/j.cell.2009.11.001 PMID:20005807

Mundy, L. M., Sahm, D. F., & Gilmore, M. (2000). Relationships between Enterococcal Virulence and Antimicrobial Resistance. *Clinical Microbiology Reviews*, *13*(4), 513–522. doi:10.1128/CMR.13.4.513-522.2000 PMID:11023953

Muniyappa, R., Hall, G., Kolodziej, T. L., Karne, R. J., Crandon, S. K., & Quon, M. J. (2008). Cocoa consumption for 2 wk enhances insulin-mediated vasodilatation without improving blood pressure or insulin resistance in essential hypertension. *The American Journal of Clinical Nutrition*, *88*(6), 1685–1696. doi:10.3945/ajcn.2008.26457 PMID:19064532

Murdoch, D. R., Corey, G. R., Hoen, B., Miró, J. M., Fowler, V. G. Jr, Bayer, A. S., & Cabell, C. H. et al. (2009). Clinical presentation, etiology, and outcome of infective endocarditis in the 21st century: The International Collaboration on Endocarditis-Prospective Cohort Study. *Archives of Internal Medicine*, *169*(5), 463–473. doi:10.1001/archinternmed.2008.603 PMID:19273776

Murray, C. J. L., Barber, R. M., Foreman, K. J., Ozgoren, A. A., Abd-Allah, F., Abera, S. F., & Vos, T. et al. (2015). Global, regional, and national disability-adjusted life years (DALYs) for 306 diseases and injuries and healthy life expectancy (HALE) for 188 countries, 1990–2013: Quantifying the epidemiological transition. *Lancet*, *386*(10009), 2145–2191. doi:10.1016/S0140-6736(15)61340-X PMID:26321261

Murray, K. P., Zhao, J. J., Davis, S. L., Kullar, R., Kaye, K. S., Lephart, P., & Rybak, M. J. (2013). Early use of daptomycin versus vancomycin for methicillin-resistant Staphylococcus aureus bacteremia with vancomycin minimum inhibitory concentration >1 mg/L: A matched cohort study. *Clinical Infectious Diseases*, *56*(11), 1562–1569. doi:10.1093/cid/cit112 PMID:23449272

Murry, C. E., Richard, V. J., Reimer, K. A., & Jennings, R. B. (1990). Ischemic preconditioning slows energy metabolism and delays ultrastructural damage during a sustained ischemic episode. *Circulation Research*, *66*(4), 913–931. doi:10.1161/01.RES.66.4.913 PMID:2317895

Myburgh, R., Hochfeld, W. E., Dodgen, T. M., Ker, J., & Pepper, M. S. (2012). Cardiovascular pharmacogenetics. *Pharmacology & Therapeutics*, *133*(3), 280–290. doi:10.1016/j.pharmthera.2011.11.002 PMID:22123178

Mylonakis, E., & Calderwood, S. B. (2001). Infective endocarditis in adults. *The New England Journal of Medicine*, *345*(18), 1318–1330. doi:10.1056/NEJMra010082 PMID:11794152

Nabel, E. G., & Braunwald, E. (2012). A tale of coronary artery disease and myocardial infarction. *The New England Journal of Medicine*, *366*(1), 54–63. doi:10.1056/NEJMra1112570 PMID:22216842

Naccarato, M., Yoong, D., & Gough, K. (2012). A potential drug-herbal interaction between Ginkgo biloba and efavirenz. *J Int Assoc Physicians AIDS Care (Chic)*, *11*(2), 98–100. doi:10.1177/1545109711435364 PMID:22323244

Nagaraj, S., Schrum, A. G., Cho, H. I., Celis, E., & Gabrilovich, D. I. (2010). Mechanism of T cell tolerance induced by myeloid-derived suppressor cells. *Journal of Immunology (Baltimore, MD.: 1950)*, *184*(6), 3106–3116. doi:10.4049/jimmunol.0902661 PMID:20142361

Nagase, T., Ishikawa, K., Miyajima, N., Tanaka, A., Kotani, H., & Nomura, N. et al.. (1998). Prediction of the coding sequences of unidentified human genes. IX. The complete sequences of 100 new cDNA clones from brain which can code for large proteins *in vitro*. *DNA Research*, *5*(1), 31–39. doi:10.1093/dnares/5.1.31 PMID:9628581

Nagato, A. C., Bezerra, F. S., Lanzetti, M., Lopes, A. A., Silva, M. A., Porto, L. C., & Valenca, S. S. (2012). Time course of inflammation, oxidative stress and tissue damage induced by hyperoxia in mouse lungs. *International Journal of Experimental Pathology*, *93*(4), 269–278. doi:10.1111/j.1365-2613.2012.00823.x PMID:22804763

Nagaya, N., Yamamoto, H., Uematsu, M., Itoh, T., Nakagawa, K., & Miyazawa, T. (2004). Green tea reverses endothelial dysfunction in healthy smokers. *Heart (British Cardiac Society)*, *90*(12), 1485–1486. doi:10.1136/hrt.2003.026740 PMID:15547040

Naghavi, M., Libby, P., Falk, E., Casscells, S. W., Litovsky, S., Rumberger, J., & Willerson, J. T. et al. (2003). From Vulnerable Plaque to Vulnerable Patient: A Call for New Definitions and Risk Assessment Strategies: Part I. *Circulation*, *108*(14), 1664–1672. doi:10.1161/01.CIR.0000087480.94275.97 PMID:14530185

Naghavi, M., Wang, H., Lozano, R., Davis, A., Liang, X., Zhou, M., & Murray, C. J. et al. (2015). Global, regional, and national age-sex specific all-cause and cause-specific mortality for 240 causes of death, 19902013: A systematic analysis for the Global Burden of Disease Study 2013. *Lancet*, *385*(9963), 117–171. doi:10.1016/S0140-6736(14)61682-2 PMID:25530442

Nagy, T., Champattanachai, V., Marchase, R. B., & Chatham, J. C. (2006). Glucosamine inhibits angiotensin II-induced cytoplasmic Ca2+ elevation in neonatal cardiomyocytes via protein-associated O-linked N-acetylglucosamine. *American Journal of Physiology. Cell Physiology*, *290*(1), C57–C65. doi:10.1152/ajpcell.00263.2005 PMID:16107505

Nahan, R., Barnes, P., Stussman, B., & Bloom, B. (2011). Costs of complementary and alternative medicine (CAM) and frequency of visits to CAM practitioners: United States, 2007. National Health Statistics Reports no. 18. Hyattsville, MD: National Center for Health Statistics; 2009.

Nahrendorf, M., Swirski, F. K., Aikawa, E., Stangenberg, L., Wurdinger, T., Figueiredo, J.-L., & Pittet, M. J. et al. (2007). The healing myocardium sequentially mobilizes two monocyte subsets with divergent and complementary functions. *The Journal of Experimental Medicine*, *204*(12), 3037–3047. doi:10.1084/jem.20070885 PMID:18025128

Naimi, T. S., Brown, D. W., Brewer, R. D., Giles, W. H., Mensah, G., Serdula, M. K., & Stroup, D. F. et al. (2005). Cardiovascular risk factors and confounders among nondrinking and moderate-drinking U.S. adults. *American Journal of Preventive Medicine*, *28*(4), 369–373. doi:10.1016/j.amepre.2005.01.011 PMID:15831343

Nakayama, H., Wilkin, B. J., Bodi, I., & Molkentin, J. D. (2006). Calcineurin-dependent cardiomyopathy is activated by TRPC in the adult mouse heart. *The FASEB Journal*, *20*(10), 1660–1670. doi:10.1096/fj.05-5560com PMID:16873889

Nannini, E. C., Stryjewski, M. E., Singh, K. V., Bourgogne, A., Rude, T. H., Corey, G. R., & Murray, B. E. et al. (2009). Inoculum effect with cefazolin among clinical isolates of methicillin-susceptible Staphylococcus aureus: Frequency and possible cause of cefazolin treatment failure. *Antimicrobial Agents and Chemotherapy*, *53*(8), 3437–3441. doi:10.1128/AAC.00317-09 PMID:19487449

Nantz, M. P., Rowe, C. A., Bukowski, J. F., & Percival, S. S. (2009). Standardized capsule of Camellia sinensis lowers cardiovascular risk factors in a randomized, double-blind, placebo-controlled study. *Nutrition (Burbank, Los Angeles County, Calif.)*, *25*(2), 147–154. doi:10.1016/j.nut.2008.07.018 PMID:18848434

Natarajan, V., Dudek, S. M., Jacobson, J. R., Moreno-Vinasco, L., Huang, L. S., Abassi, T., & Garcia, J. G. et al. (2013). Sphingosine-1-phosphate, FTY720, and sphingosine-1-phosphate receptors in the pathobiology of acute lung injury. *American Journal of Respiratory Cell and Molecular Biology*, *49*(1), 6–17. doi:10.1165/rcmb.2012-0411TR PMID:23449739

Neely, M. N., Youn, G., Jones, B., Jelliffe, R. W., Drusano, G. L., Rodvold, K. A., & Lodise, T. P. (2014). Are vancomycin trough concentrations adequate for optimal dosing? *Antimicrobial Agents and Chemotherapy*, *58*(1), 309–316. doi:10.1128/AAC.01653-13 PMID:24165176

Nelskyla, A., Parr, M. J., & Skrifvars, M. B. (2013). Prevalence and factors correlating with hyperoxia exposure following cardiac arrest - an observational single centre study. *Scan J Trauma Resusc Emerg Med*, *21*(1), 35. doi:10.1186/1757-7241-21-35 PMID:23639102

Nelson, S. K., Wong, G. H. W., & McCord, J. M. (1995). Leukemia inhibitory factor and tumor necrosis factor induce manganese superoxide dismutase and protect rabbit hearts from reperfusion injury. *Journal of Molecular and Cellular Cardiology*, *27*(1), 223–229. doi:10.1016/S0022-2828(08)80021-1 PMID:7760346

Nerbonne, J. M., & Kass, R. S. (2005). Molecular physiology of cardiac repolarization. *Physiological Reviews*, *85*(4), 1205–1253. doi:10.1152/physrev.00002.2005 PMID:16183911

Neri, I., Monari, F., Sgarbi, L., Berardi, A., Masellis, G., & Facchinetti, F. (2010). L-arginine supplementation in women with chronic hypertension: Impact on blood pressure and maternal and neonatal complications. *The Journal of Maternal-Fetal & Neonatal Medicine*, *23*(12), 1456–1460. doi:10.3109/14767051003677962 PMID:20958228

Newton-Cheh, C., & Smith, J. G. (2010). What can human genetics teach us about the causes of cardiovascular disease? *Journal of the American College of Cardiology*, *55*(25), 2843–2845. doi:10.1016/j.jacc.2009.11.097 PMID:20579541

Ng, F., & Tang, B. L. (2013). Sirtuins modulation of autophagy. *Journal of Cellular Physiology*, *228*(12), 2262–2270. doi:10.1002/jcp.24399 PMID:23696314

Nguyen, C., & Shapiro, R. (2014). New immunosuppressive agents in pediatric transplantation. *Clinics (Sao Paulo)*, *69*(Suppl 1), 8–16. doi:10.6061/clinics/2014(Sup01)03 PMID:24860853

NHLBI. (2015). *Description of high blood pressure*. Retrieved from http://www.nhlbi.nih.gov/health/health-topics/topics/hbp/

Nicholls, S. J. (2009). Relationship between LDL, HDL, blood pressure and atheroma progression in the coronaries. *Current Opinion in Lipidology*, *20*(6), 491–496. doi:10.1097/MOL.0b013e32832ec396 PMID:19593124

Nickson, P., Toth, A., & Erhardt, P. (2007). PUMA is critical for neonatal cardiomyocyte apoptosis induced by endoplasmic reticulum stress. *Cardiovascular Research*, *73*(1), 48–56. doi:10.1016/j.cardiores.2006.10.001 PMID:17107669

Nishimura, R. A., Otto, C. M., Bonow, R. O., Carabello, B. A., Erwin, J. P. III, Guyton, R. A., & Thomas, J. D. et al. (2014). 2014 AHA/ACC guideline for the management of patients with valvular heart disease: executive summary: a report of the American College of Cardiology/American Heart Association Task Force on Practice Guidelines. *Circulation*, *129*(23), 2440–2492. doi:10.1161/CIR.0000000000000029 PMID:24589852

Nishiyama, A., Ishii, D. N., Backx, P. H., Pulford, B. E., Birks, B. R., & Tamkun, M. M. (2001). Altered K(+) channel gene expression in diabetic rat ventricle: Isoform switching between Kv4.2 and Kv1.4. *American Journal of Physiology. Heart and Circulatory Physiology*, *281*(4), H1800–H1807. PMID:11557574

Nomura, F., Kurobe, N., Mori, Y., Hikita, A., Kawai, M., Suwa, M., & Okutani, Y. (2008). Multicenter prospective investigation on the efficacy and safety of carperitide as a first-line drug for acute heart failure syndrome with preserved blood pressure: COMPASS: Carperitide Effects Observed Through Monitoring Dyspnea in Acute Decompensated Heart Failure Study. *Circulation Journal*, *72*(11), 1777–1786. doi:10.1253/circj.CJ-07-0760 PMID:18832779

Novak, J., Bitsch, C., Langbehn, J., Pank, F., Skoula, M., & Gotsiou, Y. (2000). Ratios of cis-and trans-sabinene hydrate in Origanum majorana L. and Origanum microphyllum (Bentham) Vogel. *Biochemical Systematics and Ecology*, *28*(7), 697–704. doi:10.1016/S0305-1978(99)00098-8 PMID:10854745

Nurden, A.T., Pillois, X., & Nurden, P. (2012). Understanding the genetic basis of Glanzmann thrombasthenia: implications for treatment. *Expert Review of Hematology, 5*, 487-503.

Nurden, A. T., Fiore, M., Nurden, P., & Pillois, X. (2011). Glanzmann thrombasthenia: A review of ITGA2B and ITGB3 defects with emphasis on variants, phenotypic variability, and mouse models. *Blood*, *118*(23), 5996–6005. doi:10.1182/blood-2011-07-365635 PMID:21917754

Nurden, A. T., & Nurden, P. (2015). Inherited disorders of platelet function: Selected updates. *Journal of thrombosis and haemostasis*. *JTH*, *13*(Suppl 1), S2–S9. PMID:26149024

Nurden, A. T., Pillois, X., & Wilcox, D. A. (2013). Glanzmann thrombasthenia: State of the art and future directions. *Seminars in Thrombosis and Hemostasis*, *39*(06), 642–655. doi:10.1055/s-0033-1353393 PMID:23929305

Nurden, A., & Nurden, P. (2011). Advances in our understanding of the molecular basis of disorders of platelet function. *Journal of thrombosis and haemostasis*. *JTH*, *9*(Suppl 1), 76–91. PMID:21781244

Nurden, P., & Nurden, A. T. (2008). Congenital disorders associated with platelet dysfunctions. *Thrombosis and Haemostasis*, *99*, 253–263. PMID:18278172

Nyyssönen, K., Parviainen, M. T., Salonen, R., Tuomilehto, J., & Salonen, J. T. (1997). Vitamin C deficiency and risk of myocardial infarction: Prospective population study of men from eastern Finland. *BMJ: British Medical Journal*, *314*(7081), 634–638. doi:10.1136/bmj.314.7081.634 PMID:9066474

O'Connor, C., & Peacock, W. F. (2016). *Efficacy and safety of ularitide for the treatment of acute decompensated heart failure (TRUE-AHF)*. Retrieved on March 11, 2016 from https://clinicaltrials.gov/ct2/show/study/NCT01661634#locn

Obad, S., dos Santos, C. O., Petri, A., Heidenblad, M., Broom, O., Ruse, C., & Kauppinen, S. et al. (2011). Silencing of microRNA families by seed-targeting tiny LNAs. *Nature Genetics*, *43*(4), 371–378. doi:10.1038/ng.786 PMID:21423181

OConnor, C. M., Starling, R. C., Hernandez, A. F., Armstrong, P. W., Dickstein, K., Hasselblad, V., & Califf, R. M. et al. (2011). Effect of nesiritide in patients with acute decompensated heart failure. *The New England Journal of Medicine*, *365*(1), 32–43. doi:10.1056/NEJMoa1100171 PMID:21732835

ODriscoll, R., Davison, A., Elliott, M., Howard, L., Wedzicha, J., Mackway-Jones, K., & Hinshaw, K. et al. (2008). BTS guideline for emergency oxygen use in adult patients. *Thorax*, *63*(Supplement 6), vi1–vi68. doi:10.1136/thx.2008.102947 PMID:18838559

Oeckinghaus & Ghosh. (2009, October). The NF-κB Family of Transcription Factors and Its Regulation. *Cold Spring Harbor Perspectives in Biology*, *1*(4), a000034. PMID:20066092

Office of Disease Prevention and Health Promotion. (2015). *Social Determinants of Health*. Retrieved from http://www.healthypeople.gov/2020/topics-objectives/topic/social-determinants-health

Ofori-Acquah, S. F., King, J., Voelkel, N., Schaphorst, K. L., & Stevens, T. (2008). Heterogeneity of barrier function in the lung reflects diversity in endothelial cell junctions. *Microvascular Research, 75*(3), 391–402. doi:10.1016/j.mvr.2007.10.006 PMID:18068735

OGara, P. T., Kushner, F. G., Ascheim, D. D., Casey, D. E. Jr, Chung, M. K., de Lemos, J. A., & Zhao, D. X. et al. (2013). 2013 ACCF/AHA guideline for the management of ST-elevation myocardial infarction: executive summary: a report of the American College of Cardiology Foundation/American Heart Association Task Force on Practice Guidelines: developed in collaboration with the American College of Emergency Physicians and Society for Cardiovascular Angiography and Interventions. *Catheterization and Cardiovascular Interventions, 82*(1), E1–E27. doi:10.1002/ccd.24776 PMID:23299937

Ogita, M., Miyauchi, K., Kasai, T., Doi, S., Wada, H., Naito, R., & Daida, H. et al. (2015). Impact of preprocedural high-sensitive C-reactive protein levels on long-term clinical outcomes of patients with stable coronary artery disease and chronic kidney disease who were treated with drug-eluting stents. *Journal of Cardiology, 66*(1), 15–21. doi:10.1016/j.jjcc.2014.10.010 PMID:25572020

Ohba, T., Watanabe, H., Murakami, M., Sato, T., Ono, K., & Ito, H. (2009). Essential role of STIM1 in the development of cardiomyocyte hypertrophy. *Biochemical and Biophysical Research Communications, 389*(1), 172–176. doi:10.1016/j.bbrc.2009.08.117 PMID:19715666

Ohba, T., Watanabe, H., Murakami, M., Takahashi, Y., Iino, K., Kuromitsu, S., & Ito, H. et al. (2007). Upregulation of TRPC1 in the development of cardiac hypertrophy. *Journal of Molecular and Cellular Cardiology, 42*(3), 498–507. doi:10.1016/j.yjmcc.2006.10.020 PMID:17174323

Oh-hora, M., & Rao, A. (2008). Calcium signaling in lymphocytes. *Current Opinion in Immunology, 20*(3), 250–258. doi:10.1016/j.coi.2008.04.004 PMID:18515054

Ohta, Y., Hartwig, J. H., & Stossel, T. P. (2006). FilGAP, a Rho- and ROCK-regulated GAP for Rac binds filamin A to control actin remodelling. *Nature Cell Biology, 8*(8), 803–814. doi:10.1038/ncb1437 PMID:16862148

Oka, S., Zhai, P., Yamamoto, T., Ikeda, Y., Byun, J., Hsu, C. P., & Sadoshima, J. (2015). Peroxisome Proliferator Activated Receptor-alpha Association With Silent Information Regulator 1 Suppresses Cardiac Fatty Acid Metabolism in the Failing Heart. *Circulation: Heart Failure, 8*(6), 1123–1132. doi:10.1161/CIRCHEARTFAILURE.115.002216 PMID:26443578

Olaison, L., & Schadewitz, K. (2002). Enterococcal endocarditis in Sweden, 19951999: Can shorter therapy with aminoglycosides be used? *Clinical Infectious Diseases, 34*(2), 159–166. doi:10.1086/338233 PMID:11740702

OLeary, D. H., Polak, J. F., Kronmal, R. A., Manolio, T. A., Burke, G. L., & Wolfson, S. K. Jr. (1999). Carotid-Artery Intima and Media Thickness as a Risk Factor for Myocardial Infarction and Stroke in Older Adults. *The New England Journal of Medicine, 340*(1), 14–22. doi:10.1056/NEJM199901073400103 PMID:9878640

Olichon, A., Baricault, L., Gas, N., Guillou, E., Valette, A., & Belenguer, P. et al.. (2003). Loss of OPA1 perturbates the mitochondrial inner membrane structure and integrity, leading to cytochrome c release and apoptosis. *The Journal of Biological Chemistry, 278*(10), 7743–7746. doi:10.1074/jbc.C200677200 PMID:12509422

Oliveira, A., Barros, H., & Lopes, C. (2009). Gender heterogeneity in the association between lifestyles and non-fatal acute myocardial infarction. *Public Health Nutrition, 12*(10), 1799–1806. doi:10.1017/S1368980008004588 PMID:19161646

Ollendorf, D. A., Sandhu, A. T., Chapman, R., Heidenreich, P. A., Russo, E., Shore, K. K., …Pearson, S. D. (2015). *CardioMEMS HF System (St. Jude Medical) and sacubitril/valsartan (Entresto, Norvatis) for Management of Congestive Heart Failure: effectiveness, Value and Value Based Price Benchmarks.* Retrieved March 11, 2016, from http://ctaf.org/sites/default/files/u148/CHF_Draft_Report_091115.pdf

Ong, S., Subrayan, S., Lim, S. Y., Yellon, D. M., Davidson, S. M., & Hausenloy, D. J. (2010). Inhibiting mitochondrial fission protects the heart against ischemia/reperfusion injury. *Circulation*, *121*(18), 2012–2022. doi:10.1161/CIRCULATIONAHA.109.906610 PMID:20421521

Onohara, N., Nishida, M., Inoue, R., Kobayashi, H., Sumimoto, H., Sato, Y., & Kurose, H. et al. (2006). TRPC3 and TRPC6 are essential for angiotensin II-induced cardiac hypertrophy. *The EMBO Journal*, *25*(22), 5305–5316. doi:10.1038/sj.emboj.7601417 PMID:17082763

Oritani, K., & Kincade, P. W. (1996). Identification of stromal cell products that interact with pre-B cells. *The Journal of Cell Biology*, *134*(3), 771–782. doi:10.1083/jcb.134.3.771 PMID:8707854

Ota, H., Akishita, M., Eto, M., Iijima, K., Kaneki, M., & Ouchi, Y. (2007). Sirt1 modulates premature senescence-like phenotype in human endothelial cells. *Journal of Molecular and Cellular Cardiology*, *43*(5), 571–579. doi:10.1016/j.yjmcc.2007.08.008 PMID:17916362

Ota, H., Eto, M., Ogawa, S., Iijima, K., Akishita, M., & Ouchi, Y. (2010). SIRT1/eNOS axis as a potential target against vascular senescence, dysfunction and atherosclerosis. *Journal of Atherosclerosis and Thrombosis*, *17*(5), 431–435. doi:10.5551/jat.3525 PMID:20215708

Othman, M. (2011). Platelet-type von Willebrand disease: A rare, often misdiagnosed and underdiagnosed bleeding disorder. *Seminars in Thrombosis and Hemostasis*, *37*(05), 464–469. doi:10.1055/s-0031-1281030 PMID:22102188

Oudemans-van Straaten, H. M., Jansen, P. G., Hoek, F. J., van Deventer, S. J., Sturk, A., Stoutenbeek, C. P., . . . Eysman, L. (1996). Intestinal permeability, circulating endotoxin, and postoperative systemic responses in cardiac surgery patients. *J Cardiothorac Vasc Anesth, 10*(2), 187-194. doi: S1053-0770(96)80235-7 [pii]

Ozelo, M. C., Svirin, P., & Larina, L. (2005). Use of recombinant factor VIIa in the management of severe bleeding episodes in patients with Bernard-Soulier syndrome. *Annals of Hematology*, *84*(12), 816–822. doi:10.1007/s00277-005-1080-y PMID:16044315

Pai, M. P., Neely, M., Rodvold, K. A., & Lodise, T. P. (2014). Innovative approaches to optimizing the delivery of vancomycin in individual patients. *Advanced Drug Delivery Reviews*, *77*, 50–57. doi:10.1016/j.addr.2014.05.016 PMID:24910345

Pallauf, K., Giller, K., Huebbe, P., & Rimbach, G. (2013). Nutrition and healthy ageing: Calorie restriction or polyphenol-rich "MediterrAsian" diet? *Oxidative Medicine and Cellular Longevity*, *707421*. doi:10.1155/2013/707421 PMID:24069505

Palloshi, A., Fragasso, G., Piatti, P., Monti, L. D., Setola, E., Valsecchi, G., & Margonato, A. et al. (2004). Effect of oral L-arginine on blood pressure and symptoms and endothelial function in patients with systemic hypertension, positive exercise tests, and normal coronary arteries. *The American Journal of Cardiology*, *93*(7), 933–935. doi:10.1016/j.amjcard.2003.12.040 PMID:15050504

Pal, S., Khossousi, A., Binns, C., Dhaliwal, S., & Radavelli-Bagatini, S. (2012). The effects of 12-week psyllium fibre supplementation or healthy diet on blood pressure and arterial stiffness in overweight and obese individuals. *The British Journal of Nutrition*, *107*(5), 725–734. doi:10.1017/S0007114511003497 PMID:21787454

Palty, R., Raveh, A., Kaminsky, I., Meller, R., & Reuveny, E. (2012). SARAF inactivates the store operated calcium entry machinery to prevent excess calcium refilling. *Cell*, *149*(2), 425–438. doi:10.1016/j.cell.2012.01.055 PMID:22464749

Panama, B. K., Latour-Villamil, D., Farman, G. P., Zhao, D., Bolz, S. S., Kirshenbaum, L. A., & Backx, P. H. (2011). Nuclear factor kappaB downregulates the transient outward potassium current I(to,f) through control of KChIP2 expression. *Circulation Research*, *108*(5), 537–543. doi:10.1161/CIRCRESAHA.110.229112 PMID:21252158

Panguluri, S. K., Tur, J., Chapalamadugu, K. C., Katnik, C., Cuevas, J., & Tipparaju, S. M. (2013). MicroRNA-301a mediated regulation of Kv4.2 in diabetes: Identification of key modulators. *PLoS ONE*, *8*(4), e60545. doi:10.1371/journal.pone.0060545 PMID:23573265

Panguluri, S. K., Tur, J., Fukumoto, J., Deng, W., Sneed, K. B., Kolliputi, N., & Tipparaju, S. M. et al. (2013). Hyperoxia-induced hypertrophy and ion channel remodeling in left ventricle. *American Journal of Physiology. Heart and Circulatory Physiology*, *304*(12), H1651–H1661. doi:10.1152/ajpheart.00474.2012 PMID:23585127

Pan, Z., Brotto, M., & Ma, J. (2014). Store-operated Ca2+ entry in muscle physiology and diseases. *BMB Rep*, *47*(2), 69–79. doi:10.5483/BMBRep.2014.47.2.015 PMID:24411466

Papademetriou, V., Narayan, P., & Kokkinos, P. (2004). Angiotensin-Converting Enzyme Inhibitors and Angiotensin Receptor Blockers in African-American Patients With Hypertension. *Journal of Clinical Hypertension*, *6*(6), 310–314. doi:10.1111/j.1524-6175.2004.03446.x PMID:15187493

Papanicolaou, K. N., Khairallah, R. J., Ngoh, G. A., Chikando, A., Luptak, I., & O'Shea, K. M. et al.. (2011). Mitofusin-2 maintains mitochondrial structure and contributes to stress-induced permeability transition in cardiac myocytes. *Molecular and Cellular Biology*, *6*(130), 9–28. PMID:21245373

Papanicolaou, K. N., Kikuchi, R., Ngoh, G. A., Coughlan, K. A., Dominguez, I., Stanley, W. C., & Walsh, K. (2012). Mitofusins 1 and 2 are Essential for Postnatal Metabolic Remodeling in Heart. *Circulation Research*, *111*(8), 1012–1026. doi:10.1161/CIRCRESAHA.112.274142 PMID:22904094

Papanicolaou, K. N., Ngoh, G. A., Dabkowski, E. R., OConnell, K. A., Ribeiro, R. F. Jr, Stanley, W. C., & Walsh, K. (2012). Cardiomyocyte deletion of mitofusin-1 leads to mitochondrial fragmentation and improves tolerance to ROS-induced mitochondrial dysfunction and cell death. *American Journal of Physiology. Heart and Circulatory Physiology*, *302*(1), H167–H179. doi:10.1152/ajpheart.00833.2011 PMID:22037195

Paria, B. C., Vogel, S. M., Ahmmed, G. U., Alamgir, S., Shroff, J., Malik, A. B., & Tiruppathi, C. (2004). Tumor necrosis factor-alpha-induced TRPC1 expression amplifies store-operated Ca2+ influx and endothelial permeability. *American Journal of Physiology. Lung Cellular and Molecular Physiology*, *287*(6), L1303–L1313. doi:10.1152/ajplung.00240.2004 PMID:15347566

Park, C. Y., Hoover, P. J., Mullins, F. M., Bachhawat, P., Covington, E. D., Raunser, S., & Lewis, R. S. et al. (2009). STIM1 clusters and activates CRAC channels via direct binding of a cytosolic domain to Orai1. *Cell*, *136*(5), 876–890. doi:10.1016/j.cell.2009.02.014 PMID:19249086

Parker, J. O., Parker, J. D., Caldwell, R. W., Farrell, B., & Kaesemeyer, W. H. (2002). The effect of supplemental L-arginine on tolerance development during continuous transdermal nitroglycerin therapy. *Journal of the American College of Cardiology*, *39*(7), 1199–1203. doi:10.1016/S0735-1097(02)01729-1 PMID:11923046

Partiseti, M., Le Deist, F., Hivroz, C., Fischer, A., Korn, H., & Choquet, D. (1994). The calcium current activated by T cell receptor and store depletion in human lymphocytes is absent in a primary immunodeficiency. *The Journal of Biological Chemistry*, *269*(51), 32327–32335. PMID:7798233

Pasterkamp, G., Van Keulen, J. K., & De Kleijn, D. P. (2004). Role of Toll-like receptor 4 in the initiation and progression of atherosclerotic disease. *European Journal of Clinical Investigation*, *34*(5), 328–334. doi:10.1111/j.1365-2362.2004.01338.x PMID:15147329

Patel, N., Pai, M. P., Rodvold, K. A., Lomaestro, B., Drusano, G. L., & Lodise, T. P. (2011). Vancomycin: We cant get there from here. *Clinical Infectious Diseases*, *52*(8), 969–974. doi:10.1093/cid/cir078 PMID:21460308

Patel, V. B., Misra, S., Patel, B. B., & Majumdar, A. P. (2010). Colorectal cancer: Chemopreventive role of curcumin and resveratrol. *Nutrition and Cancer*, *62*(7), 958–967. doi:10.1080/01635581.2010.510259 PMID:20924971

Paterson, A. D., Rommens, J. M., Bharaj, B., Blavignac, J., Wong, I., Diamandis, M., & Hayward, C. P. M. et al. (2010). Persons with Quebec platelet disorder have a tandem duplication of PLAU, the urokinase plasminogen activator gene. *Blood*, *115*(6), 1264–1266. doi:10.1182/blood-2009-07-233965 PMID:20007542

Pélissier-Alicot, A. L., Gaulier, J. M., Champsaur, P., & Marquet, P. (2003). Mechanisms underlying postmortem redistribution of drugs: A review. *Journal of Analytic Toxicolology*, *27*(8), 533–544. doi:10.1093/jat/27.8.533 PMID:14670131

Peng, X., Hassoun, P. M., Sammani, S., McVerry, B. J., Burne, M. J., Rabb, H., & Garcia, J. G. et al. (2004). Protective effects of sphingosine 1-phosphate in murine endotoxin-induced inflammatory lung injury. *American Journal of Respiratory and Critical Care Medicine*, *169*(11), 1245–1251. doi:10.1164/rccm.200309-1258OC PMID:15020292

Pepe, S., Marasco, S. F., Haas, S. J., Sheeran, F. L., Krum, H., & Rosenfeldt, F. L. (2007). Coenzyme Q10 in cardiovascular disease. *Mitochondrion*, *7*(Suppl), S154–S167. doi:10.1016/j.mito.2007.02.005 PMID:17485243

Percy, J. N., & Keppel, K. G. (2002). A Summary of Health Disparity. *Public Health Reports*, *117*(3), 273–280. doi:10.1016/S0033-3549(04)50161-9 PMID:12432138

Perez-Garcia, M. T., Lopez-Lopez, J. R., & Gonzalez, C. (1999). Kvbeta1.2 subunit coexpression in HEK293 cells confers O2 sensitivity to kv4.2 but not to Shaker channels. *The Journal of General Physiology*, *113*(6), 897–907. doi:10.1085/jgp.113.6.897 PMID:10352037

Perez, K. K., Olsen, R. J., Musick, W. L., Cernoch, P. L., Davis, J. R., Peterson, L. E., & Musser, J. M. (2014). Integrating rapid diagnostics and antimicrobial stewardship improves outcomes in patients with antibiotic-resistant Gram-negative bacteremia. *The Journal of Infection*, *69*(3), 216–225. doi:10.1016/j.jinf.2014.05.005 PMID:24841135

Perez, V. V. D. A., Mazo, T., Marchini, T., Caceres, L., Evelson, P., & Gelpi, R. J. (2016). Ischemic postconditioning confers cardioprotection and prevents reduction of Trx-1 in young mice, but not in middle-aged and old mice. *Molecular and Cellular Biochemistry*. doi:10.1007/s11010-016-2677-2

Persson, I. A., Persson, K., Hagg, S., & Andersson, R. G. (2011). Effects of cocoa extract and dark chocolate on angiotensin-converting enzyme and nitric oxide in human endothelial cells and healthy volunteersa nutrigenomics perspective. *Journal of Cardiovascular Pharmacology*, *57*(1), 44–50. doi:10.1097/FJC.0b013e3181fe62e3 PMID:20966764

Peter, J. (1997). Barnes.Nuclear Factor-κB — A Pivotal Transcription Factor in Chronic Inflammatory Diseases. *The New England Journal of Medicine*, *336*(15), 1066–1071. doi:10.1056/NEJM199704103361506 PMID:9091804

Peters, C. G., Michelson, A. D., & Flaumenhaft, R. (2012). Granule exocytosis is required for platelet spreading: Differential sorting of alpha-granules expressing VAMP-7. *Blood*, *120*(1), 199–206. doi:10.1182/blood-2011-10-389247 PMID:22589474

Peters, F. T., & Remane, D. (2012). Aspects of matrix effects in applications of liquid chromatography-mass spectrometry to forensic and clinical toxicologya review. *Analytical and Bioanalytical Chemistry*, *403*(8), 2155–2172. doi:10.1007/s00216-012-6035-2 PMID:22549818

Peterson, L. R. (2009). Bad bugs, no drugs: No ESCAPE revisisted. *Clinical Infectious Diseases*, *49*(6), 992–993. doi:10.1086/605539 PMID:19694542

Peters, S. C., & Piper, H. M. (2007). Reoxygenation-induced Ca2+ rise is mediated via Ca2+ influx and Ca2+ release from the endoplasmic reticulum in cardiac endothelial cells. *Cardiovascular Research*, *73*(1), 164–171. doi:10.1016/j.cardiores.2006.09.015 PMID:17097624

Petkova-Kirova, P. S., Gursoy, E., Mehdi, H., McTiernan, C. F., London, B., & Salama, G. (2006). Electrical remodeling of cardiac myocytes from mice with heart failure due to the overexpression of tumor necrosis factor-alpha. *American Journal of Physiology. Heart and Circulatory Physiology*, *290*(5), H2098–H2107. doi:10.1152/ajpheart.00097.2005 PMID:16339842

Petrache, I., Choi, M. E., Otterbein, L. E., Chin, B. Y., Mantell, L. L., Horowitz, S., & Choi, A. M. K. (1999). Mitogen-activated protein kinase pathway mediates hyperoxia-induced apoptosis in cultured macrophage cells. *American Journal of Physiology. Lung Cellular and Molecular Physiology*, *277*(3), L589–L595. PMID:10484467

Petti, C. A., Bhally, H. S., Weinstein, M. P., Joho, K., Wakefield, T., Reller, L. B., & Carrol, K. C. (2006). Utility of Extended Blood Culture Incubation for Isolation of Haemophilus, Actinobacillus, Cardiobacterium, Eikenella, and Kingella Organisms: A Retrospective Multicenter Evaluation. *Journal of Clinical Microbiology*, *44*(1), 257–259. doi:10.1128/JCM.44.1.257-259.2006 PMID:16390985

Phelan, J., Link, B. G., & Tehranifar, P. (2010). Social Conditions as Fundamental Causes of health Inequalities: Theory, Evidence, and Policy Implications. *Journal of Health and Social Behaviors, 51*(s), 28-40

Pibarot, P., & Dumesnil, J. G. (2009). Prosthetic heart valves: Selection of the optimal prosthesis and long-term management. *Circulation*, *119*(7), 1034–1048. doi:10.1161/CIRCULATIONAHA.108.778886 PMID:19237674

Pierrakos, C., Karanikolas, M., Scolletta, S., Karamouzos, V., & Velissaris, D. (2012). Acute respiratory distress syndrome: Pathophysiology and therapeutic options. *J Clin Med Res*, *4*(1), 7–16. doi:10.4021/jocmr761w PMID:22383921

Pignatelli, P., Carnevale, R., Di Santo, S., Bartimoccia, S., Sanguigni, V., Lenti, L., & Violi, F. et al. (2011). Inherited human gp91phox deficiency is associated with impaired isoprostane formation and platelet dysfunction. *Arteriosclerosis, Thrombosis, and Vascular Biology*, *31*(2), 423–434. doi:10.1161/ATVBAHA.110.217885 PMID:21071703

Pillarisetti, S. (2008). A review of Sirt1 and Sirt1 modulators in cardiovascular and metabolic diseases. *Recent Patents on Cardiovascular Drug Discovery*, *3*(3), 156–164. doi:10.2174/157489008786263989 PMID:18991791

Pilz, G., Graw, M., Heer, T., Klos, M., Ali, E., & Hoefling, B. (2009). Myocardial hypoperfusion due to hypoplastic coronary arteries: A cause for false-positive results during adenosine stress Cardiac Magnetic Resonance Imaging. *Journal of Cardiovascular Magnetic Resonance*, *11*(Suppl 1), 155. doi:10.1186/1532-429X-11-S1-P155

Pimple, B. P., Kadam, P. V., & Patil, M. J. (2012). Comparative antihyperglycaemic and antihyperlipidemic effect of Origanum majorana extracts in NIDDM rats. *Oriental Pharmacy and Experimental Medicine*, *12*(1), 41–50. doi:10.1007/s13596-011-0047-x

Piquereau, J., Caffin, F., Novotova, M., Prola, A., Garnier, A., Mateo, P., & Joubert, F. et al. (2012). Down-regulation of OPA1 alters mouse mitochondrial morphology, PTP function, and cardiac adaptation to pressure overload. *Cardiovascular Research*, *94*(3), 408–417. doi:10.1093/cvr/cvs117 PMID:22406748

Plotnikov, A., Zehorai, E., Procaccia, S., & Seger, R. (2011). The MAPK cascades: Signaling components, nuclear roles and mechanisms of nuclear translocation. *Biochimica et Biophysica Acta*, *1813*(9), 1619–1633. doi:10.1016/j.bbamcr.2010.12.012 PMID:21167873

Pocock, T. M., Foster, R. R., & Bates, D. O. (2004). Evidence of a role for TRPC channels in VEGF-mediated increased vascular permeability in vivo. *American Journal of Physiology. Heart and Circulatory Physiology*, *286*(3), H1015–H1026. doi:10.1152/ajpheart.00826.2003 PMID:14551041

Pohlhammer, J., Kronenberg, F., Rantner, B., Stadler, M., Peric, S., Hammerer-Lercher, A., & Kollerits, B. et al. (2014). High-sensitivity cardiac troponin T in patients with intermittent claudication and its relation with cardiovascular events and all-cause mortalitythe CAVASIC Study. *Atherosclerosis*, *237*(2), 711–717. doi:10.1016/j.atherosclerosis.2014.10.097 PMID:25463110

Porzionato, A., Sfriso, M. M., Mazzatenta, A., Macchi, V., De Caro, R., & Di Giulio, C. (2015). Effects of hyperoxic exposure on signal transduction pathways in the lung. *Respiratory Physiology & Neurobiology*, *209*, 106–114. doi:10.1016/j.resp.2014.12.002 PMID:25485998

Porzionato, A., Zaramella, P., Macchi, V., Grisafi, D., Salmaso, R., Baraldi, M., & De Caro, R. et al. (2012). Fluoxetine may worsen hyperoxia-induced lung damage in neonatal rats. *Histology and Histopathology*, *27*(12), 1599–1610. PMID:23059890

Porzionato, A., Zaramella, P., Macchi, V., Sarasin, G., Di Giulio, C., Rigon, A., & De Caro, R. et al. (2013). Cyclosporine and hyperoxia-induced lung damage in neonatal rats. *Respiratory Physiology & Neurobiology*, *187*(1), 41–46. doi:10.1016/j.resp.2013.02.018 PMID:23454024

Poston, D. Jr, & Min, H. (2008). Statistical Modeling for Causes of Death: Multinomial Logit Regression Model. *Journal of Modern Statistical Methods*, *7*(2), 597–606

Pothapragada, S., Zhang, P., Sheriff, J., Livelli, M., Slepian, M. J., Deng, Y., & Bluestein, D. (2015). A phenomenological particle-based platelet model for simulating filopodia formation during early activation. *International Journal for Numerical Methods in Biomedical Engineering*, *31*(3), e02702. doi:10.1002/cnm.2702 PMID:25532469

Potier, M., & Trebak, M. (2008). New developments in the signaling mechanisms of the store-operated calcium entry pathway. *Pflugers Archiv*, *457*(2), 405–415. doi:10.1007/s00424-008-0533-2 PMID:18536932

Poulose, N., & Raju, R. (2015). Sirtuin regulation in aging and injury. *Biochimica et Biophysica Acta*, *1852*(11), 2442–2455. doi:10.1016/j.bbadis.2015.08.017 PMID:26303641

Pounder, D. J., & Jones, G. R. (1990). Post-mortem drug redistributiona toxicological nightmare. *Forensic Science International*, *45*(3), 253–263. doi:10.1016/0379-0738(90)90182-X PMID:2361648

Pozeg, Z. I. (2003). In Vivo Gene Transfer of the O2-Sensitive Potassium Channel Kv1.5 Reduces Pulmonary Hypertension and Restores Hypoxic Pulmonary Vasoconstriction in Chronically Hypoxic Rats. *Circulation*, *107*(15), 2037–2044. doi:10.1161/01.CIR.0000062688.76508.B3 PMID:12695303

Pozo-Guisado, E., Campbell, D. G., Deak, M., Alvarez-Barrientos, A., Morrice, N. A., Alvarez, I. S., & Martin-Romero, F. J. et al. (2010). Phosphorylation of STIM1 at ERK1/2 target sites modulates store-operated calcium entry. *Journal of Cell Science*, *123*(Pt 18), 3084–3093. doi:10.1242/jcs.067215 PMID:20736304

Prabu, S. K., Anandatheerthavarada, H. K., Raza, H., Srinivasan, S., Spear, J. F., & Avadhani, N. G. (2006). Protein Kinase A-mediated Phosphorylation Modulates Cytochrome c Oxidase Function and Augments Hypoxia and Myocardial Ischemia-related Injury. *The Journal of Biological Chemistry*, *281*(4), 2061–2070. doi:10.1074/jbc.M507741200 PMID:16303765

Prakash, H., Luth, A., Grinkina, N., Holzer, D., Wadgaonkar, R., Gonzalez, A. P., & Kleuser, B. et al. (2010). Sphingosine kinase-1 (SphK-1) regulates Mycobacterium smegmatis infection in macrophages. *PLoS ONE*, *5*(5), e10657. doi:10.1371/journal.pone.0010657 PMID:20498849

Prakriya, M., & Lewis, R. S. (2006). Regulation of CRAC channel activity by recruitment of silent channels to a high open-probability gating mode. *The Journal of General Physiology*, *128*(3), 373–386. doi:10.1085/jgp.200609588 PMID:16940559

Prakriya, M., & Lewis, R. S. (2015). Store-Operated Calcium Channels. *Physiological Reviews*, *95*(4), 1383–1436. doi:10.1152/physrev.00020.2014 PMID:26400989

Prasad, A., Gossl, M., Hoyt, J., Lennon, R. J., Polk, L., Simari, R., & Lerman, A. et al. (2013). Remote ischemic preconditioning immediately before percutaneous coronary intervention does not impact myocardial necrosis, inflammatory response, and circulating endothelial progenitor cell counts: A single center randomized sham controlled trial. *Catheterization and Cardiovascular Interventions*, *81*(6), 930–936. doi:10.1002/ccd.24443 PMID:22517646

Predescu, S. A., Predescu, D. N., & Malik, A. B. (2007). Molecular determinants of endothelial transcytosis and their role in endothelial permeability. *American Journal of Physiology. Lung Cellular and Molecular Physiology*, *293*(4), L823–L842. doi:10.1152/ajplung.00436.2006 PMID:17644753

Predescu, S. A., Predescu, D. N., Timblin, B. K., Stan, R. V., & Malik, A. B. (2003). Intersectin regulates fission and internalization of caveolae in endothelial cells. *Molecular Biology of the Cell*, *14*(12), 4997–5010. doi:10.1091/mbc.E03-01-0041 PMID:12960435

Preuss, H. G., Echard, B., Polansky, M. M., & Anderson, R. (2006). Whole cinnamon and aqueous extracts ameliorate sucrose-induced blood pressure elevations in spontaneously hypertensive rats. *Journal of the American College of Nutrition*, *25*(2), 144–150. doi:10.1080/07315724.2006.10719525 PMID:16582031

Proia, R. L., & Hla, T. (2015). Emerging biology of sphingosine-1-phosphate: Its role in pathogenesis and therapy. *The Journal of Clinical Investigation*, *125*(4), 1379–1387. doi:10.1172/JCI76369 PMID:25831442

Przyklenk, K., Bauer, B., Ovize, M., Kloner, R. A., & Whittaker, P. (1993). Regional ischemic preconditioning protects remote virgin myocardium from subsequent sustained coronary occlusion. *Circulation*, *87*(3), 893–899. doi:10.1161/01.CIR.87.3.893 PMID:7680290

Psarros, C., Lee, R., Margaritis, M., & Antoniades, C. (2012). Review: Nanomedicine for the prevention, treatment and imaging of atherosclerosis. *Maturitas*, *73*, 52-60. doi:10.1016/j.maturitas.2011.12.014

Purcell, N. H., Tang, G., Yu, C., Mercurio, F., DiDonato, J. A., & Lin, A. (2001). Activation of NF-kappa B is required for hypertrophic growth of primary rat neonatal ventricular cardiomyocytes. *Proceedings of the National Academy of Sciences of the United States of America*, *98*(12), 6668–6673. doi:10.1073/pnas.111155798 PMID:11381115

Putney, J. W. (2011). The physiological function of store-operated calcium entry. *Neurochemical Research*, *36*(7), 1157–1165. doi:10.1007/s11064-010-0383-0 PMID:21234676

Putney, J. W. Jr. (1986). A model for receptor-regulated calcium entry. *Cell Calcium*, *7*(1), 1–12. doi:10.1016/0143-4160(86)90026-6 PMID:2420465

Putney, J. W. Jr. (1990). Capacitative calcium entry revisited. *Cell Calcium*, *11*(10), 611–624. doi:10.1016/0143-4160(90)90016-N PMID:1965707

Qidwai, W., & Ashfaq, T. (2013). Role of garlic usage in cardiovascular disease prevention: An evidence-based approach. *Evidence-Based Complementary and Alternative Medicine*. PMID:23690831

Qin, D., Huang, B., Deng, L., El-Adawi, H., Ganguly, K., Sowers, J. R., & El-Sherif, N. (2001). Downregulation of K(+) channel genes expression in type I diabetic cardiomyopathy. *Biochemical and Biophysical Research Communications*, *283*(3), 549–553. doi:10.1006/bbrc.2001.4825 PMID:11341759

Quarles, E. K., Dai, D. F., Tocchi, A., Basisty, N., Gitari, L., & Rabinovitch, P. S. (2015). Quality control systems in cardiac aging. *Ageing Res Rev*, *23*(Pt A), 101-115. doi:10.1016/j.arr.2015.02.003

Quiat, D., & Olson, E. N. (2013). MicroRNAs in cardiovascular disease: From pathogenesis to prevention and treatment. *The Journal of Clinical Investigation*, *123*(1), 11–18. doi:10.1172/JCI62876 PMID:23281405

Radicke, S., Cotella, D., Graf, E. M., Banse, U., Jost, N., Varro, A., & Wettwer, E. et al. (2006). Functional modulation of the transient outward current Ito by KCNE beta-subunits and regional distribution in human non-failing and failing hearts. *Cardiovascular Research*, *71*(4), 695–703. doi:10.1016/j.cardiores.2006.06.017 PMID:16876774

Raj, P., Zieroth, S., & Netticadan, T. (2015). An overview of the efficacy of resveratrol in the management of ischemic heart disease. *Annals of the New York Academy of Sciences*, *1348*(1), 55–67. doi:10.1111/nyas.12828 PMID:26227659

Rajput, C., Kini, V., Smith, M., Yazbeck, P., Chavez, A., Schmidt, T., & Mehta, D. et al. (2013). Neural Wiskott-Aldrich syndrome protein (N-WASP)-mediated p120-catenin interaction with Arp2-Actin complex stabilizes endothelial adherens junctions. *The Journal of Biological Chemistry*, *288*(6), 4241–4250. doi:10.1074/jbc.M112.440396 PMID:23212915

Rajput, C., Tauseef, M., Farazuddin, M., Yazbeck, P., Amin, M. R., Avin Br, V., & Mehta, D. et al. (2016). MicroRNA-150 Suppression of Angiopoetin-2 Generation and Signaling Is Crucial for Resolving Vascular Injury. *Arteriosclerosis, Thrombosis, and Vascular Biology*, *36*(2), 380–388. doi:10.1161/ATVBAHA.115.306997 PMID:26743170

Ramasamy, R., Trueblood, N., & Schaefer, S. (1998). Metabolic effects of aldose reductase inhibition during low-flow ischemia and reperfusion. *American Journal of Physiology. Heart and Circulatory Physiology*, *275*(1), H195–H203. PMID:9688914

Rammelkamp, C. H., & Maxon, T. (1942). Resistance of Staphylococcus aureus to the action of penicillin. *Proc Royal Soc Exper Biol Med*, *51*(3), 386–389. doi:10.3181/00379727-51-13986

Ramsey, L. B., Johnson, S. G., Caudle, K. E., Haidar, C. E., Voora, D., Wilke, R. A., & Niemi, M. et al. (2014). The clinical pharmacogenetics implementation consortium guideline for SLCO1B1 and simvastatin-induced myopathy: 2014 update. *Clinical Pharmacology and Therapeutics*, *96*(4), 423–428. doi:10.1038/clpt.2014.125 PMID:24918167

Rao, S. V., Califf, R. M., Kramer, J. M., Peterson, E. D., Gross, T. P., Pepine, C. J., . . . Kulick, D. (2010). *Coronary Balloon Angioplasty and Stents (Percutaneous Coronary Inverention, PCI)*. Retrieved from http://www.medicinenet.com/coronary_angioplasty/article.htm

Rao, A. K. (2013). Inherited platelet function disorders: Overview and disorders of granules, secretion, and signal transduction. *Hematology/Oncology Clinics of North America*, *27*(3), 585–611. doi:10.1016/j.hoc.2013.02.005 PMID:23714313

Rao, S., Tan, A., Thomas, N., & Prestidge, C. A. (2014). Review: Perspective and potential of oral lipid-based delivery to optimize pharmacological therapies against cardiovascular diseases. *Journal of Controlled Release*, *193*, 174–187. doi:10.1016/j.jconrel.2014.05.013

Rassaf, T., Totzeck, M., Hendgen-Cotta, U. B., Shiva, S., Heusch, G., & Kelm, M. (2014). Circulating Nitrite Contributes to Cardioprotection by Remote Ischemic Preconditioning. *Circulation Research*, *114*(10), 1601–1610. doi:10.1161/CIRCRESAHA.114.303822 PMID:24643960

Rea, M. E., & Dunlap, M. E. (2008). Renal hemodynamics in heart failure: Implications for treatment. *Current Opinion in Nephrology and Hypertension*, *17*(1), 87–92. doi:10.1097/MNH.0b013e3282f357da PMID:18090676

Regan, E. R., & Aird, W. C. (2012). Dynamical systems approach to endothelial heterogeneity. *Circulation Research*, *111*(1), 110–130. doi:10.1161/CIRCRESAHA.111.261701 PMID:22723222

Regar, E., Ligthart, J., Bruining, N., & van Soest, G. (2011). The diagnostic value of intracoronary optical coherence tomography. *Herz*, *36*(5), 417–429. doi:10.1007/s00059-011-3487-7 PMID:21744151

Regulations. (2015). *Electronic Code of Federal Regulations. Title 21. Part 182 -- Substances Generally Recognized As Safe*. Retrieved from http://www.accessdata.fda.gov/scripts/cdrh/cfdocs/cfcfr/CFRSearch.cfm?CFRPart=182

Relling, M. V., & Klein, T. E. (2011). CPIC: Clinical Pharmacogenetics Implementation Consortium of the Pharmacogenomics Research Network. *Clinical Pharmacology and Therapeutics*, *89*(3), 464–467. doi:10.1038/clpt.2010.279 PMID:21270786

Rendu, F., & Brohard-Bohn, B. (2001). The platelet release reaction: Granules constituents, secretion and functions. *Platelets*, *12*(5), 261–273. doi:10.1080/09537100120068170 PMID:11487378

Ren, Q., Ye, S., & Whiteheart, S. W. (2008). The platelet release reaction: Just when you thought platelet secretion was simple. *Current Opinion in Hematology*, *15*(5), 537–541. doi:10.1097/MOH.0b013e328309ec74 PMID:18695380

Rincon, F., Kang, J., Maltenfort, M., Vibbert, M., Urtecho, J., Athar, M. K., & Bell, R. et al. (2014). Association between hyperoxia and mortality after stroke: A multicenter cohort study. *Critical Care Medicine*, *42*(2), 387–396. doi:10.1097/CCM.0b013e3182a27732 PMID:24164953

Rincon, F., Kang, J., Vibbert, M., Urtecho, J., Athar, M. K., & Jallo, J. (2014). Significance of arterial hyperoxia and relationship with case fatality in traumatic brain injury: A multicentre cohort study. *Journal of Neurology, Neurosurgery, and Psychiatry*, *85*(7), 799–805. doi:10.1136/jnnp-2013-305505 PMID:23794718

Riviere, C., Richard, T., Quentin, L., Krisa, S., Merillon, J. M., & Monti, J. P. (2007). Inhibitory activity of stilbenes on Alzheimer's beta-amyloid fibrils in vitro. *Bioorg Med Chem, 15*(2), 1160-1167. doi:S0968-0896(06)00817-0 [pii] 10.1016/j.bmc.2006.09.069

Rizvi, S. I., & Pandey, K. B. (2010). Activation of the erythrocyte plasma membrane redox system by resveratrol: A possible mechanism for antioxidant properties. *Pharmacological Reports*, *62*(4), 726–732. doi:10.1016/S1734-1140(10)70330-3 PMID:20885013

Robaszkiewicz, A., Balcerczyk, A., & Bartosz, G. (2007). Antioxidative and prooxidative effects of quercetin on A549 cells. *Cell Biology International*, *31*(10), 1245–1250. doi:10.1016/j.cellbi.2007.04.009 PMID:17583542

Roberts, I. S. D., Benamore, R. E., Peebles, C., Roobottom, C., & Traill, Z. C. (2011). Diagnosis of coronary artery disease using minimally invasive autopsy: Evaluation of a novel method of post-mortem coronary CT angiography. *Clinical Radiology*, *66*(7), 645–650. doi:10.1016/j.crad.2011.01.007 PMID:21377145

Robertson, D., & Biaggioni, I. (2015). Adrenoceptor Antagonist Drugs. In B. Katzung & A. Trevor (Eds.), Basic & Clinical Pharmacology. New York, NY: McGraw-Hill.

Roberts, R., & Stewart, A. F. (2012). 9p21 and the genetic revolution for coronary artery disease. *Clinical Chemistry*, *58*(1), 104–112. doi:10.1373/clinchem.2011.172759 PMID:22015375

Rodriguez-Gonzalez, R., Martin-Barrasa, J. L., Ramos-Nuez, A., Canas-Pedrosa, A. M., Martinez-Saavedra, M. T., Garcia-Bello, M. A., & Villar, J. et al. (2014). Multiple system organ response induced by hyperoxia in a clinically relevant animal model of sepsis. *Shock (Augusta, Ga.)*, *42*(2), 148–153. doi:10.1097/SHK.0000000000000189 PMID:24978892

Roever, L., Casella-Filho, A., Dourado, P. M., Resende, E. S., & Chagas, A. C. (2014). Cardiac tumors: A brief commentary. *Front Public Health*, *2*, 264. doi:10.3389/fpubh.2014.00264 PMID:25538934

Roger, V. L., Weston, S. A., Redfield, M. M., Hellermann-Homan, J. P., Killian, J., Yawn, B. P., & Jacobsen, S. J. (2004). Trends in heart failure incidence and survival in a community-based population. *Journal of the American Medical Association*, *292*(3), 344–350. doi:10.1001/jama.292.3.344 PMID:15265849

Roleder, T., Jąkała, J., Kałuża, G., Partyka, Ł., Proniewska, K., Pociask, E., . . . Dudek, D. (2015). The basics of intravascular optical coherence tomography. *PWKI, 2*, 74-83. doi:10.5114/pwki.2015.52278

Rome, B. N., Kramer, D. B., & Kesselheim, A. S. (2014). FDA Approval of Cardiac Implantable Electronic Devices via Original and Supplement Premarket Approval Pathways, 19792012. *Journal of the American Medical Association, 311*(4), 385. doi:10.1001/jama.2013.284986 PMID:24449317

Roos, J., DiGregorio, P. J., Yeromin, A. V., Ohlsen, K., Lioudyno, M., Zhang, S., & Stauderman, K. A. et al. (2005). STIM1, an essential and conserved component of store-operated Ca2+ channel function. *The Journal of Cell Biology, 169*(3), 435–445. doi:10.1083/jcb.200502019 PMID:15866891

Rosati, B., Grau, F., & McKinnon, D. (2006). Regional variation in rnRNA transcript abundance within the ventricular wall. *Journal of Molecular and Cellular Cardiology, 40*(2), 295–302. doi:10.1016/j.yjmcc.2005.11.002 PMID:16412459

Rosenberg, E. M., & Cook, L. N. (1991). Electromechanical dissociation in newborns treated with extracorporeal membrane oxygenation: An extreme form of cardiac stun syndrome. *Critical Care Medicine, 19*(6), 780–784. doi:10.1097/00003246-199106000-00009 PMID:2055055

Rosenberg, M., Zugck, C., Nelles, M., Juenger, C., Frank, D., Remppis, A., & Frey, N. et al. (2008). Osteopontin, a new prognostic biomarker in patients with chronic heart failure. *Circulation: Heart Failure, 1*(1), 43–49. doi:10.1161/CIRCHEARTFAILURE.107.746172 PMID:19808269

Rossi, J. L., Velentza, A. V., Steinhorn, D. M., Watterson, D. M., & Wainwright, M. S. (2007). MLCK210 gene knockout or kinase inhibition preserves lung function following endotoxin-induced lung injury in mice. *American Journal of Physiology. Lung Cellular and Molecular Physiology, 292*(6), L1327–L1334. doi:10.1152/ajplung.00380.2006 PMID:17307813

Ross, S. D., & Kron, I. L. (2000, September). Attenuation of lung reperfusion injury after transplantation using an inhibitor of nuclear factor-kappaB. *American Journal of Physiology. Lung Cellular and Molecular Physiology, 279*(3), L528–L536. PMID:10956628

Ross, S. G., Bolliger, S. A., Ampanozi, G., Oesterhelweg, L., Thali, M. J., & Flach, P. M. (2014). Postmortem CT angiography: Capabilities and limitations in traumatic and natural causes of death. *Radiographics, 34*(3), 830–846. doi:10.1148/rg.343115169 PMID:24819799

Ross, S. G., Thali, M. J., Bolliger, S., Germerott, T., Ruder, T. D., & Flach, P. M. (2012). Sudden death after chest pain: Feasibility of virtual autopsy with postmortem CT angiography and biopsy. *Radiology, 264*(1), 250–259. doi:10.1148/radiol.12092415 PMID:22570504

Rostami, A., Khalili, M., Haghighat, N., Eghtesadi, S., Shidfar, F., & Heidari, I. (2015). High-cocoa polyphenol-rich chocolate improves blood pressure in patients with diabetes and hypertension. *ARYA Atheroscler, 11*(1), 21–29. PMID:26089927

Rousseau, A., Bak, Z., Janerot-Sjoberg, B., & Sjoberg, F. (2005). Acute hyperoxaemia-induced effects on regional blood flow, oxygen consumption and central circulation in man. *Acta Physiologica Scandinavica, 183*(3), 231–240. doi:10.1111/j.1365-201X.2005.01405.x PMID:15743383

Rowe, G. C., & Arany, Z. (2014). Genetic models of PGC-1 and glucose metabolism and homeostasis. *Reviews in Endocrine & Metabolic Disorders, 15*(1), 21–29. doi:10.1007/s11154-013-9273-5 PMID:24057597

Rubak, P., Nissen, P. H., Kristensen, S. D., & Hvas, A. M. (2015). Investigation of platelet function and platelet disorders using flow cytometry. *Platelets*, 1–9. PMID:25901600

Rubenfeld, G. D., Caldwell, E., Peabody, E., Weaver, J., Martin, D. P., Neff, M., & Hudson, L. D. et al. (2005). Incidence and outcomes of acute lung injury. *The New England Journal of Medicine*, *353*(16), 1685–1693. doi:10.1056/NEJMoa050333 PMID:16236739

Ruhle, B., & Trebak, M. (2013). Emerging roles for native Orai Ca2+ channels in cardiovascular disease. *Curr Top Membr*, *71*, 209–235. doi:10.1016/B978-0-12-407870-3.00009-3 PMID:23890117

Rundek, T., Naini, A., Sacco, R., Coates, K., & DiMauro, S. (2004). Atorvastatin decreases the coenzyme Q10 level in the blood of patients at risk for cardiovascular disease and stroke. *Archives of Neurology*, *61*(6), 889–892. doi:10.1001/archneur.61.6.889 PMID:15210526

Rutledge, T., Reis, S. E., Olson, M., Owens, J., Kelsey, S. E., Pepine, C. J., & Rogers, W. J. et al. (2003). Socioeconomic Status Variables Predict Cardiovascular Disease Risk Factors and Prospective Mortality Risk among Women with Chest Pain: The WISE Study. *Behavior Modification*, *27*(1), 54–67. doi:10.1177/0145445502238693 PMID:12587260

Rybak, M. J., Lomaestro, B. M., Rotschafer, J. C., Moellering, R. C. Jr, Craig, W. A., Billeter, M., & Levine, D. P. et al. (2009). Therapeutic monitoring of vancomycin in adults summary of consensus recommendations from the American Society of Health-System Pharmacists, the Infectious Diseases Society of America, and the Society of Infectious Diseases Pharmacists. *Pharmacotherapy*, *29*(11), 1275–1279. doi:10.1592/phco.29.11.1275 PMID:19873687

Sabe, A. A., Elmadhun, N. Y., Dalal, R. S., Robich, M. P., & Sellke, F. W. (2014). Resveratrol regulates autophagy signaling in chronically ischemic myocardium. *The Journal of Thoracic and Cardiovascular Surgery*, *147*(2), 792–798, Discussion 798–799. doi:10.1016/j.jtcvs.2013.06.062 PMID:24267781

Sabe, A. A., Sadek, A. A., Elmadhun, N. Y., Dalal, R. S., Robich, M. P., Bianchi, C., & Sellke, F. W. (2015). Investigating the effects of resveratrol on chronically ischemic myocardium in a Swine model of metabolic syndrome: A proteomics analysis. *Journal of Medicinal Food*, *18*(1), 60–66. doi:10.1089/jmf.2014.0036 PMID:25089828

Sackner-Bernstein, J. D., Kowalski, M., Fox, M., & Aaronson, K. D. (2005). Short-term risk of death after treatment with nesiritide for decompensated heart failure: a pooled anyalysis of randomized controlled trials. *JAMA, 293,*(15) 1900-1905.

Sackner-Bernstein, J. D., Skopicki, H. A., & Aaronson, K. D. (2005). Risk of worsening renal function with nesiritide in patients with acutely decompensated heart failure. *Circulation*, *111*(12), 1487–1491. doi:10.1161/01.CIR.0000159340.93220.E4 PMID:15781736

Sagar, S., Liu, P. P., & Cooper, L. T. Jr. (2012). Myocarditis. *Lancet*, *379*(9817), 738–747. doi:10.1016/S0140-6736(11)60648-X PMID:22185868

Sakoulas, G., Bayer, A. S., Pogliano, J., Tsuji, B. T., Yang, S. J., Mishra, N. N., & Moise, P. A. et al. (2012). Ampicillin enhances daptomycin- and cationic host defense peptide-mediated killing of ampicillin- and vancomycin-resistant Enterococcus faecium. *Antimicrobial Agents and Chemotherapy*, *56*(2), 838–844. doi:10.1128/AAC.05551-11 PMID:22123698

Sakoulas, G., Moise, P. A., Casapao, A. M., Nonejuie, P., Olson, J., Okumura, C. Y., & Nizet, V. et al. (2014). Antimicrobial salvage therapy for persistent staphylococcal bacteremia using daptomycin plus ceftaroline. *Clinical Therapeutics*, *36*(10), 1317–1333. doi:10.1016/j.clinthera.2014.05.061 PMID:25017183

Sakoulas, G., Nonejuie, P., Nizet, V., Pogliano, J., Crum-Cianflone, N., & Haddad, F. (2013). Treatment of high-level gentamicin-resistant Enterococcus faecalis endocarditis with daptomycin plus ceftaroline. *Antimicrobial Agents and Chemotherapy*, *57*(8), 4042–4045. doi:10.1128/AAC.02481-12 PMID:23689728

Sakoulas, G., Rose, W., Nonejuie, P., Olson, J., Pogliano, J., Humphries, R., & Nizet, V. (2014). Ceftaroline restores daptomycin activity against daptomycin-nonsusceptible vancomycin-resistant Enterococcus faecium. *Antimicrobial Agents and Chemotherapy*, *58*(3), 1494–1500. doi:10.1128/AAC.02274-13 PMID:24366742

Salazar, M. R., Carbajal, H. A., Espeche, W. G., Aizpurua, M., Leiva Sisnieguez, C. E., March, C. E., & Reaven, G. M. et al. (2013). Identifying cardiovascular disease risk and outcome: Use of the plasma triglyceride/high-density lipoprotein cholesterol concentration ratio versus metabolic syndrome criteria. *Journal of Internal Medicine*, *273*(6), 595–601. doi:10.1111/joim.12036 PMID:23331522

Salem, J. E., Saidel, G. M., Stanley, W. C., & Cabrera, M. E. (2002). Mechanistic model of myocardial energy metabolism under normal and ischemic conditions. *Annals of Biomedical Engineering*, *30*(2), 202–216. doi:10.1114/1.1454133 PMID:11962772

Saliba, Y., Keck, M., Marchand, A., Atassi, F., Ouille, A., Cazorla, O., & Lompre, A.-M. et al. (2015). Emergence of Orai3 activity during cardiac hypertrophy. *Cardiovascular Research*, *105*(3), 248–259. doi:10.1093/cvr/cvu207 PMID:25213556

Samani, N. J., Erdmann, J., Hall, A. S., Hengstenberg, C., Mangino, M., Mayer, B., & Schunkert, H. et al. (2007). Genomewide association analysis of coronary artery disease. *The New England Journal of Medicine*, *357*(5), 443–453. doi:10.1056/NEJMoa072366 PMID:17634449

Samapati, R., Yang, Y., Yin, J., Stoerger, C., Arenz, C., Dietrich, A., & Kuebler, W. M. et al. (2012). Lung endothelial Ca2+ and permeability response to platelet-activating factor is mediated by acid sphingomyelinase and transient receptor potential classical 6. *American Journal of Respiratory and Critical Care Medicine*, *185*(2), 160–170. doi:10.1164/rccm.201104-0717OC PMID:22246702

Sammani, S., Moreno-Vinasco, L., Mirzapoiazova, T., Singleton, P. A., Chiang, E. T., Evenoski, C. L., & Garcia, J. G. et al. (2010). Differential effects of sphingosine 1-phosphate receptors on airway and vascular barrier function in the murine lung. *American Journal of Respiratory Cell and Molecular Biology*, *43*(4), 394–402. doi:10.1165/rcmb.2009-0223OC PMID:19749179

Sanders, T. A. B., Vickers, M., & Haines, A. P. (1981). Effect on blood lipids and haemostasis of a supplement of cod-liver oil, rich in eicosapentaenoic and docosahexaenoic acids, in healthy young men. *Clinical Science*, *61*(3), 317–324. doi:10.1042/cs0610317 PMID:6266735

Sandrock, K., Nakamura, L., Vraetz, T., Beutel, K., Ehl, S., & Zieger, B. (2010). Platelet secretion defect in patients with familial hemophagocytic lymphohistiocytosis type 5 (FHL-5). *Blood*, *116*(26), 6148–6150. doi:10.1182/blood-2010-08-302943 PMID:21183701

Sandrock-Lang, K., Oldenburg, J., Wiegering, V., Halimeh, S., Santoso, S., Kurnik, K., & Zieger, B. et al. (2015a). Characterisation of patients with Glanzmann thrombasthenia and identification of 17 novel mutations. *Thrombosis and Haemostasis*, *113*(4), 782–791. doi:10.1160/TH14-05-0479 PMID:25373348

Sandrock-Lang, K., Wentzell, R., Santoso, S., & Zieger, B. (2015b). Inherited platelet disorders. *Hamostaseologie*, 35. PMID:25707719

Santel, A., & Fuller, M. T. (2001). Control of mitochondrial morphology by a human mitofusin. *Journal of Cell Science*, *114*(Pt 5), 867–874. PMID:11181170

Sato, K., Dohi, Y., Kojima, M., Miyagawa, K., Takase, H., & Katada, E. (2006). Effects of ascorbic acid on ambulatory blood pressure in elderly patients with refractory hypertension. *Arzneimittel-Forschung*, *56*(7), 535–540. doi:10.1055/s-0031-1296748 PMID:16927536

Savoia, A., Kunishima, S., De Rocco, D., Zieger, B., Rand, M. L., Pujol-Moix, N., & Lanza, F. et al. (2014). Spectrum of the mutations in Bernard-Soulier syndrome. *Human Mutation*, *35*(9), 1033–1045. doi:10.1002/humu.22607 PMID:24934643

Sawyer, D. B., Siwik, D. A., Xiao, L., Pimentel, D. R., Singh, K., & Colucci, W. S. (2002). Role of oxidative stress in myocardial hypertrophy and failure. *Journal of Molecular and Cellular Cardiology*, *34*(4), 379–388. doi:10.1006/jmcc.2002.1526 PMID:11991728

Schaar, J., Mastik, F., Regar, E., den Uil, C., Gijsen, F., Wentzel, J., . . . van der Stehen, A. (2007). Current Diagnostic Modalities for Vulnerable Plaque Detection. *CPD, 13*(10), 995-1001. doi:10.2174/138161207780487511

Scheuermann-Freestone, M., Madsen, P. L., Manners, D., Blamire, A. M., Buckingham, R. E., Styles, P., & Clarke, K. et al. (2003). Abnormal cardiac and skeletal muscle energy metabolism in patients with type 2 diabetes. *Circulation*, *107*(24), 3040–3046. doi:10.1161/01.CIR.0000072789.89096.10 PMID:12810608

Schiattarella, G. G., & Hill, J. A. (2015). Therapeutic targeting of autophagy in cardiovascular disease. *Journal of Molecular and Cellular Cardiology*. doi:10.1016/j.yjmcc.2015.11.019 PMID:26602750

Schiener, M., Hossann, M., Viola, J. R., Ortega-Gomez, A., Weber, C., Lauber, K., & Soehnlein, O. et al. (2014). Review: Nanomedicine-based strategies for treatment of atherosclerosis. *Trends in Molecular Medicine*, 20271–20281. doi:10.1016/j.molmed.2013.12.001 PMID:24594264

Schlegel, N., Burger, S., Golenhofen, N., Walter, U., Drenckhahn, D., & Waschke, J. (2008). The role of VASP in regulation of cAMP- and Rac 1-mediated endothelial barrier stabilization. *American Journal of Physiology. Cell Physiology*, *294*(1), C178–C188. doi:10.1152/ajpcell.00273.2007 PMID:17989211

Schmidt, T. T., Tauseef, M., Yue, L., Bonini, M. G., Gothert, J., Shen, T. L., & Mehta, D. et al. (2013). Conditional deletion of FAK in mice endothelium disrupts lung vascular barrier function due to destabilization of RhoA and Rac1 activities. *American Journal of Physiology. Lung Cellular and Molecular Physiology*, *305*(4), L291–L300. doi:10.1152/ajplung.00094.2013 PMID:23771883

Schmitz, G., & Orso, E. (2015). Lipoprotein(a) hyperlipidemia as cardiovascular risk factor: Pathophysiological aspects. *Clinical Research in Cardiology; Official Journal of the German Cardiac Society*, *10*(Suppl), 21–25. doi:10.1007/s11789-015-0074-0 PMID:25708587

Schork, N. J. (2015). Personalized medicine: Time for one-person trials. *Nature*, *520*(7549), 609–611. doi:10.1038/520609a PMID:25925459

Schwartz, M. D., Moore, E. E., Moore, F. A., Shenkar, R., Moine, P., Haenel, J. B., & Abraham, E. (2013). Nuclear factor-κB is activated in alveolar macrophages from patients with acute respiratory distress syndrome. *Critical Care Medicine*. PMID:8706481

Schweizer, M. L., Furuno, J. P., Harris, A. D., Johnson, J. K., Shardell, M. D., McGregor, J. C., & Perencevich, E. N. et al. (2011). Comparative effectiveness of nafcillin or cefazolin versus vancomycin in methicillin-susceptible Staphylococcus aureus bacteremia. *BMC Infectious Diseases*, *11*(1), 279. doi:10.1186/1471-2334-11-279 PMID:22011388

Scott, S. A., Sangkuhl, K., Stein, C. M., Hulot, J. S., Mega, J. L., Roden, D. M., & Shuldiner, A. R. et al. (2013). Clinical Pharmacogenetics Implementation Consortium guidelines for CYP2C19 genotype and clopidogrel therapy: 2013 update. *Clinical Pharmacology and Therapeutics*, *94*(3), 317–323. doi:10.1038/clpt.2013.105 PMID:23698643

Seals, D. R., Johnson, D. G., & Fregosi, R. F. (1991). Hyperoxia lowers sympathetic activity at rest but not during exercise in humans. *American Journal of Physiology. Regulatory, Integrative and Comparative Physiology*, *260*(5), R873–R878. PMID:2035699

Sebastian, C., Satterstrom, F. K., Haigis, M. C., & Mostoslavsky, R. (2012). From sirtuin biology to human diseases: An update. *The Journal of Biological Chemistry*, *287*(51), 42444–42452. doi:10.1074/jbc.R112.402768 PMID:23086954

Sehrt, D., Meineke, I., Tzvetkov, M., Gultepe, S., & Brockmoller, J. (2011). Carvedilol pharmacokinetics and pharmacodynamics in relation to CYP2D6 and ADRB pharmacogenetics. *Pharmacogenomics*, *12*(6), 783–795. doi:10.2217/pgs.11.20 PMID:21599570

Seiler, K. S., & Starnes, J. W. (2000). Exogenous GSH protection during hypoxia-reoxygenation of the isolated rat heart: Impact of hypoxia duration. *Free Radical Research*, *32*(1), 41–55. doi:10.1080/10715760000300051 PMID:10625216

Seligsohn, U. (2012). Treatment of inherited platelet disorders. *Haemophilia: The Official Journal of the World Federation of Hemophilia, 18*(S4), 161-5.

Selton-Suty, C., Célard, M., Le Moing, V., Doco-Lecompte, T., Chirouze, C., Iung, B., & Hoen, B. et al. (2012). Preeminence of Staphylococcus aureus in infective endocarditis: A 1-year population-based survey. *Clinical Infectious Diseases*, *54*(9), 1230–1239. doi:10.1093/cid/cis199 PMID:22492317

Semsarian, C., Ingles, J., & Wilde, A. A. (2015). Sudden cardiac death in the young: The molecular autopsy and a practical approach to surviving relatives. *European Heart Journal*. PMID:25765769

Sena, L. A., & Chandel, N. S. (2012). Physiological roles of mitochondrial reactive oxygen species. *Molecular Cell*, *48*(2), 158–167. doi:10.1016/j.molcel.2012.09.025 PMID:23102266

Shalwala, M., Zhu, S. G., Das, A., Salloum, F. N., Xi, L., & Kukreja, R. C. (2014). Sirtuin 1 (SIRT1) activation mediates sildenafil induced delayed cardioprotection against ischemia-reperfusion injury in mice. *PLoS ONE*, *9*(1), e86977. doi:10.1371/journal.pone.0086977 PMID:24466304

Shan, D., Marchase, R. B., & Chatham, J. C. (2008). Overexpression of TRPC3 increases apoptosis but not necrosis in response to ischemia-reperfusion in adult mouse cardiomyocytes. *American Journal of Physiology. Cell Physiology*, *294*(3), C833–C841. doi:10.1152/ajpcell.00313.2007 PMID:18184877

Shapiro, A.D. (2000). Platelet function disorders. *Haemophilia: The Official Journal of the World Federation of Hemophilia, 6*(S1), 120-7.

Sharma & Kwon. (2007). New applications of nanoparticles in cardiovascular imaging. *Journal of Experimental Nanoscience, 2*(1-2), 115-126. DOI: 10.1080/17458080601101176

Sharp, C. F., Gardiner, S. J., Jensen, B. P., Roberts, R. L., Troughton, R. W., Lainchbury, J. G., & Begg, E. J. (2009). CYP2D6 genotype and its relationship with metoprolol dose, concentrations and effect in patients with systolic heart failure. *The Pharmacogenomics Journal*, *9*(3), 175–184. doi:10.1038/tpj.2009.9 PMID:19365402

Shaw, P. J., & Feske, S. (2012). Physiological and pathophysiological functions of SOCE in the immune system. *Frontiers in Bioscience (Elite Edition)*, *4*(6), 2253–2268. doi:10.2741/e540 PMID:22202035

Shen, W. W., Frieden, M., & Demaurex, N. (2011). Local cytosolic Ca2+ elevations are required for stromal interaction molecule 1 (STIM1) de-oligomerization and termination of store-operated Ca2+ entry. *The Journal of Biological Chemistry*, *286*(42), 36448–36459. doi:10.1074/jbc.M111.269415 PMID:21880734

Shim, A. H., Tirado-Lee, L., & Prakriya, M. (2015). Structural and functional mechanisms of CRAC channel regulation. *Journal of Molecular Biology*, *427*(1), 77–93. doi:10.1016/j.jmb.2014.09.021 PMID:25284754

Shimizu, M., Saxena, P., Konstantinov, I. E., Cherepanov, V., Cheung, M. M., Wearden, P., & Redington, A. N. et al. (2010). Remote ischemic preconditioning decreases adhesion and selectively modifies functional responses of human neutrophils. *The Journal of Surgical Research*, *158*(1), 155–161. doi:10.1016/j.jss.2008.08.010 PMID:19540519

Shinde, A. V., Motiani, R. K., Zhang, X., Abdullaev, I. F., Adam, A. P., Gonzalez-Cobos, J. C., & Trebak, M. et al. (2013). STIM1 controls endothelial barrier function independently of Orai1 and Ca2+ entry. *Science Signaling*, *6*(267), ra18. doi:10.1126/scisignal.2003425 PMID:23512989

Shinmura, K., Tamaki, K., Ito, K., Yan, X., Yamamoto, T., Katsumata, Y., & Ishii, I. et al. (2015). Indispensable role of endothelial nitric oxide synthase in caloric restriction-induced cardioprotection against ischemia-reperfusion injury. *American Journal of Physiology. Heart and Circulatory Physiology*, *308*(8), H894–H903. doi:10.1152/ajpheart.00333.2014 PMID:25681423

Shinmura, K., Tamaki, K., Saito, K., Nakano, Y., Tobe, T., & Bolli, R. (2007). Cardioprotective effects of short-term caloric restriction are mediated by adiponectin via activation of AMP-activated protein kinase. *Circulation*, *116*(24), 2809–2817. doi:10.1161/CIRCULATIONAHA.107.725697 PMID:18040027

Shi, S., Verin, A. D., Schaphorst, K. L., Gilbert-McClain, L. I., Patterson, C. E., Irwin, R. P., & Garcia, J. G. et al. (1998). Role of tyrosine phosphorylation in thrombin-induced endothelial cell contraction and barrier function. *Endothelium*, *6*(2), 153–171. doi:10.3109/10623329809072202 PMID:9930649

Shoji, N., Iwasa, A., Takemoto, T., Ishida, Y., & Ohizumi, Y. (1982). Cardiotonic principles of ginger (Zingiber officinale Roscoe). *Journal of Pharmaceutical Sciences*, *71*(10), 1174–1175. doi:10.1002/jps.2600711025 PMID:7143220

Simons, L. A., Balasubramaniam, S., Vonkonigsmark, M., Parfitt, A., Simons, J., & Peters, W. (1995). On the effect of garlic on plasma-lipids and lipoproteins in mild hypercholesterolemia. *Atherosclerosis*, *113*(2), 219–225. doi:10.1016/0021-9150(94)05449-S PMID:7605361

Simons, S., Wollersheim, H., & Thien, T. (2009). A systematic review on the influence of trial quality on the effect of garlic on blood pressure. *The Netherlands Journal of Medicine*, *67*(6), 212–219. PMID:19749390

Singhal, A. K., Symons, J. D., Boudina, S., Jaishy, B., & Shiu, Y.-T. (2010). Role of Endothelial Cells in Myocardial Ischemia-Reperfusion Injury. *Vascular Disease Prevention*, *7*(1), 1–14. doi:10.2174/1874120701007010001 PMID:25558187

Singh, I., Knezevic, N., Ahmmed, G. U., Kini, V., Malik, A. B., & Mehta, D. (2007). Galphaq-TRPC6-mediated Ca2+ entry induces RhoA activation and resultant endothelial cell shape change in response to thrombin. *The Journal of Biological Chemistry*, *282*(11), 7833–7843. doi:10.1074/jbc.M608288200 PMID:17197445

Singh, M., Dalal, S., & Singh, K. (2014). Osteopontin: At the cross-roads of myocyte survival and myocardial function. *Life Sciences*, *118*(1), 1–6. doi:10.1016/j.lfs.2014.09.014 PMID:25265596

Singh, M., Foster, C. R., Dalal, S., & Singh, K. (2010). Role of osteopontin in heart failure associated with aging. *Heart Failure Reviews*, *15*(5), 487–494. doi:10.1007/s10741-010-9158-6 PMID:20127409

Singh, R. B., Niaz, M. A., Rastogi, S. S., Shukla, P. K., & Thakur, A. S. (1999). Effect of hydrosoluble coenzyme Q10 on blood pressures and insulin resistance in hypertensive patients with coronary artery disease. *Journal of Human Hypertension*, *13*(3), 203–208. doi:10.1038/sj.jhh.1000778 PMID:10204818

Singleton, P. A., Dudek, S. M., Chiang, E. T., & Garcia, J. G. (2005). Regulation of sphingosine 1-phosphate-induced endothelial cytoskeletal rearrangement and barrier enhancement by S1P1 receptor, PI3 kinase, Tiam1/Rac1, and alpha-actinin. *The FASEB Journal*, *19*(12), 1646–1656. doi:10.1096/fj.05-3928com PMID:16195373

Sin, T. K., Yu, A. P., Yung, B. Y., Yip, S. P., Chan, L. W., Wong, C. S., & Siu, P. M. et al. (2014). Modulating effect of SIRT1 activation induced by resveratrol on Foxo1-associated apoptotic signalling in senescent heart. *The Journal of Physiology*, *592*(Pt 12), 2535–2548. doi:10.1113/jphysiol.2014.271387 PMID:24639483

Ski, C. F., King-Shier, K. M., & Thompson, D. R. (2014). Gender, socioeconomic and ethnic/racial dispairties in cardiovascular disease: A time for change. *International Journal of Cardiology*, *170*(3), 255–257. doi:10.1016/j.ijcard.2013.10.082 PMID:24238906

Small, E. M., & Olson, E. N. (2011). Pervasive roles of microRNAs in cardiovascular biology. *Nature*, *469*(7330), 336–342. doi:10.1038/nature09783 PMID:21248840

Smirnova, E., Griparic, L., Shurland, D. L., & van der Bliek, A. M. (2001). Dynamin-related protein Drp1 is required for mitochondrial division in mammalian cells. *Molecular Biology of the Cell*, *12*(8), 2245–2256. doi:10.1091/mbc.12.8.2245 PMID:11514614

Smirnova, E., Shurland, D. L., Ryazantsev, S. N., & van der Bliek, A. M. (1998). A human dynamin-related protein controls the distribution of mitochondria. *The Journal of Cell Biology*, *143*(2), 351–358. doi:10.1083/jcb.143.2.351 PMID:9786947

Smith, S. A., & Morrissey, J. H. (2015). 2013 Scientific Sessions Sol Sherry Distinguished Lecture in Thrombosis: Polyphosphate: A Novel Modulator of Hemostasis and Thrombosis. *Arteriosclerosis, Thrombosis, and Vascular Biology*.

Smith, H., Galmes, R., Gogolina, E., Straatman-Iwanowska, A., Reay, K., Banushi, B., & Gissen, P. et al. (2012). Associations among genotype, clinical phenotype, and intracellular localization of trafficking proteins in ARC syndrome. *Human Mutation*, *33*(12), 1656–1664. doi:10.1002/humu.22155 PMID:22753090

Smith, M. L., Vorce, S. P., Holler, J. M., Shimomura, E., Magluilo, J., Jacobs, A. J., & Huestis, M. A. (2007). Modern Instrumental Methods in Forensic Toxicology. *Journal of Analytical Toxicology*, *31*(5), 237–9A. doi:10.1093/jat/31.5.237 PMID:17579968

Smith, S. A., & Morrissey, J. H. (2014). Polyphosphate: A new player in the field of hemostasis. *Current Opinion in Hematology*, *21*(5), 388–394. doi:10.1097/MOH.0000000000000069 PMID:25010799

Smyth, J. T., Petranka, J. G., Boyles, R. R., DeHaven, W. I., Fukushima, M., Johnson, K. L., & Putney, J. W. Jr et al.. (2009). Phosphorylation of STIM1 underlies suppression of store-operated calcium entry during mitosis. *Nature Cell Biology*, *11*(12), 1465–1472. doi:10.1038/ncb1995 PMID:19881501

Society of Forensic Toxicologists/American Academy of Forensic Sciences. SOFT/AAFS forensic laboratory guidelines. (2006). Available at: http://www.soft-tox.org/files/Guidelines_2006_Final.pdf Accessed June 19, 2015.

Soejima, H., Ogawa, H., Sakamoto, T., Miyamoto, S., Kajiwara, I., Kojima, S., & Kishikawa, H. et al. (2003). Increased serum matrix metalloproteinase-1 concentration predicts advanced left ventricular remodeling in patients with acute myocardial infarction. *Circulation Journal*, *67*(4), 301–304. Retrieved from http://www.ncbi.nlm.nih.gov/pubmed/12655159 doi:10.1253/circj.67.301 PMID:12655159

Solaini, G., & Harris, D. A. (2005). Biochemical dysfunction in heart mitochondria exposed to ischaemia and reperfusion. *The Biochemical Journal*, *390*(Pt 2), 377–394. doi:10.1042/BJ20042006 PMID:16108756

Soloperto, G. (2012). Progress in atherosclerotic plaque imaging. *World Journal of Radiology*, *4*(8), 353. doi:10.4329/wjr.v4.i8.353 PMID:22937215

Song, M. Y., Makino, A., & Yuan, J. X. (2011). STIM2 Contributes to Enhanced Store-operated Ca Entry in Pulmonary Artery Smooth Muscle Cells from Patients with Idiopathic Pulmonary Arterial Hypertension. *Pulm Circ*, *1*(1), 84–94. doi:10.4103/2045-8932.78106 PMID:21709766

Song, Y., Laaksonen, H., Saukko, S., Toivonen, S., & Zhu, J. (2001). Histopathological findings of cardiac conduction system of 150 Finns. *Forensic Science International*, *119*(3), 310–317. doi:10.1016/S0379-0738(00)00457-6 PMID:11390145

Son, Y., Cheong, Y.-K., Kim, N.-H., Chung, H.-T., Kang, D. G., & Pae, H.-O. (2011). Mitogen-Activated Protein Kinases and Reactive Oxygen Species: How Can ROS Activate MAPK Pathways? *Journal of Signal Transduction, 792639*. doi:10.1155/2011/792639 PMID:21637379

Soppimath, K., Kulkarni, A., & Aminabhavi, T. (2001). Development of Hollow Microspheres as Floating Controlled-Release Systems for Cardiovascular Drugs: Preparation and Release Characteristics. *Drug Development and Industrial Pharmacy*, *27*(6), 507–515. doi:10.1081/DDC-100105175 PMID:11548857

Sorensen, K. E., Celermajer, D. S., Georgakopoulos, D., Hatcher, G., Betteridge, D. J., & Deanfield, J. E. (1994, January). Impairment of endothelium-dependent dilation is an early event in children with familial hypercholesterolemia and is related to the lipoprotein(a) level. *The Journal of Clinical Investigation*, *93*(1), 50–55. doi:10.1172/JCI116983 PMID:8282821

Spassova, M. A., Soboloff, J., He, L. P., Xu, W., Dziadek, M. A., & Gill, D. L. (2006). STIM1 has a plasma membrane role in the activation of store-operated Ca(2+) channels. *Proceedings of the National Academy of Sciences of the United States of America*, *103*(11), 4040–4045. doi:10.1073/pnas.0510050103 PMID:16537481

Spear, B. B., Heath-Chiozzi, M., & Huff, J. (2001). Clinical application of pharmacogenetics. *Trends in Molecular Medicine*, *7*(5), 201–204. doi:10.1016/S1471-4914(01)01986-4 PMID:11325631

Spear, J. F., Prabu, S. K., Galati, D., Raza, H., Anandatheerthavarada, H. K., & Avadhani, N. G. (2007). β1-Adrenoreceptor activation contributes to ischemia-reperfusion damage as well as playing a role in ischemic preconditioning. *American Journal of Physiology. Heart and Circulatory Physiology*, *292*(5), H2459–H2466. doi:10.1152/ajpheart.00459.2006 PMID:17237252

Spellberg, B., Bartlett, J. G., & Gilbert, D. N. (2013). The Future of Antibiotics and Resistance. *The New England Journal of Medicine*, *368*(4), 299–302. doi:10.1056/NEJMp1215093 PMID:23343059

Spellberg, B., Guidos, R., Gilbert, D., Bradley, J., Boucher, H. W., Scheld, W. M., & Edwards, J. Jr et al.. (2008). The epidemic of antibiotic resistant infections: A call to action for the medical community from the Infectious Diseases Society of America. *Clinical Infectious Diseases*, *46*(2), 155–164. doi:10.1086/524891 PMID:18171244

Spoelstra-de Man, A. M., Smit, B., Oudemans-van Straaten, H. M., & Smulders, Y. M. (2015). Cardiovascular effects of hyperoxia during and after cardiac surgery. *Anaesthesia*, *70*(11), 1307–1319. doi:10.1111/anae.13218 PMID:26348878

St. Jude's Confirm Implantable Cardiac Monitor Wins FDA Approval. (n.d.). Retrieved from http://www.medgadget.com/2008/09/saint_judes_confirm_implantable_cardiac_monitor_wins_fda_approval.html

Stabler, S. N., Tejani, A. M., Huynh, F., & Fowkes, C. (2012a). Garlic for the prevention of cardiovascular morbidity and mortality in hypertensive patients. *Cochrane Database of Systematic Reviews*, *8*, CD007653–CD007653. doi:10.1002/14651858.CD007653.pub2 PMID:22895963

Stamler, J., Caggiula, A. W., & Grandits, G. A. (1997). Relation of body mass and alcohol, nutrient, fiber, and caffeine intakes to blood pressure in the special intervention and usual care groups in the Multiple Risk Factor Intervention Trial. *The American Journal of Clinical Nutrition*, *65*(1Suppl), 338S–365S. PMID:8988947

Stampfer, M. J., Hu, F. B., Manson, J. E., Rimm, E. B., & Willett, W. C. (2000). Primary prevention of coronary heart disease in women through diet and lifestyle. *The New England Journal of Medicine*, *343*(24), 1814–1815. doi:10.1056/NEJM200012143432415 PMID:10882764

Stathopulos, P. B., Li, G. Y., Plevin, M. J., Ames, J. B., & Ikura, M. (2006). Stored Ca2+ depletion-induced oligomerization of stromal interaction molecule 1 (STIM1) via the EF-SAM region: An initiation mechanism for capacitive Ca2+ entry. *The Journal of Biological Chemistry*, *281*(47), 35855–35862. doi:10.1074/jbc.M608247200 PMID:17020874

Stathopulos, P. B., Zheng, L., & Ikura, M. (2009). Stromal interaction molecule (STIM) 1 and STIM2 calcium sensing regions exhibit distinct unfolding and oligomerization kinetics. *The Journal of Biological Chemistry*, *284*(2), 728–732. doi:10.1074/jbc.C800178200 PMID:19019825

Stein, S., & Matter, C. M. (2011). Protective roles of SIRT1 in atherosclerosis. *Cell Cycle (Georgetown, Tex.)*, *10*(4), 640–647. doi:10.4161/cc.10.4.14863 PMID:21293192

Stenmark, K. R., & Abman, S. H. (2005). Lung vascular development: Implications for the pathogenesis of bronchopulmonary dysplasia. *Annual Review of Physiology*, *67*(1), 623–661. doi:10.1146/annurev.physiol.67.040403.102229 PMID:15709973

Stevens, T. (2011). Functional and molecular heterogeneity of pulmonary endothelial cells. *Proceedings of the American Thoracic Society*, *8*(6), 453–457. doi:10.1513/pats.201101-004MW PMID:22052919

Stiber, J., Hawkins, A., Zhang, Z. S., Wang, S., Burch, J., Graham, V., & Rosenberg, P. et al. (2008). STIM1 signalling controls store-operated calcium entry required for development and contractile function in skeletal muscle. *Nature Cell Biology*, *10*(6), 688–697. doi:10.1038/ncb1731 PMID:18488020

Stone, N. J., Robinson, J. G., Lichtenstein, A. H., Bairey Merz, C. N., Blum, C. B., Eckel, R. H., & Wilson, P. et al. (2014). 2013 ACC/AHA guideline on the treatment of blood cholesterol to reduce atherosclerotic cardiovascular risk in adults: A report of the American College of Cardiology/American Heart Association Task Force on Practice Guidelines. *Journal of the American College of Cardiology*, *63*(2525 Pt B), 2889–2934. doi:10.1016/j.jacc.2013.11.002 PMID:24239923

Streicher, J. M., Ren, S., Herschman, H., & Wang, Y. (2010). MAPK-Activated Protein Kinase-2 in Cardiac Hypertrophy and Cyclooxygenase-2 Regulation in Heart. *Circulation Research*, *106*(8), 1434–1443. doi:10.1161/CIRCRESAHA.109.213199 PMID:20339119

Suarez-Mier, M. P., & Aguiler, B. (2014). Methodological Approach to Cardiac Autopsy. In Clinico-Pathological Atlas of Cardiovascular Diseases. Springer.

Suhaj, M. (2006). Spice antioxidants isolation and their antiradical activity: A review. *Journal of Food Composition and Analysis*, *19*(6), 531–537. doi:10.1016/j.jfca.2004.11.005

Suh, W. M., Seto, A. H., Margey, R. J. P., Cruz-Gonzalez, I., & Jang, I. K. (2011). Intravascular Detection of the Vulnerable Plaque. *Circulation: Cardiovascular Imaging*, *4*(2), 169–178. doi:10.1161/CIRCIMAGING.110.958777 PMID:21406663

Sukriti, S., Tauseef, M., Yazbeck, P., & Mehta, D. (2014). Mechanisms regulating endothelial permeability. *Pulm Circ*, *4*(4), 535–551. doi:10.1086/677356 PMID:25610592

Sundivakkam, P. C., Freichel, M., Singh, V., Yuan, J. P., Vogel, S. M., Flockerzi, V., & Tiruppathi, C. et al. (2012). The Ca(2+) sensor stromal interaction molecule 1 (STIM1) is necessary and sufficient for the store-operated Ca(2+) entry function of transient receptor potential canonical (TRPC) 1 and 4 channels in endothelial cells. *Molecular Pharmacology*, *81*(4), 510–526. doi:10.1124/mol.111.074658 PMID:22210847

Sundivakkam, P. C., Natarajan, V., Malik, A. B., & Tiruppathi, C. (2013). Store-operated Ca2+ entry (SOCE) induced by protease-activated receptor-1 mediates STIM1 protein phosphorylation to inhibit SOCE in endothelial cells through AMP-activated protein kinase and p38beta mitogen-activated protein kinase. *The Journal of Biological Chemistry*, *288*(23), 17030–17041. doi:10.1074/jbc.M112.411272 PMID:23625915

Sung, M. M., Das, S. K., Levasseur, J., Byrne, N. J., Fung, D., Kim, T. T., & Dyck, J. R. et al. (2015). Resveratrol treatment of mice with pressure-overload-induced heart failure improves diastolic function and cardiac energy metabolism. *Circulation: Heart Failure*, *8*(1), 128–137. doi:10.1161/CIRCHEARTFAILURE.114.001677 PMID:25394648

Sun, X., Shikata, Y., Wang, L., Ohmori, K., Watanabe, N., Wada, J., & Garcia, J. G. et al. (2009). Enhanced interaction between focal adhesion and adherens junction proteins: Involvement in sphingosine 1-phosphate-induced endothelial barrier enhancement. *Microvascular Research*, *77*(3), 304–313. doi:10.1016/j.mvr.2008.12.004 PMID:19323978

Sun, Z., Wu, W., Liu, J., Ma, N., Zheng, Z., Li, Q., & Miao, J. et al. (2014). Influence of glucose-lowering rate on CKMB and myoglobin serum levels in type-2 diabetes patients with coronary heart disease. *Human Immunology*, *75*(12), 1182–1187. doi:10.1016/j.humimm.2014.10.006 PMID:25454625

Sureddi, R., & Mehta, J. L. (2011). Nanomedicine in Cardiovascular Diseases: Emerging Diagnostic and Therapeutic Potential. *Journal Of Nanotechnology In Engineering And Medicine*, *2*(3), 031012. doi:10.1115/1.4005490

Suwa, M., Seino, Y., Nomachi, Y., Matsuki, S., & Funahashi, K. (2005). Multicenter prospective investigation of the efficacy and safety of carperitide for acute heart failure in the real world of therapy. *Circulation Journal*, *36*(3), 283–290. doi:10.1253/circj.69.283 PMID:15731532

Suzuki, J., Umeda, M., Sims, P. J., & Nagata, S. (2010). Calcium-dependent phospholipid scrambling by TMEM16F. *Nature*, *468*(7325), 834–838. doi:10.1038/nature09583 PMID:21107324

Sventek, J. C., & Zambraski, E. J. (1988). Effects of chronic hyperoxia on the cardiovascular responses to vasoactive compounds in the rabbit. *Aviation, Space, and Environmental Medicine*, *59*(4), 314–320. PMID:3163478

Szabo, S., Lieberman, J. P., & Lue, Y. A. (1990). Unusual pathogens in narcotic-associated endocarditis. *Reviews of Infectious Diseases*, *12*(3), 412–415. doi:10.1093/clinids/12.3.412 PMID:2359905

Szegezdi, E., Duffy, A., OMahoney, M. E., Logue, S. E., Mylotte, L. A., OBrien, T., & Samali, A. (2006). ER stress contributes to ischemia-induced cardiomyocyte apoptosis. *Biochemical and Biophysical Research Communications*, *349*(4), 1406–1411. doi:10.1016/j.bbrc.2006.09.009 PMID:16979584

Tabassum, N., & Ahmad, F. (2011). Role of natural herbs in the treatment of hypertension. *Pharmacognosy Reviews*, *5*(9), 30.

Tahraoui, A., El-Hilaly, J., Israili, Z. H., & Lyoussi, B. (2007). Ethnopharmacological survey of plants used in the traditional treatment of hypertension and diabetes in south-eastern Morocco (Errachidia province). *Journal of Ethnopharmacology*, *110*(1), 105–117. doi:10.1016/j.jep.2006.09.011 PMID:17052873

Takahama, H., Minamino, T., Asanuma, H., Fujita, M., Asai, T., Wakeno, M., & Kitakaze, M. et al. (2009). Prolonged targeting of ischemic/reperfused myocardium by liposomal adenosine augments cardioprotection in rats. *Journal of the American College of Cardiology*, *53*(8), 709–717. doi:10.1016/j.jacc.2008.11.014 PMID:19232905

Tanno, M., Kuno, A., Horio, Y., & Miura, T. (2012). Emerging beneficial roles of sirtuins in heart failure. *Basic Research in Cardiology*, *107*(4), 273. doi:10.1007/s00395-012-0273-5 PMID:22622703

Tanno, M., Kuno, A., Yano, T., Miura, T., Hisahara, S., Ishikawa, S., & Horio, Y. et al. (2010). Induction of manganese superoxide dismutase by nuclear translocation and activation of SIRT1 promotes cell survival in chronic heart failure. *The Journal of Biological Chemistry*, *285*(11), 8375–8382. doi:10.1074/jbc.M109.090266 PMID:20089851

Tanno, M., Sakamoto, J., Miura, T., Shimamoto, K., & Horio, Y. (2007). Nucleocytoplasmic shuttling of the NAD+-dependent histone deacetylase SIRT1. *The Journal of Biological Chemistry*, *282*(9), 6823–6832. doi:10.1074/jbc.M609554200 PMID:17197703

Taubert, D., Berkels, R., Roesen, R., & Klaus, W. (2003). Chocolate and blood pressure in elderly individuals with isolated systolic hypertension. *Journal of the American Medical Association*, *290*(8), 1029–1030. doi:10.1001/jama.290.8.1029 PMID:12941673

Taubert, D., Roesen, R., Lehmann, C., Jung, N., & Schomig, E. (2007). Effects of low habitual cocoa intake on blood pressure and bioactive nitric oxide: A randomized controlled trial. *Journal of the American Medical Association*, *298*(1), 49–60. doi:10.1001/jama.298.1.49 PMID:17609490

Taubert, D., Roesen, R., & Schoemig, E. (2007). Effect of cocoa and tea intake on blood pressure - A meta-analysis. *Archives of Internal Medicine*, *167*(7), 626–634. doi:10.1001/archinte.167.7.626 PMID:17420419

Tauseef, M., Farazuddin, M., Sukriti, S., Rajput, C., Meyer, J. O., Ramasamy, S. K., & Mehta, D. (2016). Transient receptor potential channel 1 maintains adherens junction plasticity by suppressing sphingosine kinase 1 expression to induce endothelial hyperpermeability. *The FASEB Journal*, *30*(1), 102–110. doi:10.1096/fj.15-275891 PMID:26316271

Tauseef, M., Kini, V., Knezevic, N., Brannan, M., Ramchandaran, R., Fyrst, H., & Mehta, D. et al. (2008). Activation of sphingosine kinase-1 reverses the increase in lung vascular permeability through sphingosine-1-phosphate receptor signaling in endothelial cells. *Circulation Research*, *103*(10), 1164–1172. doi:10.1161/01.RES.0000338501.84810.51 PMID:18849324

Tauseef, M., Knezevic, N., Chava, K. R., Smith, M., Sukriti, S., Gianaris, N., & Mehta, D. et al. (2012). TLR4 activation of TRPC6-dependent calcium signaling mediates endotoxin-induced lung vascular permeability and inflammation. *The Journal of Experimental Medicine*, *209*(11), 1953–1968. doi:10.1084/jem.20111355 PMID:23045603

Tearney, G. J. (1997). In Vivo Endoscopic Optical Biopsy with Optical Coherence Tomography. *Science*, *276*(5321), 2037–2039. doi:10.1126/science.276.5321.2037 PMID:9197265

Tefre, K.L., Ingerslev, J., & Sorensen, B. (2009). Clinical benefit of recombinant factor VIIa in management of bleeds and surgery in two brothers suffering from the Bernard-Soulier syndrome. *Haemophilia: The Official Journal of the World Federation of Hemophilia, 15*, 281-4.

Teresa, A. (2007). Hopkins, Noriyuki Ouchi, Rei Shibata, Kenneth Walsh.Adiponectin actions in the cardiovascular system. *Cardiovascular Research*, 11–18.

Tessier, S. N., & Storey, K. B. (2012). Myocyte enhancer factor-2 and cardiac muscle gene expression during hibernation in thirteen-lined ground squirrels. *Gene*, *501*(1), 8–16. doi:10.1016/j.gene.2012.04.004 PMID:22513076

Testa, G., Biasi, F., Poli, G., & Chiarpotto, E. (2014). Calorie restriction and dietary restriction mimetics: A strategy for improving healthy aging and longevity. *Current Pharmaceutical Design*, *20*(18), 2950–2977. doi:10.2174/138161281 13196660699 PMID:24079773

Tester, D. J., & Ackerman, M. J. (2012). The Molecular Autopsy: Should the Evaluation Continue After the Funeral? *Pediatric Cardiology*, *33*(3), 461–470. doi:10.1007/s00246-012-0160-8 PMID:22307399

Teutsch, C., Kondo, R. P., Dederko, D. A., Chrast, J., Chien, K. R., & Giles, W. R. (2007). Spatial distributions of Kv4 channels and KChip2 isoforms in the murine heart based on laser capture microdissection. *Cardiovascular Research*, *73*(4), 739–749. doi:10.1016/j.cardiores.2006.11.034 PMID:17289005

Thébaud, B., & Abman, S. H. (2007). Bronchopulmonary Dysplasia. *American Journal of Respiratory and Critical Care Medicine*, *175*(10), 978–985. doi:10.1164/rccm.200611-1660PP PMID:17272782

Thennes, T., & Mehta, D. (2012). Heterotrimeric G proteins, focal adhesion kinase, and endothelial barrier function. *Microvascular Research*, *83*(1), 31–44. doi:10.1016/j.mvr.2011.05.004 PMID:21640127

Thiel, M., Chouker, A., Ohta, A., Jackson, E., Caldwell, C., Smith, P., . . . Sitkovsky, M. V. (2005). Oxygenation inhibits the physiological tissue-protecting mechanism and thereby exacerbates acute inflammatory lung injury. *PLoS Biol, 3*(6), e174. doi: 10.1371/journal.pbio.0030174

Thomas, N., & Walsh, K. (2015). *Ularitide received FDA Fast Track designation for the treatment of acute decompensated heart failure*. Retrieved on March 11, 2016, from http://www.cardiorentis.com/de/media/index.php

Thomson, A. J., Drummond, G. B., Waring, W. S., Webb, D. J., & Maxwell, S. R. (2006). Effects of short-term isocapnic hyperoxia and hypoxia on cardiovascular function. *J Appl Physiol (1985), 101*(3), 809-816. doi: 10.1152/japplphysiol.01185.2005

Thuerauf, D. J., Marcinko, M., Gude, N., Rubio, M., Sussman, M. A., & Glembotski, C. C. (2006). Activation of the Unfolded Protein Response in Infarcted Mouse Heart and Hypoxic Cultured Cardiac Myocytes. *Circulation Research, 99*(3), 275–282. doi:10.1161/01.RES.0000233317.70421.03 PMID:16794188

Thygesen, K., Alpert, J. S., Jaffe, A. S., Simoons, M. L., Chaitman, B. R., White, H. D., & Mendis, S et al.. (2012). Third Universal Definition of Myocardial Infarction. *Journal of the American College of Cardiology, 60*(16), 1581–1598. doi:10.1016/j.jacc.2012.08.001 PMID:22958960

Timmers, L., van Keulen, J. K., Hoefer, I. E., Meijs, M. F., van Middelaar, B., den Ouden, K., & de Kleijn, D. P. et al. (2009). Targeted deletion of nuclear factor kappaB p50 enhances cardiac remodeling and dysfunction following myocardial infarction. *Circulation Research, 104*(5), 699–706. doi:10.1161/CIRCRESAHA.108.189746 PMID:19168865

Tipparaju, S. M., Li, X. P., Kilfoil, P. J., Xue, B., Uversky, V. N., Bhatnagar, A., & Barski, O. A. (2012a). Interactions between the C-terminus of Kv1.5 and Kvbeta regulate pyridine nucleotide-dependent changes in channel gating. *Pflugers Archiv, 463*(6), 799–818. doi:10.1007/s00424-012-1093-z PMID:22426702

Tiruppathi, C., Ahmmed, G. U., Vogel, S. M., & Malik, A. B. (2006). Ca2+ signaling, TRP channels, and endothelial permeability. *Microcirculation (New York, N.Y.), 13*(8), 693–708. doi:10.1080/10739680600930347 PMID:17085428

Tiruppathi, C., Freichel, M., Vogel, S. M., Paria, B. C., Mehta, D., Flockerzi, V., & Malik, A. B. (2002). Impairment of store-operated Ca2+ entry in TRPC4(-/-) mice interferes with increase in lung microvascular permeability. *Circulation Research, 91*(1), 70–76. doi:10.1161/01.RES.0000023391.40106.A8 PMID:12114324

Tiruppathi, C., Soni, D., Wang, D. M., Xue, J., Singh, V., Thippegowda, P. B., & Malik, A. B. et al. (2014). The transcription factor DREAM represses the deubiquitinase A20 and mediates inflammation. *Nature Immunology, 15*(3), 239–247. doi:10.1038/ni.2823 PMID:24487321

Tojyo, Y., Morita, T., Nezu, A., & Tanimura, A. (2014). Key components of store-operated Ca2+ entry in non-excitable cells. *Journal of Pharmacological Sciences, 125*(4), 340–346. doi:10.1254/jphs.14R06CP PMID:25030742

Tome-Carneiro, J., Larrosa, M., Gonzalez-Sarrias, A., Tomas-Barberan, F. A., Garcia-Conesa, M. T., & Espin, J. C. (2013). Resveratrol and clinical trials: The crossroad from in vitro studies to human evidence. *Current Pharmaceutical Design, 19*(34), 6064–6093. doi:10.2174/13816128113199990407 PMID:23448440

Tong, M., & Sadoshima, J. (2016). Mitochondrial autophagy in cardiomyopathy. *Current Opinion in Genetics & Development, 38*, 8–15. doi:10.1016/j.gde.2016.02.006 PMID:27003723

Tong, X., Taylor, A. W., Giles, L., Wittert, G. A., & Shi, Z. (2014). Tea consumption is inversely related to 5-year blood pressure change among adults in Jiangsu, China: A cross-sectional study. *Nutrition Journal, 13*(1), 98. doi:10.1186/1475-2891-13-98 PMID:25311544

Toth, A., Jeffers, J. R., Nickson, P., Min, J. Y., Morgan, J. P., Zambetti, G. P., & Erhardt, P. (2006). Targeted deletion of Puma attenuates cardiomyocyte death and improves cardiac function during ischemia-reperfusion. *American Journal of Physiology. Heart and Circulatory Physiology, 291*(1), H52–H60. doi:10.1152/ajpheart.01046.2005 PMID:16399862

Touchberry, C. D., Elmore, C. J., Nguyen, T. M., Andresen, J. J., Zhao, X., Orange, M., & Wacker, M. J. et al. (2011). Store-operated calcium entry is present in HL-1 cardiomyocytes and contributes to resting calcium. *Biochemical and Biophysical Research Communications*, *416*(1-2), 45–50. doi:10.1016/j.bbrc.2011.10.133 PMID:22079292

Tran, K. A., Zhang, X., Predescu, D., Huang, X., Machado, R. F., Gothert, J. R., & Zhao, Y. Y. et al. (2015). Endothelial beta-Catenin Signaling Is Required for Maintaining Adult Blood-Brain Barrier Integrity and CNS Homeostasis. *Circulation*. doi:10.1161/CIRCULATIONAHA.115.015982

Trial, M. (1997). The effect of digoxin on mortality and morbidity in patients with heart failure. *The New England Journal of Medicine*, *336*(8), 525–533. doi:10.1056/NEJM199702203360801 PMID:9036306

Tribouilloy, C., Rusinaru, D., Sorel, C., Thuny, F., Casalta, J. P., Riberi, A., & Habib, G. et al. (2010). Clinical characteristics and outcome of infective endocarditis in adults with bicuspid aortic valves: A multicentre observational study. *Heart (British Cardiac Society)*, *96*(21), 1723–1729. doi:10.1136/hrt.2009.189050 PMID:20478858

Tripathi, D., & Bég, O. A. (2014). A study on peristaltic flow of nanofluids: Application in drug delivery systems. *International Journal of Heat and Mass Transfer*, 7061–7070. doi:10.1016/j.ijheatmasstransfer.2013.10.044

Trovato, F., & Lauris, G. (1989). Marital Status and Mortality in Canada: 1951- 1981. *Journal of Marriage and the Family*, *51*(4), 907–922. doi:10.2307/353204

Trueblood, N. A., Ramasamy, R., Wang, L. F., & Schaefer, S. (2000). Niacin protects the isolated heart from ischemia-reperfusion injury. *American Journal of Physiology. Heart and Circulatory Physiology*, *279*(2), H764–H771. PMID:10924076

Tsai, E. J., & Kass, D. A. (2009). Cyclic GMP signaling in cardiovascular pathophysiology and therapeutics. *Pharmacology & Therapeutics*, *122*(3), 216–238. doi:10.1016/j.pharmthera.2009.02.009 PMID:19306895

Tsai, M. S., Huang, C. H., Tsai, C. Y., Chen, H. W., Lee, H. C., Cheng, H. J., & Chen, W. J. et al. (2011). Ascorbic acid mitigates the myocardial injury after cardiac arrest and electrical shock. *Intensive Care Medicine*, *37*(12), 2033–2040. doi:10.1007/s00134-011-2362-6 PMID:21953354

Tsai, P.-J., Tsai, T.-H., Yu, C.-H., & Ho, S.-C. (2007). Evaluation of NO-suppressing activity of several Mediterranean culinary spices. *Food and Chemical Toxicology*, *45*(3), 440–447. doi:10.1016/j.fct.2006.09.006 PMID:17074427

Tsao, P. S., Aoki, N., Lefer, D. J., Johnson, G. III, & Lefer, A. M. (1990). Time course of endothelial dysfunction and myocardial injury during myocardial ischemia and reperfusion in the cat. *Circulation*, *82*(4), 1402–1412. doi:10.1161/01.CIR.82.4.1402 PMID:2401073

Tse, H. (2011). *Oxford desk reference*. Oxford, UK: Oxford University Press. doi:10.1093/med/9780199568093.001.0001

Tsigrelis, C., Singh, K. V., Coutinho, T. D., Murray, B. E., & Baddour, L. M. (2007). Vancomycin-resistant Enterococcus faecalis endocarditis: Linezolid failure and strain characterization of virulence factors. *Journal of Clinical Microbiology*, *45*(2), 631–635. doi:10.1128/JCM.02188-06 PMID:17182759

Turner, R. C., Millns, H., Neil, H. A. W., Stratton, I. M., Manley, S. E., Matthews, D. R., & Holman, R. R. (1998). Risk factors for coronary artery disease in non-insulin dependent diabetes mellitus: United Kingdom prospective diabetes study (UKPDS: 23). *BMJ: British Medical Journal*, *316*(7134), 823–828. doi:10.1136/bmj.316.7134.823 PMID:9549452

Twig, G., Elorza, A., Molina, A. J. A., Mohamed, H., Wikstrom, J. D., Walzer, G., & Shirihai, O. S. et al. (2008). Fission and selective fusion govern mitochondrial segregation and elimination by autophagy. *The EMBO Journal*, *27*(2), 433–446. doi:10.1038/sj.emboj.7601963 PMID:18200046

U.S. Department of Health and Human Services. (2008). *2008 Physical Activity Guidelines for Americans*. Retrieved from www.health.gov/paguidelines

Uehara, A., Yasukochi, M., Imanaga, I., Nishi, M., & Takeshima, H. (2002). Store-operated Ca2+ entry uncoupled with ryanodine receptor and junctional membrane complex in heart muscle cells. *Cell Calcium*, *31*(2), 89–96. doi:10.1054/ceca.2001.0257 PMID:11969249

Ueshima, H., Stamler, J., Elliott, P., Chan, Q., Brown, I. J., Carnethon, M. R., & Zhou, B. et al. (2007). Food omega-3 fatty acid intake of individuals (total, linolenic acid, long-chain) and their blood pressure INTERMAP study. *Hypertension*, *50*(2), 313–319. doi:10.1161/HYPERTENSIONAHA.107.090720 PMID:17548718

Uhlig, S., Yang, Y., Waade, J., Wittenberg, C., Babendreyer, A., & Kuebler, W. M. (2014). Differential regulation of lung endothelial permeability in vitro and in situ. *Cellular Physiology and Biochemistry*, *34*(1), 1–19. doi:10.1159/000362980 PMID:24977477

Ulker, S., McKeown, P. P., & Bayraktutan, U. (2003). Vitamins reverse endothelial dysfunction through regulation of eNOS and NAD(P)H oxidase activities. *Hypertension*, *41*(3), 534–539. doi:10.1161/01.HYP.0000057421.28533.37 PMID:12623955

Unger, E., Porter, T., Lindner, J., & Grayburn, P. (2014). Cardiovascular drug delivery with ultrasound and microbubbles. *Advanced Drug Delivery Reviews*, 72110–72126. doi:10.1016/j.addr.2014.01.012 PMID:24524934

Unites States White House. (2015). *National action plan for combating antibiotic-resistant bacteria*. Retrieved on 2/23/2016 from https://www.whitehouse.gov/sites/default/files/docs/national_action_plan_for_combating_antibotic-resistant_bacteria.pdf

Urban, D., Li, L., Christensen, H., Pluthero, F. G., Chen, S. Z., Puhacz, M., & Kahr, W. H. A. et al. (2012). The VPS33B-binding protein VPS16B is required in megakaryocyte and platelet alpha-granule biogenesis. *Blood*, *120*(25), 5032–5040. doi:10.1182/blood-2012-05-431205 PMID:23002115

Urivetzky, M., Kessaris, D., & Smith, A. D. (1992). Ascorbic acid overdosing: A risk factor for calcium oxalate nephrolithiasis. *The Journal of Urology*, *147*(5), 1215–1218. PMID:1569652

Usatyuk, P. V., Singleton, P. A., Pendyala, S., Kalari, S. K., He, D., Gorshkova, I. A., & Natarajan, V. et al. (2012). Novel role for non-muscle myosin light chain kinase (MLCK) in hyperoxia-induced recruitment of cytoskeletal proteins, NADPH oxidase activation, and reactive oxygen species generation in lung endothelium. *The Journal of Biological Chemistry*, *287*(12), 9360–9375. doi:10.1074/jbc.M111.294546 PMID:22219181

Vahtola, E., Louhelainen, M., Merasto, S., Martonen, E., Penttinen, S., Aahos, I., & Mervaala, E. et al. (2008). Forkhead class O transcription factor 3a activation and Sirtuin1 overexpression in the hypertrophied myocardium of the diabetic Goto-Kakizaki rat. *Journal of Hypertension*, *26*(2), 334–344. doi:10.1097/HJH.0b013e3282f293c8 PMID:18192848

van den Broek, K. C., Defilippi, C. R., Christenson, R. H., Seliger, S. L., Gottdiener, J. S., & Kop, W. J. (2011). Predictive value of depressive symptoms and B-type natriuretic peptide for new-onset heart failure and mortality. *The American Journal of Cardiology*, *107*(5), 723–729. doi:10.1016/j.amjcard.2010.10.055 PMID:21316507

Van der Heiden, K., & Cuhlmann, S. (2010). Luong le A, Zakkar M, Evans PC.Role of nuclear factor kappaB in cardiovascular health and disease. *Clinical Science (London, England)*, *118*(10), 593–605. doi:10.1042/CS20090557

van der Net, J. B., Versmissen, J., Oosterveer, D. M., Defesche, J. C., Yazdanpanah, M., Aouizerat, B. E., & Sijbrands, E. J. et al. (2009). Arachidonate 5-lipoxygenase-activating protein (ALOX5AP) gene and coronary heart disease risk in familial hypercholesterolemia. *Atherosclerosis*, *203*(2), 472–478. doi:10.1016/j.atherosclerosis.2008.07.025 PMID:18775537

Van Geet, C., Izzi, B., Labarque, V., & Freson, K. (2009). Human platelet pathology related to defects in the G-protein signaling cascade. *Journal of thrombosis and haemostasis. JTH*, *7*(Suppl 1), 282–286. PMID:19630817 van Kooten, C., Lombardi, G., Gelderman, K. A., Sagoo, P., Buckland, M., Lechler, R., & Cuturi, M. C. (2011). Dendritic cells as a tool to induce transplantation tolerance: Obstacles and opportunities. *Transplantation*, *91*(1), 2–7. doi:10.1097/TP.0b013e31820263b3 PMID:21452405

van Nieuw Amerongen, G. P., Draijer, R., Vermeer, M. A., & van Hinsbergh, V. W. (1998). Transient and prolonged increase in endothelial permeability induced by histamine and thrombin: Role of protein kinases, calcium, and RhoA. *Circulation Research*, *83*(11), 1115–1123. doi:10.1161/01.RES.83.11.1115 PMID:9831706

Vandenbroucke St Amant, E., Tauseef, M., Vogel, S. M., Gao, X. P., Mehta, D., Komarova, Y. A., & Malik, A. B. (2012). PKCalpha activation of p120-catenin serine 879 phospho-switch disassembles VE-cadherin junctions and disrupts vascular integrity. *Circulation Research*, *111*(6), 739–749. doi:10.1161/CIRCRESAHA.112.269654 PMID:22798526

Vandenbroucke, E., Mehta, D., Minshall, R., & Malik, A. B. (2008). Regulation of endothelial junctional permeability. *Annals of the New York Academy of Sciences*, *1123*(1), 134–145. doi:10.1196/annals.1420.016 PMID:18375586

Varma, K. R., Jain, T. C., & Bhattacharyya, S. C. (1962). Terpenoids—XXXIV: Structure and stereochemistry of zingiberol and juniper camphor. *Tetrahedron*, *18*(8), 979–984. doi:10.1016/S0040-4020(01)92752-8

Vasauskas, A. A., Chen, H., Wu, S., & Cioffi, D. L. (2014). The serine-threonine phosphatase calcineurin is a regulator of endothelial store-operated calcium entry. *Pulm Circ*, *4*(1), 116–127. doi:10.1086/675641 PMID:25006427

Vekich, J. A., Belmont, P. J., Thuerauf, D. J., & Glembotski, C. C. (2012). Protein Disulfide Isomerase-associated 6 is an ATF6-inducible ER Stress Response Protein that Protects Cardiac Myocytes from Ischemia/Reperfusion-mediated Cell Death. *Journal of Molecular and Cellular Cardiology*, *53*(2), 259–267. doi:10.1016/j.yjmcc.2012.05.005 PMID:22609432

Velten, M., Hutchinson, K. R., Gorr, M. W., Wold, L. E., Lucchesi, P. A., & Rogers, L. K. (2011). Systemic Maternal Inflammation and Neonatal Hyperoxia Induces Remodeling and Left Ventricular Dysfunction in Mice. *PLoS ONE*, *6*(9), e24544. doi:10.1371/journal.pone.0024544 PMID:21935422

Vendelin, M., Béraud, N., Guerrero, K., Andrienko, T., Kuznetsov, A. V., & Olivares, J. et al.. (2005). Mitochondrial regular arrangement in muscle cells: A crystal-like pattern. *American Journal of Physiology. Cell Physiology*, *288*(3), C757–C767. doi:10.1152/ajpcell.00281.2004 PMID:15496480

Viehman, G. E., Ma, X. L., Lefer, D. J., & Lefer, A. M. (1991). Time course of endothelial dysfunction and myocardial injury during coronary arterial occlusion. *The American Journal of Physiology*, *261*(3 Pt 2), H874–H881. PMID:1653539

Villalba, J. M., & Alcain, F. J. (2012). Sirtuin activators and inhibitors. *BioFactors (Oxford, England)*, *38*(5), 349–359. doi:10.1002/biof.1032 PMID:22730114

Vincent, J.-L. (2008). Understanding cardiac output. *Critical Care (London, England)*, *12*(4), 174. doi:10.1186/cc6975 PMID:18771592

Vink, A., de Kleijn, D. P., & Pasterkamp, G. (2004). Functional role for toll-like receptors in atherosclerosis and arterial remodeling. *Current Opinion in Lipidology*, *15*(5), 515–521. doi:10.1097/00041433-200410000-00004 PMID:15361786

Vinten-Johansen, J. (2004). Involvement of neutrophils in the pathogenesis of lethal myocardial reperfusion injury. *Cardiovascular Research*, *61*(3), 481–497. doi:10.1016/j.cardiores.2003.10.011 PMID:14962479

Visser, Y. P., Walther, F. J., Laghmani, E. H., Laarse, A., & Wagenaar, G. T. M. (2010). Apelin attenuates hyperoxic lung and heart injury in neonatal rats. *American Journal of Respiratory and Critical Care Medicine*, *182*(10), 1239–1250. doi:10.1164/rccm.200909-1361OC PMID:20622042

Voelkers, M., Salz, M., Herzog, N., Frank, D., Dolatabadi, N., Frey, N., & Most, P. et al. (2010). Orai1 and Stim1 regulate normal and hypertrophic growth in cardiomyocytes. *Journal of Molecular and Cellular Cardiology*, *48*(6), 1329–1334. doi:10.1016/j.yjmcc.2010.01.020 PMID:20138887

Vogel, S. M., Gao, X., Mehta, D., Ye, R. D., John, T. A., Andrade-Gordon, P., & Malik, A. B. et al. (2000). Abrogation of thrombin-induced increase in pulmonary microvascular permeability in PAR-1 knockout mice. *Physiological Genomics*, *4*(2), 137–145. PMID:11120874

Vogel, S. M., & Malik, A. B. (2012). Cytoskeletal dynamics and lung fluid balance. *Compr Physiol*, *2*(1), 449–478. doi:10.1002/cphy.c100006 PMID:23728978

Volkers, M., Dolatabadi, N., Gude, N., Most, P., Sussman, M. A., & Hassel, D. (2012). Orai1 deficiency leads to heart failure and skeletal myopathy in zebrafish. *Journal of Cell Science*, *125*(Pt 2), 287–294. doi:10.1242/jcs.090464 PMID:22302996

Von Reyn, C. F., Levy, B. S., Arbeit, R. D., Friedland, G., & Crumpacker, C. S. (1981). Infective endocarditis: An analysis based on strict case definitions. *Annals of Internal Medicine*, *94*(4_Part_1), 505–518. doi:10.7326/0003-4819-94-4-505 PMID:7011141

Voora, D., Shah, S. H., Spasojevic, I., Ali, S., Reed, C. R., Salisbury, B. A., & Ginsburg, G. S. (2009). The SLCO1B1*5 genetic variant is associated with statin-induced side effects. *Journal of the American College of Cardiology*, *54*(17), 1609–1616. doi:10.1016/j.jacc.2009.04.053 PMID:19833260

Vrolijk, M. F., Haenen, G. R., Opperhuizen, A., Jansen, E. H., Schiffers, P. M., & Bast, A. (2015). The supplement–drug interaction of quercetin with tamsulosin on vasorelaxation. *European Journal of Pharmacology*, *746*, 132–137. doi:10.1016/j.ejphar.2014.11.006 PMID:25449042

Wadgaonkar, R., Patel, V., Grinkina, N., Romano, C., Liu, J., Zhao, Y., & Natarajan, V. et al. (2009). Differential regulation of sphingosine kinases 1 and 2 in lung injury. *American Journal of Physiology. Lung Cellular and Molecular Physiology*, *296*(4), L603–L613. doi:10.1152/ajplung.90357.2008 PMID:19168577

Wainwright, M. S., Rossi, J., Schavocky, J., Crawford, S., Steinhorn, D., Velentza, A. V., & Watterson, D. M. et al. (2003). Protein kinase involved in lung injury susceptibility: Evidence from enzyme isoform genetic knockout and in vivo inhibitor treatment. *Proceedings of the National Academy of Sciences of the United States of America*, *100*(10), 6233–6238. doi:10.1073/pnas.1031595100 PMID:12730364

Waisman, D., Brod, V., Wolff, R., Sabo, E., Chernin, M., Weintraub, Z., . . . Bitterman, H. (2003). Effects of hyperoxia on local and remote microcirculatory inflammatory response after splanchnic ischemia and reperfusion. *Am J Physiol Heart Circ Physiol*, *285*(2), H643-652. doi: 10.1152/ajpheart.00900.2002

Waisman, D., Brod, V., Rahat, M. A., Amit-Cohen, B. C., Lahat, N., Rimar, D., & Bitterman, H. et al. (2012). Dose-related effects of hyperoxia on the lung inflammatory response in septic rats.[doi]. *Shock (Augusta, Ga.)*, *37*(1), 95–102. doi:10.1097/SHK.0b013e3182356fc3 PMID:21921827

Waksman, R., Mehran, R., & Krucoff, M. W. (2008). Postmarket evaluation of breakthrough technologies. *American Heart Journal*, *156*(2), 201–208. doi:10.1016/j.ahj.2008.01.036 PMID:18657647

Wallentin, L., James, S., Storey, R. F., Armstrong, M., Barratt, B. J., Horrow, J., & Becker, R. C. et al. (2010). Effect of CYP2C19 and ABCB1 single nucleotide polymorphisms on outcomes of treatment with ticagrelor versus clopidogrel for acute coronary syndromes: A genetic substudy of the PLATO trial. *Lancet*, *376*(9749), 1320–1328. doi:10.1016/S0140-6736(10)61274-3 PMID:20801498

Walsh, M. C., Szefler, S., Davis, J., Allen, M., Van Marter, L., Abman, S., & Jobe, A. et al. (2006). Summary proceedings from the bronchopulmonary dysplasia group. *Pediatrics*, *117*(3 Pt 2), S52–S56. doi:10.1542/peds.2005-0620I PMID:16777823

Wang, B., Yang, Q., Sun, Y. Y., Xing, Y. F., Wang, Y. B., Lu, X. T., & Zhao, Y. X. et al. (2014). Resveratrol-enhanced autophagic flux ameliorates myocardial oxidative stress injury in diabetic mice. *Journal of Cellular and Molecular Medicine*, *18*(8), 1599–1611. doi:10.1111/jcmm.12312 PMID:24889822

Wang, H., Qi, F., Dai, X., Tian, W., Liu, T., Han, H., & Du, C. et al. (2014). Requirement of B7-H1 in mesenchymal stem cells for immune tolerance to cardiac allografts in combination therapy with rapamycin. *Transplant Immunology*, *31*(2), 65–74. doi:10.1016/j.trim.2014.06.005 PMID:24978830

Wang, L. Y., Chan, K. W., Yuwen, Y., Shi, N. N., Han, X. J., & Lu, A. (2013). Expert consensus on the treatment of hypertension with chinese patent medicines. *Evidence-Based Complementary and Alternative Medicine*, *510146*. doi:10.1155/2013/510146 PMID:23662141

Wang, L., Wang, J., Xu, H., & Li, B. (2013). Postconditioning in patients treated with primary percutaneous coronary intervention: An updated meta-analysis. *Catheterization and Cardiovascular Interventions*, *82*(5), E662–E671. doi:10.1002/ccd.25095 PMID:23804529

Wang, Y. (2014). Molecular Links between Caloric Restriction and Sir2/SIRT1 Activation. *Diabetes Metab J*, *38*(5), 321–329. doi:10.4093/dmj.2014.38.5.321 PMID:25349818

Wang, Y., Bi, Y., Wu, K., & Wang, C. (2011). Dendritic cell co-transfected with FasL and allergen genes induces T cell tolerance and decreases airway inflammation in allergen induced murine model. *Molecular Biology Reports*, *38*(2), 809–817. doi:10.1007/s11033-010-0170-7 PMID:20373028

Wang, Z. H., Liu, J. L., Wu, L., Yu, Z., & Yang, H. T. (2014). Concentration-dependent wrestling between detrimental and protective effects of H2O2 during myocardial ischemia/reperfusion.[Original Article]. *Cell Death & Disease*, *5*(6), e1297. doi:10.1038/cddis.2014.267 PMID:24946090

Wang, Z. Y., Qin, W., & Yi, F. (2015). Targeting histone deacetylases: Perspectives for epigenetic-based therapy in cardio-cerebrovascular disease. *J Geriatr Cardiol*, *12*(2), 153–164. doi:10.11909/j.issn.1671-5411.2015.02.010 PMID:25870619

Wang, Z., Li, J., Cho, J., & Malik, A. B. (2014). Prevention of vascular inflammation by nanoparticle targeting of adherent neutrophils. *Nature Nanotechnology*, *9*(3), 204–210. doi:10.1038/nnano.2014.17 PMID:24561355

Wang, Z., Zou, J., Cao, K., Hsieh, T. C., Huang, Y., & Wu, J. M. (2005). Dealcoholized red wine containing known amounts of resveratrol suppresses atherosclerosis in hypercholesterolemic rabbits without affecting plasma lipid levels. *International Journal of Molecular Medicine*, *16*(4), 533–540. PMID:16142383

Warboys, C. M., de Luca, A., Amini, N., Luong, L., Duckles, H., Hsiao, S., & Evans, P. C. et al. (2014). Disturbed flow promotes endothelial senescence via a p53-dependent pathway. *Arteriosclerosis, Thrombosis, and Vascular Biology*, *34*(5), 985–995. doi:10.1161/ATVBAHA.114.303415 PMID:24651677

Waring, W. S., Thomson, A. J., Adwani, S. H., Rosseel, A. J., Potter, J. F., Webb, D. J., & Maxwell, S. R. (2003). Cardiovascular effects of acute oxygen administration in healthy adults. *Journal of Cardiovascular Pharmacology*, *42*(2), 245–250. doi:10.1097/00005344-200308000-00014 PMID:12883329

Watanabe, H., Murakami, M., Ohba, T., Takahashi, Y., & Ito, H. (2008). TRP channel and cardiovascular disease. *Pharmacology & Therapeutics*, *118*(3), 337–351. doi:10.1016/j.pharmthera.2008.03.008 PMID:18508125

Weber, E. W., Han, F., Tauseef, M., Birnbaumer, L., Mehta, D., & Muller, W. A. (2015). TRPC6 is the endothelial calcium channel that regulates leukocyte transendothelial migration during the inflammatory response. *The Journal of Experimental Medicine*, *212*(11), 1883–1899. doi:10.1084/jem.20150353 PMID:26392222

Webster, K. A. (2012). A sirtuin link between metabolism and heart disease. *Nature Medicine*, *18*(11), 1617–1619. doi:10.1038/nm.2983 PMID:23135512

Weeke, P., & Roden, D. M. (2013). Pharmacogenomics and Cardiovascular Disease. *Current Cardiology Reports*, *15*(7), 376. doi:10.1007/s11886-013-0376-0 PMID:23689943

Wei, J. Q., Shehadeh, L. A., Mitrani, J. M., Pessanha, M., Slepak, T. I., Webster, K. A., & Bishopric, N. H. (2008). Quantitative Control of Adaptive Cardiac Hypertrophy by Acetyltransferase p300. *Circulation*, *118*(9), 934–946. doi:10.1161/CIRCULATIONAHA.107.760488 PMID:18697823

Weir, E. K., Lopez-Barneo, J., Buckler, K. J., & Archer, S. L. (2005). Acute oxygen-sensing mechanisms. *The New England Journal of Medicine*, *353*(19), 2042–2055. doi:10.1056/NEJMra050002 PMID:16282179

Weissmann, N., Sydykov, A., Kalwa, H., Storch, U., Fuchs, B., Mederos y Schnitzler, M., & Dietrich, A. et al. (2012). Activation of TRPC6 channels is essential for lung ischaemia-reperfusion induced oedema in mice. *Nature Communications*, *3*, 649. doi:10.1038/ncomms1660 PMID:22337127

Weitz, J. (2011). Blood Coagulation and Anticoagulant, Fibrinolytic, and Antiplatelet Drugs. In L. Brunton, B. Chabner, & B. Knollmann (Eds.), Goodman & Gilman's: The Pharmacologic Basis of Therapeutics. New York, NY: McGraw-Hill.

Wei, Y. Z. H., Lin, R., Fu, Y., & Wang, W. (2014). Short-term calorie restriction activates SIRT1-4 and -7 in cardiomyocytes in vivo and in vitro. *Molecular Medicine Reports*, *9*(4), 1218–1224. doi:10.3892/mmr.2014.1944 PMID:24535021

Wellcome Trust Case Control, C. (2007). Genome-wide association study of 14,000 cases of seven common diseases and 3,000 shared controls. *Nature*, *447*(7145), 661–678. doi:10.1038/nature05911 PMID:17554300

Wenger, N. K. (2014). Prevention of cardiovascular disease: Highlights for the clinician of the 2013 American College of Cardiology/American Heart Association guidelines. *Clinical Cardiology*, *37*(4), 239–251. doi:10.1002/clc.22264 PMID:24633723

Westedt, U., Kalinowski, M., Wittmar, M., Merdan, T., Unger, F., Fuchs, J., & Kissel, T. et al. (2007). Poly(vinyl alcohol)-graft-poly(lactide-co-glycolide) nanoparticles for local delivery of paclitaxel for restenosis treatment. *Journal of Controlled Release*, 11941–11951. doi:10.1016/j.jconrel.2007.01.009 PMID:17346845

Westfall, T., & Westfall, D. (2011). Adrenergic Agonists and Antagonists. In L. Brunton, B. Chabner, & B. Knollmann (Eds.), Goodman & Gilman's: The Pharmacologic Basis of Therapeutics. New York, NY: McGraw-Hill

Whirl-Carrillo, M., McDonagh, E., Hbert, J., Gong, L., Snghkul, K., Thron, C., & Klein, T. E. et al. (2012). Pharmacogenomics Knowledge for Personalized Medicine. *Clinical Pharmacology and Therapeutics*, *92*(4), 414–417. doi:10.1038/clpt.2012.96 PMID:22992668

White, J. G. (1987). Inherited abnormalities of the platelet membrane and secretory granules. *Human Pathology*, *18*(2), 123–139. doi:10.1016/S0046-8177(87)80331-3 PMID:3542800

WHO. (2013). *WHO traditional medicine strategy: 2014-2023*. World Health Organization.

WHO. (2015, January). *Cardiovascular diseases (CVDs)*. Retrieved from http://www.who.int/mediacentre/factsheets/fs317/en/

Williams, D. R., & Jackson, P. B. (2005). Social Sources of Racial Disparities in Health. *Health Affairs*, *24*(2), 325–334. doi:10.1377/hlthaff.24.2.325 PMID:15757915

Williams, M. J. A., Sutherland, W. H. F., McCormick, M. P., Yeoman, D. J., & de Jong, S. A. (2005). Aged garlic extract improves endothelial function in men with coronary artery disease. *Phytotherapy Research*, *19*(4), 314–319. doi:10.1002/ptr.1663 PMID:16041725

Williamson, J. R., Chang, K., Frangos, M., Hasan, K. S., Ido, Y., Kawamura, T., & Tilton, R. G. et al. (1993). Hyperglycemic Pseudohypoxia and Diabetic Complications. *Diabetes*, *42*(6), 801–813. doi:10.2337/diab.42.6.801 PMID:8495803

Wilson, D. B., Link, D. C., Mason, P. J., & Bessler, M. (2014). Inherited bone marrow failure syndromes in adolescents and young adults. *Annals of Medicine*, *46*(6), 353–363. doi:10.3109/07853890.2014.915579 PMID:24888387

Wilson, S. H., Caplice, N. M., Simari, R. D., Holmes, D. R. Jr, Carlson, P. J., & Lerman, A. (2000). Activated nuclear factor-kappaB is present in the coronary vasculature in experimental hypercholesterolemia. *Atherosclerosis*, *148*(1), 23–30. doi:10.1016/S0021-9150(99)00211-7 PMID:10580167

Wingren, C. J., & Ottosson, A. (2015). Postmortem heart weight modelled using piecewise linear regression in 27,645 medicolegal autopsy cases. *Forensic Science International*, *252*, 157–162. doi:10.1016/j.forsciint.2015.04.036 PMID:26004078

Winkleby, M. A., Jatulis, D. E., Frank, E., & Fortmann, S. P. (1992). Socioeconomic status and health: How education, income, and occupation contribute to risk factors for cardiovascular disease. *American Journal of Public Health*, *82*(6), 816–820. doi:10.2105/AJPH.82.6.816 PMID:1585961

Winnik, S., Auwerx, J., Sinclair, D. A., & Matter, C. M. (2015). Protective effects of sirtuins in cardiovascular diseases: From bench to bedside. *European Heart Journal*, *36*(48), 3404–3412. doi:10.1093/eurheartj/ehv290 PMID:26112889

Witteles, R. M., & Fowler, M. B. (2008). Insulin-resistant cardiomyopathy clinical evidence, mechanisms, and treatment options. *Journal of the American College of Cardiology*, *51*(2), 93–102. doi:10.1016/j.jacc.2007.10.021 PMID:18191731

Wittnich, C., Torrance, S. M., & Carlyle, C. E. (2000). Effects of hyperoxia on neonatal myocardial energy status and response to global ischemia. *The Annals of Thoracic Surgery*, *70*(6), 2125–2131. doi:10.1016/S0003-4975(00)01756-2 PMID:11156132

Wojtovich, A. P., Nadtochiy, S. M., Brookes, P. S., & Nehrke, K. (2012). Ischemic preconditioning: The role of mitochondria and aging. *Experimental Gerontology*, *47*(1), 1–7. doi:10.1016/j.exger.2011.11.001 PMID:22100642

Wolfrum, S., Teupser, D., Tan, M., Chen, K. Y., & Breslow, J. L. (2007). The protective effect of A20 on atherosclerosis in apolipoprotein E-deficient mice is associated with reduced expression of NF-κB target gene. *Proceedings of the National Academy of Sciences of the United States of America*, *104*(47), 18601–18606. doi:10.1073/pnas.0709011104 PMID:18006655

Wolkowicz, P. E., Huang, J., Umeda, P. K., Sharifov, O. F., Tabengwa, E., Halloran, B. A., & Grenett, H. E. et al. (2011). Pharmacological evidence for Orai channel activation as a source of cardiac abnormal automaticity. *European Journal of Pharmacology*, *668*(1-2), 208–216. doi:10.1016/j.ejphar.2011.06.025 PMID:21745466

Wong, S. C., Fukuchi, M., Melnyk, P., Rodger, I., & Giaid, A. (1998). Induction of cyclooxygenase-2 and activation of nuclear factor-kappaB in myocardium of patients with congestive heart failure. *Circulation*, *98*(2), 100–103. doi:10.1161/01.CIR.98.2.100 PMID:9679714

Woodle, E. S., Walsh, R. C., Alloway, R. R., Girnita, A., & Brailey, P. (2011). Proteasome inhibitor therapy for antibody-mediated rejection. *Pediatric Transplantation*, *15*(6), 548–556. doi:10.1111/j.1399-3046.2011.01543.x PMID:21884344

Wu, S. M., Zhang, W. X., Wang, M. H., Zhang, H. Z., Wu, D. G., Zhou, Z. J., & Xiong, L. H. (2013). Proteomic analysis of the immunosuppressive effects of mesenchymal stem cells in a rat heart transplantation model. *Adv Clin Exp Med, 22*(6), 785-794. Retrieved from http://www.ncbi.nlm.nih.gov/pubmed/24431306

Wu, A. H., & French, D. (2013). Implementation of liquid chromatography/mass spectrometry into the clinical laboratory. *Clinica Chimica Acta, 420*, 4–10. doi:10.1016/j.cca.2012.10.026 PMID:23085380

Wu, G., & Meininger, C. J. (2000). Arginine nutrition and cardiovascular function. *The Journal of Nutrition, 130*(11), 2626–2629. PMID:11053497

Wu, X., Guo, R., Chen, P., Wang, Q., & Cunningham, P. N. (2009). TNF induces caspase-dependent inflammation in renal endothelial cells through a Rho- and myosin light chain kinase-dependent mechanism. *American Journal of Physiology. Renal Physiology, 297*(2), F316–F326. doi:10.1152/ajprenal.00089.2009 PMID:19420112

Wyman, J. F. (2012). Principles and procedures in forensic toxicology. *Clinics in Laboratory Medicine, 32*(3), 493–507. doi:10.1016/j.cll.2012.06.005 PMID:22939304

Xie, C., Xie, Z., Xu, X., & Yang, D. (2015). Persimmon (Diospyros kaki L.) leaves: A review on traditional uses, phytochemistry and pharmacological properties. *Journal of Ethnopharmacology, 163*, 229–240. doi:10.1016/j.jep.2015.01.007 PMID:25637828

Xiong, X. J., Wang, P. Q., Li, S. J., Li, X. K., Zhang, Y. Q., & Wang, J. (2015). Garlic for hypertension: A systematic review and meta-analysis of randomized controlled trials. *Phytomedicine, 22*(3), 352–361. doi:10.1016/j.phymed.2014.12.013 PMID:25837272

Xiong, Y., & Hla, T. (2014). S1P control of endothelial integrity. *Current Topics in Microbiology and Immunology, 378*, 85–105. doi:10.1007/978-3-319-05879-5_4 PMID:24728594

Xu, J., Murphy, S. L., Kochanek, K. D., & Bastian, B. A. (2016). *Deaths: Final Data for 2013*. Retrieved from http://www.cdc.gov/nchs/data/nvsr/nvsr64/nvsr64_02.pdf

Xu, D., Guthrie, J. R., Mabry, S., Sack, T. M., & Truog, W. E. (2006). Mitochondrial aldehyde dehydrogenase attenuates hyperoxia-induced cell death through activation of ERK/MAPK and PI3K-Akt pathways in lung epithelial cells. *American Journal of Physiology. Lung Cellular and Molecular Physiology, 291*(5), L966–L975. doi:10.1152/ajplung.00045.2006 PMID:16782756

Xu, J. Q., Murphy, S. L., Kochanek, K. D., & Bastian, B. A. (2016). *Deaths: Final data for 2013. National Vital Statistics Reports, 64(2)*. Hyattsville, MD: National Center for Health Statistics

Xu, X. H., Shah, P. K., Faure, E., Equils, O., Thomas, L., Fishbein, M. C., & Arditi, M. et al. (2001). Toll-like receptor-4 is expressed by macrophages in murine and human lipid-rich atherosclerotic plaques and upregulated by oxidized LDL. *Circulation, 104*(25), 3103–3108. doi:10.1161/hc5001.100631 PMID:11748108

Yamamoto, T., Byun, J., Zhai, P., Ikeda, Y., Oka, S., & Sadoshima, J. (2014). Nicotinamide mononucleotide, an intermediate of NAD+ synthesis, protects the heart from ischemia and reperfusion. *PLoS ONE, 9*(6), e98972. doi:10.1371/journal.pone.0098972 PMID:24905194

Yamamoto, Y., & Oue, E. (2006). Antihypertensive effect of quercetin in rats fed with a high-fat high-sucrose diet. *Bioscience, Biotechnology, and Biochemistry, 70*(4), 933–939. doi:10.1271/bbb.70.933 PMID:16636461

Yamashita, N., Hoshida, S., Otsu, K., Taniguchi, N., Kuzuya, T., & Hori, M. (2000). The involvement of cytokines in the second window of ischaemic preconditioning. *British Journal of Pharmacology, 131*(3), 415–422. doi:10.1038/sj.bjp.0703594 PMID:11015290

Yancy, C. W., Jessup, M., Bozkurt, B., Butler, J., Casey, D. E. Jr, Drazner, M. H., & Wilkoff, B. L. et al. (2013). 2013 ACCF/AHA guideline for the management of heart failure: A report of the American college of Cardiology Foundation/American Heart Association Task Force on practice guidelines. *Circulation*, *128*(16), e240–e327. doi:10.1161/CIR.0b013e31829e8807 PMID:23741058

Yancy, C. W., Jessup, M., Bozkurt, B., Butler, J., Casey, D. E. Jr, Drazner, M. H., & Wilkoff, B. L. et al. (2013). 2013 ACCF/AHA guideline for the management of heart failure: A report of the American College of Cardiology Foundation/American Heart Association Task Force on Practice Guidelines. *Journal of the American College of Cardiology*, *62*(16), e147–e239. doi:10.1016/j.jacc.2013.05.019 PMID:23747642

Yan, G.-X., & Antzelevitch, C. (1998). Cellular Basis for the Normal T Wave and the Electrocardiographic Manifestations of the Long-QT Syndrome. *Circulation*, *98*(18), 1928–1936. doi:10.1161/01.CIR.98.18.1928 PMID:9799215

Yang, B., Lin, H., Xiao, J., Lu, Y., Luo, X., Li, B., & Wang, Z. et al. (2007). The muscle-specific microRNA miR-1 regulates cardiac arrhythmogenic potential by targeting GJA1 and KCNJ2. *Nature Medicine*, *13*(4), 486–491. doi:10.1038/nm1569 PMID:17401374

Yang, C. S., & Pan, E. (2012). The effects of green tea polyphenols on drug metabolism. *Expert Opinion on Drug Metabolism & Toxicology*, *8*(6), 677–689. doi:10.1517/17425255.2012.681375 PMID:22509899

Yang, H., Kim, A., David, T., Palmer, D., Jin, T., Tien, J., & Jan, L. Y. et al. (2012). TMEM16F forms a Ca2+-activated cation channel required for lipid scrambling in platelets during blood coagulation. *Cell*, *151*(1), 111–122. doi:10.1016/j.cell.2012.07.036 PMID:23021219

Yang, Q., Zhong, Y., Ritchey, M., Cobain, M., Gillespie, C., Merritt, R., & Bowman, B. A. (2015). *Vital Signs: Predicted Heart Age and Racial Disparities in Heart Age among U.S. Adults at the State Level. Morbidity and Mortality Weekly Report 64*. Hyattsville, MD: National Center for Health Statistics

Yang, Y. K., Wang, L. P., Chen, L., Yao, X. P., Yang, K. Q., Gao, L. G., & Zhou, X.-L. (2015). Coenzyme Q10 treatment of cardiovascular disorders of ageing including heart failure, hypertension and endothelial dysfunction. *Clinica Chimica Acta*, *450*, 83–89. doi:10.1016/j.cca.2015.08.002 PMID:26254995

Yao, L. H., Jiang, Y. M., Shi, J., Tomas-Barberan, F. A., Datta, N., & Singanusong, R. (2004). Flavonoids in food and their health benefits. *Plant Foods for Human Nutrition (Dordrecht, Netherlands)*, *59*(3), 113–122. doi:10.1007/s11130-004-0049-7 PMID:15678717

Yarema, M. C., & Becker, C. E. (2005). Key concepts in postmortem drug redistribution. *Clinical Toxicology (Philadelphia, PA)*, *43*(4), 235–241. doi:10.1081/CLT-58950 PMID:16035199

Yashodhara, B. M., Umakanth, S., Pappachan, J. M., Bhat, S. K., Kamath, R., & Choo, B. H. (2009). Omega-3 fatty acids: A comprehensive review of their role in health and disease. *Postgraduate Medical Journal*, *85*(1000), 84–90. doi:10.1136/pgmj.2008.073338 PMID:19329703

Yazdanparast, R., & Shahriyary, L. (2008). Comparative effects of Artemisia dracunculus, Satureja hortensis and Origanum majorana on inhibition of blood platelet adhesion, aggregation and secretion. *Vascular Pharmacology*, *48*(1), 32–37. doi:10.1016/j.vph.2007.11.003 PMID:18069068

Ye, S., Karim, Z. A., Al Hawas, R., Pessin, J. E., Filipovich, A. H., & Whiteheart, S. W. (2012). Syntaxin-11, but not syntaxin-2 or syntaxin-4, is required for platelet secretion. *Blood*, *120*(12), 2484–2492. doi:10.1182/blood-2012-05-430603 PMID:22767500

Yildirim, F., Iskesen, I., Kurdal, A. T., Ozturk, T., Taneli, F., Gozukara, C., & Ozbakkaloglu, A. (2016). Is Attenuation of Oxidative Stress Helpful to Understand the Mechanism of Remote Ischemic Preconditioning in Cardiac Surgery? *Journal of Cardiothoracic and Vascular Anesthesia*, *30*(1), 134–140. doi:10.1053/j.jvca.2015.06.027 PMID:26411813

Yoon, Y., Pitts, K. R., Dahan, S., & McNiven, M. A. (1998). A novel dynamin-like protein associates with cytoplasmic vesicles and tubules of the endoplasmic reticulum in mammalian cells. *The Journal of Cell Biology*, *140*(4), 779–793. doi:10.1083/jcb.140.4.779 PMID:9472031

You, J. J., Singer, D. E., Howard, P. A., Lane, D. A., Eckman, M. H., Fang, M. C., & Lip, G. Y. H. (2012). Antithrombotic therapy for atrial fibrillation: Antithrombotic therapy and prevention of thrombosis, 9th ed: American college of chest physicians evidence-based clinical practice guidelines. Chest, 141(2), e531S-e575S. doi:10.1378/chest.11-2304

Young, J. B., Abraham, W. T., Stevenson, L. W., Horton, D. P., Elkayam, U., & Bourge, R. C. (2002). Intravenous nesiritide vs nitroglycerin for treatment of decompensated congestive heart failure: A randomized controlled trial. *Journal of the American Medical Association*, *287*(12), 1531–1540. PMID:11911755

Young, J. M., Florkowski, C. M., Molyneux, S. L., McEwan, R. G., Frampton, C. M., Nicholls, M. G., & George, P. M. et al. (2012). A randomized, double-blind, placebo-controlled crossover study of coenzyme Q10 therapy in hypertensive patients with the metabolic syndrome. *American Journal of Hypertension*, *25*(2), 261–270. doi:10.1038/ajh.2011.209 PMID:22113168

Young, R. W. (2012). Hyperoxia: A review of the risks and benefits in adult cardiac surgery. *The Journal of Extra-Corporeal Technology*, *44*(4), 241–249. PMID:23441567

Youngster, I., Shenoy, E. S., Hooper, D. C., & Nelson, S. B. (2014). Comparative evaluation of the tolerability of cefazolin and nafcillin for treatment of methicillin-susceptible Staphylococcus aureus infections in the outpatient setting. *Clinical Infectious Diseases*, *59*(3), 369–375. doi:10.1093/cid/ciu301 PMID:24785233

Yuan, J. P., Zeng, W., Dorwart, M. R., Choi, Y. J., Worley, P. F., & Muallem, S. (2009). SOAR and the polybasic STIM1 domains gate and regulate Orai channels. *Nature Cell Biology*, *11*(3), 337–343. doi:10.1038/ncb1842 PMID:19182790

Yuan, Z., & Seto, E. (2007). A functional link between SIRT1 deacetylase and NBS1 in DNA damage response. *Cell Cycle (Georgetown, Tex.)*, *6*(23), 2869–2871. doi:10.4161/cc.6.23.5026 PMID:18156798

Yue, Z., Xie, J., Yu, A. S., Stock, J., Du, J., & Yue, L. (2015). Role of TRP channels in the cardiovascular system. *American Journal of Physiology. Heart and Circulatory Physiology*, *308*(3), H157–H182. doi:10.1152/ajpheart.00457.2014 PMID:25416190

Yue, Z., Zhang, Y., Xie, J., Jiang, J., & Yue, L. (2013). Transient receptor potential (TRP) channels and cardiac fibrosis. *Current Topics in Medicinal Chemistry*, *13*(3), 270–282. doi:10.2174/1568026611313030005 PMID:23432060

Yu, G., Fang, M., Gong, M., Liu, L., Zhong, J., Feng, W., & Gong, F. et al. (2008). Steady state dendritic cells with forced IDO expression induce skin allograft tolerance by upregulation of regulatory T cells. *Transplant Immunology*, *18*(3), 208–219. doi:10.1016/j.trim.2007.08.006 PMID:18047928

Yu, Q., Lee, C. F., Wang, W., Karamanlidis, G., Kuroda, J., Matsushima, S., & Tian, R. et al. (2014). Elimination of NADPH Oxidase Activity Promotes Reductive Stress and Sensitizes the Heart to Ischemic Injury. *Journal of the American Heart Association: Cardiovascular and Cerebrovascular Disease*, *3*(1), e000555. doi:10.1161/JAHA.113.000555 PMID:24470522

Yu, X., Wang, H., Feng, L., & Zhu, J. (2014). Quantitative Research in Modern Forensic Analysis of Death Cause: New Classification of Death Cause, Degree of Contribution, and Determination of Manner of Death. *Journal of Forensic Research*, *5*(2), 1.

Yzydorczyk, C., Comte, B., Cambonie, G., Lavoie, J.-C., Germain, N., & Shun, T. (2008). Neonatal Oxygen Exposure in Rats Leads to Cardiovascular and Renal Alterations in Adulthood. *Hypertension, 52*(5), 889–895. doi:10.1161/HYPERTENSIONAHA.108.116251 PMID:18852387

Zagranichnaya, T. K., Wu, X., & Villereal, M. L. (2005). Endogenous TRPC1, TRPC3, and TRPC7 proteins combine to form native store-operated channels in HEK-293 cells. *The Journal of Biological Chemistry, 280*(33), 29559–29569. doi:10.1074/jbc.M505842200 PMID:15972814

Zaher, T. E., Miller, E. J., Morrow, D. M. P., Javdan, M., & Mantell, L. L. (2007). Hyperoxia-induced signal transduction pathways in pulmonary epithelial cells. *Free Radical Biology & Medicine, 42*(7), 897–908. doi:10.1016/j.freeradbiomed.2007.01.021 PMID:17349918

Zakynthinos, E., & Pappa, N. (2009). Inflammatory biomarkers in coronary artery disease. *Journal of Cardiology, 53*(3), 317–333. doi:10.1016/j.jjcc.2008.12.007 PMID:19477372

Zapotoczny, S., Szczubiałka, K., & Nowakowska, M. (2015). Review article: Nanoparticles in endothelial theranostics. *Pharmacological Reports, 67*(4), 751–755. doi:10.1016/j.pharep.2015.05.018

Zarain-Herzberg, A., Fragoso-Medina, J., & Estrada-Aviles, R. (2011). Calcium-regulated transcriptional pathways in the normal and pathologic heart. *IUBMB Life, 63*(10), 847–855. doi:10.1002/iub.545 PMID:21901815

Zeng, W., Yuan, J. P., Kim, M. S., Choi, Y. J., Huang, G. N., Worley, P. F., & Muallem, S. (2008). STIM1 gates TRPC channels, but not Orai1, by electrostatic interaction. *Molecular Cell, 32*(3), 439–448. doi:10.1016/j.molcel.2008.09.020 PMID:18995841

Zern, T. L., West, K. L., & Fernandez, M. L. (2003). Grape polyphenols decrease plasma triglycerides and cholesterol accumulation in the aorta of ovariectomized guinea pigs. *The Journal of Nutrition, 133*(7), 2268–2272. PMID:12840191

Zeymer, U., Bauer, T., Gersh, B. J., Zahn, R., Gitt, A., Junger, C., & Senges, J. (2011). Beneficial effect of reperfusion therapy beyond the preservation of left ventricular function in patients with acute ST-segment elevation myocardial infarction. *International Journal of Cardiology, 146*(2), 177–180. doi:10.1016/j.ijcard.2009.06.034 PMID:19604587

Zhang, C. L., McKinsey, T. A., Lu, J. R., & Olson, E. N. (2001). Association of COOH-terminal-binding protein (CtBP) and MEF2-interacting transcription repressor (MITR) contributes to transcriptional repression of the MEF2 transcription factor. *The Journal of Biological Chemistry, 276*(1), 35–39. doi:10.1074/jbc.M007364200 PMID:11022042

Zhang, C., Lin, G., Wan, W., Li, X., Zeng, B., Yang, B., & Huang, C. (2012). Resveratrol, a polyphenol phytoalexin, protects cardiomyocytes against anoxia/reoxygenation injury via the TLR4/NF-kappaB signaling pathway. *International Journal of Molecular Medicine, 29*(4), 557–563. doi:10.3892/ijmm.2012.885 PMID:22246136

Zhang, L., Gu, F., Chan, J., Wang, A., Langer, R., & Farokhzad, O. (2008, May). Nanoparticles in medicine: Therapeutic applications and developments. *Clinical Pharmacology and Therapeutics, 83*(5), 761–769. doi:10.1038/sj.clpt.6100400 PMID:17957183

Zhang, Q. J., Wang, Z., Chen, H. Z., Zhou, S., Zheng, W., Liu, G., & Liang, C. C. et al. (2008). Endothelium-specific overexpression of class III deacetylase SIRT1 decreases atherosclerosis in apolipoprotein E-deficient mice. *Cardiovascular Research, 80*(2), 191–199. doi:10.1093/cvr/cvn224 PMID:18689793

Zhang, S. L., Kozak, J. A., Jiang, W., Yeromin, A. V., Chen, J., Yu, Y., & Cahalan, M. D. et al. (2008). Store-dependent and -independent modes regulating Ca2+ release-activated Ca2+ channel activity of human Orai1 and Orai3. *The Journal of Biological Chemistry, 283*(25), 17662–17671. doi:10.1074/jbc.M801536200 PMID:18420579

Zhang, S. L., Yeromin, A. V., Zhang, X. H., Yu, Y., Safrina, O., Penna, A., & Cahalan, M. D. et al. (2006). Genome-wide RNAi screen of Ca(2+) influx identifies genes that regulate Ca(2+) release-activated Ca(2+) channel activity. *Proceedings of the National Academy of Sciences of the United States of America*, *103*(24), 9357–9362. doi:10.1073/pnas.0603161103 PMID:16751269

Zhang, S. Y., Xu, M. L., Zhang, C. E., Qu, Z. Y., Zhang, B. B., Zheng, Z. Y., & Zhang, L. M. (2012). Association of ALOX5AP gene single nucleotide polymorphisms and cerebral infarction in the Han population of northern China. *BMC Medical Genetics*, *13*(1), 61. doi:10.1186/1471-2350-13-61 PMID:22849376

Zhang, X., Shan, P., Sasidhar, M., Chupp, G. L., Flavell, R. A., Choi, A. M. K., & Lee, P. J. (2003). Reactive Oxygen Species and Extracellular Signal-Regulated Kinase 1/2 Mitogen-Activated Protein Kinase Mediate Hyperoxia-Induced Cell Death in Lung Epithelium. *American Journal of Respiratory Cell and Molecular Biology*, *28*(3), 305–315. doi:10.1165/rcmb.2002-0156OC PMID:12594056

Zhang, Y., Bi, Y., Yang, H., Chen, X., Liu, H., Lu, Y., & Liu, G. et al. (2014). mTOR limits the recruitment of CD11b+Gr1+Ly6Chigh myeloid-derived suppressor cells in protecting against murine immunological hepatic injury. *Journal of Leukocyte Biology*, *95*(6), 961–970. doi:10.1189/jlb.0913473 PMID:24569105

Zhang, Y., Mi, S. L., Hu, N., Doser, T. A., Sun, A., Ge, J., & Ren, J. (2014). Mitochondrial aldehyde dehydrogenase 2 accentuates aging-induced cardiac remodeling and contractile dysfunction: Role of AMPK, Sirt1, and mitochondrial function. *Free Radical Biology & Medicine*, *71*, 208–220. doi:10.1016/j.freeradbiomed.2014.03.018 PMID:24675227

Zhan, Z. Q., Nikus, K. C., & Wang, C. Q. (2015). Cocaine-induced right ventricular dysfunction: Right ventricular infarction or afterload elevation? *The American Journal of Emergency Medicine*, *33*(9), 1318–1319. doi:10.1016/j.ajem.2015.05.016 PMID:26027888

Zhao, K., Huang, Z., Lu, H., Zhou, J., & Wei, T. (2010). Induction of inducible nitric oxide synthase increases the production of reactive oxygen species in RAW264.7 macrophages. *Bioscience Reports*, *30*(4), 233–241. doi:10.1042/BSR20090048 PMID:19673702

Zhao, X., He, G., Chen, Y. R., Pandian, R. P., Kuppusamy, P., & Zweier, J. L. (2005). Endothelium-derived nitric oxide regulates postischemic myocardial oxygenation and oxygen consumption by modulation of mitochondrial electron transport. *Circulation*, *111*(22), 2966–2972. doi:10.1161/CIRCULATIONAHA.104.527226 PMID:15939832

Zhao, Y. Y., & Malik, A. B. (2009). A novel insight into the mechanism of pulmonary hypertension involving caveolin-1 deficiency and endothelial nitric oxide synthase activation. *Trends in Cardiovascular Medicine*, *19*(7), 238–242. doi:10.1016/j.tcm.2010.02.003 PMID:20382348

Zhao, Y. Y., Zhao, Y. D., Mirza, M. K., Huang, J. H., Potula, H. H., Vogel, S. M., & Malik, A. B. et al. (2009). Persistent eNOS activation secondary to caveolin-1 deficiency induces pulmonary hypertension in mice and humans through PKG nitration. *The Journal of Clinical Investigation*, *119*(7), 2009–2018. doi:10.1172/JCI33338 PMID:19487814

Zhou, S., Wan, L., Shao, Y., Ying, C., Wang, Y., Zou, D., & Chen, Y. et al. (2015). Detection of aortic rupture using post-mortem computed tomography and post-mortem computed tomography angiography by cardiac puncture. *International Journal of Legal Medicine*, 1–6. PMID:25773916

Zhu-Mauldin, X., Marsh, S. A., Zou, L., Marchase, R. B., & Chatham, J. C. (2012). Modification of STIM1 by O-linked N-acetylglucosamine (O-GlcNAc) attenuates store-operated calcium entry in neonatal cardiomyocytes. *The Journal of Biological Chemistry*, *287*(46), 39094–39106. doi:10.1074/jbc.M112.383778 PMID:22992728

Zhu, X., Liu, B., Zhou, S., Chen, Y. R., Deng, Y., Zweier, J. L., & He, G. (2007). Ischemic preconditioning prevents in vivo hyperoxygenation in postischemic myocardium with preservation of mitochondrial oxygen consumption. *American Journal of Physiology. Heart and Circulatory Physiology*, *293*(3), H1442–H1450. doi:10.1152/ajpheart.00256.2007 PMID:17513495

Zick, C. D., & Smith, K. R. (1991). Marital Transitions, Poverty, and Gender Differences in Mortality. *Journal of Marriage and the Family*, *53*(2), 327–336. doi:10.2307/352902

Zipes, D. P., & Wellens, H. J. (1998). Sudden cardiac death. *Circulation*, *98*(21), 2334–2351. doi:10.1161/01.CIR.98.21.2334 PMID:9826323

Zitt, C., Zobel, A., Obukhov, A. G., Harteneck, C., Kalkbrenner, F., Luckhoff, A., & Schultz, G. (1996). Cloning and functional expression of a human Ca2+-permeable cation channel activated by calcium store depletion. *Neuron*, *16*(6), 1189–1196. doi:10.1016/S0896-6273(00)80145-2 PMID:8663995

Zografos, T. A., Katritsis, G. D., Tsiafoutis, I., Bourboulis, N., Katsivas, A., & Katritsis, D. G. (2014). Effect of one-cycle remote ischemic preconditioning to reduce myocardial injury during percutaneous coronary intervention. *The American Journal of Cardiology*, *113*(12), 2013–2017. doi:10.1016/j.amjcard.2014.03.043 PMID:24793669

Zordoky, B. N., Robertson, I. M., & Dyck, J. R. (2015). Preclinical and clinical evidence for the role of resveratrol in the treatment of cardiovascular diseases. *Biochimica et Biophysica Acta*, *1852*(6), 1155–1177. doi:10.1016/j.bbadis.2014.10.016 PMID:25451966

Zorov, D. B., Filburn, C. R., Klotz, L. O., Zweier, J. L., & Sollott, S. J. (2000). Reactive oxygen species (ROS)-induced ROS release: A new phenomenon accompanying induction of the mitochondrial permeability transition in cardiac myocytes. *The Journal of Experimental Medicine*, *192*(7), 1001–1014. doi:10.1084/jem.192.7.1001 PMID:11015441

Zuo, P. Y., Chen, X. L., Liu, Y. W., Zhang, R., He, X. X., & Liu, C. Y. (2015). Non-HDL-cholesterol to HDL-cholesterol ratio as an independent risk factor for the development of chronic kidney disease. *Nutrition, Metabolism, and Cardiovascular Diseases*, *25*(6), 582–587. doi:10.1016/j.numecd.2015.03.003 PMID:25921842

Zweier, J. L., Flaherty, J. T., & Weisfeldt, M. L. (1987). Direct measurement of free radical generation following reperfusion of ischemic myocardium. *Proceedings of the National Academy of Sciences of the United States of America*, *84*(5), 1404–1407. doi:10.1073/pnas.84.5.1404 PMID:3029779

About the Contributors

Ashim Malhotra serves as assistant professor of pharmacology at the School of Pharmacy at Pacific University in Oregon. He is a combination pharmacist and molecular pharmacologist and an expert in mitochondrial pharmacology. He has served as a grant reviewer for the National Science Foundation (NSF) and private biomedical foundations in the United States. He has served as Chair of the national Sub-Committee on Strategic Planning for the American Association of Colleges of Pharmacy (AACP). He is the School of Pharmacy's Past Chair of Assessment, and the Chair-Elect of Diversity of the College of Health Professions, and a recipient of the 2016 Pacific University Junior Faculty Award, the 2016 AACP Teacher of the Year Award, and along with his colleagues, the 2014 AACP Innovations in Teaching Award. Before joining Pacific University, he worked at the NYU School of Medicine for five years and the New York Methodist Hospital for two years. He received his Ph.D. in 2006 from St. John's University in New York, USA and received his Bachelor of Pharmacy degree from Jamia Hamdard University in New Delhi, India in 2000.

Shivani Soni joined as a lecturer at Chapman University and California State University, Fullerton in Fall 2016. She worked as an associate professor in Department of Biological sciences at Alabama State University till July 2016. Her husband Dr. Amandeep Salhotra and 5 year old son Mr. Shivam Salhotra lives in Southern CA. Dr. Soni obtained her Bachelor's and Master's degrees in Zoology from University of Delhi, India. She completed her PhD in Molecular Parasitology in 2004 from University of Delhi, India. Her PhD thesis entitled "Selection of antimalarial resistant lines of *Plasmodium yoelii* and sporogonic studies in *Anopheles stephensi*" focused on the currently important global public health problem of emergence of resistance to existing antimalarial drugs, which is a major setback to malaria control in the developing world.She received her postdoctoral training with Dr. Manjit Hanspal at Tufts School of Medicine, Boston, Massachusetts. Later she joined as a senior postdoctoral fellow in the lab of Dr. Shiladitya Sengupta at Health Science & Technology division of Harvard Medical School-MIT, Boston, Massachusetts. Her research interests are in the area of Hematology and Oncology. Her research has focused in the field of erythropoesis (Red blood cell formation), where she demonstrated the role of a novel protein Emp (Erythroblast Macrophage Protein) in red blood cells and macrophage development. Emp was discovered by Dr. Hanspal in 1994 and Dr. Soni was the first one to characterize its function *in vivo* in 2006 This has resulted in multiple high impact publications and a prestigious travel award from American Society of Hematology. Additionally, she had also explored events preceding the release of malarial parasite from RBC's as an extension of her PhD work. Her current research work is to elucidate the role of Emp in colorectal cancer progression and to explore its value as predictive & prognostic biomarkers. She had successfully acquired NIH grant for this project. Her another project focuses on developing strategies that can be applied into clinico-pathological conditions related to abnormal erythropoiesis, cell-to-cell adhesion & migration. Another part of her research in the area of Oncology involves engineering concepts pertaining to biological systems. In collaboration, she has developed several novel polymeric hybrid nanoformulations for cancer chemotherapy and targeting aberrant signal transduction pathways which has led to many publications in peer reviewed journals as well as patents. Dr. Soni is the reviewer of many journals related to Hematology, Oncology and Biochemistry.

* * *

Madeeha Aqil obtained her PhD degree from International Center of Genetic engineering and Biotechnology (ICGEB), a highly regarded research institution in New Delhi, India. She has done her pioneering work in role of HIV-1 accessory protein Nef derived exosomes and micro RNA in HIV infection. She completed her postdoctoral training from Department of Oral Medicine and Diagnostic Sciences, College of Dentistry, University of Illinois at Chicago, US. During her postdoctoral training she investigated role of nitric oxide signaling in DNA Damage, cell cycle regulation and metastasis. Currently, she is assistant professor, in Department of Oral Medicine and Diagnostic Sciences, College of Dentistry, University of Illinois at Chicago, US. She is actively involved in writing research papers and book chapters and teaching physiology to dental students. In addition, Dr. Madeeha serves as associate editor of "Tumor Biology", the official journal of International society of oncology and biomarkers (ISOBM) published by Springer Publications. She serves scientific community by serving as a reviewer in reputed journals like Journal of Extracellular vesicles, Journal of Visualized experiments and journal of Biosciences. Dr. Madeeha has mentored many junior researchers and has received certificate of appreciation from Illinois Mathematics and Science Academy for supporting their students through the Student Inquiry and Research program. She has received travel award by Department of Science and Technology, Govt. of India to attend the meeting of Nobel Laureates and students in Lindau, Germany. Dr. Madeeha has been awarded Keystone symposia scholarship by Bill and Melinda Gates Foundation to attend the keystone symposia on HIV Evolution, Genomics and Pathogenesis held at Whistler, British Columbia, Canada. She had been awarded Travel grant by Hong Kong University, Pasteur Research Center to attend the 1st Pasteur Asia Immunology Course at Pasteur Research Center in Hong Kong. Dr Madeeha has published her research in highly reputed scientific journals like Journal of Extracellular Vesicles, PLOS ONE and Tumor Biology.

Diptiman Bose received his Ph.D in Pharmacology from the University the Pacific, Stockton in 2006. In 2012 he was hired as an Assistant Professor in Pharmacology by the Western New England University, College of Pharmacy. His research focuses on investigating the impact of xenobiotics and pharmacological agents on ion channels and proteins involved in regulating cellular calcium homeostasis. He has published extensively on studies focused on the regulation of calcium channels, calcium ion dysfunctions, and is the author of reviews and book chapter on calcium homeostasis.

John D. Bowman received his MS in Pharmacy Administration from Auburn University in 1976 and completed a hospital pharmacy residency in 1977. After working as a hospital clinical pharmacist for 15 years, John joined Samford University School of Pharmacy in 1992 as Assistant Professor. While in Alabama, he was active in the Alabama Society of Hospital Pharmacists and became President in 1987. He was promoted to Associate Professor, and in 2007 joined the new Texas A&M Rangel College of

Pharmacy. He was inducted as Fellow of the American Society of Health-System Pharmacists in 2007. He is a Board Certified Pharmacotherapy Specialist, and has written articles on a variety of subjects in pharmacy.

Mahua Choudhury earned her BS in Zoology, Botany, Chemistry and MS in Molecular Biology, Biophysics & Genetics from the University of Calcutta and her PhD (2008) in Medical Pharmacology from the University of Missouri-Columbia. From 2008 to 2011 Dr. Choudhury was an American Diabetes Association Postdoctoral Fellow and subsequently a Research Instructor in Pediatrics and Neonatology at the University of Colorado-Aurora. In 2012, Dr. Choudhury became an Assistant Professor of Pharmaceutical Sciences in the Texas A&M Health Science Center, Texas. Dr. Choudhury's research is funded by several organizations including the Bill and Melinda Gates Foundation, Mitsubishi, the American Diabetes Association, and the Morris L. Lichtenstein Foundation. With their support Dr. Choudhury's research team is working toward understanding and controlling interactions of diet and environmental chemicals on genetic control of metabolism, especially during gestation. Dr. Choudhury investigates epigenetic regulation using a variety of models using rodent, non-human primate, and human derived cells and tissues. Her lab's primary research interest is in maternal-fetal health and metabolic syndrome, with a focus on epigenetics and the biology of microRNAs. Dr. Choudhury's research team members investigate epigenetic regulation (DNA methylation, microRNA, and histone modifications) as an early step towards diminishing mortality in human populations who are at high risk with pregnancy disorders or metabolic complications.

Fawzy Elbarbry obtained a BSc in pharmacy and MSc in pharmaceutical chemistry from Tanta University College of Pharmacy, a premier pharmacy school in Egypt and the Middle East. Subsequently, he obtained a PhD in Drug Metabolism and Pharmacokinetics followed by two years of postdoctoral fellowship from College of Pharmacy and Nutrition, University of Saskatchewan, Canada. In 2008, he joined Pacific University School of Pharmacy as an Assistant Professor and promoted to Associate Professor in 2013. Additionally, and through the Foreign Pharmacy Graduate Examination Certification (FPGEC) Program, he became a registered pharmacist in the State of Washington where he practices on an on-call basis as a clinical pharmacist since 2013. As an academician and a pharmacist, he has demonstrated strong interest and ability to promote innovation in pharmacy services, practice at the advanced level, educate, conduct nationally recognized scholarship, and to provide leadership. In the past nine years, Dr. Elbarbry has been actively teaching in the pharmacy curriculum. His teaching and course coordination has been recognized in many ways by his peers, students, and administrators. For example, he has been awarded the AACP Teacher of the Year Award in 2010, 2012, and 2014; the Outstanding Faculty Member Award in 2009 and 2011; Dean's Excellence Award in 2014; and the President's Award for Excellence in Graduate Teaching in 2015. Dr. Elbarbry also maintains an active research program that focuses generally on investigating the potential effect of herbal remedies and dietary supplements on drug metabolizing enzymes and modulation of chronic illnesses such as hypertension. In the past 9 years, he mentored and trained more than 30 students from Pacific University in his research lab as part of 6-week Advanced Pharmacy Practice Experiential (APPE) rotations or summer research programs. This experience has led to more than 15 peer-review papers, 10 posters, and 6 oral presentations at local, national, and international meetings. On the professional level, Dr. Elbarbry serves as an editor and active reviewer for more than 15 journals and granting agencies. As an active member with the Global Science and Technology Forum (GSTF), he has played a key role in organizing the PHARMA 2014 conference in Singapore and PHARMA 2015 conference in Thailand. Additionally he has been involved in many services with the AACP and American Association of Pharmaceutical Scientists (AAPS) since 2008.

Sheree Finley received her M.S. degree in Biochemistry in 2000 from Auburn University in Auburn, Alabama. She is an instructor of Organic Chemistry and Biochemistry as a faculty member at Alabama State University in Montgomery, Alabama. Her research interests include studies of the microbial diversity of gravesoil of naturally decomposing corpses for forensic applications as well as biochemical and genetic studies of the internal organs of criminal cadavers. She is an active member of the American Society of Microbiology, the American Chemical Society, and the American Academy of Forensic Sciences. Her research has garnered a national award from the American Academy of Forensic Sciences.

Gulnaz T. Javan is an Assistant Professor at Alabama State University, Physical Sciences Department, and Forensic Science Program. She received her Ph.D. degree on 2003 from Istanbul University's Institute of Forensic Science in Turkey. Dr. Javan studies the human thanatomicrobiome (i.e., thanatos-, Greek for death), has endeavored to unlock the microbial secrets of death. Thanatomicrobiome is a relatively new term introduced at a recent American Academy of Forensic Science annual meeting in Seattle, Washington. Also, she is actively researching gene expression in the internal organs of cadavers obtained from homicides, suicides, over-doses, and accidental death. Other research interests of her include monitoring the microbial diversity in the soil under the decomposing cadavers at varying time intervals and forensic entomology. As a faculty member she has thought courses in Forensic Genetics/DNA Analysis, Forensic Serology, CSI, Ethics & Professional Responsibility, Forensic Biology, Population Genetics, and Microbial Forensics and there correspondent laboratories to both graduate and undergraduate students. She is a recent awardee of a National Science Foundation and a Forensic Sciences Foundation research award.

Zubair Karim is Research Assistant Professor in Pharmaceutical Sciences, School of Pharmacy, The University of Texas at El Paso (UTEP). Prior to joining UTEP in October 2016, he served at the College of Pharmacy at Western University of Health Sciences, Pomona, CA from 2013 to 2016. Dr. Karim received his Ph.D. in Biochemistry from the Banaras Hindu University, Varanasi, India in 2004 and did his post-doctoral training under Prof. Sidney Whiteheart (Department of Biochemistry, University of Kentucky College of Medicine, Lexington, KY). During his postdoctoral training at University of Kentucky, Dr. Karim was involved in the regulation of platelet SNARE machinery, were he discovered non-genomic role of I kappa kinase in platelets, thereby opening a new area of platelet research. His research interests are in the area of platelet signaling and SNARE machinery, and he is currently funded by the National Institutes of Health NHLBI.

Fadi T. Khasawneh is Associate Professor and Chair in Pharmaceutical Sciences at the School of Pharmacy at The University of Texas at El Paso (UTEP). Prior to joining UTEP in October 2016, he served at the College of Pharmacy at Western University of Health Sciences, Pomona, California from 2008 to 2016. Dr. Khasawneh received his bachelor's degree in Pharmacy (1999) from Jordan University of Science and Technology (Jordan), and his Ph.D. in Pharmacology from the University of Illinois at Chicago (UIC) in 2007. Dr. Khasawneh's research interests are in the area of thrombosis development, and the signaling pathways involved in human platelet activation, and are currently partially funded by the National Institutes of Health NHLBI, and the American Heart Association. He serves as a peer reviewer for the American Heart Association, and the Department of Veterans Affairs.

Yan Li is a Professional Staff in Cleveland Clinic, assistant professor of Molecular Medicine in Cleveland Clinic Lerner College of Medicine of Case Western Reserve University, and Cardiologist in No.1 Hospital of Lanzhou University, He has over 17 years clinical and medical research experience, Dr. Li received his M.D. degree from Sichuan University, worked as a cardiologist in the No.1 Hospital of Lanzhou University heart center from 2005-2010, he joined into Cleveland Clinic at 2010. Dr. Li has several high impact score peer-reviewed publications and many book chapters in medical clinical and research field. Dr. Li's research is focused on the identify the complement system in clinical autoimmune diseases and transplant rejection.

Yun Lu is an attending physician of the Gynaecology and Obstetrics at The First Hospital of Lanzhou University. She received her M.D. from Sichuan University and completed the training of the resident physician at The First Hospital of Lanzhou University. She also is an instructor of Lanzhou University. She is one of the authors of the book named The Countryside Practical Manual of Gynaecology and Obstetrics.

Jennifer Mathews received both her B.A. (1995; SUNY Potsdam) and M.S. (2000; University of Northern Colorado) in Biological Sciences. Before pursuing her doctoral studies she worked for Ortho-McNeil Pharmaceutical (Johnson and Johnson). Dr. Mathews has a Ph.D. in Pharmacology from the University of Rochester School of Medicine and Dentistry. She began her tenure at St. John Fisher College in 2007. Dr. Mathews teaches in the Department of Pharmaceutical Sciences with primary responsibilities in the Systems Pharmacology course sequence. In addition, she offers an elective in substances of abuse and co-coordinates the Introduction to Diversity course. She precepts fourth year pharmacy students on both service and academic APPE rotations. Dr. Mathews has been recognized as Teacher of the Year (2008; 2014) and Advisor of the Year (2013; 2014). Dr. Mathews is actively involved in service, both to the profession and community and serves on many committees and advisory panels. In 2013 she led a team of 8 students to the Blackfeet Reservation in Browning, Montana. Dr. Mathews is a member of AALHE, GLMA, AACP, and APhA.

Dolly Mehta is a professor (tenured) of Pharmacology and Medicine at the University of Illinois at Chicago, US. She conducts her cutting edge research to identify the signaling "switches" that induce endothelial cell contraction and compromise endothelial barrier function, and those that turn off endothelial contraction, promoting barrier repair. Her research projects are well funded by National Institutes of Health (NIH). She is an associate editor of American Journal of Physiology (AJP)-Lung Cellular and Molecular Physiology. She has received numerous awards for her outstanding research contributions in the field of pulmonary vascular biology, such as, Giles Filley Award for Excellency in Physiology- American Physiological Society. She served as a member of prestigious NIH NHLBI RIBT Study Section and NIH Respiratory Integrative Biology and Translational Research Study Section. She is regularly invited to deliver a talk in various national and international scientific meetings and research institution, such as Federation of American Society of Experimental Biology (FASEB), American Thoracic Society (ATS), etc. She has published high impact factor research articles, review papers and books chapters. She has trained many PhD students and postdoctoral fellows, who are now successfully placed in academia and in pharmaceutical industries.

Hosik Min is an assistant professor at University of South Alabama, and and has received his Ph.D in sociology from the Texas A&M University. His research interests are in health disparities, demography, and population aging.

Ifeyinwa Nwankwo is an M.D. candidate in the class of 2018 at Case Western Reserve University School of Medicine. After graduating from CWRU with a degree in Spanish and a minor in Chemistry, she is currently pursuing her passion for medicine by conducting public health research concerning health prevention and education through the Hunger Network's Stay Well Project. In her spare time, she enjoys cooking as well as volunteering at local clinics and nursing homes.

Sait Ozsoy received his M.D. degree on 1997 from Gulhane Military Medical Academy (GMMA) School of Medicine Ankara, Turkey. As a forensic pathologist and forensic examiner, he worked at Gazi University, Ankara, Turkey between 2003-2007. Dr. Ozsoy worked at "The Council of Forensic Medicine, Morgue Department in Ankara" in 2006.He has been working as a forensic pathologist in Department of Forensic Medicine in GMMA since 2007. Dr. Ozsoy teaches crimininology, forensic autopsy, causes of death, disaster victim identification (DVI), and natural deaths (sudden cardiac deaths, and intracranial pathologies etc.) to graduate and undergraduate students at GMMA.

Catherine A. Powell received her B.S. in Cellular Biology and Molecular Genetics from University of Maryland (2009). She earned her Ph.D. in Biomedical Sciences from Ohio State University in 2015. Her doctoral thesis work focused on the role of metabolic regulator fatty acid binding protein 5 in the development and progression of triple negative breast cancer. Dr. Powell is currently a postdoctoral researcher at Texas A&M Health Science Center. Her research focus is on the epigenetic regulation of metabolic disorder. Dr. Powell's interests focus on understanding the epigenetic mechanisms to develop novel therapeutic targets for the treatment of metabolic disorders.

Jacqueline Schwartz is an alumnus of Loyola Marymount University where she received a Bachelors of Science degree in Biology, and University of the Pacific, where she received her Doctorate of Pharmacy degree in 2010. She completed a first-year General Medicine Pharmacy Residency at Kingsbrook Jewish Medical Center in Brooklyn, New York. Subsequently, she also completed a second-year Infectious Disease Pharmacy Residency at State University of New York Downstate Medical Center in Brooklyn, New York. With the completion of her training she served as a clinical pharmacist at Bellevue Hospital Center, New York's largest public hospital. During her time at Bellevue Hospital Center she was also adjunct faculty at Long Island Univeristy School of Pharmacy and St. Johns University School of Pharmacy. She is currently an Assistant Professor of Pharmacy Practice at the School of Pharmacy at Pacific University.

Anne Schweighardt received her Pharm.D. from the University of Utah in 2009. She completed an integrated two-year pharmacotherapy residency at Texas Tech University Health Sciences Center in Lubbock, Texas. In August of 2011 she joined the faculty of Wegmans School of Pharmacy.

Poulomi Sengupta is currently a DST Women scientist in the CSIR-National Chemical Laboratory, Pune, India. She has received her Bachelor's in Chemistry honours from Presidency college Calcutta India in the year 2000 followed by M.Sc. from IIT Kanpur in Chemistry. She got another master's degree from Washington University in St. Louis, Missouri USA in the year 2005. Later she worked in the same school as RA (research assistant) from 2005 to 2008 and RAII in Brigham and Women's Hospital from 2009-2011. She is currently registered as a Ph.D. student under the supervision of Dr. BLV Prasad.

Alison Shafer is currently a candidate for a PharmD, with graduation set for May 2016.

Aymen Shatnawi is an Assistant Professor of Pharmacology and Pharmacogenomics at University of Charleston, School of Pharmacy. Prior joining the department of Pharmaceutical and Administrative Sciences, he worked as a Research Associate at both Duke University, Department of Pharmacology and McGill University Goodman Cancer Center. Dr. Shatnawi is currently teaching Pharmacology and pharmacogenomics courses. In addition, his research is mainly focused on identifying the mechanisms by which androgen receptor and its co-regulators involved in prostate cancer development and progression. His research mainly consists of multidisciplinary approaches that incorporate biochemistry, molecular and cellular biology, plant chemistry, pharmacology and bioinformatics to identify the signaling pathways involved in the disease state. Dr. Shatnawi has a bachelor degree in Pharmacy, a master degree in Pharmaceutical Technology, and a doctorate degree in biomedical sciences from Medical University of Ohio.

Mohammad Tauseef completed his Pharmacy School from Jamia Hamdard, New Delhi, and PhD in Cardiovascular Pharmacology from Faculty of Medical Sciences, University of Delhi, India. Later, he joined department of pharmacology, college of medicine, The University of Illinois, Chicago, US, as a postdoctoral research associate. After completing his postdoctoral training in vascular endothelial pharmacology, he was appointed as a research assistant professor in department of pharmacology, The University of University, Chicago. Currently, Dr. Tauseef is an assistant professor of pharmacology (tenure track), at Department of Pharmaceutical Sciences, college of pharmacy, Chicago State University, Chicago IL. He is actively engaged in teaching Pharmacology, Physiology and Pathophysiology courses to PharmD students. He performs his biomedical research to investigate the role of calcium signaling in the regulation of vascular endothelial hyperpermeability and inflammation. Increase in endothelial permeability is the earliest sign in the initiation of serious cardio-pulmonary disorders during septic conditions, such as acute respiratory distress syndrome (ARDS) and thrombosis. Tauseef is trying to identify molecular signaling mechanisms, activated during vascular inflammation to develop potential therapeutics against vascular inflammatory diseases. He utilizes array of techniques such as gene silencing technology in endothelial cells and genetic knockout mice models to answer his research questions. He regular presents his research findings in national and international scientific meetings and received awards from American Society of Pharmacology and Experiential therapeutics (ASPET), American Heart Association (AHA) and American Physiological Society (APS). He is an active member of American Association of College of Pharmacy (AACP), American Association of Immunologists (AAI) and Member, Editorial Board, The Journal of Clinical Research. Tauseef has published his research work in top tier, peer reviewed international journals, such as Circulation Research, Journal of experimental Medicine, The FASEB Journal, etc.

Srinivas M. Tipparaju contributed research and understanding in the field of cardiovascular disease and ion channels. As research investigator Dr. Tipparaju published extensively in high impact research journals and received extramural funding. In addition, Dr. Tipparaju contributed to fields of drug delivery and formulation development.

R. Brigg Turner is an assistant professor in the School of Pharmacy at Pacific University. He completed a first-year pharmacy residency at West Virginia University Hospitals and subsequently completed a second-year specialty in infectious diseases at the same institution. Currently, he practices at the Legacy Health System in the area of infectious diseases and helps coordinate the antimicrobial stewardship program.

Yali Yao is a Professor of Lanzhou University, Chief Physician, Ph.D. and M.D. mentor. She successively held the director of Department of cardiology, member of Heart Failure Professional Committee of the Chinese Medical Doctor Association, the vice-chairman of Integrative Cardiovascular Association of Gansu Province. She has been engaged in the profession of cardiovascular research for more than 30 years and has profound academic theoretical attainments and rich clinical experience. She is well-versed in diagnosis and interventional treatment of arrhythmia.

Jian Zhang received his Ph. D degree from Department of Nutrition in Auburn University in 2012. Zhang then worked as Research Associate in the same department. Dr. Zhang is currently a postdoctoral research associate at the Texas A&M University Health Science Center. He is involved in studying epigenetics in metabolic disorder. Dr. Zhang has more than ten years' experience in anti-diabetic and anti-obesity mechanisms of dietary agents, natural products, and their metabolites.

Index

www.ingramcontent.com/pod-product-compliance
Lightning Source LLC
LaVergne TN
LVHW060356300926
849162LV00006B/1281